Primary Care of the OLDER ADULT

A Multidisciplinary Approach

Primary Care of the OLDER ADULT

A Multidisciplinary Approach

Mary M. Burke, RN, DNSc, GNP-C
Gerontologic Nursing Consultant
Washington, DC

Joy A. Laramie, MSN, CNP
Assistant Clinical Professor of Health Care Sciences
George Washington University
Washington, DC

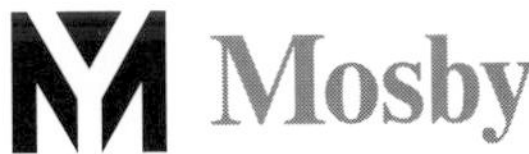

A Harcourt Health Sciences Company
St. Louis Philadelphia London Sydney Toronto

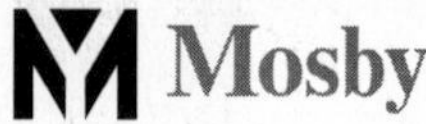

A Harcourt Health Sciences Company

Vice President, Nursing Editorial Director: Sally Schrefer
Senior Editor: Michael S. Ledbetter
Senior Developmental Editor: Laurie K. Muench
Project Manager: Deborah Vogel
Project Specialist: Mary Drone
Designer: Bill Drone

FIRST EDITION

NOTICE

Pharmacology is an ever-changing field. Standard safety precautions must be followed, but as new research and clinical experience broaden our knowledge, changes in treatment and drug therapy may become necessary or appropriate. Readers are advised to check the most current product information provided by the manufacturer of each drug to be administered to verify the recommended dose, the method and duration of administration, and contraindications. It is the responsibility of the appropriately licensed health care provider, relying on experience and knowledge of the patient, to determine dosages and the best treatment for each individual patient. Neither the publisher nor the editor assumes any liability for any injury and/or damage to persons or property arising from this publication.

Mosby, Inc.
A Harcourt Health Sciences Company
11830 Westline Industrial Drive
St. Louis, Missouri 63146

Printed in the United States of America

International Standard Book Number: 0-8151-8916-8

00 01 02 03 04 GW/FF 9 8 7 6 5 4 3 2 1

In memory of my mother,
Laura Bianchini McLaughlin, a wonderful woman.

Mary M. Burke

To my mom, Betty J. Laramie,
who gives me endless love, support, and encouragement.
All my successes I owe to you.

Joy A. Laramie

Contributors

Thomas Berryman, DPM
Podiatrist
Advanced Footcare Practice
East Stroudsburg, Pennsylvania

Cleo A. Boulter, MSN, RN
Vice President, PPS
Centennial HealthCare
Atlanta, Georgia

Janice T. Brown, RN, MSN, GNP-C, ANP-C
Instructor
Georgetown University Medical School
Washington, DC

Elizabeth Burgraff, RN, C, MS
Family Nurse Practitioner
St. Elizabeth's Medical Center
Boston, Massachusetts

Georges Catinis, MD
Assistant Professor
Gastroenterology and Transplant Hepatology
Louisiana State University
New Orleans, Louisiana

Charles Cefalu, MD, MS
Professor and Chief of Geriatric Medicine
Department of Family Medicine
Louisiana State University Medical Center
New Orleans, Louisiana

Mary Corcoran, OTR, PhD
Associate Research Professor
George Washington University
Washington, DC

Jill C. Cunningham, MSN, CANP
Adult Nurse Practitioner
Georgetown University Medical Center
Orthopaedics and Rheumatology
Washington, DC

Mary T. Delaney, RN, PhD
Senior Lecturer, College of Nursing
Wayne State University
Detroit, Michigan

Vaunette P. Fay, RN-CS, GNP, FNP, PhD
Associate Professor, School of Nursing
University of Texas—Houston Health Science Center
Houston, Texas

Janet Feldman, RN, PhD
Vice President
Qualatas Associates
Downers Grove, Illinois

Kathleen French, MSN, MPH, CRNP, CDE
Family Nurse Practitioner
20th Medical Group
Shaw Air Force Base, South Carolina

Kimberly H. Groner, MSN, CANP
Adult Nurse Practitioner—Rheumatology
Georgetown University Medical Center
Washington, DC

Mary Marmoll Jirovec, RN, BSN, MSN, PhD, FAAN
Associate Professor
Wayne State University
Detroit, Michigan

Sr. Mary Paul McLaughlin, BS, MSN, CNP
Gerontologic Nurse Practitioner
St. Gertrude Monastery
Ridgely, Maryland

M. Eletta Morse, RN, BA, MSN, CRNP
Nurse Practitioner
FutureCare, Inc.
Glen Burnie, Maryland

Cheryl B. Moxley, BS, BBA, RD
Clinical Nutrition Specialist
Washington Hospital Center
Washington, DC

Carine M. Nassar, MS, RD, LD, CNSD
Senior Clinical Nutrition Specialist
Washington Hospital Center
Washington, DC

Christina M. Puchalski, MD, MS
Assistant Professor of Medicine and Geriatrics
George Washington University Medical Center
Washington, DC

Karen Reilly, ScD
Associate
Abt Associates
Cambridge, Massachusetts

Verna E. Reynolds, MD, CMD
Medical Director/Physician
Sentara Life Care
Norfolk, Virginia

Anita Rothwell, MSN
Nurse Practitioner
Kaiser Permanente
Kensington, Maryland

David A. Sayles, MD
Director, Division of Geriatric Psychiatry
George Washington University Medical Center
Washington, DC

Mohamad Sidani, MD, MS
Assistant Professor, School of Medicine
Department of Family Medicine
Louisiana State University Health Sciences
New Orleans, Louisiana

Eleanor Stewart, MD
Assistant Director of Geriatric Medicine
Providence Hospital
Washington, DC

Carol Taylor, CSFN, RN, MSN, PhD
Director, Center for Clinical Bioethics
Assistant Professor of Nursing
Georgetown University
Washington, DC

Kevin Young, MPH, LPT
Physical Therapist
Health Care Financing Administration
Baltimore, Maryland;
Maryland Orthopedics
Endicott City, Maryland

Preface

Primary Care of the Older Adult: A Multidisciplinary Approach provides primary practitioners with current scientific knowledge and innovative clinical insights from a variety of practitioners. It is our belief that the ongoing transition in health care delivery systems will diminish rigid practice boundaries that have existed among disciplines. Shared knowledge and collaboration in primary care practices between disciplines is an underlying principle that guided the development of this book.

We have sought experts from many fields to share their knowledge and practice acumen. Among the contributors are gerontologic nurse practitioners, adult nurse practitioners, family nurse practitioners, a clinical specialist, a geriatrician, a family practice physician, an internist, a psychiatrist, a podiatrist, a nutritionist, a physical therapist, an occupational therapist, and health policy specialists.

This book is primarily for students who have completed foundational courses and are now in their clinical rotation in primary care settings with older adults as their patients. The book is also intended for practicing primary care providers who wish to have an available reference with updated information and interventions. The material in the book is presented as succinctly as possible and includes relevant and timely content for primary care practitioners. The content focus is on conditions, problems, and illnesses that primary care providers encounter when treating older adult patients.

The book is organized into five units. Unit 1, Health Maintenance, includes four chapters of basic knowledge for health assessment, health promotion, and disease prevention. Unit II, Clinical Management, focuses on frequently experienced illnesses and conditions in the older adult and on bringing together fundamental knowledge and practical experienced-based information for the practicing primary care provider. Unit III, Common Syndromes, and Unit IV, Vulnerabilities, together comprise 12 chapters that capture the art of care by addressing the common and at times seemingly insurmountable conditions that every provider at times will encounter when providing care to older adults. The final section, Unit V, is called Foundation of Care. Many times these chapters are found at the beginning of a textbook and, although we value this information, our emphasis is on clinical practice. Our hope is that after students and practitioners have had their clinical questions answered, they will find in this last section of the book important and thoughtful information. Certainly we hope that students and many practitioners will be encouraged by the material in the book to further develop a research study that answers some of the perplexing questions that will always remain a critical aspect of primary care of older adults.

We have tried to convey our deep concern for the dignity, personal integrity, and autonomy of each older patient that we serve. All of us as primary care providers have a responsibility to meet the needs of the patient above and beyond the needs of the health care organization in which we function.

Acknowledgments

As with any endeavor, we owe much to many, first and foremost to our contributors. We are indebted to your willingness and the sacrifice of time that we know it took to produce the quality chapters that mark this book. We express our sincere appreciation and hope that all will experience a satisfaction in seeing the results of their work.

We would like to extend a special thanks to two individuals. Charles Cefalu is a leader in multidisciplinary care of older adults; his assistance was more than that of an ordinary contributor. His chapters are excellent, and he was instrumental in extending invitations to potential contributors. We also thank Jamie Nicholas, an invaluable resource, who came to our rescue with outstanding graphics for a portion of the exercise chapter. Special thanks to Deborah Chyun, RN, MSN, PhD; Sheila Dunn, RN, MSN, C-ANP; Courtney Lyder, RN, MS, ND, C-GNP; and Mariah Snyder, RN, PhD, FAAN, for their many helpful suggestions to this edition.

The production of this book occurred during a time of merger mania within the economy of the nation, and the publishing business was no exception. Our editor, Michael Ledbetter, who has been a personable supporter throughout this undertaking from the very beginning, deserves special kudos for keeping us on track and managing all the intricacies of this long and, at times, arduous process. Our thanks also go to other people at Mosby, most notably Laurie Muench, for her good-natured assistance, Barbara Cullen, Eric Ham, and Mary Drone. A special thanks to Mike McConnell. We are grateful to all of you for your support.

We want to thank all of our colleagues and students present and past for sharing your knowledge and your professional lives with us. A special acknowledgment goes to those we love as family, since nothing is possible without the unconditional love we receive from those with whom we share our lives.

Mary M. Burke

Joy A. Laramie

Contents

Introduction to the Text

The health care delivery system in the United States strives to provide two fundamental rights: the right to access to care and the right to quality in services delivered. The current United States health care delivery system is not perfect, but this fact should never seriously impede health care professionals in the continuous pursuit of providing optimal care to their elderly patients.

Older adults are an extremely diverse population in abilities, life experiences, social resources, and ethnicity. Widely held generalizations and stereotypical images of older adults threaten the primary care provider's ability to conduct appropriate interviews and objective assessments. It is the responsibility of each person working with older adults to introspectively review these negative views of older people and work diligently to view each person as unique.

All older people have multiple talents and virtues. The primary provider needs to always be aware of the strengths of an older person and not view him or her as a failing organ system. Many times family members, friends, or paid caregivers will be important informants regarding the daily life and condition of the older patient. It is wise to ask the older person's permission before questions are asked of these supportive people. Dignity is many times closely related to autonomy. To be treated with dignity and kindness is a treasured commodity, but it is also a human right, and it is the responsibility of the practitioner to ensure that the right is respected.

Theories of aging reflect the complexities of the process, but none are comprehensive. Theories that attempt to explain only the physiologic changes that occur during the aging process include genetic theories, cellular theories, and organ system theories (autoimmune). Other physiologic concepts of aging that are proposed are nutrient deprivation, lipofuscin, wear and tear theory, and cross-linking theory. Psychologic theories abound and include disengagement theory, activity theory, life course theory, and continuity theory. None of these theories or constructs can claim sufficient evidence to account for aging effects that are experienced by older people. The majority of theorists and practitioners agree that with advanced age come factors such as increased vulnerability, increased susceptibility to disease, decrease in vitality, and slowed response to and recovery from stress.

Biologic principles that are paramount for understanding the diversity of older people are

1. Older people age at different rates from one another; chronologic age is not always a reflection of physiologic age.
2. Within each older person, organ systems age at different rates; a person with severe congestive heart failure may write a great symphony, thereby exhibiting a high level of cognitive function.

Generalizations concerning typical pain syndrome such as chest pain in myocardial infarction do not hold for most older adults. A symptom as benign as slight confusion in a frail older adult may well be the alarm for an impeding infarction. Pneumonia often will not present with any fever, and the x-rays may be negative. The primary provider must always be alert and respond to a patient or family member who reports, "I don't know what it is, but something is wrong."

The common comorbidities of age cloud the diagnostic process. The process of diagnosing is also made difficult by iatrogenic complexities of adverse response to treatments. It is well known that older people are at increased risk for complications related to multiple drug use. Every primary care visit should include a review of all prescription and over-the-counter drug use. Many times a symptom that is the result of one drug is treated by adding another drug to the regimen. A potassium supplement may be added because of a diuretic, an H_2 blocker may be added because of a nonsteroidal antiinflammatory drug, a laxative may be added because of the constipation from a calcium channel blocker. There is no easy and universal solution to this problem, but the first step is to recognize the existence of problems associated with multiple drug use and then work toward a solution.

There is a never-ending influx of new and redesigned old drugs that are marketed extensively to primary care providers, with nurse practitioners as a new and expanding customer. New drugs play an important role in many fields of health care when used appropriately, but there should be a note of caution when considering a newly marketed drug for use in the older population because of the increased risk for adverse drug reactions in this population. Listed below are drugs that the Food and Drug Administration (FDA) has taken off the market within the 1990 decade.

Bromfenac sodium, marketed as Duract capsules, associated with fatal hepatic failure, voluntarily withdrawn from the market June 22, 1998

Dexfenfluramine dihydrochloride, marketed as Redux capsules, associated with valvular heart disease, voluntarily withdrawn from the market September 1997

Encainide hydrochloride, marketed as Enkaid, associated with death rates after recent heart attack, voluntarily withdrawn from the market December 16, 1991

Flosequian, marketed as Manoplax, associated with adverse effects on survival, voluntarily withdrawn from the market July 1993

Mibefradil dihydrochloride, marketed as Posicor, associated with harmful interactions with other drugs voluntary withdrawn from the market on June 6, 1998

Temafloxacin hydrochloride, marketed as Omniflox, associated with hypoglycemia in elderly patients, frequently associated with renal failure and markedly abnormal liver tests, voluntarily withdrawn from the market September 25, 1997

Ticrynafen, marketed as Seacryn, associated with liver toxicity, voluntarily withdrawn from the market May 20, 1996 (FDA, 1999).

One drug that has not been taken off the market is the controversial diabetes drug troglitazone (Rezulin). The drug maker Warner-Lambert reported that it has linked 43 cases of acute liver failure to the use of the drug since its approval; 28 of these patients died, and 7 had liver transplants (Schwartz, Washington Post, March 27, 1999). New warning information concerning monitoring recommendations has been added to the labeling package (American Diabetes Association, 1999). It is the responsibility of all primary care providers to stay informed about FDA action and recommendations concerning drug products. The internet has made this feasible.

As authors of this book, we have sought contributors from many disciplines who are experts in the field of geriatrics and gerontology to provide the reader with a multidisciplinary focus. The book is primarily written for nurse practitioner students in gerontology, adult and family masters programs, and nurse practitioners working in primary care settings who are providing care for older adults. Primary care providers of other disciplines will find a great deal of material that we know is helpful. We continue to believe that the most complex but highly rewarding challenge of the field of nursing is the provision of primary health care to older people.

References

American Diabetes Association, http://www.diabetes.org/publications/adasearch, 1999.
Food and Drug Administration, http://www.fda.gov
Schwartz J: *Washington Post,* March 27, 1999.

Unit I

1

Health Assessment and Health Maintenance Screening

The traditional problem-focused medical assessment is often ineffectual in assessing the multiple, complex needs of the older patient. A practitioner who attempts to identify or focus on one specific diagnosis will often fail to recognize the real issue that prompted the patient to seek medical attention: the impact of the "diagnosis" on his or her daily functioning. The recognition of the complex medical, social, and mental health problems and resulting functional disabilities of many frail elderly persons has led to the development of a multidimensional, interdisciplinary approach to the evaluation of this population. The Comprehensive Geriatric Assessment (CGA) is often viewed as "the procedure" that defines geriatric care (Gudmundsson and Carnes, 1996). CGA helps providers diagnose and prioritize problems and develop short- and long-term plans for prevention, treatment, and rehabilitation strategies that emphasize improving or maintaining patient function, reducing unnecessary utilization of health care resources, and prolonging survival of elderly patients (Reuben, Yoshikawa, and Besdine, 1996). Improvement in function, rather than a cure for disability, is often the goal of comprehensive geriatric assessment (Gudmundsson and Carnes, 1996). Function may be impacted by biologic, psychologic, and social issues experienced by the individual. Findings such as multiple chronic medical problems, depression, cognitive impairment, or lack of adequate social supports or financial assets, either alone or in combination will significantly impact an older person's ability to carry out daily functions. In a survey performed by the National Center for Health Statistics in the 1980s, 45% of persons age 65 years and older not living in institutions were found to have some degree of limitation in daily activities (Williams, 1983). By incorporating multidisciplinary perspectives into a systematic assessment, CGA evaluates the "whole patient" (Rubenstein, 1996).

The process of CGA begins following identification of the patient in need—most commonly an elderly person who has experienced deteriorations in health and function (Williams, 1983). Patients most likely to benefit include:

- Persons over the age of 75
- Persons with mild to moderate disabilities
- Persons who may be at risk of nursing home placement
- Persons with a poor social network (Gudmundsson and Carnes, 1996)

Age may be irrelevant if a person is coping with functional impairments and/or such "geriatric syndromes" as immobility, incontinence, use of multiple or inappropriate medications, cognitive impairment, weight loss, or depression or if the older person has been recently discharged from a hospital, is recently widowed, or is living alone. Therefore a chronically ill 50-year-old with no family supports may be a more appropriate candidate for CGA than a healthy, active 75-year-old with a strong social support system.

The Assessment Environment

CGA exists as a continuum and therefore may occur in a variety of settings. The first reports of geriatric assessment programs came from a British geriatrician named Marjory Warren who created specialized geriatric assessment units during the 1930s (Williams, 1983). Depending on the individual patient's level of disability, cognition, access to transportation, and social supports, CGA may occur in the hospital, nursing facility, outpatient clinic, or home. Each of these sites presents challenges and benefits to performing the CGA. For example, in a hospital setting one has the benefit of time (the duration of the hospitalization) and, usually, opportunities to gain information from family and friends who visit. However, because the patient is sick, the hospital setting does not offer the opportunity to assess him or her at baseline. In a nursing facility, many of the same benefits and challenges as the inpatient setting may be found. One benefit, however, is the Minimum Data Set (MDS) (see Appendix A). The MDS is an exhaustive assessment tool required for every patient in the long-term setting that is completed mostly by the nursing staff and provides information regarding medical diagnoses, disabilities, and level of functioning; it is updated regularly. This is an important and underused tool in the comprehensive assessment of a patient in this setting.

The outpatient clinic setting is probably where the most CGAs take place. This setting can be a challenging one in which to fully assess the functional capabilities of the older person. Pressures of tight schedules, tight space, and looming productivity reports are not conducive to the investment of the time and skill required of a thorough comprehensive assessment. In addition, most clinic settings are not designed with the older person in mind. Although laws requiring handicapped accessibility have brought about major improvements, issues such as inappropriate lighting, sound, office design, and decor may still create challenges for the older person trying to access his health care provider. Poor sound barriers between examination rooms or background music may make it difficult for the person with a hearing impairment to understand what is being said to him by the examiner in the same room. Poor lighting that casts shadows or solid colors and vertical lines in the decor may hinder depth perception. A desk in front of a sunny window may cause the person with macular degeneration to see only an outline of the person to whom he or she is speaking. Although some of these issues may be out of the nurse practitioner's control, there are some simple techniques that may help to overcome some of these barriers. Sitting close to and directly in front of the patient and speaking in low and even tones can help to accommodate communication with persons with visual or hearing impairment. A portable amplifying device for persons without a hearing aid can be invaluable in facilitating communication with the hearing-impaired person. Appointments for older persons may be scheduled at a time when the office is less crowded, hectic, and overwhelming for the frail elderly patient and should routinely be of longer duration than the standard 10- or 15-minute follow-up appointment.

The average time spent per new patient in outpatient geriatric assessment units in one study was 2.7 hours (Gudmundsson and Carnes, 1996). Fortunately, the assessment of the older person can occur over several visits, with the initial visit focused on any urgent concerns and needs. The gathering of information from a new patient is often facilitated by mailing a preappointment questionnaire to the patient's home to be completed and brought in to the first appointment. The use of such a questionnaire, however, does not negate the need for discussing the information with the patient in the office. The use of a problem list that is updated at each visit offers an efficient way to track a patient's often multiple medical issues. It may be designed to include not only diagnoses, but a medication list, advance directive information, and health screening information for quick reference at each visit. Although CGA is ideally performed by a multidisciplinary team, in reality the assessment may be performed by the primary health care provider alone. Nurse practitioners have the distinct advantage of a biopsychosocial background in approaching patients of all ages and therefore are well equipped to perform the comprehensive assessment of the frail older person.

The home is the ideal setting for CGA, allowing observation of the actual living situation, barriers, and resources with which the patient lives. Unfortunately, practitioners who have the time and desire to make home visits are rare.

Use of Assessment Tools

Many standardized tools have been developed to facilitate assessment of various aspects of functioning. These tools are an important first step in the gathering of information regarding a person's biologic, psychological, and social functional abilities. They provide fairly objective and standardized means for health care professionals to communicate findings. They can save time, facilitate the process of assessment, and improve accuracy and reliability; and they are particularly helpful in screening for problems that often go unsuspected, even after clinical examination. However, it is important that the person administering the instrument have a working knowledge of its proper application to protect the reliability and validity of the test. Abnormal results on screening tools alone do not provide a diagnosis, but rather indicate the need for further evaluation. One caveat: Assessment instruments are important for data collection, but relying too heavily on numeric scores can oversimplify a situation and shift attention away from the individual patient and his or her functional abilities within the patient's particular situation (Gudmundsson and Carnes, 1996).

Values

One cannot approach the assessment of the biopsychosocial issues that may affect function without gleaning an appreciation of the individual's values. In this context, value goes beyond defining what the individual considers to be important in his life to determining what traits, roles, and activities a person feels identifies himself to the world as an individual and what gives that person meaning in his life. These values are developed over the course of a lifetime and are influenced by family, culture, religion, and life experiences. The primary care provider cannot develop a plan to meet the needs of an individual until he or she understands what the priorities and goals of the individual are. This requires actively seeking, acknowledging, and respecting this information.

As the U.S. population ages, it is becoming more diverse in terms of culture and ethnicity. Non-Hispanic whites accounted for 80% of the 65 and older population in 1980, but this figure dropped to 74% in 1995 and is projected to be only about 67% by the year 2050. Although the black elderly population is the largest component of the minority elderly population, this segment is projected to show only modest increases in numbers in the foreseeable future. Furthermore, the composition of elderly minorities will change, with one in six elderly Americans expected to be of Hispanic origin by the year 2050. The fastest growing segments of the elderly population are Asian and Pacific Islanders, who are expected to grow from 2% of the older population in 1995 to 7% by 2050 (Markides and Rudkin, 1996).

The cultural background of an individual will influence not only the practitioner's assessment and teaching regarding language, diet, and disease risks, but will also necessitate consideration of other issues that may impact functional status, either negatively or positively. The great diversity in economic status within and among ethnic origins, as well as the patient's status regarding health insurance, necessitates consideration of a patient's ability to pay for a diagnostic test, treatment, or service the practitioner may order. On the other hand, many black, Hispanic, Asian-American, and Native American elderly have been found to benefit from higher rates of co-residence with adult children and from social support from their extended families. Although this situation may exist out of necessity for economic survival, the availability of family members in the household or in close proximity can be a great support to ethnic and minority elderly who have few other resources (Markides and Rudkin, 1996).

Another important cultural consideration is the individual's feelings regarding effective and desirable practices and outcomes of health care. It is important to remember that some Hispanic persons may utilize traditional American medicine in conjunction with faith healing or other traditional practices. The practitioner may be unaware of other practices unless the patient is asked. These beliefs must be recognized and respected if the maximum benefit for the patient is to be achieved. Education regarding medicine and diet may need to be tailored to the cultural beliefs and values of each individual patient. The primary care provider must recognize and respect an individual's cultural viewpoints and discover effective methods to provide health care and teaching in a manner that will be acceptable to the individual patient. As with all patients, it is critical to ascertain that instructions are understood. The nurse practitioner should not assume that a polite nod indicates understanding of what has been said. The patient or family member should be asked to repeat or explain instructions given. If a language barrier exists, a translator should be found.

Religious considerations play an important role in the assessment of most older individuals, whether or not they are of a culturally diverse group. Practices associated with and attitudes toward diet, medications, family roles, and decisions regarding health care may be dictated by one's religious beliefs. Again, the nurse practitioner must learn to provide care to patients with respect for and consideration of these firmly held beliefs.

Advance Directives

Decisions regarding health care may result in any one of many different outcomes. Each individual holds his or her own beliefs concerning what constitutes a desirable or "quality" outcome. A health care provider cannot assist a patient or family to make decisions that will work toward the desired outcome unless he or she has taken the time to ascertain what the goals of the patient or family are. This process is known as advance care planning. A patient with end-stage congestive heart failure desires no "heroic measures" to prolong her life, and her only desire is to see her grandson graduate from college, even if the possibility exists that she may not survive the long trip. A healthy 60-year-old man has no medical problems, takes no medication, and jogs 3 miles a day. Last year he watched his father die after months on a ventilator and vows never to allow that to happen to himself. A frail elderly man wishes only to have a peaceful death in his own home with his family by his side and does not care to undergo aggressive medical evaluations that may prolong his life by a few months. A healthy and active 90-year-old woman is looking forward to celebrating her 100th birthday, as did her mother and grandmother before her. Each of these individuals will require a different approach to his or her care if the goals are to be met, but chances are that, without the help of their health care provider, none of them will succeed.

Although advance care planning is especially relevant for persons facing life-threatening illnesses, it is impossible to predict when a previously healthy person may suffer an acute, life-threatening event. Thus it is important to discuss preferences regarding health care and desired outcomes with everyone. The best time to initiate these discussions is during a routine visit when a patient is healthy, but it is wise to remember that decisions should be reviewed and updated at regular intervals throughout the provider's relationship with the patient and family.

Although a critical aspect of advance care planning is the provider's knowledge of the patient's and family's values and goals, two documents have traditionally been used in the advance care planning process to guide patients and provide written documentation regarding their wishes. The living will is a document that allows a patient to specify preferences for health care in a variety of hypothetic situations. However, most of these scenarios are described in the setting of terminal illness or persistent vegetative state. This situation may not apply for all patients who wish to execute these documents. Therefore conversations regarding advance directives need to be centered on the conceivable medical possibilities that may arise within the patient's current situation.

The other document commonly used is the durable power of attorney (DPOA) for health. This is a legal document that requires legal assistance and is specifically designed to allow a person to designate a proxy to make decisions regarding health care on his or her behalf in the event of incapacitation. It is critical that the person designated understands the patient's values and wishes so that appropriate decisions are made on behalf of the patient.

Often it is clear to the health care provider and family that the patient is not able to participate in the decision-making process (e.g., the patient with advanced dementia). However, there are times when the patient's ability to make decisions may not be clear. In these situations it becomes necessary for the provider to formally assess the patient's capacity to make decisions regarding his or her own health care. Every health care decision does not require the same degree of decision-making capacity to make an appropriate decision. An individual may be capable of performing some tasks adequately (i.e., have the capacity to make some decisions) but not others. This "decision-specific capacity" assumes that an individual has or lacks capacity for a particular decision at a particular time and under a particular set of circumstances. The determination that a patient has sufficient decision-making capacity to consent to or refuse a particular treatment is based on observation of a specific set of abilities:

- The patient understands that he or she has the right to make a choice.
- The patient understands the medical situation, prognosis, risks, benefits, and consequences of treatment (or no treatment).
- The patient can communicate the decision.
- The patient's decision is stable and consistent over a period of time (Mezey, Mitty, and Ramsey, 1997).

A patient who has had a stroke that has left him aphasic may understand the choices, but if he is not able to communicate his wishes verbally, in writing, or in any other fashion, he is not able to participate in the decision-making process.

The requirements for who may perform the capacity assessment (i.e., one physician vs. a physician *and* a psychiatrist) vary between states. The nurse practitioner can play an important role in this process. All documentation of a patient's ability, or lack thereof, to communicate meaningfully may be taken into account. If a patient is certified as lacking capacity, the documentation should include the following:

- The cause and nature of the mental incapacity
- The extent of the incapacity
- The probable duration of the incapacity

The mental status of a patient with a delirium due to a pneumonia will most likely clear on treatment of the underlying infection, and his or her capacity to make health care decisions must be reevaluated following treatment. However, a patient with moderate to advanced Alzheimer's disease can be expected to have a permanent incapacity due to the progressive course of the disease process.

If a patient that has been certified as lacking capacity has previously executed a DPOA for health, the person appointed becomes the decision maker for the patient. If no DPOA has been identified, the authority to make decisions goes to one of the following (order of priority varies somewhat from state to state):

- Court-appointed guardian/conservator (if none of the following is available)
- Spouse
- Adult child
- Parent

- Adult sibling
- Nearest living adult relative

Advance care planning and execution of a DPOA can spare the patient, family, provider, (and courts!) a great deal of anxiety and grief. It is imperative that the primary provider, be it a physician or nurse practitioner, be comfortable in addressing these issues. It is one of the most valuable services providers can offer their patients.

Biopsychosocial Assessment

Medical Assessment

Figure 1-1 illustrates the approach to the comprehensive geriatric assessment. The individual's values impact his or her individual biopsychosocial traits, which in turn interact to determine his or her functional ability, which is the "target" of the comprehensive assessment.

All of the areas of assessment must be approached with consideration for the current or planned living situation, be it independent in a home or apartment, assisted living, or long-term care. The assessment, diagnosis, and plan for a patient in a long-term care facility will probably differ greatly from an individual living independently in the community because the presentation of disease, the differential diagnoses, the availability of resources, and the goals of care will probably vary significantly among various settings. The biologic component of the assessment includes such issues as the medical history and physical examination, current status regarding presence or absence of disease states, risk behaviors, preventive health practices, nutrition, and medication use. Other important aspects to be evaluated are nutritional status, the presence of pain (which may impact function and quality of life), and the potential for or actual existence of abuse or neglect by caregivers (all of which will be covered in later chapters).

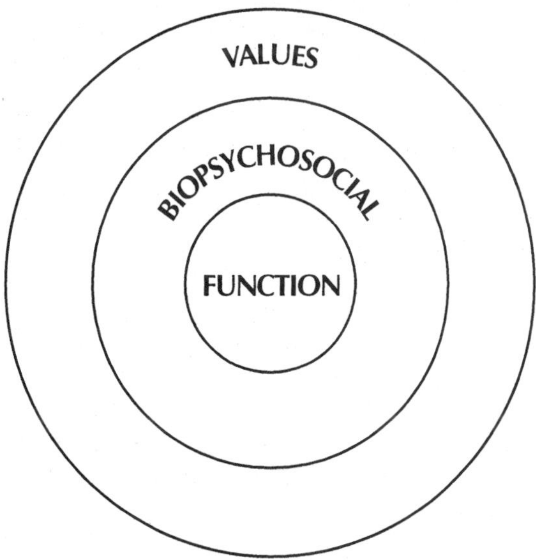

Figure 1-1 Approach to comprehensive geriatric assessment.

The assessment begins with first contact with the patient. Did the patient call to schedule an appointment herself? Was the patient able to communicate her needs on the phone and indicate understanding of information given to her such as date and time of appointment and location of office? Or did a family member make the call? The physical examination begins on first visualization of the patient. Did the patient walk into the office independently? Is she able to follow instructions such as, "Follow me to the examination room," or "Step up on the scale"? If not, is it because of hearing impairment, cognitive impairment, or physical disability? Is there an intention tremor when you shake the patient's hand in greeting? Is the patient in the long-term care setting bedridden or ambulatory? The health care provider does not derive information solely by formal examination and assessment; even a social encounter can reveal volumes about a patient's functional abilities.

The approach to assessment of the various organ systems and disease processes will be addressed in later chapters. However, there are a few "pearls" of assessment that should be routine (in any setting) and therefore are worth mentioning separately:

1. Patients or families should always be asked to "brown bag" (i.e., to bring in) the bottles of *all* medications the patient is taking, including over-the-counter medications, to *each* visit. The medication list in the chart may not always be reliable; medications may have been stopped or started by the patient or other health care providers.
2. Blood pressure and pulse should always be measured in the lying, sitting, and standing positions to determine the presence of orthostatic hypotension, an often overlooked cause of frequent falls.
3. Weight should be checked and recorded at each visit, with drops or increases addressed appropriately.
4. Hearing aids should always be removed and inspected, and the ear canals inspected for cerumen to ensure optimal hearing function.
5. An oral examination must always be performed to assess dentition and oral mucosa. Dentures must also be assessed for fit, then removed and inspected for rough edges that may irritate or injure the oral mucosa.
6. Abdominal examinations should always include a digital rectal examination. Although testing for fecal occult blood may not always be appropriate, examination of the prostate and assessment for the presence of impacted stool almost always is.
7. The musculoskeletal examination should not only cover assessment of muscle strength and range of motion but should include a thorough assessment of the feet; presence of ulcers or painful callouses, excessively long toenails, and inappropriate footwear can all impact ambulatory status.
8. Whether an assessment is comprehensive or focused will depend on the presenting complaint of the patient. Keep in mind the following "pearls" in assessment of an acute problem:
   a. Infection may present as vague changes from baseline rather than fever and localizing symptoms. A change in appetite, recurrent falls, or a nurse's report that a patient "just isn't himself" warrants investigation.
   b. The three most common sites of infection, especially in the long-term care setting, are denoted by the mnemonic *PUS*: *P*neumonia, *U*rine, *S*kin.
   c. Providers should have a low threshold of suspicion for fractures when presented with a limb that is swollen or painful.

Although screening and preventive care recommendations vary somewhat between professional health organizations, they still offer some guidance in determining issues to be addressed. Table 1-1 (Hayward, Steinberg, and Ford, 1991) outlines recommendations by organization. Although age 85 has been proposed as a general cutoff range beyond which conventional screening tests are unlikely to be of continued benefit (Goldberg and Chavin, 1997), it is always important to consider these recommendations in the context of the individual patient's current health status, ability to participate in the screening process, potential for benefit from screening and treatment of a particular disease, and goals of care. Immunization status is one area that is almost always appropriate to address. Persons of all ages should receive the tetanus-diphtheria (Td) vaccine every 10 years. Some individuals, especially women who have not served in the military, may have never received the vaccine and will need the primary series of three toxoid doses over 6 to 12 months. Patients with pressure ulcers are an often overlooked population of persons for whom Td vaccine is especially important. Annual influenza vaccination, usually given in October, is a vital preventive measure against the "flu" in all settings. The vaccine is important not only for older persons who may be susceptible to developing pneumonia following a case of the flu, but for persons such as health care workers and frequent visitors to the long-term care or other care delivery setting who may bring the virus into the facility. Finally, the American College of Physicians recommends the pneumococcal vaccine for all adults after the age of 65; persons who received the vaccine before age 65 should be reimmunized at 65 if more than 6 years have passed since the initial vaccine (Goldberg and Chavin, 1997). Persons for whom hospice-type care is desired may decline to receive the pneumococcal vaccine, preferring instead comfort-oriented symptom management and acceptance of death as a potential outcome of an infection. This may only be challenged if there is serious concern regarding the potential for pneumonia epidemic within a facility. Other preventive measures such as aspirin therapy, estrogen replacement, and vitamin and mineral supplementation are covered in other chapters.

Polypharmacy is an all too common and potentially critical issue in the care of older persons. Many of these patients see several health care providers simultaneously: (e.g., a primary physician, a cardiologist, an orthopedist, an endocrinologist, a psychiatrist) and may never think to inform each of the treatments and medications prescribed by the others. This can lead to the prescribing of multiple medications, some of which may not be compatible. In addition, the confusion caused by trade and generic drug names may lead a person to take two forms of the same medication without even being aware of it! It is for this reason that the "brown bag" method for maintaining an updated medication list is recommended. The old adage in geriatric medicine of, "Start low, go slow" is still sage; introduce new medications at the lowest possible dose and titrate up cautiously.

Nutritional Assessment

Nutritional assessment requires special attention to the individual's cultural and ethnic background. The following nutritional assessment questions take into account cultural issues (Lueckenotte, 1996):

1. What is the meaning of food and eating to the patient?
2. What does the patient typically eat during:
   a. A typical day?
   b. Special events such as secular or religious holidays?

TABLE 1-1 Screening and Preventive Care Recommendations for Asymptomatic, Low-risk Older Adults

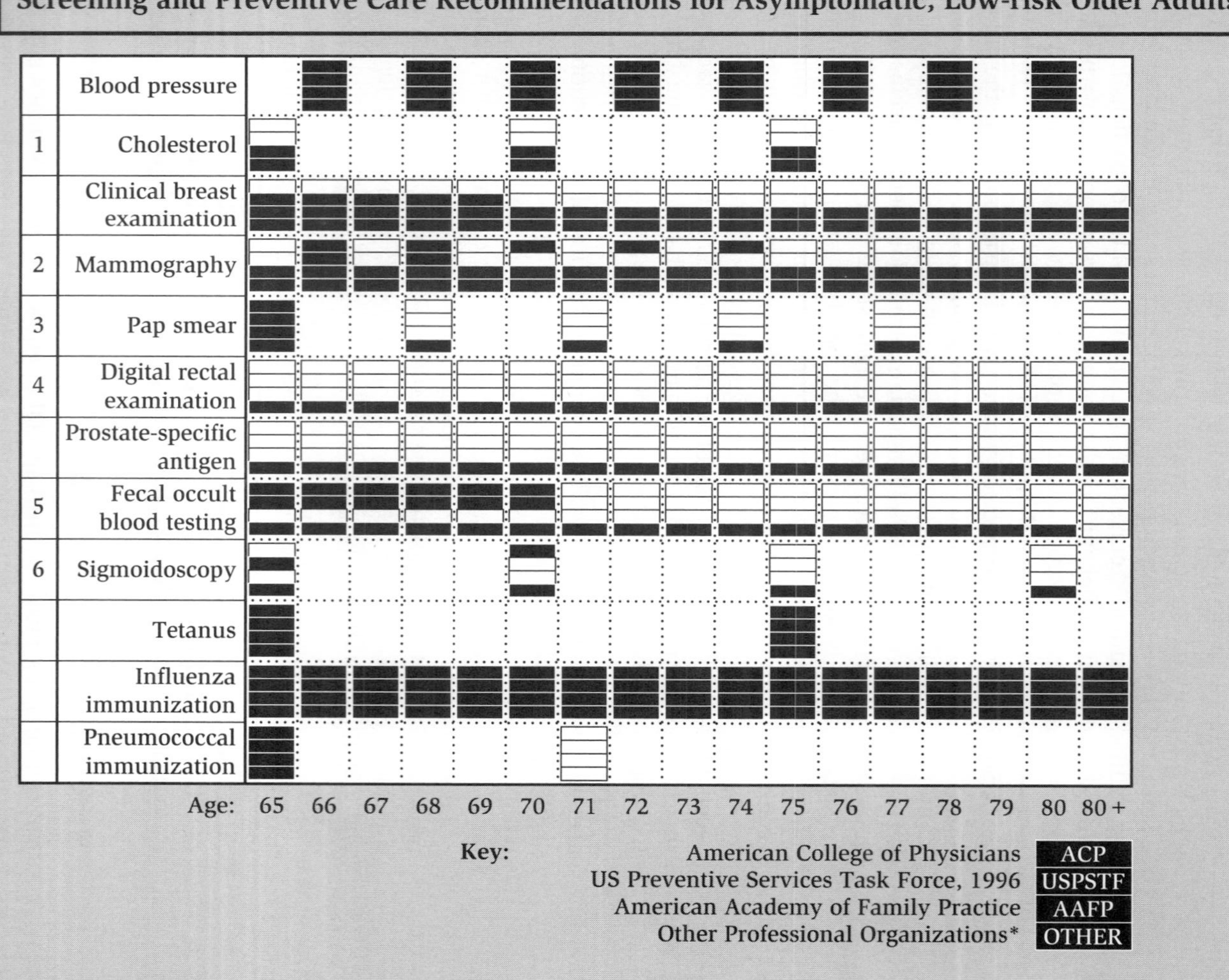

This table shows selected, age-specific preventive care services recommended by professional health organizations, which should be offered to persons who do not have a family history, symptoms, signs, or other diseases that place them at increased risk for preventable conditions. All authorities stress the importance of assessing each person's unique risks in order to tailor preventive care.

ACP, USPSTF, and AAFP emphasize that all adults should be routinely counseled about tobacco use, nutrition, exercise, substance abuse, injury prevention, sensory loss, and dental care.

1. The USPSTF finds insufficient evidence for or against screening over age 65, but does recommend screening healthy individuals between 65 and 75 *with* coronary heart disease risk factors such as smoking, hypertension, and diabetes. The ACP concurs, but advises against screening after age 75.
2. The AGS recommends discontinuation at age 85; the ACP recommends age 75. The USPSTF states that benefit may exist for women over age 70 since there is a high burden of suffering and lack of evidence for differences in the test characteristics for mammography in older women. AAFP and ACS recommend annual screening with no definitive age to discontinue screening.
3. ACP, AAFP, and USPSTF recommend no further Papanicolaou smears for women over 65 years of age who have had consistently normal smears in the previous decade.
4. The AAFP, ACP and USPSTF report that the digital rectal examination is not a good screening tool for either colorectal or prostate cancer. However the ACS recommends this procedure; the USPSTF states that there is insufficient evidence to recommend for or against DRE.
5. USPSTF and ACS recommend annual screening after age 50 with no recommended discontinuation date. The AAFP recommendations are under review. The ACP recommends fecal occult blood testing for those who decline invasive screening.
6. ACP recommends sigmoidoscopy, colonoscopy, or air-contrast barium enema every 10 years, age 50-70. The USPSTF recommends sigmoidoscopy but does not recommend an interval for screening. Guidelines are under review by the AAFP.

*Includes the Advisory Committee on Immunization Practices; National Cholesterol Education Program Panel on Detection, Evaluation, and Treatment of High Blood Cholesterol in Adults; Joint National Committee on Detection, Evaluation, and Treatment of High Blood Pressure; American Cancer Society; and American Geriatrics Society.

Modified from Hayward RSA et al: Preventive care guidelines: 1991, *Ann Intern Med* 114(9):761-762, 1991. Modified with permission. The American College of Physicians is not responsible for the accuracy of the adaptation.

3. How does the patient define food (e.g., unless rice is served, many from India do not consider the ingestion of food to be a meal)?
4. What is the timing and sequence of meals?
5. With whom does the patient usually eat (alone, with a spouse)?
6. What does the patient believe comprises a "healthy" vs. "unhealthy" diet? Any hot/cold or yin/yang beliefs?
7. From what sources does the patient obtain food items (e.g., ethnic grocery store, home garden, restaurant)? Who usually does the grocery shopping?
8. How are foods prepared (type of preparation; cooking oils used; length of time foods are cooked; amount and type of seasoning added before, during, or after preparation)?
9. Has the patient chosen a particular nutritional practice such as vegetarianism or abstinence from alcoholic beverages?
10. Do religious beliefs and practices influence the patient's diet or eating habits (e.g., amount, type, preparations, or designation of acceptable food items or combinations)?

Because the consumption of alcohol can affect so many different aspects of health, it is very important to accurately ascertain a patient's alcohol intake. "Occasionally" or "socially" may mean very different things to different people. It is important to determine the actual intake (i.e., 3 beers or 5 ounces of liquor) in an average week or month, as well as the average amount in a single episode. A patient who drinks only "on weekends" may actually be drinking alcohol continuously from Friday night through Sunday evening. A patient who only drinks "once a month" may actually drink close to an entire case of beer or liter of whiskey in one evening; This phenomenon known as "binge-drinking" is not a benign "social" intake of alcohol, and, unless patients and families are specifically asked, this information may not be revealed. One of the quickest, yet effective oral screening tools for problematic alcohol intake is the CAGE (Mayfield, McLeod, and Hall, 1974):

- Have you ever felt you could *C*ut down on your drinking?
- Have people *A*nnoyed you by criticizing your drinking?
- Have you ever felt bad or *G*uilty about your drinking?
- Have you ever had a drink first thing in the morning (an *E*ye-opener) to steady your nerves or to get rid of a hangover?

If at least two of the questions are answered affirmatively, the probability of alcoholism is high. Further investigation is also needed if only one of the questions is answered affirmatively. See Chapter 27 for an older age-specific alcohol questionnaire.

Psychologic Assessment

Cognitive Assessment. Unlike the physical examination in which one may learn a great deal from an informal social encounter, evaluation of cognitive status often requires formal focused assessment. Highly developed social graces or advanced education may easily cover the signs of an early cognitive impairment. A superficial and genial conversation will probably not reveal an underlying disorientation to time and place or a deficit in short-term memory. The most extensively used tool for assessment of mental status in geriatrics is the Folstein Mini-Mental State Examination (MMSE) (Figure 1-2). The score is reported as the patient's score/the highest possible score (e.g., 24/30).

Mini-Mental State Examination (MMSE)

Add points for each correct response.

		Score	Points
Orientation			
1. What is the:	Year	___	1
	Season	___	1
	Date	___	1
	Day	___	1
	Month	___	1
2. Where are we?	State	___	1
	County	___	1
	Town or city	___	1
	Hospital	___	1
	Floor	___	1
Registration			
3. Name three objects, taking one second to say each. Then ask the patient to repeat all three after you have said them. Give one point for each correct answer. Repeat the answers until patient learns all three.		___	3
Attention and calculation			
4. Serial sevens. Give one point for each correct answer. Stop after five answers. Alternate: Spell WORLD backwards.		___	5
Recall			
5. Ask for names of three objects learned in question 3. Give one point for each correct answer.		___	3
Language			
6. Point to a pencil and a watch. Have the patient name them as you point.		___	2
7. Have the patient repeat "No ifs, ands, or buts."		___	1
8. Have the patient follow a three-stage command: "Take a paper in your right hand. Fold the paper in half. Put the paper on the floor."		___	3
9. Have the patient read and obey the following: "CLOSE YOUR EYES." (Write it in large letters.)		___	1
10. Have the patient write a sentence of his or her choice. (The sentence should contain a subject and an object and should make sense. Ignore spelling errors when scoring.)		___	1
11. Have the patient copy the design. (Give one point if all sides and angles are preserved and if the intersecting sides form a quadrangle.)		___	1
		___ =	Total 30

In validation studies using a cut-off score of 23 or below, the MMSE has a sensitivity of 87%, a specificity of 82%, a false-positive ratio of 39.4%, and a false-negative ratio of 4.7%. These ratios refer to the MMSE's capacity to accurately distinguish patients with clinically diagnosed dementia or delirium from patients without these syndromes.

Figure 1-2 Mini-Mental State Examination (MMSE). (From Folstein MJ, Folstein S, McHugh PR: Mini-mental state: a practical method for grading the cognitive state of patients for the clinician, *J Psych Res* 12:189-198, 1975. Reprinted with permission of Elsevier Science.)

(A question may be omitted for some reason, thereby decreasing the highest possible score.) The MMSE takes approximately 10 to 15 minutes to administer, and each section of the tool assesses a different aspect of cognitive function: orientation, registration, attention and calculation, recall, and language. A score of 25/30 and above is generally considered to reflect only minimal cognitive impairment, whereas a patient with mid to late-stage Alzheimer's disease may score 15/30 and below. It is important to keep in mind that factors such as level of education, language barrier, and physical disabilities may affect performance.

Another tool for the assessment of cognitive function and "executive function" (i.e., planning and sequencing) is the "clock test" in which a patient is asked to draw a clock, put the numbers on it, and then draw hands indicating the time 11:15. The clock drawing is scored from 10 to 1 in the following manner:

10 to 6: Drawing of clock face with circle and numbers is generally intact

10: Hands are in correct position.
9: There are slight errors in placement of the hands.
8: There are more noticeable errors in the placement of hour and minute hands.
7: Placement of hands is significantly off course.
6: There is inappropriate use of clock hands (i.e., use of digital display/circling of numbers).

5 to1: Drawing of clock face with circle and numbers is NOT intact

5: Crowding of numbers at one end of the clock or reversal of numbers.
4: There is further distortion of number sequence; the integrity of clock face is now gone (i.e., numbers are missing or placed outside the boundaries of the clock face).
3: The numbers and clock face are no longer obviously connected in the drawing; hands are not present.
2: The drawing reveals some evidence of instructions being received, but only a vague representation of a clock.
1: Either no attempt or an uninterpretable effort is made.

Affective Assessment. Depression is probably the most common example of the nonspecific and atypical presentation of illness in the elderly (Kane, Ouslander, and Abrass, 1994). Nonspecific physical complaints such as fatigue, weight loss, diffuse pain, memory or sleep disturbance, and constipation may represent a variety of treatable *physical* illnesses, as well as depression. Frequently depression and physical illness coexist in elderly patients. Therefore it is not surprising that treatable depressions are often overlooked in patients with physical illness and that treatable physical illnesses are often not optimally managed in patients diagnosed as having depression (Goldberg and Chavin, 1997). The rate of suicide is higher among elderly males than any other segment of the population. A variety of biologic, physical, psychologic, and social factors predispose the elderly to depression, which is discussed further in a later chapter. However, there are also some very useful screening tools that can be used to assess the presence of depression in elderly persons. The most commonly used is the short form of the Geriatric Depression Scale (GDS) developed by Yesavage and Brink (Figure 1-3). A score between 5 and 9 suggests depression, whereas scores above 9 generally indicate depression. Another helpful tool in screening for depression is the mnemonic SIGECAPS: (Shua-Haim et al, 1997):

S: Changes in *Sleep* patterns or *Sexual* activities
I: Loss of *Interest* in activities
G: Feelings of *Guilt* or remorse
E: Lack of *Energy*
C: Difficulty *Concentrating*
A: Change in *Appetite* (increased or decreased)
P: *Psychomotor* agitation or retardation
S: Thoughts of *Suicide*

Geriatric Depression Scale (short form)

Choose the best answer for how you felt over the past week.

1.	Are you basically satisfied with your life?	yes/no
2.	Have you dropped many of your activities and interests?	yes/no
3.	Do you feel that your life is empty?	yes/no
4.	Do you often get bored?	yes/no
5.	Are you in good spirits most of the time?	yes/no
6.	Are you afraid that something bad is going to happen to you?	yes/no
7.	Do you feel happy most of the time?	yes/no
8.	Do you often feel helpless?	yes/no
9.	Do you prefer to stay home rather than go out and do new things?	yes/no
10.	Do you feel you have more problems with memory than most?	yes/no
11.	Do you think it is wonderful to be alive now?	yes/no
12.	Do you feel pretty worthless the way you are now?	yes/no
13.	Do you feel full of energy?	yes/no
14.	Do you feel that your situation is hopeless?	yes/no
15.	Do you think that most people are better off than you are?	yes/no

This is the scoring for the scale. One point for each of these answers. Cut-off: normal (0-5), above 5 suggests depression.

1. no	6. yes	11. no
2. yes	7. no	12. yes
3. yes	8. yes	13. no
4. yes	9. yes	14. yes
5. no	10. yes	15. yes

Figure 1-3 Geriatric Depression Scale (short form). (From Sheikh JI, Yesavage JA: Geriatric depression scale: recent evidence and development of a shorter version, *Clin Gerontol* 5:165-172, 1986.)

The Yale Task Force on Geriatric Assessment also found that the single question, "Do you often feel sad or depressed?" had approximately the same sensitivity and specificity as the GDS. Therefore, even if time does not allow for administration of an entire screening tool, it is still possible to assess for the presence of this very important treatable problem.

Social Assessment

Social Supports. The availability and quality of social resources such as family or other social support, housing, and income are key ingredients of social function that can greatly influence overall functional capacity. This becomes especially important for patients who depend on the help of others to maintain an independent living situation.

Box 1-1

OARS Social Resource Scale

Now I'd like to ask you some questions about your family and friends.

Are you single, married, widowed, divorced, or separated?

1 Single   3 Widowed   5 Separated
2 Married   4 Divorced   ___ Not answered

If "2" ask following
Does your spouse live here also?
1 yes
0 no
___ Not answered

Who lives with you?
(Check "yes" or "no" for each of the following.)

Yes	No	
______	______	No one
______	______	Husband or wife
______	______	Children
______	______	Grandchildren
______	______	Parents
______	______	Grandparents
______	______	Brothers and sisters
______	______	Other relatives (does not include inlaws covered in the above categories)
______	______	Friends
______	______	Nonrelated paid help (includes free room)
______	______	Others (specify)

____

In the past year about how often did you leave here to visit your family and/or friends for weekends or holidays or to go on shopping trips or outings?
1 Once a week or more
2 1-3 times a month
3 Less than once a month or only on holidays
4 Never
___ Not answered

How many people do you know well enough to visit with in their homes?
3 Five or more
2 Three to four
1 One to two
0 None
___ Not answered

About how many times did you talk to someone—friends, relatives, or others—on the telephone in the past week (either you called them or they called you)? (If subject has no phone, question still applies.)
3 Once a day or more
2 Twice
1 Once
0 Not at all
___ Not answered

How many times during the past week did you spend some time with someone who does not live with you, that is, you went to see them, or they came to visit you, or you went out to do things together?

How many times in the past week did you visit with someone, either with people who live here or people who visited you here?
3 Once a day or more
2 Two to six
1 Once
0 Not at all
___ Not answered

Do you have someone you can trust and confide in?
1 Yes
0 No
___ Not answered

Do you find yourself feeling lonely quite often, sometimes, or almost never?
0 Quite often
1 Sometimes
2 Almost never
___ Not answered

Do you see your relatives and friends as often as you want to, or not?
1 As often as wants to
0 Not as often as wants to
___ Not answered

Is there someone *(outside this place)* who would give you any help at all if you were sick or disabled, for example, your husband/wife, a member of your family, or a friend?
1 Yes
0 No one willing and able to help
___ Not answered

Modified from Duke University Center for the Study of Aging and Human Developments. *OARS multidimensional functional assessment: questionnaire,* Durham, NC, 1988, Duke University.

Box 1-1
OARS Social Resource Scale—cont'd

If "yes" ask A and B

A. Is there someone *(outside this place)* who would take care of you as long as needed, or only for a short time, or only someone who would help you now and then (taking you to the doctor, or fixing lunch occasionally)?
   3 Someone who would take care of subject indefinitely (as long as needed)
   2 Someone who would take care of subject for a short time (a few weeks to 6 months)
   1 Someone who would help subject now and then (e.g., taking him to the doctor or fixing lunch)
   ___ Not answered

B. Who is this person?
   Name ____________________
   Relationship ____________________

Rating scale

Rate the current social resources of the person being evaluated along the six-point scale presented below. Circle the *one* number that best describes the person's present circumstances.

1. *Excellent social resources:* Social relationships are very satisfying and extensive; at least one person would take care of him (her) indefinitely.
2. *Good social resources:* Social relationships are fairly satisfying and adequate and at least one person would take care of him (her) indefinitely, *or*
   Social relationships are very satisfying and extensive, and only short-term help is available.
3. *Mildly socially impaired:* Social relationships are unsatisfactory, of poor quality, few; but at least one person would take care of him (her) indefinitely, *or*
   Social relationships are fairly satisfactory and adequate, and only short-term help is available.
4. *Moderately socially impaired:* Social relationships are unsatisfactory, of poor quality, few; and only short-term care is available, *or*
   Social relationships are at least adequate or satisfactory, but help would only be available now and then.
5. *Severely socially impaired:* Social relationships are unsatisfactory, of poor quality, few; and help would be available only now and then, *or*
   Social relationships are at least satisfactory or adequate, but help is not available even now and then.
6. *Totally socially impaired:* Social relationships are unsatisfactory, of poor quality, few; and help is not available even now and then.

The relationship between social function and health becomes evident when one examines the use of health services by elderly people. Studies have shown that, regardless of marital status, elderly persons who live with others are less likely to use health services than those who live alone (Yoshikawa, Cobbs, and Brummel-Smith, 1993). It is equally important to assess the social supports of a family caregiver who may be providing full-time care to an elderly parent or relative. Family caregivers are a precious resource who bear many physical, emotional, and often financial burdens; it is in the best interest of the patient that they be supported in every way possible. The simple question, "Are you feeling overwhelmed?" can be an critical one. Caregiver stress can lead not only to illness and frustration for the caregiver but can progress to abuse and neglect of a vulnerable elderly person. It is important to remember that an elderly patient's support system may not be a "traditional" one, yet it is no less important or valuable. An elderly person living in his or her home may rely on neighbors, church members, or a building maintenance worker for assistance, support, and friendly conversation. The Older Adults Resources and Services (OARS) Social Resource Scale (Box 1-1) developed at Duke University extract data about family structure, patterns of friendship and visiting, availability of a confidant, satisfaction with the degree of social interaction, and availability of a helper in the event of illness or disability (Lueckenotte, 1996). The results are rated using a six-point scale ranging from

Box 1-2
Family APGAR

1. I am satisfied that I can turn to my family (friends) for help when something is troubling me. (*adaptation*)
2. I am satisfied with the way my family (friends) talks over things with me and shares problems with me. (*partnership*)
3. I am satisfied that my family (friends) accepts and supports my wishes to take on new activities or directions. (*growth*)
4. I am satisfied with the way my family (friends) expresses affection and responds to my emotions, such as anger, sorrow, or love. (*affection*)
5. I am satisfied with the way my family (friends) and I share time together. (*resolve*)

Scoring:
Statements are answered *always* (2 points), *some of the time* (1 point), *hardly ever* (0 points).

Reprinted with permission from Appleton & Lange. From Smilkstein G, Ashworth C, Montano D. Validity and reliability of the Family APGAR as a test of family function, *J Fam Pract* 15:303-311, 1982.

"excellent social resources" to "totally socially impaired." Different questions are used for patients who live in institutions (italicized). A shorter screening tool, the Family APGAR, assesses the family's *a*daptation, *p*artnership, *g*rowth, *a*ffection, and *r*esolve (Box 1-2). A score of less than 3 suggests a highly dysfunctional family; a score of 4 to 6, a moderately dysfunctional family. When assessing the social support system, it is also important to ask if the patient or family has received (or are receiving) services from any community resources such as social work, case management, or home health.

The asexual image of aging and the elderly has ancient origins reinforced by culture, ignorance, religion, families, and peers through the centuries (Weg, 1996). Sexuality, sensuality, and intimacy among older persons have been acknowledged more recently. The practitioner should not assume that simply because a person is elderly and may be single, divorced, or widowed, that he or she is not in a significant intimate relationship (nor, for that matter, should one assume that all elderly patients are heterosexual). The Duke Center for the Study of Aging and Human Development found that earlier interest, frequency, and enjoyment of sexual expression were reliable indicators of active sexuality in later years. Furthermore, any decline with age appeared related to death or illness of a partner rather than lack of interest. This also applies to patients living in their own homes. Sexual desires and needs do not evaporate on institutionalization. See Box 1-3 for a list of questions useful in assessing sexuality concerns in older adults.

Environmental Assessment

An elderly patient's functional ability may be significantly helped or hindered by his living environment. An individual with limited mobility in a wheelchair may be far more dependent in a small, poorly lit, cluttered apartment than in the wide, well-lit hallways of a care facility. While the environment of a hospital, assisted living or long-term care facility may be somewhat predictable, it is still important to consider these environments with the individual's particular needs and limitations in mind. A patient with chronic obstructive pulmonary disease who must travel a long hallway to reach the elevator to the dining room may find the trip too difficult and miss meals and social interaction. The

Box 1-3
Suggested Questions for Assessing Sexual Concerns

Sexual Satisfaction

- Have you experienced any changes in your sexual relationships lately?
- To what do you attribute this change?
- What types of sexual activities have you usually enjoyed the most, including things such as hugging, kissing, sleeping together, intercourse, masturbation, and so on?
- Do you or your partner take any prescription medications? What are they? How often do you take them? Have you experienced any changes in your level of energy since you started them? What about overall feelings of well-being? Any changes in sexual desire or activity?

For Men

- Have you noticed any changes in the intensity of your ejaculations, orgasms, or ability to attain or maintain an erection?
- Have you ever had orgasms without ejaculations?
- Has your level of enjoyment from sexual relations altered as a result of these changes?
- Have you ever had any problems with urethral discharge or urination?

For Women

- Have you ever experienced any vaginal soreness or irritation after sexual intercourse? How long does it last? Any problems with urgency or with burning on urination after intercourse? Have you experienced abdominal contractions or back pain after intercourse?
- Have you had any problems with vaginal discharge or itching?
- Have any of these problems interfered with your sexual pleasure?
- Have you or your partner experienced any changes in your health status recently? How have these changes affected your sexual relationship?

Alterations in Self-perception

- How has growing older changed your lifestyle or things you enjoy doing?
- How has the change in your health or your partner's health altered your lifestyle or goals?
- How do you rate your general health?
- On a scale of 1 to 10, how would you describe your satisfaction with your life?
- On a scale of 1 to 10, how would you describe your satisfaction with your sexual relationships?

Relationships with Others

- Have you ever discussed sexual topics with your spouse, friends, family, or health care professional?
- Whom do you talk to when you have problems of any kind or just want someone to talk to?

Environment

- With whom do you live?
- Do you have a chance for privacy? To be alone? To talk with others privately if you want to?

From Burke M, Sherman S: Sexuality. In Burke M, Walsh M: *Gerontologic nursing*, St Louis, 1997, Mosby.

assessment of a frail elderly patient's environment becomes especially important when he is living in his own home. Safety factors to be assessed are identified in Box 1-4. The Home Safety Checklist developed by the National Safety Council is a thorough instrument used to identify fall hazards in the home (see Chapter 23). Although the tool is long and may be too time consuming to administer during a visit, it may be included in the previsit questionnaire for the patient and family to complete before the visit. It may then be

Box 1-4

Environmental Assessment

1. Poorly lighted stairwells, halls, or bathrooms
2. Stairs with weak or absent banisters
3. Absence of grab bars near bathtub
4. Glare in hallways
5. Absence of a working smoke alarm
6. Wet floors and/or waxed floors
7. Poorly placed extension cords
8. Throw rugs
9. Clutter
10. Inappropriate footwear and long clothing
11. High beds
12. Improper use of walking aids
13. Restraints and protective devices

From Burke MM, Walsh MB: *Gerontologic nursing: wholistic care of the older adult,* ed 2, St Louis, 1997, Mosby.

reviewed by the practitioner at the time of the appointment. After identification, hazards should be eliminated or reduced. One point is allowed for every NO answer. A score of 1 to 7 is excellent, 8 to 14 is good, 15 or higher is hazardous (Reuben, Yoshikawa, and Besdine, 1996). Although some of this information may be obtained from the patient, family or friends, the value of a home visit can not be overstated. If the provider is not able to do this himself or herself, a visit by a home care agency may be arranged.

Economic Assessment

In 1989, 11.4% of people 65 and over lived in poverty (Burke and Walsh, 1997). The primary source of income for older adults is social security, although there are several other sources: property, pensions, personal savings, investments, earnings, and a variety of financial assets (Figure 1-4). However, most persons do not benefit from all or even many of these resources. In 1985, older persons spent approximately 15% of their income on health care (Reuben, Yoshikawa, Besdine, 1996).

Many providers are not comfortable discussing economic issues with patients and will instead rely on the expertise of a social worker to explore these matters. However, it is very important to be aware of a patient or family's ability to pay for treatments prescribed. Some basic information may help the provider make choices and recommendations for patients that are within their means. A simple question such as, "Do you usually have money available to cover the 'little extras' that come up?" will open the door to discussing available finances and provide at least basic information that will be important for the provider to consider. The type of insurance a patient has is very basic and often determined at the time the appointment is scheduled. Providers must have at least a basic working knowledge of services and equipment covered by various insurance plans. For example, Medicare offers no prescription medication benefit. However, a secondary or Medigap insurance program may cover prescription medications with only a minimal copayment by the patient. There are many persons over the age of 65 who choose to

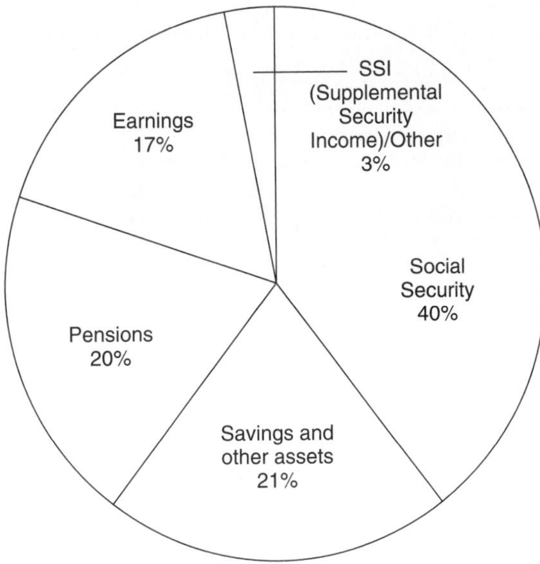

Figure 1-4 Sources of income for people 85 years old and older. (From U.S. Department of Health and Human Services, Social Security Administration, and Office of Research and Statistics: *Income of the aged chartbook, 1992,* SSA Pub. No. 13-11727, Washington, DC, 1994, U.S. Government Printing Office.)

participate in an HMO or health plan. These plans may dictate which medications, consultants, and even laboratory and radiology service the patient may use. A provider who is unaware of these requirements will do his or her patients a great disservice by inadvertently sending them to an unauthorized facility for laboratory work or x-rays for which they will be forced to pay out of pocket. Services or equipment for which the patient has no coverage should be discussed in terms of its costs and benefits. For example, hearing aids, which are not covered by any insurance programs, including Medicare, may not be a priority for an individual with hearing loss and a limited income. However, some persons may consider them vital and be willing to adjust their budget for the anticipated benefits derived from obtaining these assistive devices. It is important to become familiar with free or low-cost alternatives to care recommendations that may be available through public or private agencies.

Functional Assessment

Activities of Daily Living. It is often impossible to know that a patient requires assistance with specific tasks without formal questioning. It is not uncommon to hear family members say that a parent never needed help with dressing until the death of the spouse, when in reality, the parent had indeed required assistance, but the functional deficit (or cognitive impairment) was not realized until the caregiver was no longer available. Functional abilities involving self-care are discussed in terms of activities of daily living (ADLs), which are typically divided into the following categories (ABCDETT):

*A*mbulation: Mobility with or without an assistive device
*B*athing: Sponge baths, traditional baths, or showers

Box 1-5

Katz Index of Activities of Daily Living*

1. **Bathing (either sponge bath, tub bath, or shower)**
   a. Receives no assistance (gets in and out of tub by self if tub is usual means of bathing)
   b. Receives assistance in bathing only one part of body such as the back or a leg
   c. Receives assistance in bathing more than one part of body or is not bathed

2. **Continence**
   a. Controls urination and bowel movement completely by self
   b. Has occasional "accidents"
   c. Needs supervision to keep urine or bowel control, uses catheter, or is incontinent

3. **Dressing (gets clothes from closets and drawers, including underclothes, outer garments; uses fasteners, including braces, if worn)**
   a. Gets clothes and gets completely dressed without assistance
   b. Gets clothes and gets dressed without assistance except in tying shoes
   c. Receives assistance in getting clothes or getting dressed or stays partly or completely undressed

4. **Eating**
   a. Feeds self without assistance
   b. Feeds self except for assistance in cutting meat or buttering bread
   c. Receives assistance in feeding or is fed partly or completely by using tubes or intravenous fluids

5. **Toileting (going to the "toilet room" for bowel and urine elimination; cleaning self after elimination and arranging clothes)**
   a. Goes to "toilet room," cleans self, and arranges clothes without assistance (may use object for support such as cane, walker, or wheelchair and may manage night bedpan or commode and emptying same in morning)
   b. Receives assistance in going to "toilet room," cleaning self, or arranging clothes after elimination or receives assistance in using night bedpan or commode
   c. Does not go to room termed "toilet" for the elimination process

6. **Transferring**
   a. Moves in and out of bed or chair without assistance (may use object for support such as cane or walker)
   b. Moves in and out of bed or chair with assistance
   c. Does not get out of bed

*Response a., 3 points; b., 2 points; c., 1 point; maximum score, 18 points.

Continence: Sphincter control (bowel and bladder) (not the ability to get to a commode)
Dressing: Selecting and getting clothes, as well as the act of dressing
Eating: The ability to feed oneself (not the ability to prepare meals)
Toileting: Getting to the commode, undressing and redressing, and cleaning oneself
Transferring: Getting in and out of a bed or chair

The Katz index of ADL is a tool to assess a patient's ability to perform these functions (Box 1-5). Each function is rated on a three-point scale, with a maximum score of 18. It is important that the task classification be based on what the patient is *actually* doing, not

TABLE 1-2 Barthel Index

Action	With Help	Independently
1. Feeding (if food needs to be cut up = help)	5	10
2. Moving from wheelchair to bed and return (includes sitting up in bed)	5-10	15
3. Personal toilet (washing face, combing hair, shaving, cleaning teeth)	0	5
4. Getting on and off toilet (handling clothes, wiping, flushing)	5	10
5. Bathing self	0	5
6. Walking on level surface (or if unable to walk, propelling wheelchair)	0*	5*
7. Ascending and descending stairs	5	10
8. Dressing (includes tying shoes, fastening fasteners)	5	10
9. Controlling bowels	5	10
10. Controlling bladder	5	10

A patient scoring 100 BDI is continent, feeds himself, dresses himself, gets up out of bed and chairs, bathes himself, walks at least a block, and can ascend and descend stairs. This does not mean that he is able to live alone—he may not be able to cook, keep house, and meet the public—but he is able to get along without attendant care.

Definition and Discussion of Scoring

1. Feeding
   - 10 = Independent. The patient can feed himself a meal from a tray or table when someone puts the food within his reach. He must put on an assistive device if this is needed, cut up the food, use salt and pepper, spread butter, etc. He must accomplish this in a reasonable time.
   - 5 = Some help is necessary (e.g., with cutting up food, as listed previously).
2. Moving from wheelchair to bed and return
   - 15 = Independent in all phases of this activity. Patient can safely approach the bed in his wheelchair, lock brakes, lift footrests, move safely to bed, lie down, come to a sitting position on the side of the bed, and change the position of the wheelchair, if necessary, to transfer back into it safely and return to the wheelchair.
   - 10 = Either some minimal help is needed in some step of this activity or the patient needs to be reminded or supervised for safety of one or more parts of this activity.
   - 5 = Patient can come to a sitting position without the help of a second person but needs to be lifted out of bed, or he transfers with a great deal of help.
3. Doing personal toilet
   - 5 = Patient can wash hands and face, comb hair; clean teeth, and shave. He may use any kind of razor, but he must put in blade or plug in razor without help, as well as get it from the drawer or cabinet. Female patients must put on own makeup, if used, but need not braid or style hair.

From Mahoney FI, Barthel DW: Functional evaluation: the Barthel Index. *Maryland State Med J* 14:62, 1965. Reprinted with permission.

*Score only if unable to walk.

Continued

what he or she is *capable* of doing (Yoshikawa, Cobbs, and Brummel-Smith, 1993). Another functional assessment tool that focuses on ADL performance is the Barthel Index (Table 1-2). A patient scoring 100 on this tool is continent; feeds, dresses, and bathes himself; gets up out of bed and chairs; walks at least a block; and can ascend and descend stairs.

TABLE 1-2 Barthel Index—cont'd

4. Getting on and off toilet
   - 10 = Patient is able to get on and off toilet, fasten and unfasten clothes, prevent soiling of clothes, and use toilet paper without help. He may use a wall bar or other stable object for support if needed. If it is necessary to use a bed pan instead of toilet, he must be able to place it on a chair, empty it, and clean it.
   - 5 = Patient needs help because of imbalance or in handling clothes or in using toilet paper.
5. Bathing self
   - 5 = Patient may use a bathtub, shower, or take a complete sponge bath. He must be able to do all the steps involved in whichever method is employed without another person being present.
6. Walking on a level surface
   - 15 = Patient can walk at least 50 yards without help or supervision. He may wear braces or prostheses and use crutches, canes, or a walkerette, but not a rolling walker. He must be able to lock and unlock braces if used, assume the standing position and sit down, get the necessary mechanical aids into position for use, and dispose of them when he sits. (Putting on and taking off braces is scored under dressing.)

6a. Propelling a wheelchair
   - 5 = Patient cannot ambulate but can propel a wheelchair independently. He must be able to go around corners, turn around, maneuver the chair to a table, toilet, etc. He must be able to push a chair at least 50 yards. Do not score this item if the patient gets a score for walking.

7. Ascending and descending stairs
   - 10 = Patient is able to go up and down a flight of stairs safely without help or supervision. He may and should use handrails, canes, or crutches when needed. He must be able to carry canes or crutches as he ascends or descends stairs.
   - 5 = Patient needs help with or supervision of any one of the above items.
8. Dressing and undressing
   - 10 = Patient is able to put on and remove and fasten all clothing, and tie shoelaces (unless it is necessary to use adaptations for this). This activity includes putting on and removing and fastening corset or braces when these are prescribed. Such special clothing as suspenders, loafer shoes, or dresses that open down the front may be used when necessary.
   - 5 = Patient needs help in putting on and removing or fastening any clothing. He must do at least half the work himself. He must accomplish this in a reasonable time. Women need not be scored on use of a brassiere or girdle unless these are prescribed garments.
9. Continence of bowels
   - 10 = Patient is able to control his bowels and have no accidents. He can use a suppository or take an enema when necessary (as for spinal cord injury patients who have had bowel training).
   - 5 = Patient needs help in using a suppository or taking an enema or has occasional accidents.
10. Controlling bladder
   - 10 = Patient is able to control his bladder day and night. Spinal cord injury patients who wear an external device and leg bag must put them on independently, clean and empty bag, and stay dry day and night.
   - 5 = Patient has occasional accidents or cannot wait for the bed pan or get to the toilet in time or needs help with an external device.

The total score is not as significant or meaningful as the breakdown into individual items, since these indicate where the deficiencies are.

Any applicant to a chronic hospital who scores 100 BDI should be evaluated carefully before admission to see whether such hospitalization is indicated. Discharged patients with 100 BDI should not require further physical therapy but may benefit from a home visit to see whether any environmental adjustments are indicated.

The instrumental activities of daily living (IADLs) are higher-level abilities that allow a person to function independently in the home and community. They are:

- Using the telephone
- Shopping
- Preparing meals
- Doing laundry
- Housekeeping
- Taking medications
- Managing money
- Traveling

Some clinicians also include reading, writing, climbing stairs, and paid employment. The five-item questionnaire for IADLs allows the practitioner to assess the patient's skills in these areas (see Box 1-6).

Loss of ability in any of these areas may signify the beginning of a more severe functional decline. When a patient states that he does not perform a particular task, it is important to determine whether this reflects a functional inability or a "social norm" (e.g., a husband may have never done the grocery shopping or prepared meals). These deficits may indeed exist but do not become apparent until he is required to perform these tasks (e.g., after the death of the spouse) (Reuben, Yoshikawa, and Besdine, 1996).

Box 1-6

Five-Item Instrumental Activities of Daily Living Screening

1. **Can you get to places out of walking distance**
   a. Without help (can travel alone on bus, taxi, or drive own car)
   b. With some help (need someone to help or go with you when traveling)
   c. Or are you unable to travel unless emergency arrangements are made for a specialized vehicle such as an ambulance
2. **Can you go shopping for groceries or clothes (assuming that you have transportation)**
   a. Without help (can take care of all your shopping needs yourself)
   b. With some help (need someone to go with you on all shopping trips)
   c. Or are you completely unable to do any shopping
3. **Can you prepare your own meals**
   a. Without help (can plan and cook meals yourself)
   b. With some help (can prepare some things but unable to cook full meals yourself)
   c. Or are you unable to do any meal preparation
4. **Can you do your housework**
   a. Without help (can scrub floors, etc.)
   b. With some help (can do light housework but need help with heavy work)
   c. Or are you unable to do any housework
5. **Can you handle your own money**
   a. Without help (can write checks, pay bills, etc.)
   b. With some help (can manage day-to-day buying but need help with managing your checkbook and paying your bills)
   c. Or are you completely unable to handle money

Gait and Mobility. The formal assessment of gait and mobility does not take long and is important to assess the patient's ability to ambulate safely. The performance-oriented mobility assessment examines both the balance and gait components and is particularly useful in assessing the patient's risk of falling (Table 1-3). Another tool is the Tinetti Balance and Gait Evaluation instrument (Figure 1-5). The Rancho functional assessment screen (Table 1-4) focuses on the patient's upper extremity strength, range of motion, and ambulatory status. Each test correlates with a particular function and provides the practitioner with insight into the patient's ability to carry out routine daily activities and identifies areas in which therapies may be beneficial to enhance function.

Safety. In gathering information regarding safety, the practitioner must explore factors other than the patient's gait and balance. Many safety risks, especially in the home, can be corrected, which will enhance the patient's ability to safely remain in a more independent setting while avoiding injury. In an epidemiologic model, safety risks are considered as an interrelationship between three factors: the agent (e.g., electricity, chemicals, gravity); the person (e.g., health and cognitive status, knowledge, biologic defense mechanisms); and the environment (e.g., space, lighting, sanitation, furnishings,

TABLE 1-3 Performance-oriented Mobility Assessment

Position Change or Balance Maneuver	Observations
Balance Component	
Getting up from chair*	Potential risk of fall if patient does not get up with single movement; pushes up with arms or moves forward in chair first; unsteady on first standing
Sitting down in chair	Plops in chair; does not land in center
Withstanding nudge on sternum	Moves feet; grabs object for support
Romberg test (eyes closed)	Same as above; tests patient's reliance on visual input for balance
Neck turning	Moves feet; grabs object for support; complains of vertigo, dizziness, or unsteadiness
Reaching up	Unable to reach up to full shoulder flexion standing on tiptoes; unsteady; grabs object for support
Bending over	Unable to bend over to pick up small object (e.g., pen) from floor; grabs object to pull up on; requires multiple attempts to arise
Gait Component	
Initiation	Hesitates; stumbles; grabs object for support
Step height	Does not clear floor consistently (scrapes or shuffles); raises foot too high (more than two inches)
Step continuity	After first few steps, does not consistently begin raising one foot as other foot touches floor
Step symmetry	Step length not equal; pathologic side usually has longer step length (problem may be in hip, knee, ankle, or surrounding muscles)
Path deviation	Does not walk in straight line; weaves side to side
Turning	Stops before initiating turn; staggers; sways; grabs object for support

*Use hard, armless chair.

BALANCE

Instructions: Subject is seated in hard armless chair. The following maneuvers are tested.

1. Sitting balance	Leans or slides in chair	= 0	
	Steady, safe	= 1	____
2. Arises	Unable without help	= 0	
	Able but uses arms to help	= 1	
	Able without use of arms	= 2	____
3. Attempts to arise	Unable without help	= 0	
	Able but requires more than 1 attempt	= 1	
	Able to arise with 1 attempt	= 2	____
4. Immediate standing balance (first 5 sec)	Unsteady (staggers, moves feet, marked trunk sway)	= 0	
	Steady but uses walker or cane or grabs other objects for support	= 1	
	Steady without walker, cane, or other support	= 2	____
5. Standing balance	Unsteady	= 0	
	Steady but wide stance (medial heels more than 4 in. apart) or uses cane, walker, or other support	= 1	
	Narrow stance without support	= 2	____
6. Nudged (subject at maximum position with feet as close together as possible, examiner pushes lightly on subject's sternum with palm of hand 3 times)	Begins to fall	= 0	
	Staggers, grabs, but catches self	= 1	
	Steady	= 2	____
7. Eyes closed (at maximum position No. 6)	Unsteady	= 0	
	Steady	= 1	____
8. Turning 360 degrees	Discontinuous steps	= 0	
	Continuous	= 1	____
	Unsteady (grabs, staggers)	= 0	
	Steady	= 1	____
9. Sitting down	Unsafe (misjudged distance, falls into chair)	= 0	
	Uses arms or not a smooth motion	= 1	
	Safe, smooth motion	= 2	____

Balance score: ____ /16

Figure 1-5 Tinetti Balance and Gait Evaluation. (From Tinetti M: Performance-oriented assessment of mobility problems in elderly patients, *J Am Geriatr Soc* 34:119-126, 1986.) *Continued*

GAIT

Instructions: Subject stands with examiner; walks down hallway or across room, first at his "usual" pace, then back at "rapid, but safe" pace (using usual walking aid such as cane, walker).

10. Initiation of gait (immediately after told to "go")

Any hesitancy or multiple attempts to start	= 0	
No hesitancy	= 1	____

11. Step length and height

a. Right swing foot

Does not pass left stance foot with step	= 0	
Passes left stance foot	= 1	
Right foot does *not* clear floor completely with step	= 0	
Right foot completely clears floor	= 1	____

b. Left swing foot

Does not pass right stance foot with step	= 0	
Passes right stance foot	= 1	
Left foot does *not* clear floor completely with step	= 0	
Left foot completely clears floor	= 1	____

12. Step symmetry

Right and left step length not equal (estimate)	= 0	
Right and left step appear equal	= 1	____

13. Step continuity

Stopping or discontinuity between steps	= 0	
Steps appear continuous	= 1	____

14. Path (estimated in relation to floor tiles, 12-in. diameter; observe excursion of 1 foot over about 10 ft of the course)

Marked deviation	= 0	
Mild/moderate deviation *or* uses walking aid	= 1	
Straight without walking aid	= 2	____

15. Trunk

Marked sway or uses walking aid	= 0	
No sway but flexion of knees or back or spreads arms out while walking	= 1	
No sway, no flexion, no use of arms, and no use of walking aid	= 2	____

16. Walking stance

Heels apart	= 0	
Heels almost touching while walking	= 1	____

Gait score: ____ /12
Total score: ____ /28

Figure 1-5, cont'd For legend see p. 27.

TABLE 1-4 Rancho Functional Assessment Screen

Test	Functions Tested	Normal	Limited	Unable
Put both hands together behind head	Combing hair; washing back, etc.			
Put both hands together in back of waist	Managing clothing; washing lower back			
Sitting, touch great toe with opposite hand	Lower extremity dressing; hygiene			
Squeeze examiner's two fingers with each hand	Grasp strength (approximately 20 lb of pressure needed for functional activities)			
Hold paper between thumb and lateral side of index finger while examiner tries to pull it out	Pinch strength (approximately 3 lb of pressure needed for functional activities)			
Stand from chair without using hand	Transfer ability; fall risk			
Walk 15-30 m	Velocity; household ambulatory status			

pets, other people) (Burke and Walsh, 1997). Each of these factors must be considered in the evaluation of safety risk. Cognitive impairment and memory deficit, poor vision, and impaired sensation may place a person at risk for burns in the kitchen or bath. Impaired hand strength and coordination may place a person at risk of injury when cutting food with a sharp knife. Falls are a particularly common risk that older persons face.

Summary

The comprehensive geriatric assessment is a multi-faceted process that plays a critical role in the quality of life of older persons. The information obtained can be used in many ways to maintain or improve the person's health and function. Health promotion, disease prevention, and diagnosis are only the beginning. Referral to appropriate community resources such as case management, physical, occupational and speech therapies, and assistance with facility placement, if necessary, can dramatically improve the quality of life of both the patient and the family who may be coping with a difficult situation. A practitioner who is knowledgeable of available resources and support agencies will always be able to offer assistance and guidance to patients and families, even if there are limited medical and nursing interventions to be offered. Finally, not all providers who care for elderly patients have been trained in the skills and expertise of geriatric clinicians. It serves the medical and nursing community as a whole for those with these skills to share them with others, providing assistance and insights that may make a difference in that provider's ability to best manage the elderly patient's complicated needs.

Resources

AGENET Information Network
AGENET LLC 644-A
West Washington Ave.
Madison, WI 53703
(608) 256-4242
http://www.agenet.com

U.S. Department of Health and Human Services Healthfinder (Age Pages)
http://www.healthfinder.org

References

Burke M, Walsh M: *Gerontologic nursing: wholistic care of the older adult*, ed 2, St Louis, 1997, Mosby.

Goldberg T, Chavin S: Preventive medicine and screening in older adults, *J Am Geriatr Soc* 45:345-354, 1997.

Gudmundsson A, Carnes M: Geriatric assessment: making it work in primary care practice, *Geriatrics* 51(3):53-57, 1996.

Hayward RSA, Steinberg EP, Ford DE: Preventive care guidelines, *Ann Intern Med* 111(9):761-762, 1991.

Kane R, Ouslander J, Abrass I: *Essentials of clinical geriatrics*, ed 3, New York, 1994, McGraw-Hill.

Lueckenotte A: *Gerontologic nursing*, St Louis, 1996, Mosby.

Markides K, Rudkin L: Racial and ethnic diversity. In Birren J, editor: *Encyclopedia of gerontology: age, aging, and the aged,* Los Angeles, 1996, Academic Press.

Mayfield D, McLeod G, Hall P: The CAGE questionnaire: validation of a new alcoholism screening instrument, *Am J Psychiatry* 131:1121-1123, 1974.

Mezey M, Mitty E, Ramsey G: Assessment of decision-making capacity: nursing's role, *Gerontological Nurs* 23(3):28-35, 1997.

Reuben D, Yoshikawa T, Besdine R, editors: *Geriatric review syllabus: a core curriculum in geriatric medicine*, ed 3, Dubuque, Iowa, 1996, Kendall/Hunt Publishing.

Rubenstein L: Geriatric assessment: physical. In Birren J, editor: *Encyclopedia of gerontology: age, aging, and the aged,* Los Angeles, 1996, Academic Press.

Schiavenato M: The Hispanic elderly: implications for nursing care, *J Gerontologic Nurs* 23(6):10-15, 1997.

Shua-Haim J et al: Depression in the elderly, *Hosp Med* 33(7):44-58, 1997.

Weg R: Sexuality, sensuality, and intimacy. In Birren J, editor: *Encyclopedia of gerontology: age, aging and the aged,* Los Angeles, 1996, Academic Press.

Williams T: Comprehensive functional assessment: an overview, *J Am Geriatr Soc* 31:637-641, 1983.

Yoshikawa T, Cobbs E, Brummel-Smith K: *Ambulatory geriatric care,* St Louis, 1993, Mosby.

2

Exercise

The extent to which exercise can delay the normal decline in physical performance associated with aging is unknown. However, what is known is that two thirds of all adults age 65 and older are either irregularly active or completely sedentary. With this inactivity comes an increased risk of chronic disease, including coronary heart disease, hypertension, diabetes, obesity, back problems, constipation, osteoporosis, and depression. Findings in gerontology and sports science suggest that regular physical activity and exercise can help to maintain and enhance the functioning, health, and psychologic well-being of elderly people. Even national public health directives support the routine prescription of physical activity for the older adult (Centers for Disease Control and Prevention, 1989; Public Health Service, 1990). Experts recognize that physical activity can prevent or delay many of the physical and psychologic problems that commonly occur with aging (Shephard, 1990; Vorhies & Riley, 1993). Studies have demonstrated the direct beneficial relationships that specific types of physical activity and exercise have on the chronic conditions of aging (Table 2-1). In addition, some authors indicate that physical exercise may have broader significance for the overall well-being of elderly people, such as improvement or positive associations of moods, a sense of well-being, control of hypertension, lower occurrence of depressive symptoms, better cognitive functioning, and maintenance of bone mineralization (Emery and Gatz, 1990; Ruuskanen and Ruoppila, 1995).

Experts suggest that loss of muscle mass and strength has less to do with aging than with chronic inactivity (Brown and Coggan, 1990; Morey et al., 1989). Researchers have examined flexibility, strength, and cardiovascular fitness in the elderly and found that, regardless of age, the musculoskeletal and cardiovascular systems respond to both resistance and aerobic training (Morey et al., 1996, 1989). Studies have also demonstrated that older men and women's participation in an appropriate exercise program can increase their physical activity by as much as 25% (Hagberg et al., 1989; Kort et al., 1991). Other studies have shown that strength training can counteract muscle weakness in very elderly people (Brown and Holloszy, 1991; Posner et al., 1992). Resistance exercises especially appeared to significantly increase muscle strength. Moreover, most study participants significantly improved their functional levels of gait, transfers, and general independent living.

TABLE 2-1 Beneficial Effects of Exercise on Chronic Conditions of Aging

Condition	Exercise	Effect(s)
Coronary heart disease	Aerobic, endurance type	Reduction of BP Increase in HDL and reduction in body fat Increased cardiac output Increased maximal oxygen consumption Increased insulin sensitivity
Hypertension	Aerobic, endurance type	Decreased systolic BP and total peripheral resistance
Osteoarthritis	Stretching and strengthening	Maintain range of motion and muscle mass Increased muscle strength
Osteoporosis	Strengthening, weight bearing	Strengthening postural muscles Stimulated bone growth Decreased rate of bone loss
Diabetes mellitus	Aerobic, endurance type	Fat loss Increased insulin sensitivity Decreased glucose intolerance risk
Cognitive dysfunction	Aerobic	Improved cerebral function Increased cerebral perfusion Increased beta-endorphin secretion

Modified from Kligman E, Pepin E: Prescribing physical activity for older patients, *Geriatrics* 47(8):34, 1992. (Reproduced with permission from *Geriatrics* 47(8):34, 1992.
BP, Blood pressure; *HDL,* high-density lipoprotein.

Studies suggest that exercise training in elders is a potential means of reducing the burden of impairments and ultimately improving function and quality of life (Nichols et al., 1993; Shephard, 1990). However, not all older adults are candidates for regular physical activity. For example, people with diagnosed contraindications to acute exercise, such as severe seizure disorders, severe cardiovascular disease, and severe obstructive pulmonary diseases, require close attention and physician-directed involvement. Individuals with extreme motor, neurologic (e.g., spasticity, plegia), or musculoskeletal (e.g., joint inflammation, chronic subluxation) limitations also require a specialized approach to exercise and careful intervention by the practitioner. In general, regular physical activity and exercise are appropriate for healthy older adults with evidence of diminished flexibility, strength, and functional capacity because of chronic inactivity. This chapter focuses on exercise for the functionally independent, community-dwelling, older well adult.

Perspectives on Exercise in the Elderly

A typical exercise program includes activities aimed at increasing musculoskeletal flexibility and strength and at improving cardiovascular fitness. All of these components are important, and different types of activity are required for each.

TABLE 2-2 Physiologic Effects of Various Types of Exercise

Type of Exercise	Description	Physiologic Effect(s)
Stretching	Stretching exercise routine moving joint beyond initial point of resistance	Reduction of contractures in periarticular tissues
Strengthening		
Isometric	Contraction of muscle *without* moving the joint (muscle length does not change)	Reduction of blood flow to contracting muscle, increase in BP
Isotonic	Contraction of muscle *with* ROM (muscle length changes) Work is generated by resistance and repetitions	Increase in blood flow to contracting muscles, decrease in BP High resistance, low repetition for maximal strength and hypertrophy; low resistance, high repetitions for maximal endurance
Isokinetic	Machine controls speed of movement and offers accommodating resistance to movement	Increase in BP, increases blood flow to muscles
Endurance		
Aerobic	Sustained reciprocal motion of large muscle groups to induce metabolic and circulatory stress	Increases endurance capacity of skeletal and cardiac muscle for work

Modified from Ytterberg SR, Mahowald ML, Krug HE: Exercise for arthritis, *Bailliere's Clin Rheumatol* 8:1, 1994.
BP, Blood pressure; *ROM,* range of motion.

Exercise objectives can be either therapeutic or preventive in nature. Accomplishing these objectives can be related to specific types of exercise. Table 2-2 describes types of exercise and the associated physiologic effects.

Stretching

Clinical experience shows that stretching exercise is often overlooked. In sporting and recreational activities, many musculoskeletal injuries can be associated with an oversight in stretching. Stretching exercises are intended to maintain or improve joint range of motion (ROM) and flexibility and to prepare individuals for activity and function. It can also be used during an exercise cool-down period.

In the older adult lack of flexibility usually limits an activity, rather than decreases strength. The lack of flexibility imposed by years of inactivity can yield an enormous degree of joint and motor limitation. This physiological limitation can cause burdensome functional limitations and, in the extreme, serious subsequent dependency. Activities such as grooming, dressing, sitting at a standard-height toilet or in a straight-back chair, reaching, and even stair climbing can be impaired by the joint limitation caused by lack of flexibility.

Stretching exercises are the only exercises that will increase flexibility. Stretching exercises do not increase strength or cardiovascular fitness. Static stretching (a controlled, sustained stretch of the muscle tendon unit to the point of mild discomfort) is generally recommended as the best way of maintaining muscle length and correcting muscle imbalance. Stretching exercises should always be part of a strengthening or cardiovascular fitness program in the form of the warm-up and cool-down segments of an exercise program. Generally, stretches should be focused on the low back, hamstrings, quadriceps, pelvic, and shoulder girdle muscle groups. Figure 2-1 provides examples of stretching exercises that can be used by the older well adult. The correct position is important; however, each patient's position may vary a little according to the individual's own available degree of flexibility. The patient should feel mild tension in the muscle tendon group that is targeted to be stretched. The stretching action should be performed slowly and carefully, maintaining tension on the muscle for 10 to 20 seconds and then slowly releasing the stretch. A stretch is never to the point of pain. A stretching session usually centers around 15 to 20 minutes of stretching exercises per day. When used as the warm-up and cool-down segments of an exercise program, the stretching session can be limited to 5 to 8 minutes. The optimal duration and intensity of stretching and the effects of temperature are still being questioned in the literature. Local or national professional associations can provide information on acquiring patient education material, such as simple pictorials and techniques. Supply and medical equipment vendors who support hospital and medical clinics are also an excellent resource.

Strengthening

The musculoskeletal system protects vital organs and governs an individual's mobility. Normal age-related changes in the musculoskeletal and neurologic systems result in a decline in function for the older patient. For example, signs and symptoms of osteoarthritis, especially in weight-bearing joints, limit joint motion, flexibility, and overall mobility. Coordination, dexterity, proprioception, and vestibular integrity also show signs of decline with aging. Certainly, for the elderly the risk of functional loss is heightened when disease or a sedentary lifestyle accompanies the normal age-related changes.

Strength is essential in maintaining an individual's mobility and functional independence. Strengthening exercises should focus on the shoulder girdle and upper extremities and on the pelvic girdle and lower extremities. Studies support strength, particularly lower extremity strength, as a strong predictor of success for functionally impaired older adults (Schenkman et al., 1996; Wolfson et al., 1995). Strength can also contribute to preventing joint and muscle injury and to sustaining bone strength (Prince et al., 1991; Ytterberg, Mahowald, and Krug, 1994).

A main ingredient in building strength is to force the muscle to work. As explained later in the chapter, requiring a muscle to work against a load (e.g., dumbbell weights), through an arc of motion, and for a number of repetitions builds strength. The amount of rest taken between exercise intervals also contributes to strengthening. Another important requirement is that, in the course of exercising, enough work must be accomplished to reach a point of "fatigue." If the exercise does not achieve fatigue, the muscles are not working sufficiently to gain a training response. Fatigue can be generally described as a "tired feeling, in the body part being exercised, that makes the last 2 to 3 repetitions difficult to perform." No pain should be experienced during the last couple of exercise repetitions.

As an individual gains strength, more work (e.g., increasing the resistance, the

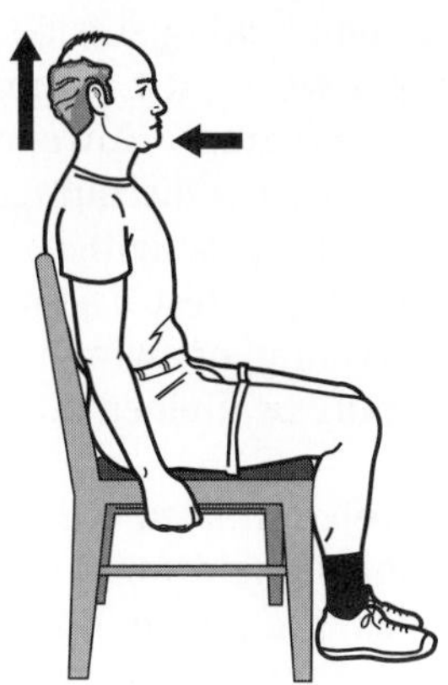

A Gently pull chin in while lengthening back of neck. Hold 10 seconds.

Repeat:_______Times
_______Times a day.

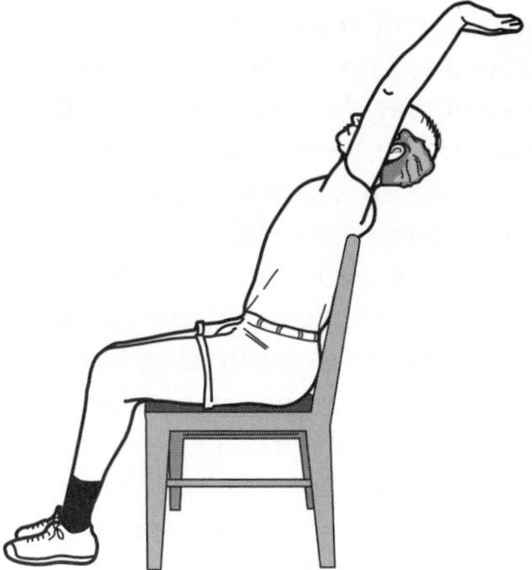

B Bring arms straight up over head and back as far as possible, causing back to arch gently. Hold 10 seconds.

Repeat:_______Times
_______Times a day.

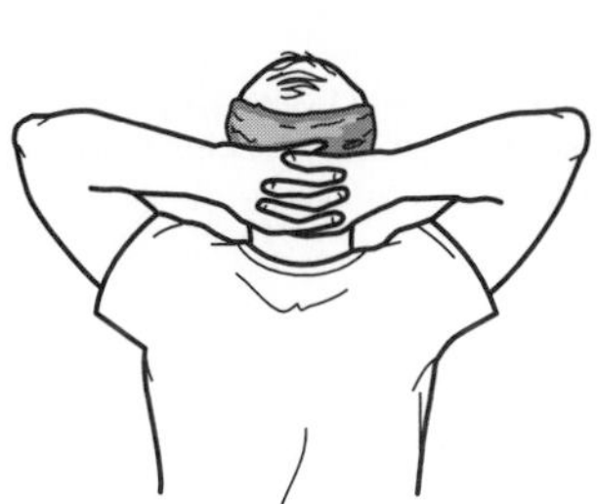

C Place hands behind your head and pull elbows back as far as possible. Hold 10 seconds.

Repeat:_______Times
_______Times a day.

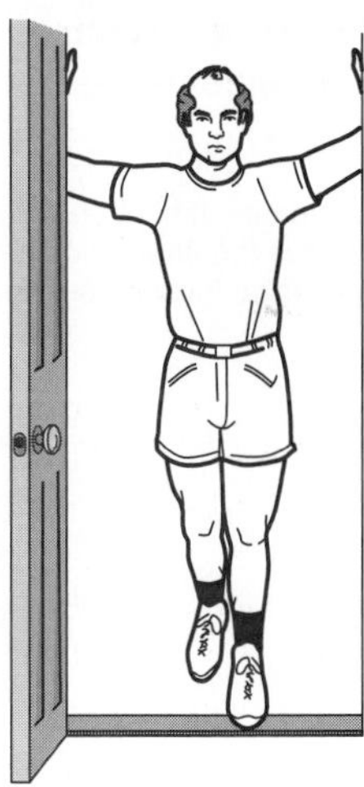

D With arms behind doorjamb, gently lean forward. Hold for _____ seconds. Stretch is felt across chest.

Repeat:_______Times
_______Times a day.

Figure 2-1 Examples of stretching exercises.

number of repetitions, or the number of exercise sessions per week) is progressively added to repeat the strengthening scenario. Vigorous strengthening sessions require "a day of rest" between sessions; therefore, three sessions per week (at a minimum) would usually be viewed as a typical frequency for an exercise program. However, with less vigorous strengthening programs, 4 to 5 sessions per week are not discouraged. Combining vigorous strengthening exercises with cardiac conditioning activities can also progress an exercise program. In this situation the scheduled "day of rest" can be substituted with such aerobic activities as brisk walking, stationary cycling, or swimming.

Types of Strengthening Exercise. Exercises can generally be divided into three types: isometric, isotonic, and isokinetic.

Isometric Exercises. In isometric exercises muscles are contracted *without* changing their length or causing joint movement. The contraction is held for a specified time, relaxed, and repeated for a specified number of times (i.e., repetitions). Isometric exercises are useful when pain or deformity restricts joint movement or as warm-up exercises for more strenuous exercises. Figure 2-2 illustrates an isometric exercise used for a painful knee(s). A combination of hip adduction and quadricep muscle contraction is being used to maintain strength. Isometric exercises do not build strength and only delay a muscle's decline in strength. If acute pain inhibits joint movement or an extremity is immobilized (e.g., casted), isometric exercises are usually the patient's only source of exercise.

Isotonic Exercises. In isotonic exercises muscle contraction *with* muscle shortening and lengthening occurs, causing the joint to move through an arc of motion. Resistance, caused by the weight of the body part and added resistance (e.g., cuff weight) that loads the muscle being exercised, makes the muscle work and build strength. Guided resistance equipment (e.g., Cybex or Nautilus machine) or free weights are typically used

Sit or lie on a flat surface with your legs straight out. With a rolled towel between your knees, push knees together. Then, still keeping your knees together, tighten the muscles in the front of your thighs by forcing your knees backwards. Hold for 10 seconds.

Repeat:______Times
______Times a day

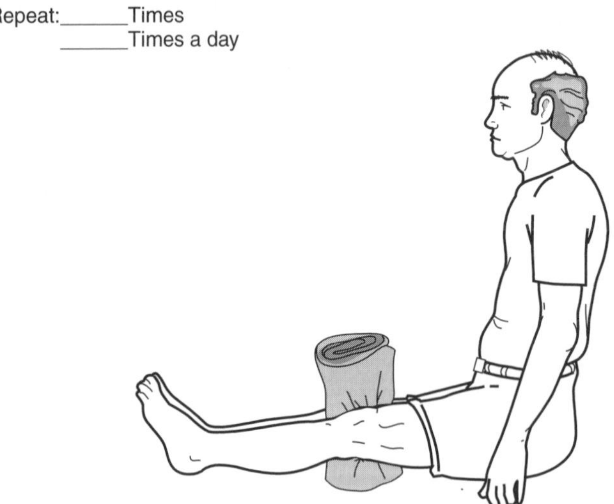

Figure 2-2 Example of an isometric exercise for the knees. (Modified from Lewis CB, Bottomley JM: *Geriatric physical therapy: a clinical approach,* Norwalk, Conn, 1994, Appleton & Lange.)

to offer resistance during isotonic exercise. Figure 2-3 illustrates a set of dumbbells, an example of free weights. Free weights are inexpensive, versatile, and easy to organize for a home program. Figure 2-4 provides an example of guided resistance equipment. The gear uses gravity-loading systems (e.g., a stack of weighted plates) to offer resistance through particular movement patterns. The equipment is easy to use and generally considered safer and more comfortable to use than free weights because there are no weights to drop, the exercise movements are guided, and solid support is provided during exercise. The equipment is popular and usually found in private health clubs or community activity-oriented organizations (e.g., YMCA).

Isotonic exercise is usually the choice for physical activity prescribed to increase and maintain strength. The usual exercise format is a set number of repetitions with sufficient weight to cause the patient to sense fatigue in the exercised extremity toward the last few repetitions of the exercise routine. The program may be progressed by adding weight or by increasing the number of repetitions. Of extreme importance is the practitioner's responsibility for determining the most appropriate weight for the patient at the start of exercising. By keeping in the office a few cuff weights ranging between 1 and 5 pounds, the practitioner can generally find a weight that a patient can safely move throughout the arc of joint motion. Clinical experience recommends starting the older patient at half the weight found suitable during the patient's office visit. Then, attaching the selected weight to an extremity, instructing the patient to continue joint motion for 12 to 15 repetitions, listening to verbal feedback, and observing the quality of joint motion will assist the practitioner in determining a suitable work level for the patient's exercise program. If the practitioner needs further expertise (e.g., paresis, joint contracture), a referral to a physical therapist for an exercise program is certainly indicated.

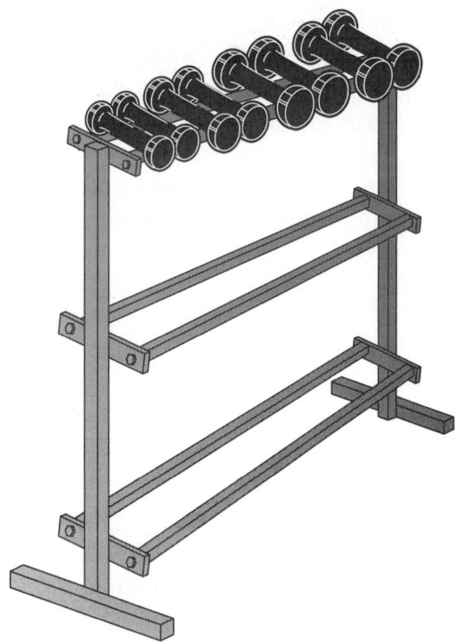

Figure 2-3 Graduated dumbbell weights. (Courtesy Sammons Preston; An AbilityOne Company, Bolingbrook, Ill.)

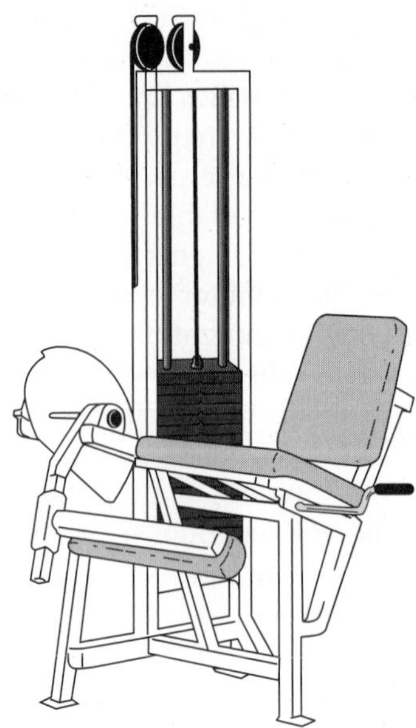

Figure 2-4 Weight-stacked, guided-resistance machine that can be used for knee extension exercises. (Redrawn from Cook BB, Stewart GW: *Strength basics: your guide to resistance training for health and optimal performance,* Champaign, Ill, 1996, Human Kinetics.)

Although there are numerous exercise progression techniques, one simple approach is to alter the following basic exercise variables: *resistance, repetitions, sets,* and the *rest interval.*

Resistance is the weight or load against which a muscle works. A *repetition* (rep) is the single, complete action of an exercise from start position to completion and back to the start position. A *set* is a given number of complete and continuous repetitions of an exercise. The *rest interval* is the amount of rest or recovery taken between sets of an exercise or between different exercises in a program. For example, 12 uninterrupted repetitions of an exercise equal one set of 12. The patient rests a minute, does 12 more repetitions performing two sets of 12, and so on. A written description of this format is as follows:

Shoulder shrugs	2	×12	3 lb	2 min
(exercise)	(sets)	(reps)	(resistance)	(rest interval)

Manipulating any of these variables alters the intensity of an exercise. The patient can be instructed to gradually increase the weight by half a pound (i.e., resistance) over a period of 2 weeks (Figure 2-5). The workload can also be gradually increased by adding sets or repetitions or by shortening the rest intervals. If the patient encounters joint pain, any of these variables can be adjusted to accommodate the patient's level of work.

Strength gains can be further accelerated by practicing an exercise pattern of faster concentric (muscle-shortening) movements and slower eccentric (muscle-lengthening) movements. For example, while performing an exercise pattern, the patient should complete a concentric contraction (elbow bending) within 2 seconds and then take 4 seconds to complete the subsequent eccentric contraction (elbow straightening). The exercise session can occur once a day for three to four times per week.

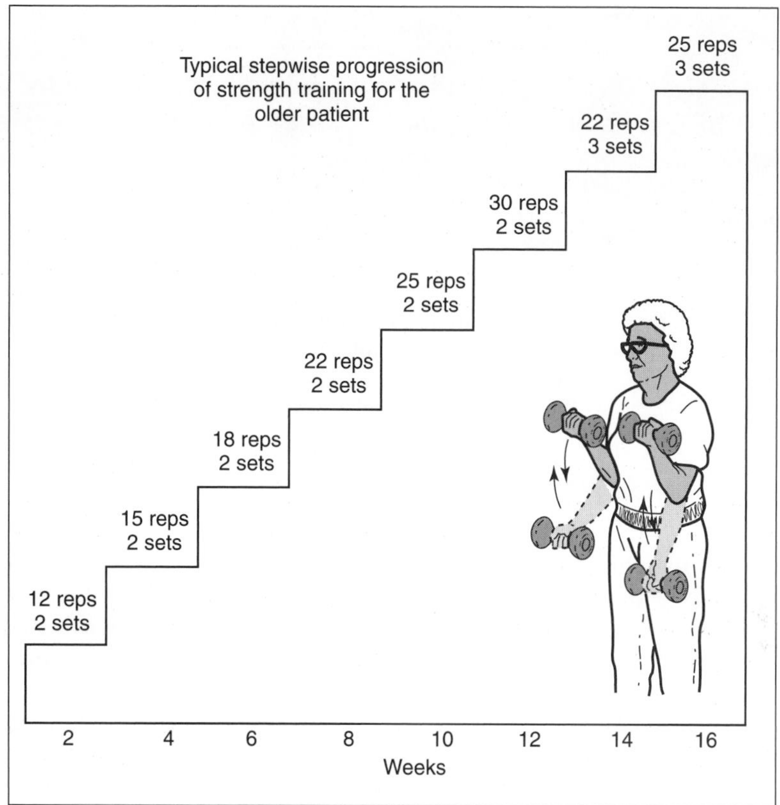

Figure 2-5 An approach used in progressing an older patient's dumbbell exercise program. The approach can be applied to other forms of strengthening programs. (Reproduced with permission from *Geriatrics* 47(8):34, 1992. Copyright by Advanstar Communications Inc. Advanstar Communications Inc. retains all rights to this article.)

Isokinetic Exercises. The third type of exercise is isokinetic, which is a form of isotonic exercise. Basically the difference between the two types is that isokinetic exercise is performed on specialized equipment designed to control the speed of movement and offer accommodating resistance to an isotonic exercise. Generally, isokinetic equipment is found in specialized orthopedic training clinics and used in the rehabilitation of severe musculoskeletal injuries. Isokinetic exercise is not discussed in this chapter.

Cardiovascular Training

Cardiovascular training should be considered the foundation of any fitness program (Posner et al., 1990). Flexibility and strength exercises support this critical component of a balanced fitness program, as the patient must be able to physically perform cardiovascular training. However, of greater importance is the impact of cardiovascular training. Not only does the activity offer extremely beneficial health and longevity outcomes (Gorman and Posner, 1988; Paffenarger et al., 1986) but also it substantially improves aerobic and overall functional capacity (Schenkman et al., 1996). Cardiovascular training

Box 2-1

American College of Sports Medicine Position Stand: Recommended Quantity and Quality of Exercise for Developing and Maintaining Cardiorespiratory and Muscular Fitness in Healthy Adults

1. ***Frequency of training***—3 to 5 days per week.
2. ***Intensity of training***—60% to 90% of maximum heart rate (HRmax) or 50% to 85% of maximum oxygen uptake (Vo_{2max}) or HRmax reserve.
3. ***Time of training***—20 to 60 minutes of continuous aerobic activity. Duration is dependent on the intensity of the activity; lower-intensity activity should be conducted over a longer period of time.
4. ***Mode of activity***—any activity that uses large muscle groups, can be maintained continuously, and is rhythmic and aerobic in nature.
5. ***Resistance training***—strength training of a moderate intensity should be an integral part of an adult fitness program.

From American College of Sports Medicine: *Med Sci Sport Exerc* 22:265-275, 1990.

increases the ability to deliver oxygen to working muscle and increases the capacity of muscle to extract oxygen and eliminate metabolic by-products. From a functional perspective, this statement means that for every given functional task there should be less relative work. In other words, for the older adult, performing the usual daily living activities should no longer be such a challenge.

For years aerobic exercise has been prescribed according to the *FIT model*. The acronym is defined as follows: *F (frequency)* is the number of times a patient exercises a week, *I (intensity)* is how hard a patient works while exercising, and *T (time)* is the duration of each exercise session. For example, a typical cardiovascular exercise program is designed according to a "traditional" exercise model developed in 1978 by the American College of Sports Medicine (ACSM). Box 2-1 shows the ACSM position on cardiovascular training, which frames the amount of exercise that is required to increase aerobic fitness and strength in a reasonable amount of time. The ACSM guidelines focus on working large muscle groups in a repetitive manner, elevating the resting heart rate, and requiring continuous activity for at least 20 minutes (time) at least three times per week (frequency). Sixty to 90% of maximal heart rate or 50% to 85% of maximum oxygen uptake (Vo_{2max}) is the recommended target range (intensity). With any less duration or frequency in training, the cardiovascular benefit of the workouts is highly questionable. For sedentary elderly people, however, 40% of their Vo_{2max} may be sufficient intensity to significantly improve aerobic fitness (Hoppenfeld, 1976). At this level, there should be no harm in encouraging the older well adult to increase the aerobic activity to more than three times a week (Watkins and Kligman, 1991). Warm-up and cool-down periods should also help to reduce the incidence of cardiac rhythm disturbances during cardiovascular exercise.

New Perspective on Physical Fitness

Today, experts recognize that forms and amounts of activity outside the "traditional" exercise model outlined by the ACSM also have the potential to increase health. Although

TABLE 2-3 Comparison of *Traditional* vs. *New* Quantity and Quality of Exercise for Developing and Maintaining Cardiorespiratory and Muscular Fitness in Healthy Adults

	Traditional Aerobic Program	New Aerobic Program
Frequency	Three times per week	Every day or nearly every day
Intensity	Within the training zone (60%-90% of predicted maximum heart rate)	Moderate intensity of perceived exertion
Time	Minimum of 20 minutes per session	Total of 30 minutes over a day period

those parameters still hold, for the most part, experts have recognized that compliance with the model has been generally inadequate. With this in mind, the ACSM has adopted different standards designed to connect a greater number of people to a healthier lifestyle.

In 1995, the ACSM and the CDC issued a joint statement that was published in the *Journal of the American Medical Association.* The February 1995 article, entitled "Physical Activity and Public Health," recommended an alternative plan for those who have not been successful with the 3- to 5-days a week, 20-minute regimen. The new recommendation is moderate-intensity exercise (Feeney, 1996) for 30 minutes most days of the week. Those 30 minutes could be broken into smaller segments; for instance, a 10-minute walk taken three times a day will produce the same basic health benefit as a 30-minute walk. Table 2-3 provides a snapshot comparison of the traditional vs. new recommendation on the quantity and quality of exercise required for developing and maintaining cardiorespiratory and muscular fitness in healthy adults.

For many years, exercise scientists have recognized that fitness is related to enhanced health. Certainly, future studies are necessary to determine whether loosening the model to make it more achievable and practical is actually going to promote activity. However, this new alternative in cardiovascular training is an encouraging approach for sedentary older adults or those with a poor fitness level who want to engage in a healthier lifestyle.

Designing an Exercise Program

The design of an exercise program for the older well adult should focus on prevention, restoration, and maintenance, with three primary objectives in mind: (1) determining an adequate, challenging, and safe activity; (2) sustaining an effective level of habitual physical activity; and (3) ensuring that the fitness activity selected remains safe and effective.

Determining an Adequate Challenging and Safe Activity

Pre-exercise Office Assessment. Before prescribing physical activity for an older adult, the practitioner should conduct a pre-exercise assessment. Typically, the well older adult will have some form of chronic disease with factors that may limit the activity or narrow the range of possibilities for exercise (e.g., medications, severe osteoarthritis, coronary artery disease, diabetes, orthostatic hypotension, painful feet, neuropathies,

Box 2-2

Factors to Consider During Preexercise Office Assessment of the Older Patient

I. History

Previous exercise programs
Present exercise programs
Chronic or acute diseases
Medications
Symptoms (e.g., chest pain, shortness of breath, joint pain or limitation, incontinence, excessive fatigue, palpitations, faint or light-headedness)
Family history (e.g., heart disease, diabetes, stroke)
Cardiovascular risk factors (e.g., obesity, hypertension, smoking, stress, elevated lipids)

II. Limited Physical Examination

Height and weight
Blood pressure
Resting pulse
Cardiac examination (based on results of cardiovascular stress test)
Pulmonary examination (FVC and FEV_1)
Musculoskeletal examinations (e.g., flexibility, strength, balance)

---

obesity, osteoporosis, incontinence, or restrictive pulmonary conditions). These factors certainly challenge the practitioner in designing a safe and effective exercise program. Therefore an assessment is imperative for providing the practitioner with adequate information to avoid injury or a worsening of underlying chronic diseases and for determining an appropriate level of activity that will be enjoyable and practical for the older adult.

The assessment should include cardiac risk, potential physical limitations, painful conditions, contraindications, and other medical complications. Box 2-2 suggests areas that should be assessed in a pre-exercise office assessment of the older adult. The history should include previous experience with exercise, an assessment of lifestyle risk factors potentially modifiable through exercise, previous activity levels to help set realistic goals, and a medication review. Table 2-4 lists medications commonly used by older patients that have pharmacologic effects interfering with physical activity. The medications include antihistamines, anticholinergics, antipsychotics, beta blockers, diuretics, insulin, and oral hypoglycemic agents. These medications may require a careful cardiovascular and neurologic evaluation and necessitate modifications of your patient's exercise prescription.

The physical examination should include vital signs and evaluation of the patient's cardiac function. Most risk of morbidity or mortality related to regular physical exercise has been associated with preexisting cardiac conditions. Accordingly, a cardiovascular stress test is recommended before vigorous exercise (i.e., exercise intensity >60% of maximal oxygen uptake) for all older men and women with or without symptoms suggestive of or known cardiovascular, pulmonary, or metabolic disease (American College of Sports Medicine, 1990; Fardy, Yanowitz, and Wilson, 1988). The exercise stress

TABLE 2-4 Medications That May Require Modification of the Exercise Prescription

Medication	Effect	Recommended Modification
Antihistamines	Drowsiness Decreased sweating Increased body core temperature Decrease duration and intensity of exercise by 25%	Increase fluid intake Caution against exercising in high ambient temperature and humidity
Anticholinergics	Decreased sweating Increased body core temperature	Same as above
Antipsychotics	Drowsiness Decreased sweating Increased body core temperature	Same as above
Beta blockers	Decrease heart rate Decreased maximal heart rate Bronchoconstriction	To gauge intensity, use rate of perceived exertion (able to talk to partner) rather than target heart rate
Diuretics	Increased risk of dehydration and electrolyte imbalance	Same as with antihistamines
Insulin	Exercise improves glucose tolerance; may alter insulin requirements	Be aware of glucose levels before exercise and of glucose needs
Oral hypoglycemic	Exercise improves glucose tolerance; may alter need for medication	Be aware of glucose levels before exercise Have sugar candy ready to ingest if symptoms of hypoglycemia occur

Reproduced with permission from *Geriatrics* Vol. 47, Number 8, August 1992, page 34. Copyright by Advanstar Communications Inc. Advanstar Communications Inc. retains all rights to this article.

testing can be used to screen high-risk patients and also to set the optimal target intensity of the fitness program. Respiratory function should also be assessed, which can be performed by simply checking (i.e., spirometry) the patient's forced vital capacity (FVC) and forced expiratory volume in 1 second (FEV_1) (Kligman and Pepin, 1992; American Thoracic Society, 1979).

Quick Assessment Tools for the Neuromusculoskeletal System. The assessment should also include a gross assessment of flexibility and joint motion, muscle strength, and balance. In the office, immediate observations of the patient's behavior should cue the practitioner on areas to focus the assessment. For example, simple observations such as a slow nonantalgic gait, labored breathing, difficulty in turning, and problems in mounting the examination table should provide a sense that strength, balance, gait, and aerobic capability must be examined. Other information that may help the practitioner design a safe and effective exercise program may include the patient's use of an assistive device, quality of vision or hearing, and ability to follow directions.

Flexibility. Flexibility in the older adult should be assessed functionally. Asking your patient to sit and rise in a standard-height chair, reach for an object overhead, clasp hands behind the head and the small of the back, climb on and off the examination table, and rise from lying on the floor provides tests of functional activities that can be used in assessing your patient's flexibility. For example, your findings would be based on the patient's ability to fully reach behind the head or the small of the back when clasping hands. An inability to reach behind either body area usually indicates a marked limitation in shoulder range of motion. Another concern would be the patient's inability to bend forward when rising from a chair, which usually indicates a lack of adequate hip flexion. Certainly, if the need arises, goniometric measurements of joints identified as limited in motion can be recorded (American Academy of Orthopedic Surgeons, 1996).

Always important but often overlooked is testing the flexibility of the hip, hamstring, and lower back. Lack of flexibility in the hip, knee, and ankle can be an indicator for gait and balance problems. Also, physical activity in patients with moderate tightness in these areas, whether young or old, usually promotes complaints of low back pain. Interestingly, some authors have recently noted a strong relationship between hip flexor tightness (i.e., greater than 10 degrees) and limited ankle dorsiflexion (i.e., at least zero degrees) causing hip and low back pain in more than 60% of their walking and jogging exercise participants (Brown, 1993). Therefore, if an older adult is a candidate for walking or jogging, the practitioner should assess hip flexor tightness (Figure 2-6) and ankle dorsiflexion range. Accordingly, testing should also include the sit and reach test to grossly assess hamstring, hip, and lower back flexibility (Chandler and Duncan, 1993). In this simple test the patient is asked to sit in a stable chair, reach forward, and then reach to each side, with the practitioner noting the patient's ability to perform the task. An object to be picked up can be placed at a reasonable distance from the patient to facilitate reach and gross trunk movements.

The sit and cross-uncross leg test is a quick test of hip flexibility. While sitting in a chair, the patient is asked to cross one thigh over the other. The patient is then asked to uncross his or her thigh and place the lateral side of his or her foot on the opposite knee. This simple test determines whether gross restriction is present.

Strength. Strength can be assessed with a number of sophisticated methods, such as manual muscle testing (Kendall and McCreary, 1983), dynamometer testing (e.g., strain gauges, hand-grip dynamometers), and progressive mobility testing (Chandler and Duncan, 1993; Tinetti, 1986). These tests are very appropriate for definitive testing, especially after a significant strength deficiency is identified. However, for the office, a gross strength assessment can be adequate in assessing the physical capability of the older adult and reliable enough to quickly and easily identify particular problems that the practitioner may wish to self-investigate more intently or refer to a specialist for a definitive assessment and prescribed treatment. The following are examples of gross strength tests that the practitioner can use in an office or clinic environment.

Rising on Toes Test. The rising on toes test can be used to determine the strength of the gastrocnemius-soleus muscle group. The quick test involves asking the patient to hold onto the back of a chair and rise up onto the toes, one leg at a time, 10 times. The patient must be able to complete the 10 repetitions with full ankle excursions. Inability to complete the test indicates moderate weakness, and strengthening must be accomplished if the patient is considering a fitness program of walking, jogging, tai chi, or dance aerobics. For the agile older patient, the test can be enhanced by having the patient walk (supported by the practitioner's hand or unsupported) on his or her toes for a short distance (e.g., 8 to 10 feet).

Walking on Heels Test. The walking on heels test can be used to quickly examine the patient's ability to dorsiflex at the ankle. The test has the patient walk in place on his or her heels (10 steps for each leg). Again, the patient must be able to complete the 10 repetitions with full ankle excursions. Like the rising on toes test, this test also can be

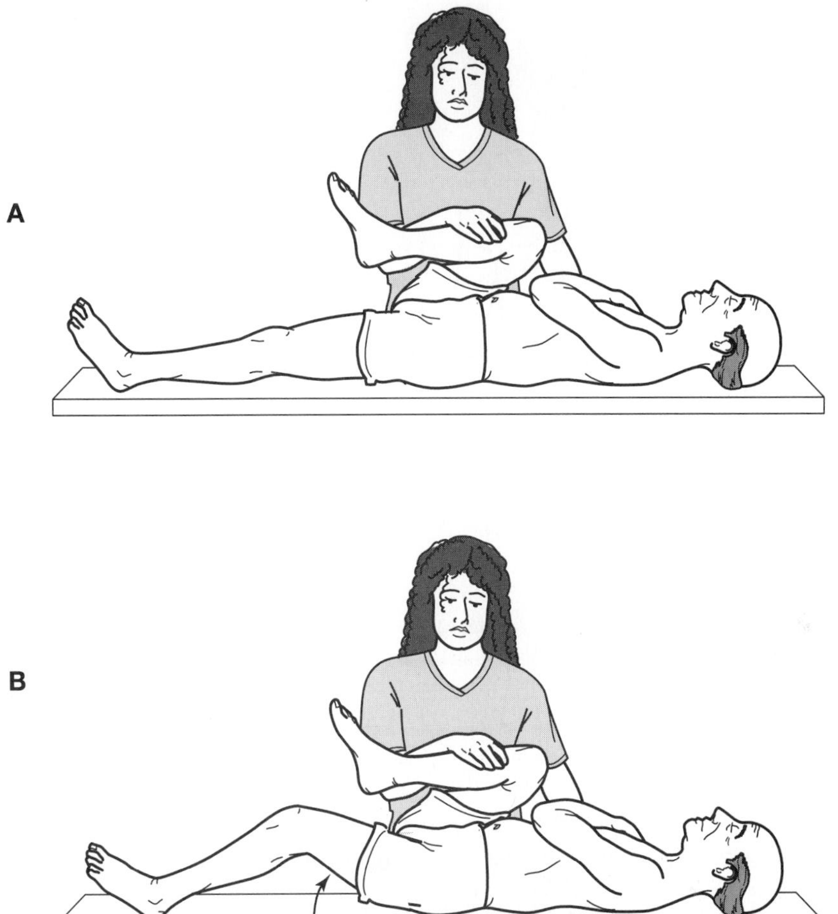

Figure 2-6 Thomas test for flexion contracture of the hip. **A,** Normal range of hip flexion. **B,** Hip flexion demonstrating flexion contracture. (Redrawn from Seidel HM et al: *Mosby's guide to physical therapy,* St Louis, 1987, Mosby.)

enhanced by having the patient walk (supported by the practitioner's hand or unsupported) on his or her heels for a short distance (e.g., 8 to 10 feet). Inability to complete the test indicates moderate weakness, and strengthening must be accomplished if the patient is considering a fitness program of walking, jogging, tai chi, or dance aerobics.

To a lesser extent, ankle inversion and eversion can be tested by having the patient walk on the lateral borders of his or her feet to test eversion and, to test inversion, by instructing the patient to walk on the medial borders of his or her feet. Besides strength, the test can determine whether there is any gross restriction in a patient's range of ankle and foot motion.

Hip Drop Test. The hip drop test shown in Figure 2-7 can be used to grossly assess gluteus medius strength. The integrity of this hip stabilizer muscle is essential in weight-bearing activities because the pelvis drops every time the patient takes a step. In this test the practitioner stands behind the patient and uses as landmarks the skin dimples overlying the posterior superior iliac spines. Normally, the skin dimples should

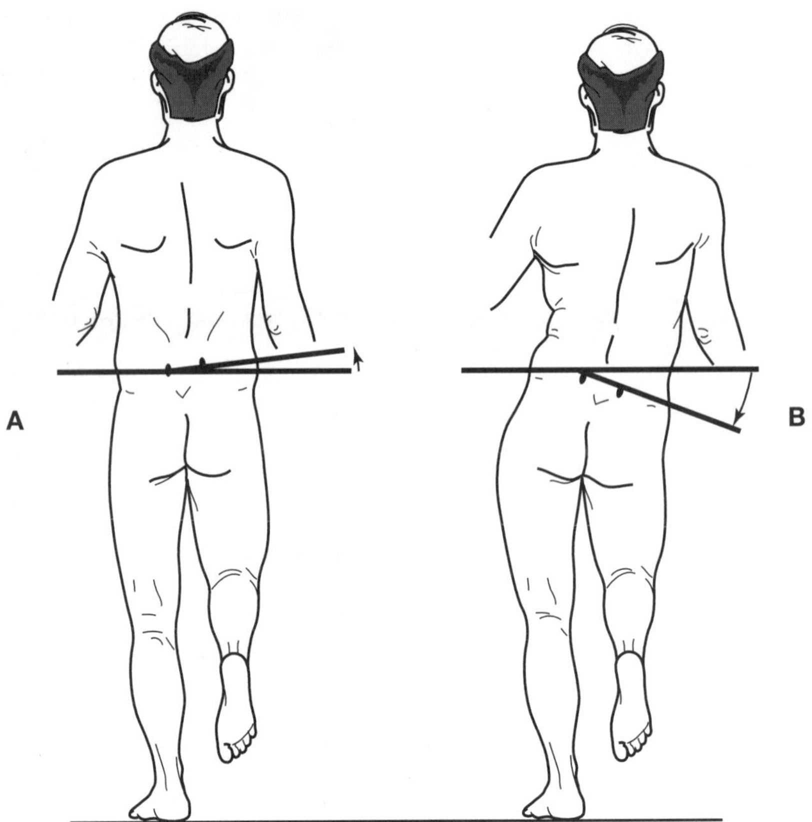

Figure 2-7 Hip drop test. **A,** Normal. **B,** Abnormal. (Redrawn from Seidel HM et al: *Mosby's guide to physical therapy,* St Louis, 1987, Mosby; and Hoppenfield S: *Physical examination of the spine and extremities,* Norwalk, Conn, 1976, Appleton & Lange.)

appear level when the patient bears weight equally on both legs. The patient is then asked to stand on one leg. The skin dimple and pelvis on the nonweight-bearing side should elevate, indicating that the gluteus medius muscle on the weight-bearing side is functioning properly (negative Trendelenburg sign). If the dimple and pelvis on the non–weight-bearing side remain in position or actually drop, the gluteus medius muscle on the weight-bearing side is weak (positive Trendelenburg sign), and a strengthening program is indicated before a weight-bearing exercise program can begin.

Hip Extension Test. The hip extension test is used to determine hip extension strength. Figure 2-8 illustrates the test. The patient is asked to lie prone and raise the entire lower extremity, against gravity, through the full range of motion (i.e., zero to 30 degrees). If the patient is unable to raise even his or her leg though the arc of motion, a strengthening program is indicated. If the patient accomplishes the hip extension, the practitioner then offers manual resistance to determine if the position can be maintained. Again, if weakness is detected, a strengthening program is necessary before a weight-bearing exercise program can begin. This test can also be performed by asking the patient to rise from a chair with arms folded across the chest and back straight. Take care to guard the patient from falling, which might happen to patients with weak hip extensors. Most

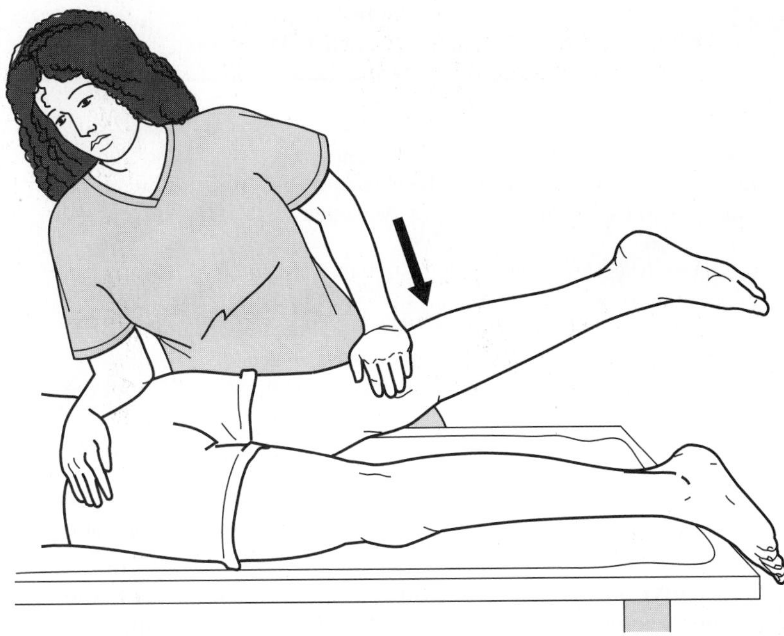

Figure 2-8 Hip extension test. The normal limit for hip extension is approximately 30 degrees. (Redrawn from Seidel HM et al: *Mosby's guide to physical therapy,* St Louis, 1987, Mosby.)

patients with "weak hip extensors" tend to stand and walk with an exaggerated lurch. Some may exhibit a forward trunk. In any case, the poor posture held during sustained physical activity will promote low back pain. The practitioner should be cautioned in strength testing the hip in older adults with a history of hip fracture. This caution can be extended to strength testing the trunk for older adults with strong history of vertebral fractures. Strength assessments under these conditions should be performed under the supervision of a rehabilitation physician or physical therapist.

Balance. Balance is a major determinant of functional independence. A patient's ability to balance can be compromised by disease or injury, medication, and the process of aging. Impaired balance poses a threat to physical safety and can lead to self-imposed restrictions on activities. Therefore an exercise program for the older adult should include activities that improve balance control.

Balance can be considered to have three basic properties: maintenance of a stable position, stabilization during voluntary movements, and reaction to external disturbance. Basically, the body does its best to keep its center of gravity close to the center of the base of support. The body's ability to maintain this stable position is supported by postural reactions and subsequent adjustments that occur before, during, and after voluntary movement or external perturbations.

Balance is usually thought of as either static or dynamic in nature. Static balance can be viewed as the patient's ability to maintain a stable upright position in unsupported sitting or standing and to withstand reasonable perturbations such as the external force of a sternal nudge. In dynamic balance the same patient's ability is determined by adding the dimension of movement in space, such as walking, bending, or reaching.

TABLE 2-5 Sharpened Romberg for Testing Balance

Task	Activity	Performance	
Circle "able" or "not able" in completing the requested task.			
1.	Standing with feet together with the eyes open for 10 seconds	able	not able
2.	Standing with feet together with the eyes open for 10 seconds and with eyes closed	able	not able
3.	Standing with feet in a semitandem (one foot ahead of the other by a half a foot length) position for 10 seconds, eyes open	able	not able
4.	Standing with feet in a semitandem (one foot ahead of the other by a half a foot length) position for 10 seconds, eyes closed	able	not able
5.	Standing in full tandem position (one foot immediately in front of the other, heel to toe), eyes open	able	not able
6.	Standing in full tandem position (one foot immediately in front of the other, heel to toe), eyes closed	able	not able

Adapted from Chandler JM, Duncan PW: In Guccione AA: *Geriatric physical therapy,* St Louis, 1993, Mosby.

Quantitative performance-oriented scales for assessing static and dynamic balance have been developed and tested (Tinetti, 1986). In addition, a posturography evaluation can be achieved by use of sophisticated movable platforms (Nashner, 1977), which are extremely expensive and somewhat large pieces of equipment that require extensive operating space not normally found in the usual office or clinic environment. Certainly, there are clinical situations when referring the patient to a local posturography testing center is appropriate. In an office setting, however, the practitioner may want to choose certain simple and relatively quick tests to assess balance. For example, static balance can be evaluated by the stand on one leg test, the sharpened Romberg, and the reach test. For dynamic balance, tests can include the get-up-and-go test, imaginary balance beam test, and walking through a simple office setting obstacle course.

STATIC BALANCE. Standing on one leg (Chandler and Duncan, 1993) with eyes open for a period of time is an easy and simple test to quickly assess significant deficits in static balance. Although there appears to be no generally accepted standard for time values associated with the one-leg stand test, the inability of a patient to stand on one leg for less than 5 seconds is certainly indicative of a significant deficit. The practitioner should conduct several patient trials to account for a patient's learning curve and ensure reliable findings. The practitioner is cautioned from allowing the patient to place the non–weight-bearing leg on the stance leg, shifting the position of the stance leg, or hopping, because these alterations are considered cheating.

The sharpened Romberg (Bannister, 1985) can also be used to quickly assess static balance. Table 2-5 illustrates the test, which involves six segments with a simple grading of either "able or not able" to complete the requested task. Figure 2-9 should clarify the patient's foot placements for testing. This relatively comprehensive test is easy to administer and a reliable assessment tool.

The reach test (Chandler and Duncan, 1993) is a must add-on for assessing static balance (Figure 2-10). The test requires the practitioner to use a yardstick to measure the distance the patient is able to reach before losing his or her balance. To perform the test, the practitioner places the flat side of a yardstick on a wall. The patient is asked to comfortably stand, with the reaching shoulder, sideways next to the wall and yardstick.

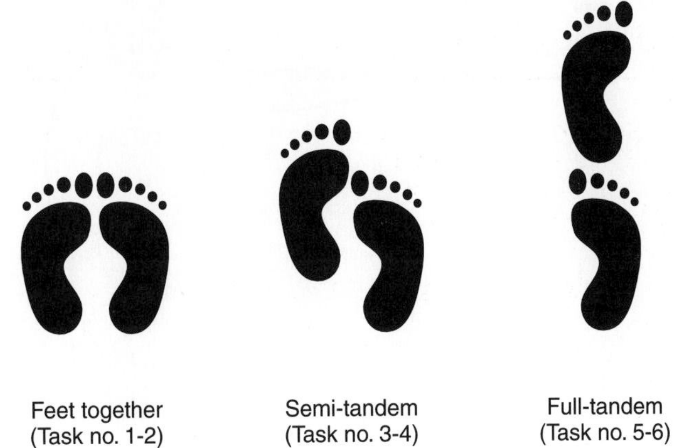

Figure 2-9 Foot placements for sharpened Romberg test. (From Guccione AA: *Geriatric physical therapy,* St Louis, 1993, Mosby.)

The patient is then asked to reach forward as far as possible along the yardstick until the practitioner notes the patient's loss of balance. The distance reached is recorded. The practitioner should be cautioned to ensure that he or she is in a position to catch the patient, should balance be completely lost.

DYNAMIC BALANCE. The get-up-and-go test (Mathias, Nayak, and Isaacs, 1987) has the patient rise from a chair and proceed, as quickly as possible, toward a preplanned destination (e.g., use of a particular clinic hallway that has been measured for distance). The complexity of the test can be upgraded by incorporating turns, controlling the patient's base of support, and adding simple functionally driven tasks into the test protocol. For example, the patient can be asked to rise from a chair and walk down a 30-foot hallway. While walking, the patient is asked to walk for 15 feet with one foot immediately in front of the other, heel to toe (i.e., imaginary balance beam test). The patient is then asked to turn around, return to the chair, and sit. Stepping over obstacles such as a telephone book(s) can be added to the protocol (i.e., obstacle course test). The trial is timed, and any difficulties recorded. Several trials are recommended to ensure testing reliability.

Obviously, depending on the patient's capabilities, the practitioner may want to take into account in the pre-exercise assessment other considerations, such as the patient's gait, speed of movement, and skills in the activities of daily living, that are not elaborated here. Nevertheless, this chapter has presented a number of options to assist the practitioner in determining a safe activity and an appropriate fitness level for the well older adult. Once the information gathered during the assessment is integrated into the patient's overall medical and physical condition, a fitness plan with commonsense goals that addresses personal needs will emerge.

The Exercise Prescription

An exercise prescription should be designed to meet the exercise history, functional status, painful conditions, medical problems, and health needs of an individual patient. Clinical traits found during the office pre-exercise assessment can also assist the

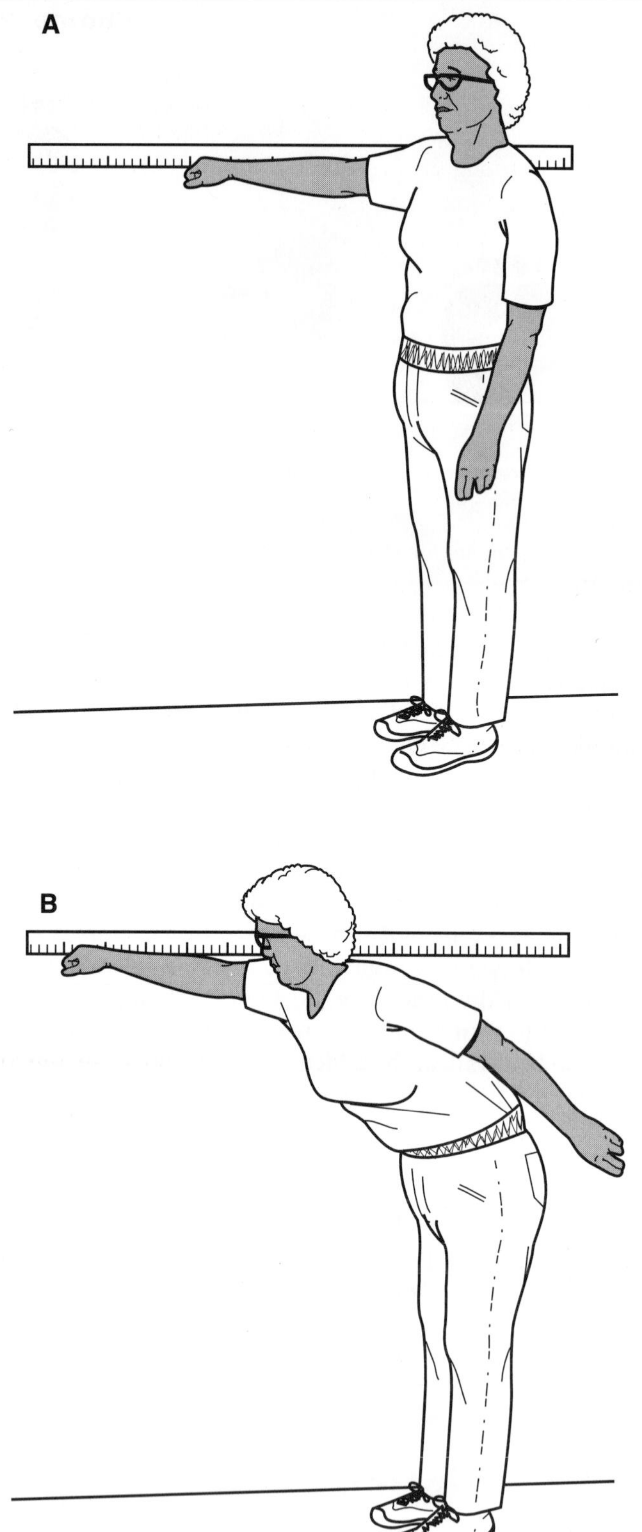

Figure 2-10 Functional reach. A, Starting position. B, Ending position. (From Guccione AA: *Geriatric physical therapy,* St Louis, 1993, Mosby.)

practitioner in determining the type of exercise and an appropriate activity level for a particular older patient. For example, patients who have a lengthy history of being sedentary or frail may drive the prescription design toward a stretching, strengthening, and balance fitness program (e.g., vs. aerobic training). Also, patients with such complications as orthostatic hypotension, impaired equilibrium, and gait disturbances may need to begin their exercise program in a supervised setting. For the apparent healthy and active older adult, however, the prescription may be immediately directed toward a moderate aerobic conditioning program. The individual's specific goals also help to design the parameters of the exercise prescription (e.g., decrease cardiovascular risk, reduce weight, improve physical function or cardiovascular fitness). All patients should be counseled to be aware of the development of signs or symptoms of cardiac risk.

The prescription for any type of exercise activity should always include the frequency of the activity, the intensity, and the time (FIT model). As discussed earlier, when setting ranges for these parameters, the settings should be sufficient to generate a training response (e.g., for strengthening, the training response can be a sense of muscle fatigue encountered during the last few exercise repetitions). For aerobic activities the target heart rate within an established training zone is the training response benchmark. The training zone is defined as 60% to 90% of a patient's maximum heart rate. The maximum heart rate is the highest rate at which the heart can safely pump (beats per minute) during exercise. Box 2-3 illustrates a common method for determining maximum and target heart rates. However, this layperson's approach should be used with caution in designing an aerobic exercise program for the elderly patient. Clinical experience encourages the use of cardiovascular stress testing to assess cardiovascular fitness in the older adult. The information obtained from a referred cardiovascular stress test can provide such parameters as safe resting and maximum heart rates, an effective exercise target zone, and a target heart rate. This pertinent data can guide the practitioner in prescribing a practical and prudent aerobic exercise program for the older adult.

As discussed earlier, aerobic exercise program progresses by slowly increasing the exercise frequency, intensity, and time. However, the practitioner should also keep in mind that, although progression is important to maintain an adequate training response, progressive increases in vigorous exercise levels also raise the risk of physical and medical complications such as musculoskeletal sprains, painful joints, and tendinitis.

Box 2-3

Determining Maximum and Target Heart Rates

Maximum heart rate = 220 beats/minute minus age

Example: Patient is 65 years old

220
−65 age
155 maximum heart rate

Target heart rate = maximum heart rate multiplied by 60%

Example:

155 maximum heart rate
×60%
93 target heart rate

Therefore the key in setting these exercise parameters is to set an optimal range for each of these components without maximizing the high risk of complications.

In addition to prescribing a conditioning phase, the exercise prescription should also include activities for a warm-up and cool-down phase. For example, the warm-up and cool-down phases can be stretching or slowed walking, and the conditioning phase necessitates a brisk walk (i.e., the actual vigorous activity). Both the warm-up and cool-down phases are essential components of an exercise program. Including such information on the prescription as aerobic exercise for 20 minutes with 5 minutes of warm-up and 5 minutes of cooldown, for a total of 30 minutes, is sufficient to remind the patient and (if applicable) the community program of the need for warm-up and cool-down periods. The frequency in this example can be three to five times a week, with a duration of 20 minutes and intensity to target heart rate.

As discussed earlier, for strength training, the appropriate intensity is generally 50% to 80% of the patient's maximum repetitive lifting ability, as estimated during the pre-exercise office assessment. Duration can start at two sets of 12 repetitions and gradually increase as the patient begins to feel no training response. The prescribed frequency should be no less often than three times a week. Elastic tubing can be substituted for a weight program. Weight or tubing tensile resistance can be gradually increased over a period of weeks. Ensure that 5 minutes of warm-up and 5 minutes of cooldown are included in the strengthening program, just as they are in aerobic training. For the older adult, some form of aerobic activity should always be part of a strengthening program. Suggesting a simple 15- to 20-minute walk or even the use of a stationary cycle for most sedentary older adults would not be unreasonable.

Examples of Typical Exercise Activities. Clinical experience suggests that the older adult's exercise program should include multiple forms of activities aimed at increasing musculoskeletal flexibility, strength, and cardiovascular endurance. Stretching should be part of every exercise session as warm-up and cooldown from the conditioning period. The following are examples of typical exercise activities that may be modified for the older well adult.

Walking. Walking is a form of total body exercise that can be considered the most prescribed exercise by practitioners. Walking is appropriate for 80% of healthy older adults and has the additional benefit of improving performance in important activities of daily living. The walk can be brisk walking, hill walking, or treadmill walking. Mall walking has become a popular type of exercise among the well elderly. It must be stressed, however, that exercise walks must be performed at a higher intensity than a normal walking pace. Figure 2-11 illustrates a typical walking program. Intensity is increased by slowly adding time and the number of walking sessions while maintaining at least 60% of a patient's maximal heart rate. The activity can improve the efficiency of the heart and lungs, burn fat and calories, build musculoskeletal strength and endurance, and improve balance and coordination. Certainly, aerobic dancing and running can also accomplish the same benefits; however, walking is easier on the joints and spine. For instance, running or aerobic dance movements exert a force equal to three to four times body weight during weight bearing. Walking transmits forces of only one to one and a half times the patient's weight on the joints and spine, which is approximately 60% to 75% less than the force transmitted in high-impact sports such as running and aerobics. Moreover, walking is accessible; that is, no special equipment except comfortable shoes and clothing is necessary. The activity is inexpensive and can be incorporated into a patient's daily routine. It also has variety; that is, it can be social (e.g., group walking) or

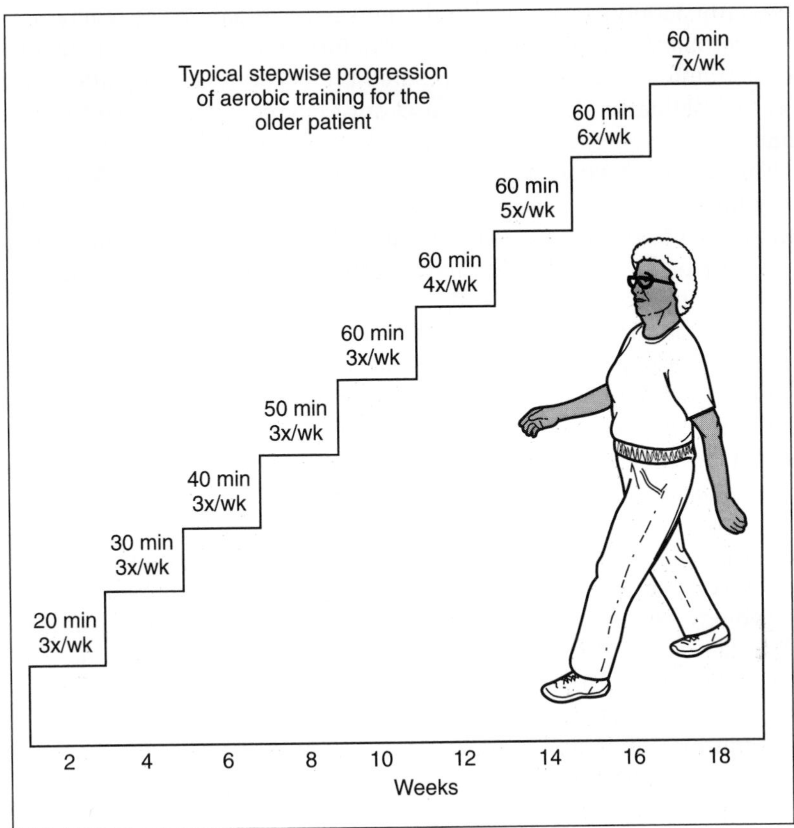

Figure 2-11 An approach used in progressing an older patient's walking program. The approach can be applied to other types of aerobic programs. (Reproduced with permission from *Geriatrics* 47(8):34, 1992. Copyright by Advanstar Communications Inc. Advanstar Communications Inc. retains all rights to this article.)

individual. It is appropriate for all fitness levels and all ages, especially the older adult. Walking programs can be a fitness model for patients with obesity, arthritis, heart disease and hypertension, type 2 diabetes, osteoporosis, and certain pulmonary disorders.

Multiple Endurance Programs. Multiple endurance exercise programs are activity programs less likely to cause muscle and joint overuse and fatigue (Brown 1993). Endurance exercises may include walking, brisk walking, treadmill walking, stationary cycling, indoor rowing and ski machines, swimming, and calisthenics. Running, bicycling, cross-country skiing, and ice-skating are also activities that build aerobic capacity but have a higher tendency for falls and should carefully be considered, especially for elderly women. One 60-minute exercise session may include a warm-up; brisk walking, riding a stationary bicycle, and rowing, while maintaining a comparable heart rate for all three activities; and a cooldown. Substituting for the conditioning activity with an aerobic videotape, stair climbing, and a stationary bike can be just as adequate for an indoor exercise program.

Aquatic Programs. Aquatic programs are also popular with the elderly. An aquatic program can be designed to help a broad range of people achieve fitness and function, especially patients with such limitations as joint pain from severe osteoarthritis, painful feet, coronary artery disease, obesity, lung disease, postural deformities, and severe deconditioning. Studies have validated the usefulness of aquatic programs in cardiovascular rehabilitation following infarct and ischemic heart disease (McMurray et al., 1986) and in musculoskeletal rehabilitation for patients with joint disease.

The relaxation effect produced by water is not understood. Mood state has been found to improve following land exercise but has not been as well studied in any aquatic environment (Connelly et al., 1990). Similarly, anxiety and depression are reduced following land exercise, although research to test these effects after aquatic exercise has not been done.

Community-based aquatic fitness programs are popular, and access is relatively simple. These programs are especially helpful to those older adults who migrate according to the change in seasons. Community aquatic programs are geographically widespread, which lessens the occurrence of "a break in training." Aquatic programs are usually group sessions, which can promote socialization and lead to a level of habitual physical activity.

Tai Chi. Tai chi has been used for centuries in Asian cultures as an old form of Chinese exercise. Although health benefits have not been fully established in Western scientific literature, evidence suggests that it is a safe form of moderate exercise that can provide physiologic benefits and enhance balance and body awareness (Lan et al., 1996; Schaller, 1996; Lai et al., 1995). For example, recent evidence encourages the use of tai chi as weight-bearing exercise for patients with rheumatoid arthritis (Kirstein, Dietz, and Hwang, 1991). Recent studies conducted by S. Wolf and colleagues at the Atlanta Frailty and Injuries Cooperative Studies on Intervention Techniques found that tai chi delayed the onset of first or multiple falls 47.5% longer than computerized platform balance training or education (Wolf et al., 1997). It also reduced the subjects' fear of falling. This finding is extremely relevant, as falls in the elderly population constitute a major risk in physical safety and an obstacle to maintaining their independence. Although other studies have demonstrated that a combined strengthening and weight-training program has a favorable impact on balance (Schaller, 1996; Wolfson et al., 1996) and that exercise for elderly patients reduces the risk of falls (Wolf et al., 1996), tai chi can serve as a favored alternative to the traditional exercise programs aimed at reducing falls in the elderly. Like aquatic fitness programs, tai chi can be a group activity that promotes socialization. Unlike aquatic programs, however, this form of fitness requires no special equipment or space. Tai chi programs have become so popular that they can be accessed through local community organizations and senior citizen groups.

Elastic Therapy. Elastic therapy can also be used to strengthen muscle groups. Commonly referred to as elastic bands (e.g., Theraband) or tubes (e.g., surgical tubing), these popular and widely used elastic tools can add resistance (as does using weights) in an isotonic exercise program. The bands come in different widths that are color coded for specific resistance (i.e., elastic tensile resistance) levels. When using surgical tubing, practitioners can select different tube diameters to match the available strength and endurance of the muscle being exercised. Such accommodation reduces the risk of overloading the patient. The smaller the tube diameter, the lower the resistance for the patient. Selection of the tensile strength of the elastic tube actually comes down to what muscle is being addressed and how strong that muscle is at the present time. A good rule is to pick a tubing size that will continually resist the muscle yet allow full (or available) motion around the joint in a controlled manner. For example, in weak muscles thin elastic tubing, which offers very little resistance, can be used. The patient who becomes stronger graduates to a thicker, more resistive type of tubing. A person should not be unstable or unable to complete the exercise.

Figure 2-12 illustrates exercise movements that use elastic material. A typical elastic exercise program consists of 12 to 15 repetitions with the appropriate size of tubing for three to five sets per exercise session. As the patient becomes stronger, tubing can be upgraded to provide more resistance. Although no aerobic capability benefit is obtained from tubing programs, the activity can be prescribed for the homebound older adult who may need strengthening of particularly large muscle groups. A general practitioner should contact a physical therapist to design an effective and safe tubing program for the older adult.

Functional Programs. Strengthening programs can also be functional in nature. Activities usually focus on certain dynamic components of a particular functional activity. Figures 2-13 and 2-14 are examples of exercises used to encourage such functional components as reaching overhead and to the side, bending forward while sitting, and pushing. The exercise program can be performed solo or with a partner, such as a family caregiver. Exercises may also include upper extremity lateral raises, shoulder shrugs, bicep curls, tricep presses, side bends, rising and sitting from a chair, wall slides, marching in place, stair climbing, and stool step-ups. A pair of cuff weights can be used to add more effort to the activity. Functional strengthening programs are usually moderate to low-level types of exercise. Nevertheless, modest physiologic benefits can occur at these lower-end exercises (Badenhop et al., 1983; Foster et al., 1989), and even for many slightly impaired elders, exercise may forestall further declines in physiologic reserves.

Sustaining an Effective Level of Habitual Physical Activity

Researchers have shown that the greatest improvements in flexibility, strength, and cardiovascular fitness occur within the first few months of an exercise program, with performance plateauing shortly thereafter (Cunningham, Imgram, and Rechnitzer, 1979; Sidney and Shephard, 1978). Improvements in cardiovascular function and flexibility achieved in the early stages of an exercise program can be maintained for at least 2 years (Morey et al., 1991). Findings indicate that exercise, when performed in the course of everyday life situations, may have a significant role and meaning for elderly individuals. However, many factors affect the older adult's continued commitment to adopting and sustaining an effective level of habitual physical activity. A change in environment due to a geographic move, poor access to equipment or services, cost, and an exacerbation of a chronic ailment are only a few of the circumstances faced by everyone in real life. Any of these interruptions may contribute to "a break in training"; however, emphasis must be placed on continuous training, which is necessary to maintain the health benefits from exercise.

Although self-paced exercise protocols have shown promise as a safe, effective, and acceptable exercise model for primary and secondary prevention in the general population of community-dwelling older adults (Morey et al., 1991; Rooks et al., 1997), experts suggest that more than 50% of patients drop out of recommended exercise programs within the first 6 months (Kligman and Pepin, 1992). Experts note that exercise is unique among all health behaviors because it takes more time and effort than any other health behavior. For instance, a 30-minute exercise session is really not limited to just

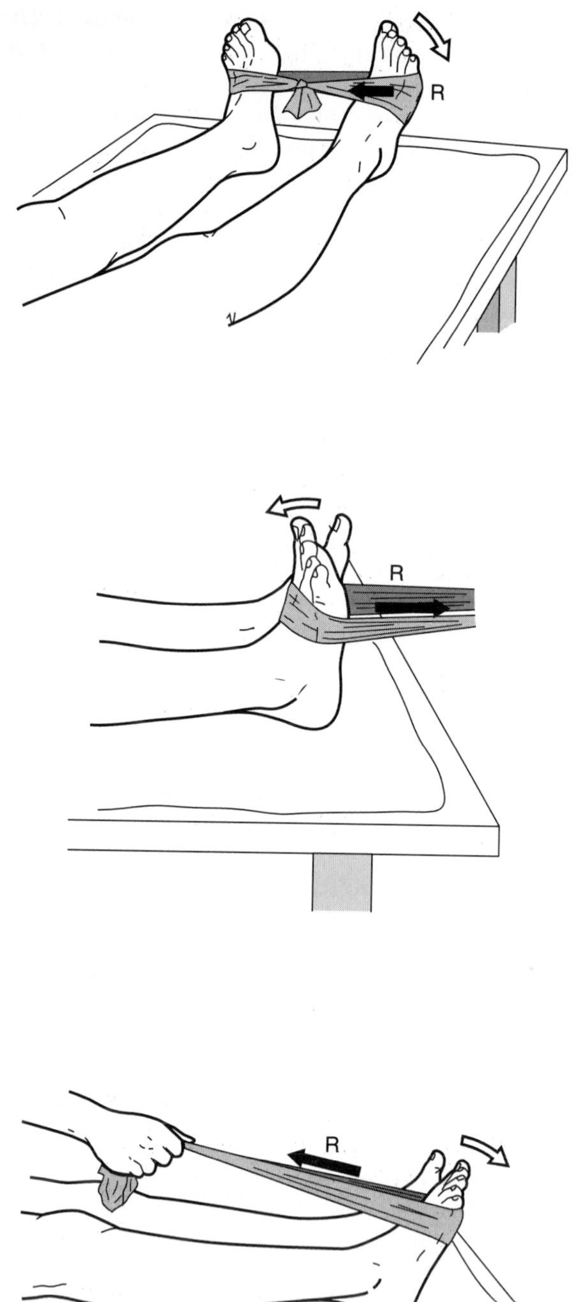

Figure 2-12 Examples of exercise using elastic bands. **R** and **dark arrow** indicate direction of resistance. **Light arrow** indicates direction of foot movement while exercising. (Redrawn from Kisner C, Lynn AC: *Therapeutic exercise: foundations and techniques,* ed 2, Philadelphia, 1990, FA Davis.)

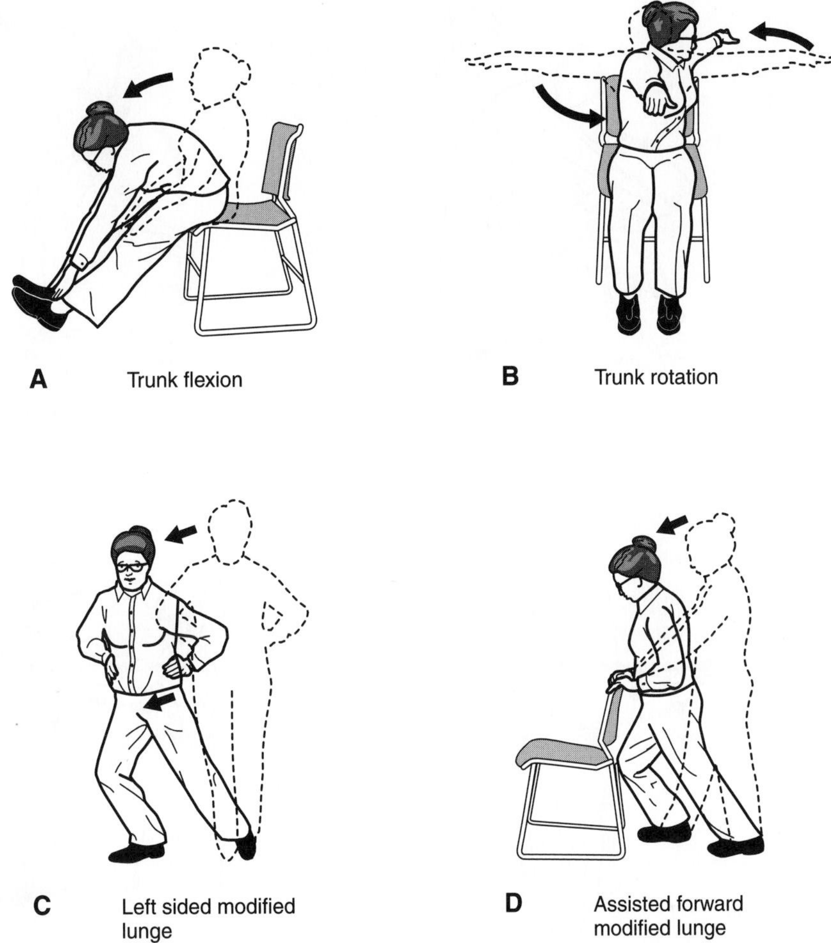

Figure 2-13 Functional solo exercise patterns. **A,** Trunk flexion. **B,** Trunk rotation. **C,** Left-sided modified lunge. **D,** Assisted forward modified lunge. (Redrawn from Lewis CB, Bottomley JM: *Geriatric physical therapy: a clinical approach,* Norwalk, Conn, 1994, Appleton & Lange.)

half an hour. The individual may have to travel somewhere, change clothes, and shower afterwards, adding up to a very big portion of time in a person's day. Exercise is a complex set of acts that includes planning for participation, initial adoption of physical activity, and continued participation or maintenance. Experts estimate that beginning exercisers probably spend 2 minutes of preparation to exercise 1 minute; thus the burden on a person's schedule is significant. With that in mind, if people are not enjoying themselves, the risk of discontinuing exercise is quite high.

Practitioners can enhance exercise compliance by clearly defining the expected health benefits of exercise for the individual patient and by selecting a type of activity the patient enjoys. The exercise, whether it is walking for 10 minutes three times a day, stepping up and down on benches or stools, or simply dancing to music in the living room, must not be simply repetitive, meaningless exercise but purposeful and engaging for the person on more than just a muscular level. Patients should be encouraged to exercise regularly,

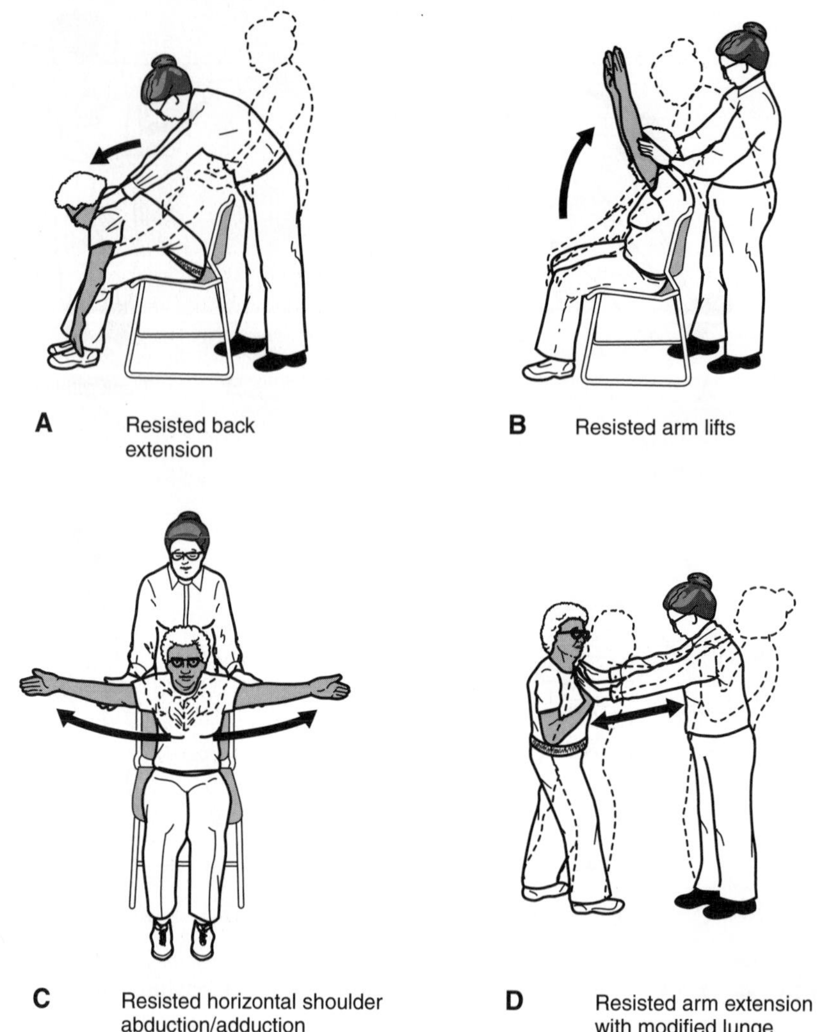

Figure 2-14 Functional partnered exercise patterns. **A,** Resisted back extension. **B,** Resisted arm lifts. **C,** Resisted horizontal shoulder abduction/adduction. **D,** Resisted arm extension with modified lunge. (Redrawn from Lewis CB, Bottomley JM: *Geriatric physical therapy: a clinical approach,* Norwalk, Conn, 1994, Appleton & Lange.)

increase their pace gradually, and vary their activity to maximize both compliance and enjoyment. Recommending simple modifications of routine daily activities can be instrumental in reaching fitness goals. If the recommended activities fit into the patient's daily schedule and lifestyle, an exercise program is more likely to be followed.

Ensuring That Fitness Activity Remains Safe and Effective

Periodic assessment is critical, given the normal age-related changes in the musculoskeletal, neurologic, and cardiopulmonary systems that, over time, result in patient-specific declines in function for the older patient. Physical fitness programs must accommodate these age-associated changes to remain safe and effective. Therefore the practitioner must periodically assess and, if applicable, modify the exercise program to fit normal age-related changes or the insult of a new disability.

Providing routine follow-up visits after the initial assessment is also important to encourage patients to continue with their fitness program. Without encouragement, many patients discontinue the exercise and lose the progress made in slowing the decline associated with the normal aging process. Suggested follow-up intervals include quarterly for the first year, every 6 months for the next 2 years, and annually in the fourth and fifth years. The follow-up, with measurements compared with the initial assessment, can provide a feeling of accomplishment and motivate patients.

Follow-up by the practitioner or office staff is recommended. Maintaining a simple list, in an office personal computer, of patients with care plans that include exercise can prompt occasional telephone calls to verify compliance. Telephone contact should be made 2 weeks and then 3 months after the evaluations to ensure patient compliance with the exercise program. Follow-up testing can be performed at 6 months or 1 year to assess improvement in physical fitness and provide further motivation to continue the exercise program. This visit is a good time to repeat an exercise stress test to assess the impact of the exercise program.

Special Considerations for the Older Adult

Pain and discomfort, such as angina pectoris, dyspnea, intermittent claudication, or joint pain, are likely to be observed in the elderly and are reasons for decreasing or even stopping an exercise session. Skin color, changes in coordination, cognition, equilibrium, and blood pressure should be monitored, especially within the first 5 minutes of recovery after exercise; older adults may tend to have blood pool in the lower extremities, which limits the adequacy of regional blood flow. The exercise intensity needs to be decreased if these complications occur.

Some clinicians who deal with exercise and injury in the older adult have reported relatively no complaints of orthopedic discomfort in the majority of their deconditioned exercisers who completed 3 months of low-intensity flexibility and strengthening activities (Brown, 1993). On the other hand, these same clinicians did report pain complaints in a significant percentage of their patients who completed 6 months of high-intensity training. Most painful episodes were classified as nonspecific joint pain, probably of osteoarthritic origin and usually at the knee or ankle-foot. The point is that some form of orthopedic discomfort should be expected when older adults do endurance training. The clinicians recommend that patients should be told up front to expect the potential discomfort and pain and that the practitioner is there to provide needed care for such problems. Conservative measures such as icing, rest, elastic wrapping, nonsteroidal antiinflammatory drugs, and modification of the exercise program succeeded in managing almost all pain.

At times, pain complaints may be attributed to musculotendinous injuries. Muscle injuries include strains, sprains, overuse, contusions, and compartment syndrome. The injured muscle or tendon is placed at significant risk for complete rupture of the muscle or tendon if subjected to high tensile force. Therefore premature return to activity may magnify the risk of rupture. If the injury is not addressed adequately and the patient continues to perform at a higher level of activity, a cycle of repetitive tissue failure develops.

Osteoporosis is common in older adults, especially in women. The risk of osteoporotic fractures in older adults, especially of the wrist, spine, or hip, is also prevalent. Exercise programs to help delay loss of bone mass should include flexibility and strength training in the major (large) muscle groups, weight-bearing activities, and certain aerobic activities that can increase flexibility, strength, and static and dynamic balance (e.g., tai chi, stair-climbing, or walking). However, patients who have severe osteoporosis should exercise caution.

- Avoid high-impact activities such as jogging.
- Avoid activities in which participants tend to fall (e.g., ice-skating, bicycling).
- Gradually increase the intensity and complexity of activities, especially those that exert sudden ballistic movements of the extremities (e.g., tennis, golf).
- Adapt weight-bearing activities to patients' movement abilities.

Back pain is also prevalent, and for most patients, a simple treatment approach of rest and reduction of the activities that cause the pain should be the first intervention. Heat or cold and nonsteroidal antiinflammatory medication can also reduce pain. For acute periods, muscle relaxants and oral pain medication used for short periods can be beneficial in managing the symptoms.

For patients experiencing cervical pain, home cervical traction (over the door) and an isometric program with gradual progression to isotonic cervical exercises may be useful. Swimming with a face mask and snorkel, to limit cervical range of motion and take advantage of the water buoyancy, can be done to continue a moderate level of physical fitness.

For thoracolumbar pain, traditional back exercises such as Williams' flexion exercises and MacKenzie extension exercises may encourage thoracolumbar flexibility and strength. If the patient is overweight, weight reduction is mandatory to reduce loading of the spine. Fitness activities for patients who have a propensity for thoracolumbar pain include walking (level surfaces), swimming, and aquatic exercise. If sitting is tolerated, sessions of 15 minutes twice to three times a day on a stationary bike can also be beneficial. Chronic thoracolumbar pain patients should avoid high-impact and vigorous anaerobic types of activities and focus on aerobic activities.

Wearing shoes for exercising is important. The selection of an appropriate shoe depends on the type of exercise and the patient's foot profile (e.g., rigid cavus foot, pes planus, hammer toes). The following characteristics should be considered:

- Cushioning is the resilient property of the midsole, shoe tongue, collar of the shoe, and heel. The purpose of cushioning is to protect the feet from pressure and friction.
- Firm heel counters that aid in rear foot stability are quite important during gait.
- Choose a wide and high toe box that is wide enough to allow the foot and toes to splay outward when the person is standing. The toe box should be high enough so that the toes are not touching the top of the box.
- Flexibility is important at the ball of the foot with the forefoot.
- Shock absorption is usually found at the heel and sometimes at the ball of the foot. Shoes with no shock absorption can promote muscle fatigue and pain in the feet and legs.

- Variable lacing systems allow fitting the shoe to the foot and accommodate structural irregularities, swelling or contracting from the weather or the time of day, and shoe wear.

Summary

Regular physical exercise for the older adult delays many physical and psychologic problems that commonly occur with aging. It can provide the foundation to support an older adult's ability to achieve daily activities of living and ultimately to improve overall function and quality of life. National recognition of a new training alternative in cardiorespiratory and muscular fitness should certainly encourage greater participation by older well adults and inspire engagement in a healthier lifestyle.

Designing an appropriate physical exercise program is a complex task. A pre-exercise assessment is a required step that the practitioner must take before prescribing a program for the well elderly. By including a limited physical examination, cardiovascular stress test, and assessments of flexibility, strength, and balance, the practitioner will be able to prescribe a safe, effective and individualized program that will help ensure continued patient participation. Taking this opportunity to record baseline information and establishing an office habit of contacting patients at a later time (i.e., follow-up contacts) will not only encourage continued participation but also ensure that the patient's physical exercise program remains safe and effective in meeting the changing health needs that occur with aging. Routine physical exercise is an inexpensive approach toward maintaining a healthier lifestyle and overall well-being for the older well adult.

Resources

American Physical Therapy Association
http://www.geriatricspt.org

Senior Site Web Page
http://www.senior-infosite.com

References

American Academy of Orthopedic Surgeons: *Joint motion: method of measuring and recording,* Edinburgh, 1996, Churchill Livingstone.

American College of Sports Medicine: Position stand on the recommended quantity and quality of exercise for developing and maintaining cardiorespiratory and muscular fitness in adults, *Med Sci Sports Exerc* 22:265-274, 1990.

American Thoracic Society: ATS statement: snowbird workshop on standardization of spirometry, *Am Rev Respir Dis* 119:831, 1979.

Badenhop DT et al: Physiological adjustments to higher- or lower-intensity exercise in elders, *Med Sci Sports Exerc* 15:496, 1983.

Bannister R: *Brain's clinical neurology,* ed 6, New York, 1985, Oxford University Press.

Brown M: In A Guccione, editor: *Geriatric physical therapy,* St Louis, 1993, Mosby.

Brown M, Coggan A: Is muscle wasting inevitable with aging? *Med Sci Sports Exerc* 22:434, 1990.

Brown M, Holloszy JO: Effects of a low intensity exercise program on selected physical performance characteristics of 60 to 71 year olds, *Aging* 3:129-139, 1991.

Centers for Disease Control and Prevention: Surgeon General's workshop on health promotion and aging: summary recommendations of the Physical Fitness and Exercise Working Group, *MMWR* 38(41):700-707, 1989.

Chandler JM, Duncan PW: In A Guccione, editor: *Geriatric physical therapy,* St Louis, 1993, Mosby.

Connelly TP et al: Effect of increased central blood volume with water immersion on plasma catecholamines during exercise, *J Appl Physiol* 69:651-656, 1990.

Cunningham DA, Imgram KJ, Rechnitzer PA: The effect of training: physiological responses, *Med Sci Sports Exerc* 11:379, 1979.

Emery GF, Gatz M: Psychological and cognitive effects of an exercise program for community-residing older adults, *Gerontologist* 30:184-188, 1990.

Fardy PS, Yanowitz FG, Wilson PK: *Cardiac rehabilitation, adult fitness and exercise testing,* ed 2, Philadelphia, 1988, Lea & Febiger.

Feeney T: Walking vs. running: setting the pace for an active America, *Advance for Physical Therapists* 21, July 1996.

Foster VL et al: Endurance training for elderly women: moderate vs. low intensity, *J Gerontol* 44:184, 1989.

Gorman KM, Posner JD: Benefits of exercise in old age, *Clin Geriatr Med* 4:181-192, 1988.

Hagberg JM et al: Cardiovascular responses of 70 to 79 yr-old men and women to exercise training, *J Appl Physiol* 66:2589, 1989.

Hoppenfeld S: *Physical examination of the spine & extremities*, Norwalk, Conn, 1976, Appleton-Lange.

Kendall FP, McCreary EK: *Muscle testing and function*, ed 2, Baltimore, 1983, Williams & Wilkins.

Kirstein AE, Dietz F, Hwang SM: Evaluating the safety and potential use of a weight-bearing exercise, tai-chi chuan, for rheumatoid arthritis patients, *Am J Phys Med Rehabil* 3:136-141, 1991.

Kligman EW, Pepin E: Prescribing physical activity for older patients, *Geriatrics* 47(8):34, 1992.

Kort WM et al: Effects of gender, age, and fitness level on response of V_{O2} max to training in 60 to 70 yr.-olds, *J Appl Physiol* 71:2004-2011, 1991.

Lai JS et al: Two year trends in cardiorespiratory function among older tai chi chuan practitioners and sedentary subjects, *J Am Geriatr Soc* 43:1222-1227, 1995.

Lan C et al: Cardiorespiratory function, flexibility, and body composition among geriatric tai chi chuan practitioners, *Arch Phys Med Rehabil* 77:612-616, 1996.

Magee DJ: *Orthopedic physical assessment,* ed 2, Philadelphia, 1992, WB Saunders.

Mathias S, Nayak U, Isaacs B: Balance in elderly patients: the get-up and go test, *Arch Phys Med Rehabil* 68:305, 1987.

McMurray RG et al: Exercise hemodynamics in water and on land in patients with coronary artery disease, *Cardiopulmonary Rehabilitation* 8:69-75, 1986.

Morey MC et al: Five-year performance trends for older exercises: a hierarchical model of endurance, strength, and flexibility, *J Am Geriatr Soc* 44(10):1226-1231, 1996.

Morey MC et al: Two-year trends in physical performance following supervised exercise among community-dwelling older veterans, *J Am Geriatr Soc* 39:986-992, 1991.

Morey MC et al: Evaluation of a supervised exercise program in a geriatric population, *J Am Geriatr Soc* 2(4):348-354, 1989.

Nashner LM: Fixed patterns of rapid postural responses among leg muscles during stance, *Exp Brain Res* 26:59-72, 1977.

Nichols JF et al: Efficacy of heavy-resistance training for active women over sixty: muscular strength, body composition, and program adherence, *J Am Geriatr Soc* 41:205-210, 1993.

Paffenarger RS et al: Physical activity, all caused mortality, and longevity of college alumni, *N Engl J Med* 314:605-613, 1986.

Posner JD et al: Low to moderate intensity endurance training in healthy older adult: physiological responses after four months, *J Am Geriatr Soc* 40:1-7, 1992.

Posner JD et al: Effects of exercise training in the elderly on the occurrence and time to onset of cardiovascular diagnosis, *J Am Geriatr Soc* 38:205-210, 1990.

Prince RL et al: Prevention of postmenopausal osteoporosis. a comparative study of exercise, calcium supplementation, and hormone-replacement therapy, *N Engl J Med* 325:1189-1195, 1991.

Public Health Service: *Healthy People 2000: national health promotion and disease prevention objectives*. Washington, DC, 1990, US Dept. of Health and Human Services.

Rooks DS et al: Self-paced resistance training and walking exercise in community-dwelling older adults: effects on neuromotor performance, *J GerontolA Biol Sci Med Sci* 52(3):161-168, 1997.

Ruuskanen JM, Ruoppila I: Physical activity and psychological well-being among people aged 65 to 84 years, *Age Ageing* 24:292-296, 1995.

Schaller K: Tai chi: an exercise option for older adults, *Journal of Gerontology Nursing* 10:12-17, 1996.

Schenkman M et al: The relative importance of strength and balance in chair rise by functionally impaired older individuals, *J Am Geriatr Soc* 44:1441-1446, 1996.

Shaw LW: National Exercise and Heart Disease Project: effects of a prescribed, supervised exercise program on mortality and cardiovascular morbidity in patients after myocardial infarction, *Am J Cardiol* 48:39-46, 1981.

Shephard RJ: The scientific basis of exercise prescribing for the very old, *J Am Geriatr Soc* 38:62-70, 1990.

Sidney KH, Shephard RJ: Frequency and intensity of exercise training for elderly subjects, *Med Sci Sports Exerc* 10:125, 1978.

Tinetti M: Performance-oriented assessment of mobility problems in elderly patients, *J Am Geriatr Soc* 34:119, 1986.

Vorhies D, Riley B: Deconditioning, *Clin Geriatr Med* 9(4):745-763, 1993.

Watkins AJ, Kligman EW: Comparison of profiles of high attendees and low attendees of a community-based health promotion program for older adults, *Gerontologist* 31:759, 1991.

Wolf S et al: The effect of tai chi quan and computerized balance training on postural stability in older subjects, *Phys Ther* 77:371-381, 1997.

Wolf S et al: Reducing frailty and falls in older persons: an investigation of tai chi and computerized balance training, *J Am Geriatr Soc* 44:489-497, 1996.

Wolfson L et al: Balance and strength training in older adults: intervention gains and tai chi maintenance, *J Am Geriatr Soc* 44:498-506, 1996.

Wolfson L et al: Strength is a major factor in balance, gait, and the occurrence of falls, *J Gerontol* 50:64-67, 1995.

Ytterberg SR, Mahowald ML, Krug HE: Exercise for arthritis, *Baillieres Clin Rheumatol* 8:1, 1994.

3

Nutrition

Numerous studies of the prevalence of malnutrition in hospitals have been conducted in the past 25 years. They indicate that the incidence of malnutrition ranges from 30% to 50% (Butterworth, 1974; Coats et al., 1993). Nutrition screening programs of geriatric populations in both institutional and community settings report malnutrition risk rates ranging from 25% to 85% (Wellman et al., 1997). Malnutrition may not be identified in the elderly because the changes that occur with malnutrition may instead be attributed to the changes that occur with aging. Those mildly or moderately malnourished may go undiagnosed (Mitchell and Chernoff, 1992). The consequences of malnutrition can be dramatic. Malnourished patients experience 2 to 20 times more complications and have up to 100% longer hospital stays, which can cost $2000 to $10,000 more per stay. Along with these longer and more expensive hospitalizations, malnourished patients have more frequent readmissions, riskier surgeries, delayed recovery times, and premature nursing home admissions. All of these factors contribute to a decreased quality of life and significantly increased health care costs (Wellman et al., 1997).

Age-related Changes

A number of body composition changes accompany aging. They include a decrease in lean body mass (which results in a decline in the basal metabolic rate), an increase in the relative amount of adipose tissue, a decline in total body water, and a decrease in bone density. Physiologic function of organs may change with age. Gastrointestinal motility and digestive or absorptive capacity may decrease. Maintenance of bowel function through exercise, adequate fluids, and fiber will be an important goal. Oral health may decline; typically dentition decreases, and cavities increase. Finally, there are declines in thirst, taste, and smell sensitivity (Baden, Karkeck, and Chernoff, 1993).

Risk Factors and Indicators of Poor Nutritional Status

Risk factors and indicators of poor nutritional status have been defined by the Nutrition Screening Initiative, a joint project of the American Academy of Family Physicians, the American Dietetic Association, and the National Council on Aging (Nutrition Screening Initiative, 1992).

Risk Factors

Nutrition risk factors are characteristics that increase the likelihood that a patient has or will have problems with nutritional status. They include an inappropriate food intake, poverty, social isolation, dependency or disability, acute or chronic diseases or conditions, chronic medication use, and advanced age.

Indicators of poor nutrition status provide evidence that poor nutritional status is present. They are broken down into major and minor indicators as follows.

Major Indicators of Poor Nutritional Status

- Weight loss of 10 + pounds
- Underweight or overweight
- Serum albumin below 3.5 g/dl
- Nutrition-related disorders
- Inappropriate food intake
- Triceps skinfold <10th percentile or >95th percentile
- Change in functional status
- Mid-arm muscle circumference <10th percentile

Minor Indicators of Poor Nutritional Status

- Alcoholism
- Cognitive impairment
- Chronic renal insufficiency
- Multiple concurrent medications
- Malabsorption syndromes
- Anorexia, nausea, dysphagia
- Change in bowel habit
- Fatigue, apathy, memory loss
- Poor oral or dental status
- Dehydration
- Poorly healing wounds
- Loss of subcutaneous fat or muscle mass
- Fluid retention
- Reduced iron, ascorbic acid, zinc

The presence of these risk factors or indicators should serve as a warning that the patient's nutritional status may be poor and further assessment is warranted. The

Determine Your Nutritional Health checklist (Figure 3-1), developed by the Nutrition Screening Initiative, is a good educational tool for increasing patients' and their families' awareness of nutrition risk factors. It enables early identification of potential nutrition-related problems and timely intervention to correct these problems (Sahyoun et al., 1997).

Assessment of Nutritional Status

A number of parameters are used in assessing a patient's nutrition status.

Weight

An ideal weight can be estimated by using the following formula:

For men	106 lb for the first 5 ft + 6 lb for each additional inch
For women	100 lb for the first 5 ft + 5 lb for each additional inch

Because the elderly can vary greatly from such estimations of ideal body weight or from standard weights from the Metropolitan Life Insurance tables, a comparison of current to usual body weight is the most revealing on an individual basis (Posthauer and Russell, 1997). Significant involuntary weight loss is considered 5% in 1 month, 7.5% in 3 months, or 10% in 6 months. Weight loss is considered severe with losses greater than these percentages in the time frame specified (Hopkins, 1993; Posthauer and Russell, 1997). If actual weights are impossible to obtain, question whether clothes are now looser or observe for signs of weight loss such as loose, sagging skin or temporal wasting. In clinic or office settings, an actual weight should be obtained at each visit, with a note on whether clothes and shoes were worn.

Biochemical Assessment

The biochemical assessment is another valuable element in a nutrition assessment. Interpretation levels of the following laboratory values may vary slightly from institution to institution.

Albumin. Albumin is a carrier protein that is needed for the maintenance of oncotic pressure. Levels correlate well with degree of malnutrition and risk of mortality and morbidity (Spiekerman, 1993; Karkeck, 1993). It is one of the most reliable biochemical indexes of malnutrition in older adults (Baden, Karkeck, and Chernoff, 1993).

Interpretation (Hopkins, 1993):
2.8 to 3.5 g/dl: Mild depletion
2.1 to 2.7 g/dl: Moderate depletion
<2.1 g/dl: Severe depletion

There are limitations in using albumin. It has a long half-life of 21 days, which makes it insensitive to acute changes in nutrition status. It can be low because of nonnutritional factors such as liver disease, infection, fluid imbalances (edema, overhydration), nephrotic syndrome, postoperative states, and metabolic stress. It can be falsely elevated because of dehydration (Hopkins, 1993). If any of these factors are currently an issue for

The Warning Signs of poor nutritional health are often overlooked. Use this checklist to find out if you or someone you know is at nutritional risk.

DETERMINE YOUR NUTRITIONAL HEALTH

Read the statements below. Circle the number in the yes column for those that apply to you or someone you know. For each yes answer, score the number in the box. Total your nutritional score.

	YES
I have an illness or condition that made me change the kind and/or amount of food I eat.	2
I eat fewer than 2 meals per day.	3
I eat few fruits or vegetables, or milk products.	2
I have 3 or more drinks of beer, liquor or wine almost every day.	2
I have tooth or mouth problems that make it hard for me to eat.	2
I don't always have enough money to buy the food I need.	4
I eat alone most of the time.	1
I take 3 or more different prescribed or over-the-counter drugs a day.	1
Without wanting to, I have lost or gained 10 pounds in the last 6 months.	2
I am not always physically able to shop, cook and/or feed myself.	2
TOTAL	

Total Your Nutritional Score. If it's —

0-2 **Good!** Recheck your nutritional score in 6 months.

3-5 **You are at moderate nutritional risk.** See what can be done to improve your eating habits and lifestyle. Your office on aging, senior nutrition program, senior citizens center or health department can help. Recheck your nutritional score in 3 months.

6 or more **You are at high nutritional risk.** Bring this checklist the next time you see your doctor, dietitian or other qualified health or social service professional. Talk with them about any problems you may have. Ask for help to improve your nutritional health.

These materials developed and distributed by the Nutrition Screening Initiative, a project of:

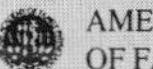
AMERICAN ACADEMY OF FAMILY PHYSICIANS

THE AMERICAN DIETETIC ASSOCIATION

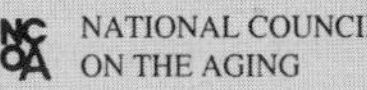
NATIONAL COUNCIL ON THE AGING

Remember that warning signs suggest risk, but do not represent diagnosis of any condition. Turn the page to learn more about the Warning Signs of poor nutritional health.

The Nutrition Screening Initiative is funded in part by a grant from Ross Laboratories, a division of Abbott Laboratories.

Figure 3-1 Checklist to determine your nutritional health. (Reprinted with permission by the Nutrition Screening Initiative, a project of the American Academy of Family Physicians, the American Dietetic Association, and the National Council on the Aging, Inc., and funded in part by a grant from Ross Products Division, Abbott Laboratories, Inc.)

Continued

The Nutrition Checklist is based on the Warning Signs described below. Use the word DETERMINE to remind you of the Warning Signs.

DISEASE

Any disease, illness or chronic condition which causes you to change the way you eat, or makes it hard for you to eat, puts your nutritional health at risk. Four out of five adults have chronic diseases that are affected by diet. Confusion or memory loss that keeps getting worse is estimated to affect one out of five or more of older adults. This can make it hard to remember what, when or if you've eaten. Feeling sad or depressed, which happens to about one in eight older adults, can cause big changes in appetite, digestion, energy level, weight and well-being.

EATING POORLY

Eating too little and eating too much both lead to poor health. Eating the same foods day after day or not eating fruit, vegetables, and milk products daily will also cause poor nutritional health. One in five adults skip meals daily. Only 13% of adults eat the minimum amount of fruit and vegetables needed. One in four older adults drink too much alcohol. Many health problems become worse if you drink more than one or two alcoholic beverages per day.

TOOTH LOSS/ MOUTH PAIN

A healthy mouth, teeth and gums are needed to eat. Missing, loose or rotten teeth or dentures which don't fit well or cause mouth sores make it hard to eat.

ECONOMIC HARDSHIP

As many as 40% of older Americans have incomes of less than $6,000 per year. Having less--or choosing to spend less--than $25-30 per week for food makes it very hard to get the foods you need to stay healthy.

REDUCED SOCIAL CONTACT

One-third of all older people live alone. Being with people daily has a positive effect on morale, well-being and eating.

MULTIPLE MEDICINES

Many older Americans must take medicines for health problems. Almost half of older Americans take multiple medicines daily. Growing old may change the way we respond to drugs. The more medicines you take, the greater the chance for side effects such as increased or decreased appetite, change in taste, constipation, weakness, drowsiness, diarrhea, nausea, and others. Vitamins or minerals when taken in large doses act like drugs and can cause harm. Alert your doctor to everything you take.

INVOLUNTARY WEIGHT LOSS/GAIN

Losing or gaining a lot of weight when you are not trying to do so is an important warning sign that must not be ignored. Being overweight or underweight also increases your chance of poor health.

NEEDS ASSISTANCE IN SELF CARE

Although most older people are able to eat, one of every five have trouble walking, shopping, buying and cooking food, especially as they get older.

ELDER YEARS ABOVE AGE 80

Most older people lead full and productive lives. But as age increases, risk of frailty and health problems increase. Checking your nutritional health regularly makes good sense.

Figure 3-1, cont'd For legend see p. 67.

the patient, it may be helpful to recheck the value as the condition resolves. For instance, a severely dehydrated patient may present with a normal albumin, but once the patient is hydrated, obtaining an additional albumin will provide a more accurate interpretation of protein stores.

Prealbumin. Prealbumin is a more sensitive indicator of visceral protein status because of its short half-life of 2 to 3 days. An upward trend is a good indicator of appropriate intake and improving nutritional status.

Interpretation (Hopkins, 1993):
10 to 15 mg/dl: Mild depletion
5 to 10 mg/dl: Moderate depletion
<5 mg/dl: Severe depletion

Prealbumin increases by 4 to 5 mg/dl a week with adequate nutritional support. An increase of less than 2 mg/dl a week reflects either an inadequate intake of protein and/or kcalories or an inadequate protein response (Spiekerman, 1993). As with albumin, prealbumin can be low because of nonnutritional factors, including acute metabolic states, postsurgery status, liver disease, infection, and dialysis. Prealbumin can be falsely elevated because of steroids, acute or chronic renal failure, and dehydration (Hopkins, 1993; Spiekerman, 1993). In the case of steroids or renal failure, trends should be monitored rather than looking at a single value (Spiekerman, 1993).

Nitrogen Balance. Nitrogen balance is one of the most widely used nutritional indicators for patients receiving enteral or parenteral nutrition support.

The desired N_2 balance for anabolism is +2 to +6. For the N_2 balance to be accurate, the following is needed: an accurate 24-hour urine collection (e.g., 24-hour urine urea nitrogen [UUN]), a minimal creatinine clearance of 50 ml/minute, and adequate caloric intake (Hopkins, 1993). N_2 balance is not an optimal nutritional indicator immediately following surgery or injury, for patients with acute sepsis or severe stress (Spiekerman, 1993) or acute or chronic renal failure (because of decreased creatinine clearance), or following spinal cord injury (Rodriguez et al., 1991).

Patient Interview

The patient interview is perhaps the most important component of assessing a patient's nutrition status and devising a plan of care. All possible barriers to a person's food intake must be identified. The following areas should be reviewed with the patient or caregiver:

Oral health examination: Does the patient have loose or lost teeth? Dentures? Mouth Pain? Dry Mouth? Is there any evidence of difficulty in swallowing (drooling, coughing after swallows, hoarseness, wet gargly voice, repeated cases of pneumonia)?

Presence of gastrointestinal complaints: Does the patient complain of anorexia? Nausea? Vomiting? Diarrhea? Constipation? Is the patient lactose intolerant?

Disabilities and function: Is there loss of vision or hearing or taste or smell changes? Is the patient able to feed herself or himself? Is assistance needed for tray setup vs. total feed? Are modified utensils needed? Does cognitive impairment affect eating?

Dietary history: What is the patient's usual intake? Who cooks the meals and shops for food? Are there specific diet restrictions? Ethnic or religious considerations? How much alcohol is consumed?

Social history: Is the patient isolated or depressed? Are support systems adequate? Is a fixed or low income preventing the purchase of adequate, nutritious food?

The development of a care plan will directly result from what is obtained in the patient interview and assessed via the weight and biochemical data.

Nutritional Requirements of the Geriatric Patient

A variety of calculations are available to estimate Calorie and protein requirements.

Energy

The *Harris-Benedict equation* is often used for calculating basal energy expenditure (BEE) because it takes into account the person's height, weight, age, and activity level (American Dietetic Association, 1992). Individualization for the variable geriatric population is necessary in applying stress factors (Baden, Karkeck, and Chernoff, 1993).

$$\text{Male: } 66 + (13.8 \times \text{weight in kg}) + (5 \times \text{height in cm}) - (6.8 \times \text{age})$$
$$\text{Female: } 655 + (9.6 \times \text{wt in kg}) + (1.8 \times \text{ht in cm}) - (4.7 \times \text{age})$$
$$\text{Total Caloric needs} = \text{BEE} \times \text{activity factor} \times \text{injury factor}$$

Activity factors include: in bed, 1.2; out of bed, 1.3.

Examples of injury factors include: mild infection, 1 to 1.2; moderate infection, 1.2 to 1.4; severe infection, 1.4 to 1.8; minor surgery, 1 to 1.1; major surgery, 1.1 to 1.2 (American Dietetic Association, 1992).

If the patient is above 125% ideal body weight, use adjusted body weight for calculations:

$$\text{Adj. wt.} = [(\text{Actual wt.} - \text{Ideal wt.}) \times 0.25] + \text{Ideal wt.}$$

The Harris-Benedict equation was developed with normal-weight, healthy adults; therefore it may not be as accurate for assessing critically ill or injured patients (Ireton-Jones et al., 1998).

An alternate method is the *Ireton-Jones formula* to determine estimated energy expenditure or EEE (Ireton-Jones et al., 1998). For the ventilated patient:

$$\text{EEE} = 1784 - 11(A) + 5(W) + 244(G) + 239(T) + 804(B)$$

For the spontaneously breathing patient:

$$\text{EEE} = 629 - 11(A) + 25(W) - 609(O)$$

where A = age in years, W = actual body weight in kilograms, G = gender (male = 1, female = 0), T = diagnosis of trauma (present = 1, absent = 0), B = diagnosis of burn (present = 1, absent = 0), and O = presence of obesity >30% above ideal body weight (present = 1, absent = 0).

A factor of 1.0 to 1.5 can be used to multiply the EEE, depending on stress level.

Perhaps the easiest method to estimate needs is the *calorie per kilogram method* (Cerra, 1986):

Maintenance needs for a well-nourished, low-stress patient: 20 to 25 kcal/kg
Caloric needs for a high-stress patient: 30 kcal/kg
Caloric needs for a very high-stress patient: 35 kcal/kg

Protein

Evidence exists for slightly increased protein requirements in the elderly of 1 to 1.1 g/kg as compared with the recommended daily allowance (RDA) of 0.8 g/kg (Baden, Karkeck, and Chernoff, 1993). Needs are higher for conditions that cause an increased metabolic rate or increased protein losses such as wound healing or fighting infection. For example, a stage IV pressure ulcer may require 2 g of protein per kilogram.

Consider the preceding calculations as merely estimations of calorie and protein requirements. Continued observance of trends in weights, laboratory values, and food intake is essential in determining whether these estimations are adequate.

Fluid

Dehydration is the most common fluid and electrolyte disturbance in the elderly. Conditions that increase the risk of dehydration include the following:

- Natural response to thirst decreased
- Mental or physical incapacities that reduce the ability to recognize thirst, create an inability to express thirst, or decrease access to water
- Self-restriction for convenience
- Increased fluid output due to less efficient kidneys
- Some drugs such as diuretics that increase urine output

Most people require 30 ml of fluid per kilogram of body weight unless a fluid restriction is indicated (Kerstetter, Holthausen, and Fitz, 1992). In general, 1 kcal/cc formulas provide approximately 85% water, 1.2 to 1.5 kcal/cc formulas provide approximately 80% water, and 2 kcal/cc formulas provide approximately 70% water. Water not provided by the formula should be provided via water flushes. Additional water may be needed in cases of fever, elevated environmental temperature, low environmental humidity, dry oxygen, and air-fluidized bed therapy, all of which cause evaporative water loss. Losses from vomiting, diarrhea, excessive ostomy drainage, and other gastrointestinal fluid losses should be replaced with an oral or intravenous rehydration solution because of the loss of water and electrolytes (Posthauer and Russell, 1997).

Diet Recommendations

General Guidelines

For the healthy geriatric patient, diet guidelines are similar to those for younger age groups. Encourage a varied diet, with an emphasis on high-fiber, low-fat foods. The Food Guide Pyramid is an educational tool that illustrates the Dietary Guidelines for Americans issued by the U.S. Department of Health and Human Services and the U.S. Department of Agriculture. Box 3-1 and Figure 3-2 illustrate how to use the guidelines and pyramid together (Nutrition Screening Initiative, 1992):

Fiber: An intake of 25 to 35 g/day is recommended to reduce constipation, improve carbohydrate tolerance, and lower serum lipids. A variety of sources such as fresh fruits, vegetables, legumes, and whole-grain products should be used.

Box 3-1

The Food Guide Pyramid: Putting the Dietary Guidelines into Action

Learning to eat right is now made simpler with the new Food Guide Pyramid by the U.S. Department of Agriculture (USDA). The Pyramid is a graphic description of what registered dietitians and other nutrition experts have been advising for years: Build your diet on a base of grains, vegetables, and fruits. Add moderate quantities of lean meat (poultry, fish, eggs, legumes) and dairy products, and limit the intake of fats and sweets.

The Food Guide Pyramid illustrates how to turn the Dietary Guidelines for Americans (issued by USDHHS/USDA in 1990) into real food choices.

The Dietary Guidelines—and their relationship to the Food Guide Pyramid—are as follows:

- **Eat a variety of foods.** The body needs more than 40 different nutrients for good health, and since no single food can supply all these nutrients, variety is crucial. Variety can be assured by choosing foods each day from the five major groups shown in the Pyramid: (1) Breads, Cereals, Rice & Pasta (6-11 servings); Vegetables (3-5 servings); (3) Fruits (2-4 servings), (4) Milk, Yogurt & Cheese (2-3 servings); (5) Meat, Poultry, Fish, Dry Beans, Eggs & Nuts (2-3 servings) and (6) Fats, Oils and Sweets (use sparingly).
- **Maintain healthy weight.** Being overweight or underweight increases the risk of developing health problems, so it is important to consume the right amount of calories each day. The number of calories needed for ideal weight (which varies according to height, frame, age, and activity) will generally determine how many servings in the Pyramid are needed.
- **Choose a diet low in fat, saturated fat, and cholesterol.** As shown in the Pyramid, fats and oils should be used sparingly, since diets high in fat are associated with obesity, certain types of cancer, and heart disease. A diet low in fat also makes it easier to include a variety of foods, because fat contains more than twice the calories of an equal amount of carbohydrates or protein.
- **Choose a diet with plenty of vegetables, fruits, and grain products.** Vegetables, fruits, and grains provide the complex carbohydrates, vitamins, minerals, and dietary fiber needed for good health. Also, they are generally low in fat. To obtain the different kinds of fiber contained in these foods, it is best to eat a variety.
- **Use sugars only in moderation.** Sugars, and many foods containing large amounts of sugars, supply calories but are limited in nutrients. Thus, they should be used in moderation by most healthy people and sparingly by those with low calorie needs. Sugars, as well as foods that contain starch (which breaks down into sugars), can also contribute to tooth decay. The longer foods containing sugars or starches remain in the mouth before teeth are brushed, the greater the risk for tooth decay. Some examples of foods that contain starches are milk, fruits, some vegetables, breads, and cereals.
- **Use salt and sodium only in moderation.** Table salt contains sodium and chloride, which are essential to good health. However, most Americans eat more than they need. Much of the sodium in people's diets comes from salt they add while cooking and at the table. Sodium is also added during food processing and manufacturing.
- **If you drink alcoholic beverages, do so in moderation.** Alcoholic beverages contain calories but little or no nutrients. Consumption of alcohol is linked with many health problems, causes many accidents, and can lead to addiction. Therefore alcohol consumption is not recommended.

Adapted from *At the Center,* National Center for Nutrition and Dietetics, Chicago, Summer 1992.

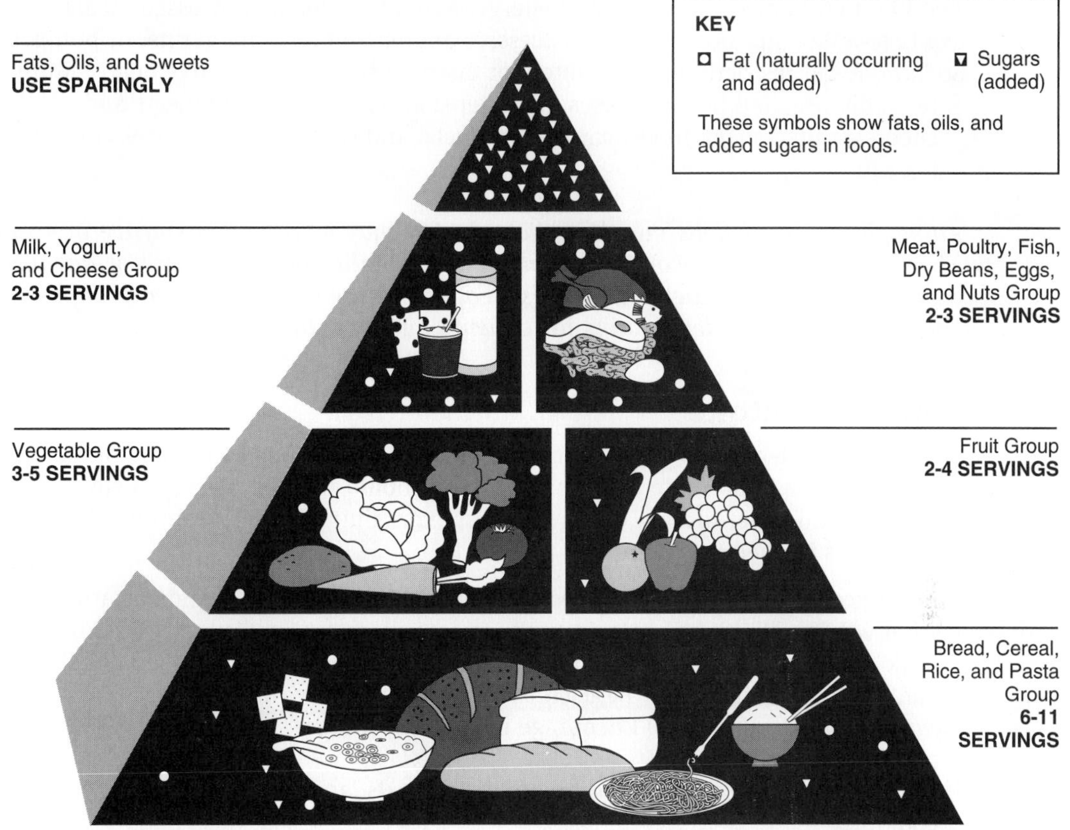

What Counts as a Serving?

With the Food Guide Pyramid, what counts as a "serving" may not always be a typical "helping" of what you eat. Here are some examples of servings:

Bread, Cereal, Rice and Pasta - 6-11 servings recommended
Examples of one serving:
1 slice of bread
1 oz. of ready-to-eat cereal
1/2 cup of cooked cereal, rice, or pasta
3 or 4 small plain crackers

Vegetables - 3-5 servings recommended
Examples of one serving:
1 cup of raw leafy vegetables
1/2 cup of other vegetables, cooked or chopped raw
3/4 cup of vegetable juice

Fruits - 2-4 servings recommended
Examples of one serving:
1 medium apple, banana, or orange
1/2 cup of chopped, cooked, or canned fruit
3/4 cup of fruit juice

Milk, Yogurt, and Cheese - 2-3 servings recommended
Examples of one serving:
1 cup of milk or yogurt
1 1/2 oz. of natural cheese
2 oz. of process cheese

Meat, Poultry, Fish, Dry Beans, Eggs, and Nuts - 2-3 servings recommended
Examples of one serving:
2-3 oz. of cooked lean meat, poultry, or fish
1/2 cup of cooked dry beans, 1 egg, or 2 tablespoons of peanut butter = 1 oz. of lean meat

How Much Is an Ounce of Meat?

Here's a handy guide to determining how much meat, chicken, fish, or cheese weigh:
1 ounce is the size of a **match box.**
3 ounces are the size of a **deck of cards.**
8 ounces are the size of a **paperback book.**

Figure 3-2 Food Guide Pyramid. (Source: U.S. Department of Agriculture.)

Fat: Limit fat intake to 30% of total energy. Avoid fried foods, processed meats, whole-milk dairy products, and excessive amounts of oils, margarine, or butter.

Sodium: A salt restriction is warranted for diseases such as congestive heart failure, renal disease, and in some cases, hypertension. Limit processed meats and cheeses, salted snack foods, canned products, and seasonings or sauces containing salt.

Although diet restrictions may be indicated, they may be counterproductive in debilitated individuals with a poor intake and limited quality of life because of advanced disease. Assess whether a diet restriction is an appropriate goal and whether its implementation would improve or detract from the patient's quality of life.

Optimizing Intake

For patients with debilitating conditions, the goal of the diet may be to maximize calorie and protein intake to promote healing. Emphasis should then be placed on substituting lower-calorie and lower-protein foods with those containing higher quantities. Examples of food choices include the following:

Dairy: Encourage whole milk, cheeses, cottage cheese, puddings, and custards made from whole milk; use cheese or cream sauces on entrees and vegetables. Fortified milk can be made by adding dry milk powder to milk for an increased nutrition content. Lactaid milk may be used by those with lactose intolerance.

Meats and meat substitutes: Encourage meats (all varieties), fish, eggs, peanut butter, and beans.

Fats: Add margarine or butter on breads, hot cereals, and vegetables; use oils in cooking.

Soups: Substitute cream soups for broth-based varieties.

Supplements: Commercial nutrition supplements can be used but may be expensive for many; a lower-cost alternate is powdered breakfast mix (use with whole milk).

It may also be helpful to encourage multiple small meals and snacks throughout the day in place of three larger meals, especially if early satiety or poor appetite is a problem.

Nutrition Support Issues

Do Not Resuscitate Status and Patient Prognosis

If food intake is deemed inadequate, consider the ramifications of initiating nutrition support. Determine whether an advance directive addresses the issue. Consider whether artificial feedings will help the patient regain useful function and improved quality of life. Also try to determine whether the possible benefits from nutrition support may be outweighed by the burdens. Benefits may include increased life span, increased ability to recover, increased possibility of returning to useful functioning, improved quality of life, improved psychologic and physiologic state, increased resistance to infection, and improved healing of skin and wounds. Burdens may include physical pain, spiritual and emotional pain and suffering, denial of a peaceful death, invasive procedures, indignity, and emotional and financial burden on the family (Dorner et al., 1997). Assessing benefits and burdens may be especially important for those patients with terminal illnesses. For example, using restraints in order to keep a nasogastric tube in place may not be an acceptable trade-off for an end-stage Alzheimer's patient with anorexia. Once initiated, it is ethically permissible for nutrition support to be discontinued (Dunn, 1994). Placing feeding tubes in the demented elderly does not necessarily improve their survival rates (Mitchell, Kiely, and Lipsitz, 1997).

Monitoring

If nutrition support is initiated, monitor trends in weight and laboratory values (weekly UUN and prealbumin, if appropriate) to ensure that the nutrition support is appropriately meeting the patient's needs.

A number of complications can result from underfeeding: muscle wasting, including loss of diaphragmatic mass (Arora and Rochester, 1982); decreased vital capacity and minute ventilation (Grant, 1994); delayed wound healing (Dickhaut, Delee, and Page, 1984; Kay, Moreland, and Schmitter, 1987); skin breakdown (Ferrell and Osterweil, 1990); decreased immune function (Shronts, 1993); and a longer hospital stay resulting from these complications. Complications can also result from overfeeding: hyperglycemia, increased CO_2 production and respiratory rate, electrolyte imbalances, uremia, fatty liver, abdominal distention, and vomiting (Klein, Stanek, and Wiles, 1998).

Refeeding Syndrome

A word of caution is in order regarding the initiation of nutrition support. In severely depleted individuals, refeeding syndrome may occur if the patient is refed too quickly. This syndrome is characterized by acute decreases in serum potassium, phosphorus, and magnesium secondary to intracellular electrolyte shifting related to carbohydrate intake. Heart and respiratory failure can result. Patients with prolonged periods of poor intake and weight loss are possible candidates. In suspected cases, initiate enteral or parenteral nutrition support at 20 cal/kg and monitor potassium, phosphorus, and magnesium for a minimum of 3 days and as the feedings progress toward the final goal (Solomon and Kirby, 1990).

Strategies for Improving a Patient's Nutritional Status

- Assess all possible barriers to an adequate intake.
- Enlist family assistance. Use home health services. If available, consult experts in nutrition, physical therapy, occupational therapy, speech, or social work as indicated to address barriers.
- Use snacks and supplements to boost intake. Encourage smaller, more frequent meals and high-calorie, high-protein foods wherever possible.
- Monitor weight on a regular basis.
- Supplement daily with a multivitamin and mineral supplement. It is often difficult for the elderly to consume adequate amounts of nutrients from food alone (Tripp, 1997).

Look at the overall medical picture when prescribing diet therapy. The optimal method for nutritionally supporting patients who are at risk for malnutrition is to feed them a nutritionally dense, well-balanced diet. Liberalizing diet restrictions may lead to a more palatable diet and more interest in food.

Summary

This chapter has addressed a fundamental physiologic need that many times is ignored by primary care providers to the detriment of the older person's health and well-being. It is an astute practitioner who always assesses the nutritional status and everyday practices of the older patient. This chapter provides an important knowledge base and practical considerations for potential risk factors, normal nutritional requirements for a healthy life, and assessment and treatment of malnutrition.

Resources

Administration on Aging
Nutrition in the Elderly
http://www.fiu.edu/~nutreldr

American Academy of Family Physicians
Nutrition Screening Initiative
http://www.aafp.org/nsi

References

American Dietetic Association: *Handbook of clinical dietetics*, ed 2, New Haven, 1992, Yale University Press.

Arora NS, Rochester DF: Effect of body weight and muscularity on human diaphragm mass, thickness, and area, *J Appl Physiol* 52:64-70, 1982.

Baden A, Karkeck J, Chernoff R: Geriatrics. In Gottschlich MM, Matarese LE, Shronts EP, editors: *Nutrition support dietetics core curriculum*, ed 2, Silver Spring, Md, 1993, Aspen.

Butterworth CE Jr: The skeleton in the hospital closet, *Nutrition Today* 9:4-8, 1974.

Cerra FB: The role of nutrition in the management of metabolic stress, *Crit Care Clin* 2(4):807-819, 1986.

Coats KG et al: Hospital malnutrition: a reevaluation 12 years later, *J Am Diet Assoc* 93:27-33, 1993.

Dickhaut SC, Delee JC, Page CP: Nutrition status: importance in predicting wound healing after amputation, *J Bone Joint Surg Am* 60:71, 1984.

Dorner B et al: The "to feed or not to feed" dilemma, *J Am Diet Assoc* Supp2: S172-S176, 1997.

Dunn H: *Hard choices for loving people*, ed 3, Herndon, Va, 1994, A & A Publishers.

Ferrell BA, Osterweil D: Pressure sores and nutrition. In Morley JE, Glick Z, Rubenstein LZ, editors: *Geriatric nutrition*, New York, 1990, Raven.

Grant JP: Nutrition care of patients with acute and chronic respiratory failure, *Nutrition in Clinical Practice* 9:11-17, 1994.

Hopkins B: Assessment of nutritional status. In Gottschlich MM, Matarese LE, Shronts EP, editors: *Nutrition support dietetics core curriculum*, ed 2, Silver Spring, Md, 1993, Aspen.

Ireton-Jones C et al: Should predictive equations or indirect calorimetry be used to design nutrition support regimens? Point–Counterpoint, *Nutr Clinical Practice* 13:141-145, 1998.

Karkeck JM: Nutrition support for the elderly, *Nutr Clinical Practice* 8:211-219, 1993.

Kay SP, Moreland JR, Schmitter E: Nutritional status and wound healing in lower extremity amputations, *Clin Orthop* 217:253, 1987.

Kerstetter JE, Holthausen BA, Fitz PA: Malnutrition in the institutionalized older adult, *J Am Diet Assoc* 92:1109-1116, 1992.

Klein CJ, Stanek GS, Wiles CE: Overfeeding macronutrients to critically ill adults: metabolic complications, *J Am Diet Assoc* 98:795-806, 1998.

Mitchell CO, Chernoff R: Nutritional assessment of the elderly. In Chernoff R, editor: Geriatric nutrition: the health professional's handbook, Gaithersburg, Md, 1991, Aspen.

Mitchell SL, Kiely DK, Lipsitz LA: The risk factors and impact on survival of feeding tube placement in nursing home residents with severe cognitive impairment, *Arch Intern Med* 157:327-332, 1997.

Nutrition Screening Initiative: *Nutrition interventions manual for professionals caring for older Americans,* Washington, DC, 1992.

Phillips PA et al: Reduced thirst after water deprivation in healthy elderly men, *N Engl J Med* 311:753-759, 1984.

Posthauer ME, Russell C: Ensuring optimal nutrition in long-term care, *Nutrition in Clinical Practice* 12:247-255, 1997.

Rodriguez DJ et al: Obligatory negative nitrogen balance following spinal cord injury, *JPEN J Parenter Enteral Nutr* 15: 319-322, 1991.

Sahyoun NR et al: Nutritional screening initiative checklist may be a better awareness/educational tool than a screening one, *J Am Diet Assoc* 97:760-764, 1997.

Shronts EP: Basic concepts of immunology and its application to clinical nutrition, *Nutr Clinical Practice* 8:177-183, 1993.

Solomon SM, Kirby DF: The refeeding syndrome: a review, *JPEN J Parenter Enteral Nutr* 14:90-97, 1990.

Spiekerman AM: Proteins used in nutritional assessment, *Clin Lab Med* 13:353-369, 1993.

Tripp F: The use of dietary supplements in the elderly: current issues and recommendations, *J Am Diet Assoc* 97(suppl 2): S181-S183, 1997.

Wellman NS et al: Elder insecurities: poverty, hunger, and malnutrition, *J Am Diet Assoc* 97(suppl 2): S120-S122, 1997.

4

Stroke Prevention

Stroke is the third most common cause of death and a major cause of disability in the industrialized world among persons age 70 years and older. In the United States 750,000 individuals suffer a stroke every year; 158,000 will die within the year, and 350,000 will be left with moderate to severe disabilities. It is estimated that at any one time 4 million Americans are disabled as a consequence of stroke (Ramirez-Lassepas, 1998).

Stroke is the leading cause of brain damage in adults. The damage results from destroyed neurons following either disruption of cerebral blood supply or hemorrhage into or around the brain. This destruction of brain tissue results in decreased brain function and, for the patient, reduced independence, a loss of self, and even death.

Dramatic decreases in stroke morbidity and mortality over the past 25 years have been largely due to hypertension control, atherosclerosis prevention, therapy for cardiac disease to eliminate sources of emboli, and surgical therapy for stroke prevention (National Stroke Association, 1998).

Cost refers to all resources consumed by the disease and its treatment in monetary terms. Costs can be divided into direct and indirect components. Direct costs include the dollar burden of all medical care received in response to a stroke, as well as nonmedical costs such as those for caregiver services and home modification. Indirect costs include the dollar value of lost productivity due to stroke (Matchar, 1998). The annual health costs of stroke are estimated at $18.6 billion. The total cost, including lost wages and care of the disabled, approximates $45 billion (Ramirez-Lassepas, 1998). The average cost per case of stroke is approximately $50,000. From a Medicare perspective, the largest proportion of the cost is hospital readmission, reflecting the co-morbidities associated with stroke. A major cost not reflected directly in Medicare data (because it is typically not covered) is nursing home care. This cost is especially great for stroke patients with more severe disability (Matchar, 1998). Stroke prevention is one of the most effective ways to reduce this public health and economic burden.

Because treatment of acute stroke has improved greatly in recent years, there is great effort by leaders in the field to instill in the minds of persons the need for urgent evaluation and treatment at the first onset of stroke symptoms. One method of achieving this goal is by renaming stroke "brain attack." This is being done in an effort to attach the same urgency in seeking treatment that has been achieved with heart attack over the years.

Age-Related Changes

Cerebral blood flow decreases with advancing age. This is caused in part by loss of neuronal connections that results in loss of neurons and glial cells with resulting brain atrophy. Atherosclerosis of extracranial and intracranial arteries, heart disease, and hypertension further decrease cerebral blood flow (Ramirez-Lassepas, 1998). The major determinants of cerebral perfusion are age and status of the vascular system (Shaw et al, 1984).

Pathophysiology

There are two basic mechanisms for stroke: occlusion and hemorrhage. Of these, arterial occlusion resulting in ischemia accounts for 80% to 86%, intraparenchymal (intracerebral) hemorrhage for 6% to 8%, and subarachnoid hemorrhage from aneurysmal rupture for 8% to 12% (Wolf, Kannel, and McGee, 1986).

When a major artery to the brain is occluded, the occurrence of ischemic symptoms depends on collateral circulation. If collateral circulation is immediately available, symptoms do not occur or are only short-lived; if it is not immediately available, the occurrence of cerebral infarction will depend of whether collateral circulation can be established in time to prevent irreversible neuronal damage (Sokoloff, 1997). The clinical result of an episode of transient focal cerebral ischemia is a transient ischemic attack, or TIA, and is defined as episodes of focal neurologic deficit of sudden onset that last minutes, rarely hours, and always subside in less than 24 hours (American Heart Association, 1994). A TIA is a warning of the possibility of a major stroke in the future.

Risk Factors

Everyone is at risk of stroke, regardless of age. However, advancing age is a major risk factor for ischemic stroke and intracerebral hemorrhage. It is estimated that the risk of stroke doubles every 10 years after the age of 55 (Ramirez-Lassepas, 1998). Risk factors are categorized as modifiable or nonmodifiable. Nonmodifiable risk factors are characteristics inherent in a particular individual and cannot be changed. Modifiable risk factors have the potential to be controlled through lifestyle change or by medical intervention. See Box 4-1 for categories of risk factors.

Men are at greater risk for stroke than women; however, the number of women who have had a stroke exceeds that of men because women survive longer than men. The incidence of stroke is more than double for blacks compared with white people, except among those over 75 years of age (Sacco, 1998). Hispanic-American populations also have an increased incidence of stroke compared with white populations (Sacco et al, 1998).

Box 4-1

Risk Factors for Ischemic Stroke

Nonmodifiable	Modifiable
Age	Hypertension
Gender	Atrial Fibrillation
Race/ethnicity	Cigarette smoking
Heredity	Hypercholesterolemia
Geographic location	Heavy alcohol use
	Asymptomatic carotid stenosis
	Transient ischemic attack
	Diabetes
	Physical inactivity
	Obesity
	Cardiovascular disease
	Hypercoagulability
	High-dose contraceptives
	Dietary factors
	Stress

Among the modifiable risk factors, hypertension is extremely important, as well as atrial fibrillation, which becomes more prevalent with increasing age. Additional factors that have been associated with risk of first stroke include diabetes, physical inactivity, obesity, cardiovascular diseases (coronary artery diseases, myocardial infarction, cardiomyopathy, congestive heart failure [CHF]), aortic arch atheroma, hypercoagulability, and the use of high-dose contraceptives in younger women (Sacco, 1998).

The most common mechanism by which heart disease causes stroke is cardioembolism, most frequently caused by cardiac arrhythmia. Atrial fibrillation is the most common arrhythmia.

With alcohol consumption, nondrinkers and, to a greater extent, heavy drinkers are at greater risk for first stroke than are mild to moderate drinkers. There is evidence to suggest that one to two drinks per day may actually provide some protection against stroke. This benefit rapidly disappears when alcohol consumption exceeds two drinks per day (Sacco, 1998). Of course, the other risks of alcohol consumption need to be weighed for each individual.

A high degree of carotid stenosis, even if asymptomatic, correlates with a high risk of stroke. In a study by Chambers and Norris (1986), patients with 70% to 99% carotid stenosis were followed for 23 months with the following results: 14% had TIAs, 22% had myocardial ischemia, 15% had fatal myocardial infarction and/or sudden death, 6% had ischemic stroke, 3% had nonfatal myocardial infarction, and 3% experienced other vascular deaths. After 8 years of follow-up with asymptomatic carotid bruits in the Framingham study, 48% experienced atherothrombotic stroke, 28% TIAs, and 14% cardioembolic stroke (Wolf et al., 1981).

Transient ischemic attacks (TIAs) are associated with an 8% risk for first stroke in the first month after a TIA and a 12% risk within the first year after diagnosis of TIA. This risk of stroke may reach 30% within 5 years after a first TIA (Sacco, 1998). The risk is higher in the first month and highest in patients with hemispheric TIA and >70% carotid stenosis (American Heart Association, 1998). Most TIAs have a duration of less than

TABLE 4-1 Occurrence of Ischemic Stroke in High-Risk Patients

Risk	Stroke Rate (%/y)
General population, aged 70	0.6
Prior myocardial infarction	1.5
Asymptomatic bruit	1.5
Asymptomatic carotid stenosis	2.0
Nonvalvular atrial fibrillation (after TIA)	5.0 (12.0)
Transient ischemic attack (with >70% carotid stenosis)	6.0 (13.0)
Prior ischemic stroke	9.0

Data from Feinberg WM: Anticoagulation for prevention of stroke, *Neurology* 51(Suppl 3):S20-22, 1998.

1 hour, with a median duration of 14 minutes in carotid-distribution ischemia and 8 minutes in vertebrobasilar ischemia. Atherosclerosis of cerebrovascular arteries is the most common cause of transient ischemia in older patients with risk factors for stroke. A TIA should be promptly evaluated to institute therapy as soon as possible to decrease the risk of stroke. See Table 4-1 for rates of occurrence of ischemic stroke in high-risk patients.

Recently, elevated levels of total plasma homocysteine (tHcy) have been shown to increase the risk for atherosclerotic vascular disease and stroke, although this is not yet being used routinely. Accumulation of tHcy occurs with certain enzyme deficiencies or with dietary deficiency of vitamin B_6, B_{12}, or folic acid and can be treated with dietary supplements (Perry et al, 1995; Wolf, 1998). In current practice, tHcy levels are most commonly drawn in the evaluation of a low B_{12} level, rather than as a primary assessment of stroke risk.

Care of certain patients in the primary care setting may be focused on prevention of a second, or recurrent, stroke. Atherosclerotic stroke, hypertension, and hyperglycemia have been documented as important predictors of early stroke recurrence. For late stroke recurrence, some studies have found age, hypertension, atrial fibrillation, CHF, and diabetes to be risk factors, as well as prior TIA or stroke (Sacco, 1998).

Assessment

The most important aspect of the assessment for stroke risk is a thorough history to assess for any of the potential contributing factors discussed, both modifiable and nonmodifiable (e.g., family history, smoking, alcohol use, activity level, hypertension, diabetes).

In the clinical setting the practitioner can order a variety of imaging procedures for the evaluation of patients at risk of stroke. New procedures have improved accuracy and lessened invasiveness but increased the complexity of decision making. When all of the standard imaging techniques are available, a sequential choice must be made to optimize diagnostic yield, reduce the risk of harm to the patient, and minimize cost. The goals of imaging are to identify candidates for specific surgical or medical therapeutic modalities, determine prognosis, and exclude rare nonvascular causes (American Heart Association, 1998).

Box 4-2

Physical Examination in Assessment of Stroke Risk

Weight
Blood pressure (annually)
Cardiovascular examination to include auscultation of carotids for bruits and assessment of peripheral circulation
Abdominal examination to assess for aortic bruit
Neurologic examination to establish any baseline deficits

Box 4-3

Diagnostic Studies for the Assessment of Stroke Risk (As Appropriate for Individual Patients)

- Complete blood count
- Lipid profile
- Electrocardiogram
- Echocardiogram
- Carotid Doppler study
- Computed tomography (CT)
- Magnetic resonance imaging
- Magnetic resonance angiography
- CT Angiography

Physical and diagnostic evaluation should include the areas listed in Boxes 4-2 and Box 4-3, respectively.

Noninvasive techniques allow study of carotid arteries with no risk to the patient. Carotid Doppler ultrasonography should be performed whenever carotid stenosis is suspected, as when carotid bruit is present or when cerebrovascular episodes have already occurred in the distribution of the carotid circulation.

Head computed tomography (CT) is useful in detection of cerebral infarction in patients who have had a TIA and in exclusion of other lesions that may simulate stroke such as subdural hematoma, brain tumor, arteriovenous malformation (AVM), or aneurysm.

Magnetic resonance imaging (MRI) of the head is used less often than CT for initial evaluation because it is more expensive, time-consuming, and less available (American Heart Association, 1998). However, MRI has certain advantages, such as the ability to detect acute and small infarcts and "flow voids" in the carotid arteries. MRI may not be performed on patients with aneurysm clips, otic or cochlear implants, old prosthetic heart valves, pacemakers, or neurostimulators or when agitation and claustrophobia cannot be resolved.

Magnetic resonance angiography (MRA) is a generic name for different approaches and variations of vascular imaging by MRI. MRA is useful in detecting arterial narrowing and, sometimes, the source vessel of ischemic attacks. Sensitivity and specificity of MRA is improved when used in conjunction with other studies such as ultrasound and CT.

CT angiography is a high-resolution, contrast-enhanced CT scan of the cervical vessels that visualizes the arterial lumen wall, providing information about changes in the carotid artery that might precipitate a TIA. CT angiography reveals enough vascular detail to be useful as a diagnostic screening method in patients with presumed atherosclerosis of the carotid bifurcation (American Heart Association, 1998).

Interventions

An important aspect with any risk factor modification program is that a given patient may have multiple risk factors that may lead to cumulative risks for stroke that require multi-targeted interventions (Sacco, 1998). An emerging issue in stroke prevention and stroke treatment is that therapies shown to be effective in clinical trials are not being used or are being used suboptimally (Matchar, 1998).

Hypertensive individuals need to reduce blood pressure to under 140 mm Hg systolic and under 90 mm Hg diastolic. (Refer to Chapter 8.) Weight reduction in obese patients and a program of moderate physical activity may be generally recommended (Wolf, 1998). (Refer to Chapters 2 and 3.)

The use of the HMG-CoA-reductase inhibitors or statin medications for the reduction of total cholesterol and low-density lipoprotein (LDL)–cholesterol concentrations has been shown to have some benefit for reduction of stroke. In addition to reducing LDL-cholesterol, HMG-CoA-reductase inhibitors prevent precipitation of vascular events by stabilizing atherosclerotic plaque and exerting beneficial effects of clotting (Wolf, 1998).

The benefit of antiplatelet therapy with aspirin in preventing vascular outcomes is well established. It reduces relative risk for stroke, myocardial infarction, and vascular death by about 25% compared with placebo (Easton, 1998). While debate continues regarding the best dosing for prophylaxis, it is generally adequate to start with a small dose ("baby aspirin," 81 mg). The dose may be increased (325 mg or 650 mg per day) in patients with high risk or who have experienced minor cerebrovascular episodes while on lower doses. Another agent that inhibits platelet aggregation is ticlopidine, which is useful for patients with TIA in whom aspirin therapy has not successfully eliminated occurrence of symptoms or who are not able to take aspirin. Patients who have had an embolic stroke or are at very high risk may require anticoagulation with warfarin (Coumadin).

Patients with atrial fibrillation who are at high risk for stroke should receive warfarin (Feinberg, 1998). Warfarin therapy is monitored via the International Normalization Ratio (INR), which is now reported with the prothrombin time. Used for many years in other countries, the INR has recently been adopted in the United States to monitor anticoagulation therapy with warfarin because of less variability in results. The usual target range for the INR is 2 to 3, although this may vary for the individual patient and is usually monitored monthly once the correct dose is determined.

Some elderly patients with atrial fibrillation may not be considered good candidates for anticoagulation. These may include patients who have a tendency to fall, patients who may not be able to manage medication regimens reliably (and have no assistance), or those who refuse or are unable to have blood drawn frequently. For these patients the priority is adequate control of the heart rate. This may be accomplished with diltiazem or digoxin, which a cardiologist or other physician may administer intravenously with cardiac monitoring until initial control is achieved. Another option includes cardioversion with medication maintenance. These patients may also benefit from aspirin therapy at the 325-mg daily dose (Wolf, 1998).

Patients with carotid stenosis of 70% to 99% should be evaluated by a vascular surgeon for possible endarterectomy. Several studies have evaluated this intervention and found benefits in certain populations, although the potential risks of the procedure must be weighed carefully (Wolf, 1998). Although many surgeons may delay surgery until stenosis is 90% to 99%, it is beneficial to obtain the input of the vascular surgeon in the management of the patient whenever significant stenosis is present. It has been established that successful outcomes for this procedure depend on low rates of stroke and death within 30 days of the surgery for the hospital and the surgeon performing the procedure (Bratzler, 1998).

Smoking causes 417,000 deaths each year (American Heart Association, 1998). The risk for stroke decreases among those who quit smoking and approaches that of nonsmokers in about 5 years (Sacco, 1998). Practitioners need to be familiar with various smoking cessation programs and tools to be prepared to help the patient with this difficult task. There are two addictions associated with smoking: the response behavior and the nicotine. A patient who has smoked less than half a pack a day (10 cigarettes) may not require much more than moral support and assistance in substituting a different, healthier habit when the smoking "trigger" occurs. These triggers often include first thing on arising in the morning, commuting in the car, and after a meal. Substituting other behaviors such as going for a walk, brushing the teeth, or chewing gum may help to "break the habit" for lighter smokers. Heavier smokers will probably require a tapered nicotine replacement in addition to behavioral modifications. There are several nicotine replacement systems currently on the market. These include gum and titrated patches. When considering a nicotine replacement patch, one must consider the number of cigarettes smoked in an average day. The patient who smokes irregularly, or less than half a pack per day, may actually be increasing the nicotine dose by using a patch and may benefit from one of the other replacements. A recent tool in smoking cessation is Zyban (Glaxo Wellcome), a short-term, low-dose buproprion course that helps to alleviate the craving for tobacco.

Patient Education

It is critical to educate patients regarding the devastating effects of stroke and especially their individual risk factors. At each visit the patient should be asked about smoking cessation, exercise, and attention to other modifiable risk factors, as appropriate. Patients and caregivers must also be educated regarding the signs of a TIA or stroke, and the importance of immediate care ("Call 911!") must be emphasized. See Box 4-4 for warning signs of a stroke.

Summary

Prevention of stroke is a very important task for those caring for persons of all ages because so many high-risk behaviors begin early in life. However, because strokes tend to

Box 4-4
Warning Signs of a Stroke

- Sudden numbness or weakness or face, arm, or leg, especially on one side of the body
- Sudden confusion, trouble speaking or understanding
- Sudden trouble seeing in one or both eyes
- Sudden trouble walking, dizziness, loss of balance or coordination
- Sudden, severe headache with no known cause

Source: American Heart Association Web Site (http://www.americanheart.org/Stroke/Warning_Signs)

occur in the elderly population, this seems to be the time most providers and patients focus on the issue. Fortunately, interventions aimed at reducing risk are still effective and beneficial. In addition, many interventions such as smoking cessation, exercise, and aspirin therapy are neither difficult nor expensive. However, the practitioner must identify patients with risk factors so that appropriate education and intervention can begin before the first stroke causes disability and possibly death.

Resources

American Heart Association Stroke Connection
(800) 553-6321

Brain Attack Coalition
http://www.stroke-site.org

National Stroke Association
(800)-STROKES
http://www.stroke.org

American Heart Association
http://www.americanheart.org

References

American Heart Association Medical/Scientific Statement: Guidelines for the management of transient ischemic attacks, *Stroke* 25:1320-1335, 1994.

American Heart Association Web Site http://www.americanheart.org/Stroke/Warning_Signs, 1998.

Bratzler DW: *Carotid endarderectomy and prevention of stroke,* http://preventstroke.org/strokeseries/carotid.html, 1998.

Chambers BR, Norris JW: Outcome in patients with asymptomatic neck bruits, *N Engl J Med* 315:860-865, 1986.

Easton JD: What have we learned from recent antiplatelet trials? *Neurology* 52(3 suppl 3):s36-s38, 1998.

Feinberg WM: Anticoagulation for prevention of stroke, *Neurology* 1(suppl 3):s20-s22, 1998.

Matchar DB: The value of stroke prevention and treatment, *Neurology* 51(suppl 3):s31-s35, 1998.

National Stroke Association Web Site http://www.stroke.org/First_Few_Hours.html, 1998.

Perry IJ et al: Prospective study of serum total homocysteine concentration and risk of stroke in middle-aged British men, *Lancet* 346:1395-1398, 1995.

Ramirez-Lassepas M: Stroke and the aging of the brain and arteries, *Geriatrics* 53 (suppl 1): s44-s48, September, 1998.

Sacco RL: Identifying patient populations at high risk for stroke, *Neurology* 51(3 suppl 3):s27-s30, September, 1998.

Sacco RL et al: Stroke incidence among white, black, and Hispanic residents of an urban community: the northern Manhattan stroke study, *Am J Epidemiol* 147:259-268, 1998.

Shaw TJ et al: Cerebral blood flow changes in benign aging and cerebrovascular disease, *Neurology* 34:855-862, 1984.

Sokoloff L: Anatomy of cerebral circulation. In Welch KMA et al: *Primer of cerebrovascular disease,* New York, 1997, Academic Press.

Wolf PA et al: Asymptomatic carotid bruit and risk of stroke: the Framingham study, *JAMA* 245:1442-1445, 1981.

Wolf PA, Kannel WB, McGee DL: Epidemiology of strokes in North America. In Barnett HJM et al: *Stroke pathophysiology, diagnosis, and management,* New York, 1986, Churchill Livingstone.

Wolf PA: Prevention of stroke, *Stroke* 352:SIII 15-18, October, 1998.

Unit II

5

Clinical Pharmacology

Prescribing drugs appropriately for the elderly is an important component of both day-to-day primary care evaluation and comprehensive assessment of the elderly patient. The basic concepts of prescribing drugs appropriately differ significantly from those used for other age groups because the effects of a drug on the elderly patient may be magnified by certain changes that occur during the aging process. Changes may be secondary to an alteration of drug absorption, metabolism, or excretion of the drug; to structural and physiologic changes of aging organ systems; or to blunting of immune defenses (Hazzard et al., 1994).

Because of these changes and because older patients in general have significantly more illnesses, they take more prescription and over-the-counter drugs than other age groups. The average older American takes 4.5 prescription and 3.5 over-the-counter medications at any given time. That same individual may refill about 15 prescriptions per year. As would be expected, the highest incidence of polypharmacy is in the nursing home population burdened with advanced age and chronic disease, averaging 8 medications per patient.

The elderly are at greater risk for and severity of adverse drug reactions (ADRs) (Table 5-1). An ADR is "the development of unwanted symptoms, signs, changes in laboratory values, or death directly related to the use of a medication" (Beck, 1991-1992). It may occur secondary to alterations in drug absorption, metabolism, or elimination. It may also occur in the form of drug-drug or drug-disease interactions. This increased risk is not independently related to age, however. Two of the most common factors associated with ADRs involve a reduction in renal or hepatic function requiring dosage adjustment (Lesar, Briceland, and Stein, 1997). In a 1997 case-control study of 21,777 patients in a community hospital in Salt Lake City, patients admitted to the hospital with ADRs had higher mortality, longer lengths of stay, and higher costs than those patients without (Pestonik et al., 1997). Another study showed that the most common drugs involved in ADRs in older hospitalized inpatients were cardiovascular and psychotropic medications (Doucet et al., 1996). Of 444 ADRs reported in 333 nursing home patients over a 4-year period, the most common organ systems involved in ADRs were, in decreasing frequency, the cardiovascular (188), nervous (129), gastrointestinal (82), endocrine (41), immune (17), hematopoietic (7), pulmonary (6), and renal (4) systems. The most common drugs

TABLE 5-1 Classes of Drugs Associated with Frequent Adverse Drug Reactions by Mechanism and Body System

Body System	Drug Class	Mechanism of ADR	Adverse Drug Reaction (ADR)
Cardiovascular	Diuretics	Fluid contraction, hypokalemia, hyponatremia	Lethargy; inappropriate antidiuretic syndrome; postural hypotension, falls, hip and other fractures
	Alpha-blocker drugs	Arterial vasodilation	Presyncopal light-headedness and falls, especially in high doses
	Beta-blocker drugs	Nonselective blockade of beta receptors	Precipitation or exaggeration of congestive heart failure, masking of hypoglycemia, postural hypotension, masking of symptoms of endocrine disease, reduction in exercise capacity, exacerbation of chronic lung disease or bronchospasm, memory loss, depression, arthropathy
Central nervous system	Anticholinergic agents (antihistamines, antispasmodics, phenothiazine and tricyclic antidepressants)	Stimulation of parasympathetic nervous system, central anticholinergic disruption	Sedation, cognitive dysfunction, lethargy, acute confusion; postural hypotension, falls, hip fracture; constipation, fecal impaction, worsening of glaucoma, urinary retention, dry mouth
	Benzodiazepine tranquilizers, barbiturates, hypnotics	Depression of central nervous system	Sedation, cognitive dysfunction, lethargy, acute confusion; postural hypotension, falls, hip and other fractures
	Central-acting antihypertensive agents (methyldopa, reserpine, clonidine)	Depression of central nervous system	Sedation, cognitive dysfunction, lethargy, acute confusion; postural hypotension
	Nonsteroidal antiinflammatory drugs		Sedation, cognitive dysfunction, lethargy, acute confusion
	Fluoroquinolones		Seizures, blurred vision, diplopia, headache, drowsiness

Gastrointestinal system	H_2 blocking agents, sucralfate	Reduction in acid secretion leading to achlorhydria	Increased risk of aspiration pneumonia in the presence of swallowing dysfunction in bed-bound patients
	Nonsteroidal antiinflammatory drugs	Direct irritation of gastric and duodenal mucosa (inhibition of surface prostaglandin)	Diarrhea or constipation; malabsorption
	Antacids, iron preparations, tetracyclines	Binding between agents	
Liver	Anticoagulant (warfarin) Antiseizure medications (carbamazepine, phenytoin, barbiturates, meperidine)	Reduction in protein levels secondary to decreased intake, malabsorption decreased production, increased catabolism	Increased bleeding time (warfarin); sedation, lethargy, acute confusion, cognitive dysfunction (phenytoin, carbamazepine, barbiturates, meperidine); ataxia and incoordination (phenytoin)
	Barbiturates, meperidine, diphenhydramine, lidocaine, theophylline, ibuprofen, tolbutamide, salicylates, long-acting benzodiazepine tranquilizers (diazepam, chlordiazepoxide, flurazepam)	Reduction in phase 1 metabolism with normal aging	Increased risk of gastrointestinal or other bleeding (salicylates, ibuprofen); sedation, lethargy, acute confusion, cognitive dysfunction, postural hypotension, falls, hip fracture (barbiturates, meperidine, diphenhydramine, ibuprofen, diazepam, chlordiazepoxide, flurazepam); hypoglycemia (tolbutamide); postural hypotension, falls, anorexia, nausea, arrhythmias
Kidney	H_2 blocker drugs antibiotics (penicillins, aminoglycosides, fluoroquinolones)	Reduction in creatinine clearance	Confusion, irritability, drowsiness, lethargy, dizziness
	Digoxin	Reduction in creatinine clearance	Anorexia, decreased appetite, nausea; cardiac conduction problems; confusion, irritability, anxiety
	Nonsteroidal antiinflammatory drugs	Inhibition of prostaglandin-mediated renal vasodilation	Fluid retention, worsening hypertension, aggravation of congestive heart failure
	Fluoroquinolones		Hematuria
Skin	Tetracyclines	Photosensitivity	Dermatitis
	Fluoroquinolones	Photosensitivity	Pruritus, urticaria, rash

involved, in decreasing frequency, were diuretics, antipsychotics, anxiolytics, potassium supplements, digoxin, nonsteroidal antiinflammatory drugs (NSAIDs), insulin, theophylline, H_2 receptor antagonists, antiinfectives, anticonvulsants, and thyroid supplements (Cooper, 1996).

The elderly are also at greater risk for both polypharmacy and ADRs because they tend to be referred to or visit more specialist physicians. Further, they visit pharmacies more often and at more different sites. Their regular pharmacy may not have the drug in stock, and an apparent perceived urgent need to be taking the drug as soon as possible may encourage them to go elsewhere. Various family members serving as caregivers for an elderly loved one may use their own respective pharmacies when refilling the drug, which may also add to the confusion and the number of pill bottles. An elderly patient may not know that he or she is taking several different forms of aspirin or acetaminophen because he or she may not be aware of the basic ingredients of different brand names. The elderly patient may make the automatic but wrong assumption that it is appropriate to take all of the various forms of a prescription or over-the-counter drug such as aspirin prescribed by all the specialists (rheumatologist, cardiologist, primary care physician).

The elderly, especially the advanced elderly (those at least 85 years old), have blunted immune defense systems to fight infection, leading to a greater risk of pneumonia and influenza and less chance of recovery. This change is due to inadequate antibody production in many cases (Hazzard et al., 1994). Manifestations of this blunted response may be seen in the gastrointestinal (junction of the esophagus and the stomach-cardiac sphincter of the stomach) and genitourinary systems (junction of the urinary sphincter and urethra), where bacteria may tend to reflux beyond otherwise "sterile" areas proximal to these sphincters. Thus older patients may have a greater risk of aspiration pneumonia or bladder infection in the presence of disease, as is explained later in this chapter. These patients lose the margin of reserve that allows the human body to fight off stresses, whether physiologic, psychologic, or physical. In the presence of various disease processes, this loss of reserve plays a significant role. An example is precipitation of congestive heart failure in a patient with angina and cardiomegaly who is challenged with a "few" grams of extra dietary salt intake, failure to take a morning dose of fluid medication or digoxin after a mild upper respiratory tract infection, or slight excesses of physical exertion (Beck, 1991-1992).

Normal changes of aging include reduction in total body water, reduction in muscle mass, and an increase in total body fat. These changes may translate into a greater risk of adverse drug reactions. Water-soluble drugs such as digoxin, theophylline, and alcohol are distributed in a smaller compartment than at other age groups. These drugs may accumulate at toxic levels at the same dose. Fat-soluble, long-acting benzodiazepines accumulate in body fat to a greater extent, which may lead to greater sedation, lethargy, and risk of falls than in younger patients with less body fat. Reduction in muscle mass with "normal" aging translates into reductions in renal clearance, especially in the advanced elderly. This difference holds true for drugs dependent on renal clearance, such as digoxin, H_2 blocking agents, fluoroquinolones, penicillins, and aminoglycosides (Calkins, Ford, and Katz, 1992).

The normal aging process is also accompanied by the following reductions: the total number of receptors (the nervous system) and the number of functioning receptors (the pancreas); the responsiveness of organ-specific receptors to a stimulus and the responsiveness of specific organ systems to stimuli; a reduction in blood supply (liver); and mass of the organ (kidneys, liver, brain) (Calkins, Ford, and Katz, 1992). An example of reduction of responsiveness of a specific organ (central nervous system) to stimuli is increased refractory time between responses and difficulty learning new material with advancing age. An example of reduction of responsiveness of organ-specific receptors to a stimulus is reduction in maximum heart rate or "blunted" heart rate increase, initiated by the carotid baroreceptors sensing an acute change in blood pressure. It is likely to occur when the patient stands or sits from a supine position (Calkins, Ford, and Katz, 1992). Normally the expected increase in heart rate would neutralize the negative effects of any transient reduction in blood pressure and prevent any symptoms of dizziness or light-headedness. The "blunted" process may precipitate postural hypotension in an otherwise "normal elderly" patient in 10% to 15% of instances. *Postural hypotension* is defined as a reduction in systolic blood pressure of 15 mm Hg or more on standing or sitting from the supine position (Calkins, Ford, and Katz, 1992). In addition, the presence of various disease processes and drugs may potentiate these responses. An example of drug-induced exaggeration of normal aging responses is the development of cognitive dysfunction secondary to alcohol and other drugs, including central-acting antihypertensive agents, psychotropics in high doses or with high anticholinergic activity, long-acting minor tranquilizers, anticholinergic agents, high doses of certain antibiotics (aminoglycosides, fluoroquinolones, penicillins), high doses of H_2 blocking agents, and NSAIDs. These agents might cause reduction in response time to stimuli, leading to confusion, sedation, or lethargy. An example of drug-induced exaggeration of reduced responsiveness of an organ-specific receptor to a stimulus is the use of cardiovascular agents that might cause heart block at high doses in the elderly, including digoxin, antiarrhythmic drugs, and calcium channel blockers.

Drug Metabolism

Five body systems deserve mention in the absorption, metabolism, and excretion of drugs in the elderly and in the development of adverse drug reactions. The least important system from this standpoint is the integumentary system. In the outer layers of the skin, 7-dehydrocholesterol is converted by ultraviolet light of the sun to vitamin D_3 (Hazzard et al., 1994). Although sunlight is not the only source of vitamin D production, institutionalized elderly patients with chronic renal or liver failure who do not get regular exercise may develop vitamin D deficiency. This deficiency may lead to the development of osteomalacia because the metabolically active form of vitamin D requires metabolism in the liver and the kidney (Hazzard et al., 1994).

The central nervous system plays an important role in the development of adverse drug reactions in the elderly, primarily because of normal structural and physiologic changes and changes secondary to Alzheimer's and related diseases. This process makes the patient more susceptible to acute confusion (delirium) and chronic confusion (cognitive dysfunction). The development of confusion syndromes is thought to be related to an anticholinergic hypothesis. (Hazzard et al., 1994; Mach et al., 1995). Drugs with significant anticholinergic or muscarinic activity—such as antihistamines, antispasmodics, tricyclic antidepressants, phenothiazines, and narcotics—should be minimized or avoided in elderly patients.

Another body system that deserves mention is the gastrointestinal tract. In the normal elderly, physiologic changes include a reduction in acid secretion, a reduction in motility, an increase in transit time, and a greater tendency toward constipation (Hazzard et al.,

1994). These changes do not usually translate into clinically significant disease. However, certain drugs dependent on an acid medium in the stomach may be absorbed to a greater or lesser degree. (Calkins, Ford, and Katz, 1992). Albumin decreases slightly with normal aging, which is of no clinical significance. However, in the presence of disease of the gastrointestinal tract (previous gastrectomy, Crohn's disease, ulcerative colitis, sprue), elderly patients may develop malabsorption syndromes leading to hypoproteinemia and hypoalbuminemia. Albumin and total protein levels may also decrease in the elderly secondary to one or a combination of three other possible mechanisms: decreased metabolism secondary to liver diseases such as cirrhosis, increased catabolism secondary to malignancy, or decreased intake secondary to socioeconomic issues or the anorexia associated with dementia or depression. Certain drugs are highly bound to protein or albumin. A reduction in total protein or albumin level may lead to a greater fraction of free drug bioavailable, leading to toxicity. Examples includes phenytoin, meperidine, digoxin, and warfarin (Calkins, Ford, and Katz, 1992). Reduction of the dose of these drugs may be necessary in the following instances: to prevent confusion and ataxia secondary to phenytoin; lethargy, drowsiness, falls, or cognitive dysfunction secondary to the meperidine; confusion, anorexia, and nausea secondary to digoxin; or bleeding secondary to warfarin. Specific formulas are available that allow dose-specific adjustments according to protein and albumin levels (Winter, 1988). Anticholinergic drugs or sucralfate may predispose the elderly patient to constipation or gastric reflux (by relaxation of the sphincter of the stomach) and subsequent aspiration risk. In addition, the use of H_2 blocking drugs to reduce acid secretion in the stomach of an elderly patient with peptic ulcer disease or hiatal hernia theoretically might seem to be a logical step in the treatment process. However, the use of such drugs would lead to further reduction in acid secretion and a neutral or basic medium. This might be an appropriate environment for bacteria refluxing from the stomach cavity to the lower esophagus. The problem is compounded when the patient develops swallowing problems from a stroke, Parkinson's disease, or other esophageal disorder and becomes bed-bound. The patient is then further predisposed to aspiration risk (Beck, 1991-1992; Cook et al., 1994).

An important system regarding the development of adverse drug reactions in the elderly is the liver. It is the most important organ for the two metabolism systems of various drugs. Phase 1 metabolism undergoes significant reduction in activity with age. Drugs metabolized in this phase are oxidized, reduced, or hydrolyzed. Their half-lives are prolonged because of this phase. These drugs include diazepam, chlordiazepoxide, flurazepam, barbiturates, meperidine, phenytoin, propranolol, quinidine, warfarin, theophylline, tolbutamide, salicylates, nortriptyline, diphenhydramine, lidocaine, and ibuprofen. Phase 2 metabolism, involving conjugation or deactivation, is not altered with age. Drugs metabolized in phase 2 include the short-acting benzodiazepines (lorazepam, oxazepam, temazepam, triazolam) with relatively short half-lives (Calkins, Ford, and Katz, 1992). This difference in metabolism and half-life is reflected clinically by studies indicating a difference in hip fracture risk between long-acting and short-acting benzodiazepines, with long-acting ones having a greater risk (Berggren et al., 1987; Cummings et al., 1995).

The most important organ system involved in the elimination of drugs dependent on renal blood flow is the kidney and subsequent creatinine clearance. Creatinine clearance decreases with advancing age, even in the presence of normal blood urea nitrogen and serum creatinine levels. Examples of affected drugs are digoxin, penicillins, aminoglycosides, H_2 blocking agents, and fluoroquinolones (Calkins, Ford, and Katz, 1992).

Significant reductions in the dosage of these drugs are necessary with reduced creatinine clearance to avoid ADRs (e.g., acute changes in mental status, cognitive dysfunction, dizziness, falls, or syncope). A formula useful for estimation of creatinine clearance is

CrCl (creatinine clearance) = 140 −
age of the patient × weight of patient in kilograms ÷
the serum creatinine (values less than 1 rounded to 1) × 72.

In the case of women, the creatinine clearance should be multiplied by 0.85 (Calkins, Ford, and Katz, 1992). A useful rule of thumb is that if the serum blood urea nitrogen or serum creatinine is elevated above the normal range, the creatinine clearance will at least be below 50 ml/minute. In such instances, the dosage of these drugs could be reduced by one half or more.

High-risk Drugs

Certain categories of drugs that present a high risk of adverse drug reactions to the elderly patient warrant special consideration and discussion. This list includes NSAIDs, H_2 blocking drugs, beta-blocking drugs, diuretics, psychotropics, central-acting alpha-blocker drugs, ganglionic antihypertensive drugs, anticholinergic drugs, antibiotics, antiarrhythmic drugs, drugs for dementia, and a miscellaneous group (Table 5-2, p. 124).

H_2 Blockers. Recent studies show a correlation between advancing age, peptic ulcer disease, and the presence of *Helicobacter pylori,* gram-negative bacteria. These bacteria colonize the lining of the stomach, especially in the presence of chronic disease (Graham et al., 1991). Excluding alcoholic and NSAID-induced causes, one study of 49 older patients with gastritis showed a high correlation with *H. pylori* (O'Riordan, Tobin, and O'Morain, 1991). In such cases H_2 blocker drugs have been shown to be inadequate for healing ulcers of the stomach and duodenum, with a greater chance of recurrence than those treated with a combination of 2 weeks of antibiotics, metronidazole, and milk of bismuth (Hentschel et al., 1993; Graham et al., 1992). This concept about the etiology of gastrointestinal disease is becoming increasingly popular. The latter regimen appears to be gaining momentum as an ideal alternative in the presence of a positive *Helicobacter* stomach biopsy, urea breath test, or positive serum antibody level (Culter et al., 1995; Peura, 1995). Both H_2 blocker drugs and sucralfate have been used nonspecifically as prophylaxis to prevent ulceration of the stomach in elderly patients with or without a history of gastrointestinal disease who are placed on salicylates or NSAIDs. This practice has become widespread among physicians, although this regimen is not an accepted indication (*Physicians Desk Reference,* 1999). However, one study indicates that high-dose famotidine (40 mg) decreases the incidence of gastric and duodenal ulceration in patients taking NSAIDs (Taha et al., 1996). A study of more than 700 nursing home patients revealed that 41% were taking H_2 blocker drugs for indications that had not been substantiated by clinical studies (Gurwitz, Noonan, and Soumerai, 1992). Another common protocol is for critically ill patients in the intensive care unit setting to receive one of these agents to prevent stress-related gastrointestinal bleeding. However, another study indicated only two conditions that warranted use of these agents in this setting to prevent this complication: respiratory failure or coagulopathy (Cook et al., 1994).

Omeprazole and lansoprazole are proton pump inhibitors, a new class of drugs to treat duodenal ulcer and gastroesophageal reflux disease. Omeprazole is indicated in the treatment of active duodenal ulcer, treatment of heartburn and other symptoms associated with gastroesophageal reflux disease, treatment of erosive esophagitis and for maintaining healing of erosive esophagitis, and long-term treatment of Zollinger-Ellison syndrome and other rare conditions that cause pathologic hypersecretion. Atrophic gastritis has been occasionally noted in long-term use. The drug should be taken before meals (*Physicians Desk Reference,* 1999).

Common side effects of anticholinergic drugs include dry mouth, constipation, mental-status changes, dry eyes, difficulty with urination, blurred vision, drying of bronchial secretions, and prevention of sweating. Medical diseases such as glaucoma, benign prostatic hyperplasia, Sjögren's syndrome (dry eyes and dry mouth), constipation, chronic bronchitis, and peripheral vascular disease may be aggravated by these drugs. They may further predispose the elderly patient to the development of fecal impaction, worsening glaucoma, urinary retention, hypothermia and hyperthermia, and exacerbations of chronic bronchitis secondary to mucus plugging (Beck, 1991-1992; Cahill et al., 1994).

Nonsteroidal Antiinflammatory Drugs. NSAIDs are a particularly hazardous category of drugs that should be avoided in the elderly if at all possible. They can cause adverse drug reactions by three different mechanisms: precipitation of confusion, gastrointestinal bleeding, and renal insufficiency or failure. In one study, NSAID use caused or exacerbated medical conditions in 86% of the 500 emergency admissions to a general hospital ward (Jones, Berman, and Doherty, 1992). In high doses all of these drugs may cause acute or cognitive dysfunction. Indomethacin, because of its high affinity for penetrating the blood-brain barrier, brings the greatest risk of central nervous system side effects such as confusion, dizziness, lethargy, restlessness, and depression (*Physicians Desk Reference,* 1999). It is inappropriate for use by the elderly (Willcox, Himmelstein, and Woolhandler, 1994). However, several recent studies, including the Baltimore Longitudinal Study of Aging, have shown an overall decreased relative risk of Alzheimer's disease or cognitive decline in patients taking NSAIDs on a regular basis. This risk reduction was the greatest for patients taking NSAIDs for at least 2 to 3 years (Stewart et al., 1997).

The NSAIDs also cause direct irritation of the gastric and duodenal mucosa, leading to gastritis, peptic ulcer, and esophagitis after first-time or sustained use. Often a patient may develop bleeding from an undiagnosed asymptomatic hiatal hernia or reflux that was precipitated by the use of these drugs. Several studies indicate that all NSAIDs in high enough dose may cause gastrointestinal bleeding, with the least risk from low doses of ibuprofen (200 to 400 mg) (Langman et al., 1994; Griffin et al., 1991). A metaanalysis of 12 studies compared the frequency of major gastrointestinal side effects among the various NSAIDs. The lowest risk again occurred with the use of ibuprofen. Comparing ibuprofen with the other NSAIDs, fenoprofen had a relative risk of 1.6, followed by aspirin (1.6), diclofenac (1.8), sulindac (2.1), diflunisal (2.2), naproxen (2.2), indomethacin (2.4), tolmetin (3.0), piroxicam (3.8), and ketoprofen (4.2) (Henry et al., 1991).

A third mechanism by which NSAIDs cause adverse drug reactions in the elderly is by prostaglandin-mediated renal vasodilation, leading to fluid retention and subsequent renal injury via several mechanisms and resulting in renal failure and glomerulopathy (Shankel et al., 1992). By causing fluid retention, they may be responsible for worsening hypertension or inability to adequately control existing hypertension or precipitating or aggravating existing congestive heart failure. Discontinuation of NSAIDs in an elderly patient with hypertension may result in a statistically significant reduction in mean blood pressure (Gurwitz et al., 1994; Gottlieb et al., 1992). The use of NSAIDs is associated with acute liver injury and a hepatitis-like syndrome (Garcia Rodriguez et al., 1992). A recent study comparing acetaminophen (4000 mg) to high (2400 mg/day) and low (1200 mg/day) doses of ibuprofen for osteoarthritis of the knee indicated no difference in relief of symptoms (Bradley et al., 1991). However, for acute flares of inflammation (swollen, warm, tender joints) for which an NSAID may be beneficial, some practical guidelines include (1) use the agent as needed, alternating it with acetaminophen; (2) use the agent in the lowest possible dose; and (3) use the agent for 5 to 7 days and then discontinue. Occasionally persistent patients will demand that they be prescribed an NSAID for continuous use. In such cases patients should be advised of the potential side effects. The patient should agree to routine (every 3 to 4 months) monitoring of the blood urea nitrogen for early signs of renal insufficiency. In addition, a hemogram should be routinely performed to monitor patients for early gastrointestinal bleeding. In these cases misoprostol, a cytoprotective agent given four times daily, may provide some protection of the mucosa from gastrointestinal problems (Levine, 1995). Disadvantages of the drug include its high cost, the necessity of administering it four times daily, and its common side effect of diarrhea. The NSAIDs should not be used concomitantly with aspirin or warfarin because of the higher risk of causing bleeding complications (*Physicians Desk Reference,* 1999).

Beta Blockers. Beta-blocker drugs should be used with caution in the elderly, particularly propranolol, which is considered in most instances an inappropriate drug because of its side effects. These include precipitation of or exacerbation of congestive heart failure, masking of hypoglycemia, development of postural hypotension, masking of symptoms of endocrine disease such as hypothyroidism, reduction in exercise capacity, exacerbation of chronic lung disease or bronchospasm, depression, memory loss, and production of arthropathy (Cahill et al., 1994; Newbern, 1991; Thiessen et al., 1990). However, some studies indicate that it may be beneficial for the treatment of anxiety in demented patients and tremor disorders in the elderly (Colenda, 1991). The drug was also used to prove efficacy of treatment of systolic hypertension (systolic blood pressure greater than 160) for the prevention of stroke and mortality (SHEP Cooperative Research Group, 1991). Use of the drug should be based on a risk-benefit ratio for the particular patient, including an evaluation of the patient's medical conditions. Beta-blocker drugs may also produce adverse effects on lipid metabolism (*Physicians Desk Reference,* 1999). Pragmatically the use of beta-blocker drugs would seem illogical because of the low incidence of high-renin, high-aldosterone hypertension and because renin and aldosterone levels decrease with normal aging (Beck, 1991-1992). They may be used as first-line agents for the elderly hypertensive patient with a previous history of angina or myocardial infarction because they can reduce overall mortality by as much as 76% in this population (Park, Forman, and Wei, 1995). However, a review of 3737 Medicare patients in New Jersey who had survived a myocardial infarction at 30 days showed that only 21% treated up to 90 days after discharge from the hospital had received a beta blocker (Soumerai et al., 1997). Beta-selective blocking drugs such as atenolol or metoprolol have fewer side effects and also have the advantage of once- or twice-daily dosing. Therefore compliance is also increased significantly. Use of atenolol as compared with placebo has been shown to decrease mortality significantly at 2-year follow-up in elderly patients (average age 68 years) who underwent cardiac surgery

(Mangano et al., 1996). They also may be particularly appropriate for the elderly patient for dual indications of atrial arrhythmias and hypertension. Beta-blocker drugs used selectively in patients with good left ventricular function have been shown to decrease the risk of congestive heart failure and death over a 2-year period (Lichstein et al., 1990). A new beta blocker, carvedilol, with alpha-blocking and antioxidant properties, was approved by the Food and Drug Administration (FDA) in mid-1997. Its approved use is for increasing left ventricular function in patients with mild to severe congestive heart failure. Its action is thought to occur by moderating the adverse effects of chronic activation of the sympathetic nervous system (Packer et al., 1996a). In one study at 1 year follow-up, ejection fraction increased significantly in these patients, with a decrease in resting and maximum heart rates as well. At 19 months follow-up, there was a 26% reduction in risk of death or hospital admission (Australia/New Zealand Heart Failure Research Collaborative Group, 1997).

Diuretics. Diuretics constitute another class of high-risk drugs that should be used with caution in the elderly, in part because of the reduction in total body water with normal aging and other factors. Side effects include hypokalemia possibly linked to sudden death, worsening renal function, left ventricular hypertrophy, and increases in total cholesterol and triglycerides. They may cause a contraction alkalosis. In addition, they may precipitate an exaggerated postural hypotensive response, leading to light-headedness, falling, and further morbidity or mortality from a hip or other fracture (Beck, 1991-1992; *Physicians Desk Reference,* 1999; Weinberger, 1992). Extreme caution is advised in administering thiazides to elderly patients with dementia or depression because of their tendency to drink less or even forget to drink fluids because of the associated memory loss. Frail and advanced elderly patients over age 85 are also at high risk because of their greater tendency to develop postural hypotension. Elderly patients on diuretics should be advised to drink lots of isotonic fluids during the summer months and especially during times of exercise and sweating. Diuretics may actually be harmful in hypertensive patients with diabetes. A recent study indicated that these patients treated on diuretics had higher cardiovascular and total mortality than untreated patients (Warram et al., 1991). Thiazides are generally not effective in the presence of renal insufficiency.

Loop diuretics (metolazone, furosemide, bumetanide) are popular drugs used to treat dependent leg edema in the elderly, but they also have the potential of exaggerating the postural hypotension caused by chronic venous insufficiency and stasis, further increasing the risk of inducing light-headedness, dizziness, falls, and fracture or other morbidity (Beck, 1991-1992). These agents should be reserved for severe edema that is refractory to leg elevation, stockings, and exercise. Loop diuretics should be reserved for patients with renal insufficiency or congestive heart failure to mobilize fluid and promote brisk diuresis. By causing calciuria, they may serve a useful purpose in the initial treatment of hypercalcemia (Beck, 1991-1992). Both loop and thiazide diuretics may be a significant cause of urinary incontinence. Removal, minimizing the dose, or changing the time of day for administration from the afternoon to midmorning may alleviate the problem in many cases (Beck, 1991-1992).

The advantages of using thiazide diuretics in the elderly for the treatment of mild hypertension include low cost and once-per-day dosing. The SHEP (systolic hypertension in the elderly) trial used a first-line drug, chlorthalidone, a long-acting diuretic. This study showed that reduction in systolic blood pressure below 160 mm Hg significantly reduced the incidence of stroke and cardiovascular disease and, to a lesser extent, cardiovascular deaths and total mortality (SHEP Cooperative Research Group, 1991). This effect was even greater for noninsulin-dependent diabetic patients than for nondiabetic patients (Curb et al., 1996). Much has been written about the adverse effects of thiazide diuretics on the lipid profile. A recent retrospective study of 9,274 Medicare and Medicaid patients in New Jersey, age 65 to 95, showed no significant effect of the use of these agents with the initiation of lipid-lowering agents (Monane et al., 1997). Recent case-control studies indicate that elderly women with hypertension using thiazides had a significantly lower risk of hip fracture than those not using thiazides, possibly secondary to reduction in excretion of calcium in the urine and the resulting retardation of osteoporosis (Heidrich, Stergachis, and Gross, 1991). Doses above 50 mg are generally not effective in achieving blood pressure control. African-American patients seem to benefit more from thiazides than Caucasian patients. For stepwise treatment of hypertension, diuretics in combination with other agents may potentiate the effect of other drugs but also have the disadvantage of being more expensive, especially in combined pill formulation.

Central-acting and Alpha-blocker Antihypertensive Drugs. Central-acting drugs such as clonidine, reserpine, and methyldopa can cause significant central nervous system side effects in the elderly. These include headache, irritability, sedation, cognitive dysfunction, and depressive symptoms (*Physicians Desk Reference,* 1999). Alpha methyldopa, an old drug because of its short half-life, is given four times per day. The drug has a number of side effects: sedation, liver involvement, and multiple drug-drug interactions (*Physicians Desk Reference,* 1999). Reserpine offers the advantage of once-per-day dosing and is cheap, but it may produce bothersome side effects, including postural hypotension, dry mouth, constipation, bradycardia, bronchospasm, and hypersecretion of the digestive tract. It causes a hypertensive crisis when used in conjunction with food and drugs that contain a monoamine oxidase (MAO) inhibitor. The use of methyldopa and reserpine is inappropriate in the elderly (Willcox, Himmelstein, and Woolhandler, 1994). Alpha-blocker drugs such as prazosin, terazosin, and doxazosin reduce blood pressure by causing vasodilation (*Physicians Desk Reference,* 1999). They have become popular because of their recent promotion as first-line agents for hypertension in the elderly patient with benign prostatic hyperplasia with associated signs and symptoms of urgency, frequency, or hesitancy. They have the added advantage of once- or twice-daily dosing. However, to achieve the dual role of blood pressure control and control of prostatic symptoms, dosages of 7 to 10 mg are often necessary. There is a risk of postural hypotension that can be minimized by taking the drug before bedtime (Guthrie, 1994).

Apresoline is an old drug that has traditionally been used for the treatment of hypertension. Its mechanism of action involves vasodilation, especially the renal arteries. Side effects of the drug include negative effects on the cardiac muscle and an increase in heart rate, thereby increasing the workload of the heart. In some cases this may contribute to the development of congestive heart failure, especially in patients with impaired left ventricular function (*Physicians Desk Reference,* 1995). Disadvantages of the drug include a short half-life and its need to be taken four times per day. The drug may also cause a lupuslike syndrome. The dual-acting alpha- and beta-blocking drugs are newer agents that combine the advantages of beta blockers with the vasodilating effects of alpha blockers. They also do not increase heart rate and may be useful antihypertensive agents in patients with a history of stable heart failure (Lessem and Weber, 1993). However, these combination drugs tend to be more expensive than other classes of drugs in general. Other classes of drugs appropriate for the treatment of hypertension in the elderly include the angiotensin-converting enzyme (ACE) inhibitor and calcium channel blocker drugs.

Antihypertensive Drugs. The ACE inhibitor drugs are a popular group of drugs used to treat hypertension. They have been shown in numerous studies to improve cardiac function in acute congestive heart failure secondary to diastolic dysfunction and to increase survival in patients with chronic severe congestive heart failure. One study using enalapril showed reduction in mortality in mild to moderate congestive heart failure at 41 months follow-up (Cohn et al., 1991; Braunwald, 1991). Captopril, the first of these agents, has been shown to reverse the reduction in renal blood flow that occurs with normal aging in healthy normotensive elderly by causing significant renal vasodilation (Hollenberg and Moore, 1994). It also has been shown to limit myocardial infarction expansion if given within 24 hours (Oldroyd et al., 1991) and to subsequently reduce short-term mortality at 5 weeks (ISIS-4 Collaborative Group, 1995). Enalapril, has also been shown to slow the progression of renal disease, proteinuria, and albuminuria when it is taken for hypertension (as compared with metoprolol), and patients are followed for 3 years (Bjorck et al., 1992). Other positive effects of ACE inhibitor drugs are a slower rate of decline of renal function and a significant reduction in albuminuria. This effect has been shown using lisinopril vs. furosemide and atenolol in hypertensive patients with moderate diabetic renal insufficiency, when followed for 18 months (Slataper et al., 1993). Captopril has been shown to slow the progression of renal disease, reduce mortality, and alleviate the need for transplantation or dialysis as opposed to placebo when patients were followed for 3 years (Lewis et al., 1993). Enalapril, as compared with beta-blocker drugs, showed a significant reduction in proteinuria at 6 months and significant reduction in end-stage renal failure in patients with nondiabetic renal insufficiency who were followed for 3 years (Hannedouche et al., 1994). In most cases they offer the added advantage of once- or twice-daily dosing. ACE inhibitor drugs are contraindicated in the presence of renal artery stenosis. Frequent side effects of these drugs include cough and angioedema (*Physicians Desk Reference,* 1999). Potassium levels should be monitored in patients prescribed ACE inhibitors because of the tendency for these patients to develop hyperkalemia.

Calcium channel blocker drugs (antagonists) are also a popular group of drugs used to treat elderly hypertensive patients by producing vasodilation and promoting loss of sodium and water. Side effects include flushing, headache, dependent edema, and constipation, depending on the specific drug. They also offer the advantage of once- or twice-daily dosing, even though they are more expensive than diuretics or beta-blocker drugs (Weinberger, 1992). However, a recent case-control study suggests increased mortality in hypertensive patients treated with these agents, with the risk increasing with increasing dosage. This risk was also increased with use of short-acting agents, particularly nifedipine. Because of the possible limitations and criticisms of the study, a clinical trial is ongoing to prove or disprove these findings, but the results are not expected until 2002. Until further findings, long-acting agents, are the preferred agents for hypertension, according to the recommendations of the National Heart, Lung, and Blood Institute (Buring, Glynn, and Hennekens, 1995; Furberg, Psaty, and Meyer, 1995; Pinkowish, 1995). An encouraging recent controlled open study compared short-acting nifedipine to diltiazem. After 5 years of follow-up, the risk of myocardial infarction, death, congestive heart failure, premature ventricular contractions, or hospitalization for worsening angina was significantly lower in patients treated with placebo or diltiazem as compared with short-acting nifedipine. This effect did not reach statistical significance (Ishikawa et al., 1997).

Calcium antagonists have also been implicated in gastrointestinal hemorrhage because they inhibit platelet aggregation. One prospective study compared calcium antagonists to beta blockers and ACE inhibitors in 1636 patients who were at least 68 years old. Compared with beta blockers, calcium antagonists had a relative risk of bleeding of 1.86, and ACE inhibitors of 1.23. After adjustment for covariables, this risk was even greater than aspirin, with a relative risk of 1.51, and NSAIDs other than ibuprofen (1.4). The risk was similar to sodium warfarin (2.2) and steroids (1.9) (Pahor et al., 1996). Another prospective study evaluated 161 elderly postoperative hip fracture patients, 70 of whom were taking calcium antagonists. Patients taking calcium antagonists showed a 74% incidence of transfusion compared to 33% for those not taking them (Zuccala et al., 1997).

Calcium antagonists can worsen heart failure or increase mortality in patients with left ventricular dysfunction. A recent randomized, double-blind, placebo-controlled multicenter trial evaluated 186 patients with dilated cardiomyopathy and ejection fractions below 50% with no evidence of coronary artery disease who were using the short-acting version of the drug. Survival was the same for both intervention and placebo groups. At 24 months' follow-up, there were no increased complications with diltiazem in patients with ejection fractions below 35%. Patients taking diltiazem had increased stroke volume and better endurance on exercise testing as compared with placebo. Patients taking diltiazem stated they felt significantly better (Figulla et al., 1996). Amlodipine vs. placebo has been shown to significantly decrease the risk of death and other end points (pulmonary edema, hypoperfusion, myocardial infarction, and sustained ventricular arrhythmia) in 1153 patients with nonischemic severe chronic heart failure (New York class IIIB or IV) with ejection fractions below 30%. Outcomes were similar in patients with ischemic disease (Packer et al., 1996b).

Verapamil, as compared with placebo, has been shown to be effective in increasing pain-free walking distance in patients with symptomatic peripheral vascular disease (Bagger et al., 1997). A recent study indicates calcium antagonists are significantly more often used than beta blockers for conditions such as previous myocardial infarction, coronary artery disease, and hypertension in older outpatients in a hospital-based academic geriatric practice (Fishkind, Paris, and Aronow, 1997).

Psychotropic Drugs. Psychotropic drugs, including minor tranquilizers, major tranquilizers, antidepressants, barbiturates, and hypnotics, are also a high-risk group. Adverse effects of these drugs in general include cognitive dysfunction, sedation, drowsiness, lethargy, and functional decline. Inappropriately high doses for the elderly patient may produce or exaggerate postural hypotension, leading to light-headedness on standing or sitting from a supine position, falls, fractures, and other morbidity (Beck, 1991-1992; Grisso et al., 1991; Cummings et al., 1995; Ray, Griffin, and Malcolm, 1991). Because of their side effect profile and their traditional overuse in institutional settings for such nonspecific conditions as insomnia, general agitation, and anxiety and for dementia syndromes, a 1987 federal law (the OBRA Act) limits their use in these settings for specific indications only and in a time-limited fashion. Proper documentation in the medical record is also required. A retrospective review of 856 older medical and surgical hospital patients showed that those receiving sedative hypnotic medications have higher hospitalization costs, longer lengths of stay, and greater severity of illness (Zisselman et al., 1996). Major and minor tranquilizers are indicated only for psychotic behavior, hallucinations, or delusions that are potentially harmful to patients or their surroundings or for the prevention of aggressive, hostile, or combative behavior. Antidepressants should be used only for depressive symptoms. Antianxiety drugs should be used only to alleviate these symptoms in a patient with anxiety that is potentially harmful to the patient's medical or social condition. Barbiturates should be used only for prevention of specific seizures. Hypnotics should be used for only occasional sleep and not on a daily basis. The first component of the law involving the use of major tranquilizers was implemented in 1994. As a result, the use of these agents has decreased significantly (Rovner et al., 1990).

The major tranquilizers, commonly known as the *phenothiazines,* can also cause a drug-induced parkinsonian syndrome consisting of bradykinesia, resting tremor, and cogwheel rigidity of the extremities (Beck, 1991-1992). It has been traditional to prescribe them prophylactically with an anticholinergic drug (diphenhydramine, benztropine, trihexyphenidyl) to prevent the nuisance side effect of tremor. However, the elderly patient presenting with this syndrome may not have the associated tremor, alleviating the need for these agents, especially considering their additional troublesome side effects mentioned previously. In many cases elderly patients are inappropriately treated for presumed Parkinson's disease instead of removing or lowering the dose of the phenothiazine (Kalish et al., 1995). The phenothiazines have a particularly disturbing and in many cases irreversible side effect of tardive dyskinesia, characterized by abnormal, involuntary, repetitious muscle movements. Increasing the dosage of the drug may temporarily suppress the involuntary movements but with subsequent breakthrough and worsening of the involuntary movements. Removal of the drug may help to alleviate the movement disorder, but there is no predictable pattern to the syndrome. Anticholinergic drugs used to treat the parkinsonian side effects of phenothiazine major tranquilizers usually are of no benefit for this condition. The risk of tardive dyskinesia in older patients may be as high as six times that of younger patients using the phenothiazine drugs (Saltz, 1992; Saltz et al., 1991; Yassa and Nair, 1992).

The choice of major tranquilizer (phenothiazine) prescribed for the elderly patient depends on the side effect of the agent matched to the signs and symptoms of the patient. All of the phenothiazine major tranquilizers cause tardive dyskinesia and varying degrees of postural hypotension, anticholinergic side effects, sedation, and potency. For instance, an elderly patient with sleep-wake cycle problems secondary to sundowning from Alzheimer's disease may benefit from the sedative properties of chlorpromazine, 10 to 25 mg, or thioridazine, 25 mg at bedtime. In dosage range, they produce sleep without inducing postural hypotension or significant anticholinergic disruption. The latter may lead to the development of delirium, worsening cognitive dysfunction, or other anticholinergic or parkinsonian side effects. By contrast, haloperidol, in a dose of 0.5 to 1 mg, may be an appropriate drug to treat aggressive, hostile, combative, or psychotic behavior in an agitated, demented patient during the day. It is the least sedating and least hypotensive, and it has the fewest anticholinergic side effects of these agents, yet it is the most potent. However, the use of haloperidol at night for sleep might be counterproductive. These agents, especially in high doses, may reduce the older demented patient's self-care activities. Functional decline may develop, manifested by reduction in independent mobility, bathing, feeding, dressing, eating, and toileting. It may further lead to fecal and urinary incontinence and subsequent hygiene problems (Beck, 1991-1992).

The tricyclic antidepressants should be used with caution because of their side-effect profile, which is similar to that of the phenothiazines. Side effects include postural hypotension, anticholinergic side effects (dry mouth, blurred vision, tachycardia, constipation, urinary retention), sedation, cognitive dysfunction, and differing potency (Beck, 1991-1992; Calkins, Ford, and Katz, 1992; *Physicians Desk Reference,* 1999; Sheikh, 1995). They nonselectively block the reuptake of various neurotransmitters, including norepinephrine, serotonin, and dopamine. In low doses these agents promote a "quieting" or quinidine-like effect on the myocardium and, in high doses, an arrhythmogenic effect. These drugs can cause significant risk to some elders because of cardiac involvement. Suicide as a risk is related to antidepressants in general but not to the specific class but rather the dose, with higher doses associated with increased risk (Jick, Dean, and Jick, 1995). Tricyclic drugs with the fewest anticholinergic properties should be used over those with high anticholinergic side effects to limit the risk of precipitating acute confusion or precipitating or worsening cognitive dysfunction, especially at high doses. Desipramine and nortriptyline should be given during the morning because of their nonsedating properties. They also offer the safest profile; imipramine and amitriptyline offer the worst. The latter is considered an inappropriate drug for the elderly in a majority of cases (Willcox, Himmelstein, and Woolhandler, 1994). Amitriptyline should not be given during the day because of its high risk of sedation and postural hypotension, and it should be avoided in doses exceeding 25 mg. Few current indications exist for its use, except to treat chronic pain syndromes in association with depressed mood or depression associated with both insomnia and anorexia. A beneficial effect is its ability to stimulate appetite. It should be used with caution in patients with Alzheimer's disease.

The most popular class of agents to treat depression in the elderly is the selective serotonin reuptake inhibitors (SSRIs). They achieve the same efficacy as the tricyclic agents but may be tolerated better because of their selectivity (Sheikh, 1995). Studies indicate that depression may be mediated primarily by a deficiency of serotonin, among other chemical agents in the brain. These agents offer an advantage over traditional tricyclic antidepressants because of their lack of significant anticholinergic side effects. Theoretically, their use in patients with Alzheimer's disease would seem appropriate to avoid worsening the structural anticholinergic disruption that typically occurs in these patients as the disease process worsens (Hazzard et al., 1994; Mach et al., 1995). This concept is especially important because Alzheimer's disease accounts for 93% of causes of dementia, either in the pure form (51%) or in the combined form with vascular causes (42%) (Calkins, Ford, and Katz, 1992). However, side effects of these agents include insomnia, agitation, decreased appetite, and nausea (Sheikh, 1995). Fluoxetine, the first of these agents, and its metabolite have a combined half-life of 4 to 16 days. It is less selective in its side-effect profile. Newer agents such as sertraline and paroxltyline (*Physicians Desk Reference,* 1999) have half-lives approximating 24 to 48 hours. Being more selective for serotonin receptors, they are more appropriate for the elderly patient. The SSRIs are strong inhibitors of the cytochrome P-450 system, which is involved in the metabolism of many medications. Because of their tendency to cause withdrawal side effects, the dosage should be tapered before discontinuance of the drug. Used with other agents such as the tricyclic agents, antihistamines, theophylline, erythromycin, benzodiazepines, and steroids, they can double or triple the levels of these agents, leading to a greater risk of adverse drug reactions (Sheikh, 1995). Fluoxetine has been shown to be an independent factor related to higher suicide risk but probably related to its multiple antidepressant use (Jick, Dean, and Jick, 1995). A recent randomized study of 68 patients showed it to be superior to placebo in the treatment of seasonal affective disorder (Lam et al., 1995). Caution should be exercised when using these drugs to treat depressive symptoms with or without dementia and in the malnourished patient because these drugs may magnify the symptoms of weight loss, nausea, and anorexia related to the disease process itself. This class of drugs also has the advantage of once-daily dosing and rapid onset of action as compared with the slower-onset tricyclic antidepressants. These drugs should be administered in the morning because of their side-effect profile.

Because of its direct serotonergic effects, trazodone, in an initial dose of 25 to 50 mg at bedtime, provides an excellent option for the dual purpose of treatment of the demented or depressed patient exhibiting insomnia or sundowning. Side effects include postural hypotension and rarely priapism, usually in much higher doses than normally used in the elderly, 150 to 300 mg. (Beck, 1991-1992; *Physician's Desk Reference,* 1999). The SSRIs are also used in combination with trazodone for the treatment of depression. This is referred to as augmentation therapy. Patients on this combination should be monitored for signs and symptoms of the so-called serotonin syndrome, which is associated with restlessness and increased anxiety (Hazzard et al., 1994); this is due to the fact that both classes of drugs cause the accumulation of serotonin, even though by different mechanisms.

Atypical antidepressants include venlafaxine and bupropion. Venlafaxine has a chemical structure unrelated to tricyclic, tetracyclic, or other agents. Its side-effect profile is similar to that of the SSRIs, with the additional possibility of increasing diastolic blood pressure with increasing dose. It has a broader spectrum of reuptake of neurotransmitters than serotonin but does not inhibit the cytochrome P-450 system. Therefore there may be less risk of adverse drug reactions in combination with other drugs (Sheikh, 1995). Bupropion is a relatively safe drug with low anticholinergic and antiadrenergic side effects that is useful for the treatment of depression. However, it should be used with caution in patients with a history of seizure disorder because it lowers the seizure threshold (Beck, 1991-1992).

Methylphenidate is an old drug that is regaining popularity for the treatment of retarded depression associated with psychomotor slowing, excessive sleepiness, and increased appetite. It should be administered in the morning because of its side effect of insomnia (Beck, 1991-1992). Because of its short half-life and quick onset of action, the drug can serve an equally useful purpose in hospitalized elderly with recent unexplained confusion. In such cases a major question is whether the patient's mental status is secondary to dementia or depression. The protocol involves a dose of 5 to 10 mg (the Ritalin challenge) and doubling the dose every day for up to 5 days. The mental status of the patient in whom confusion is mostly secondary to depression will improve in mood and orientation, and the patient primarily affected with dementia will become more confused. Results can be seen as early as the second or third day of administration. Because of its side effect of anorexia, patients taking this drug should be monitored for appetite problems. It should be used with caution for patients with a history of malnutrition or dementia. It should be used with caution for patients with significant cardiovascular disease because of its basic properties as an alpha stimulant and its tendency to worsen hypertension and anxiety and cause arrhythmias (Frierson, Wey, and Tabler, 1991).

Lithium is used to treat bipolar (manic-depressive) disorder. Regular monitoring of serum levels are recommended because of the frequency of adverse side effects with this drug, especially when used with other agents. Because the drug is distributed in the total body water content of the body, excretion depends on adequate renal function. Dosages should be reduced for renal insufficiency. Levels of the drug may be increased for patients taking an ACE inhibitor and NSAIDs. Other agents such as acetazolamide, urea, xanthine preparations (theophylline), and alkalinizing agents may decrease serum levels. Lithium may interfere with blood monitoring for thyroid disease. Use with calcium channel blocker drugs can increase the risk of nervous system toxicity. Use of lithium with diuretics or in patients with restricted sodium diets for treatment of congestive heart failure or hypertension decreases sodium resorption by the renal tubules, which may lead to an increased risk of hyponatremia and lithium toxicity (*Physicians Desk Reference,* 1999). Other agents that may interfere with lithium metabolism include antipsychotics, calcium channel blockers, and medications containing iodine. Early symptoms of toxicity include diarrhea, drowsiness, loss of appetite, muscle weakness, nausea or vomiting, slurred speech, or trembling. Late symptoms include confusion, unsteadiness, blurred vision, convulsions, dizziness, and increased urination. Less common side effects include postural hypotension, weight gain, bradycardia, cardiac arrhythmias, and heart block.

The benzodiazepine minor tranquilizers are useful agents for the treatment of agitation, anxiety, and insomnia in the elderly. In this category, short-acting ones such as lorazepam (0.5 to 1 mg) and oxazepam (15 mg) are the recommended drugs of choice to prevent the worrisome side effects encountered with the long-acting agents, as mentioned previously (Beck, 1991-1992; *Physicians Desk Reference,* 1999). For this reason, flurazepam, chlordiazepoxide, and diazepam are inappropriate for elderly patients (Willcox, Himmelstein, and Woolhandler, 1994). Alprazolam is a short-acting benzodiazepine that requires metabolism by the liver. It should be used in a low dose (0.25 mg) twice or three times daily. It has minor antidepressant effects in addition to its antianxiety effect (*Physicians Desk Reference,* 1999). Other relatively short-acting benzodiazepines (triazolam and temazepam) serve a useful purpose for the occasional treatment of insomnia. Triazolam has a half-life of 4 to 6 hours. Temazepam has a half-life of 6 to 8 hours. Triazolam is useful to induce sleep, and temazepam will maintain sleep. Triazolam, in doses higher than 0.125 mg and used on a regular basis, has been implicated as a cause of delayed recall of tasks in elderly patients. For this reason, it should be used only occasionally in a dose of 0.125 mg (Bixler et al., 1991; Greenblatt et al., 1991). The benzodiazepines in general are known to cause short-term impairment in memory, even though their long-term effect is unknown (Rummans et al., 1993).

Meprobamate is an older drug used to treat anxiety. However, its use in the elderly is inappropriate because of the risk of causing sedation, confusion, and lethargy (Willcox, Himmelstein, and Woolhandler, 1994). Buspirone is a useful agent to treat chronic anxiety but must be given on a regular basis to be effective. Because onset of action requires 7 to 10 days, use of a short-acting benzodiazepine for this period of time may be necessary to relieve anxiety.

Zolpidem tartrate is a short-acting, nonbenzodiazepine hypnotic with a chemical structure unrelated to the benzodiazepines, barbiturates, or other hypnotic drugs. It interacts with GABA receptor sites. Therefore, it shares some of the properties of the benzodiazepines, including the potential to depress the central nervous system and impair motor and cognitive performance in the elderly. Like the benzodiazepines, it also has been associated with signs and symptoms of withdrawal with abrupt cessation of therapy. It is indicated for the occasional use of insomnia. Although experience in the elderly is limited, 5-mg dose is recommended for elderly patients (*Physicians Desk Reference,* 1999).

Agents useful for the treatment of agitation and anxiety associated with dementia syndromes include trazodone and buspirone (Colenda, 1991). Carbamazepine in lower doses that traditionally have been used to treat seizure disorder (i.e., 100 to 200 mg twice daily) has also recently become a popular agent for the treatment of agitation and aggressive, hostile, and combative behavior in these patients. It offers a safer side-effect profile than the traditional psychotropic agents, with little toxicity. However, regular laboratory monitoring (every 4 to 6 months) of the liver and bone marrow (hemogram) are advisable because the drug can cause liver and bone marrow depression (Tariot et al., 1994, 1995).

These psychotropic agents (major and minor tranquilizers, antidepressants, and hypnotics) should be withdrawn slowly because abrupt withdrawal may cause side effects. Common ones include agitation, anxiety, confusion, tachycardia, hypertension, and diaphoresis, depending on the specific category. A rare side effect is seizure. A good rule of thumb for tapering the benzodiazepines is to taper with a long-acting agent. In addition, for every year that the patient has been using the drug, the dosage should be tapered over a month time frame.

Levodopa is a dopaminergic agent useful for treating the symptoms of Parkinson's disease. Large doses of this drug are necessary, causing nausea as a major side effect. It is rapidly metabolized in the peripheral tissues to dopamine, and only a small amount gets to the central nervous system unchanged and metabolically active. In addition, the ingestion of protein can inhibit its absorption. Therefore carbidopa is administered with levodopa. The former inhibits the degradation of peripheral levodopa and does not cross the blood-brain barrier. The preparation is available in a convenient single oral dose form. Other side effects of carbidopa-levodopa include involuntary (choreiform, dystonic) movements, depression, paranoid or psychotic behavior, cognitive dysfunction, and suicidal ideation. Less common side effects include cardiac irregularities, postural hypotension, urinary retention, and bradykinetic episodes (on-off phenomena) (*Physicians Desk Reference,* 1997). Selegiline is a selective MAO inhibitor that has been used in recent years to treat early symptoms of Parkinson's disease to delay the need to start levodopa. A British multicenter study randomized 520 patients to either levodopa or levodopa and selegiline. At 4 years' follow-up, disability was the same in both groups, even though the dosage of levodopa steadily increased in the levodopa group but remained stable in the combined treatment group. However, at 2.5 years' follow-up, the mortality rate from Parkinson's disease was higher for the combined treatment group than with levodopa alone (Lees, 1995).

Drugs for Dementia. Various agents have been recommended for the treatment of Alzheimer's disease since the recognition that lecithin and acetylcholine deficiencies may play a role in its development. These agents include lecithin-containing health foods and megadoses of other vitamins. Even though popularly used, clinical trials do not prove their efficacy. Ergonorine (Ergoloid Mesylates), an old drug, has been used for the treatment of dementia but has shown no clinically significant effects (Beck, 1991-1992). Cerebral vasodilators were a popular group of drugs for the treatment of organic brain syndrome, Alzheimer's disease, or vascular dementia in the past. The theory behind the use of these agents was to increase vascular and oxygen supply to the brain. These drugs are contraindicated because of their risk of causing postural hypotension or "steal syndrome" (diverting blood from the brain to other tissues). This may further lead to dizziness, causing falls, fractures, and other morbidity (Willcox, Himmelstein, and Woolhandler, 1994; Ham and Sloane, 1992). Pentoxifylline, a drug approved for use in treating peripheral vascular insufficiency, has been shown to slow the cognitive deterioration in patients with multiinfarct dementia, but it has little effect on memory (Black et al., 1992).

Tacrine, an acetylcholinesterase inhibitor, is the first of a new class of drugs approved for Alzheimer's disease. Studies prove its effectiveness for mild cases of the disease and only for short-term benefit (up to 30 weeks). Long-term studies are not available. In addition to cost, its disadvantages include the need for regular blood monitoring because the drug causes asymptomatic elevation of the liver function tests. This toxicity is usually associated with higher doses of the drug. Removal of the drug usually resolves the problem. Another disadvantage is a high frequency of other side effects, including diarrhea and nausea, occurring in up to 74% of patients, with 59% of patients stopping the drug (Knapp et al., 1994; Maltby et al., 1994). Donepezil is a reverse inhibitor of the enzyme acetylcholinesterase that slows the degradation of acetylcholine. The drug is useful for mild cases of Alzheimer's disease and also has been proven to be helpful for short-term benefit only (up to 30 weeks). It should be used in a patient with a Mini-Mental status of between 10 and 26. In such cases, it has been shown to slow the progression of the disease. A major advantage over tacrine is that regular blood monitoring of liver function studies is not necessary (Rogers and Friedhoff, 1996).

Antibiotics. Classes of antibiotics for which the dosage should be reduced in the elderly consistent with creatinine clearance, as mentioned earlier, include oral and parenterally administered penicillins and fluoroquinolones because of their risk of causing confusion, sedation, and lethargy (Beck, 1991-1992; Calkins, Ford, and Katz, 1992). Aminoglycosides, used in high doses and on a regular basis, may cause hearing loss, vestibular damage, and acute and chronic renal failure. In addition, appropriate use of antibiotics in the elderly is important to prevent the development of resistant strains of bacteria, an increasingly alarming concern among health care and public health officials. This includes penicillin-resistant pneumococci *(Streptococcus pneumoniae)* secondary to inappropriate use of penicillin for treatment of viral upper respiratory infection and allergic or chronic sinusitis. In addition, vancomycin-resistant *Enterococcus* and methicillin-resistant *Staphylococcus aureus* have emerged in increasing numbers, secondary to inappropriate use of vancomycin as a first-line agent for broad coverage of suspected sepsis and for general surgical prophylaxis. Fluoroquinolones have been inappropriately used as first-line agents for the treatment of community-acquired pneumonia in the healthy elderly, with resultant overwhelming sepsis and death in occasional cases. Appropriate general indications for the use of antibiotics include a productive colored sputum, evidence of bacteria and leukocytes in the urine if symptomatic, evidence of cellulitis or suspected osteomyelitis or bacterial meningitis, or abscess formation.

The indiscriminate use of these agents can lead to diarrhea secondary to *Clostridium difficile* and related morbidity and mortality from pseudomembranous colitis (Beck, 1991-1992). Mild cases should be treated with oral metronidazole 250 mg three times daily for 10 days. Moderate to severe cases with systemic symptoms of fever and leukocytosis should be treated with intravenous vancomycin (Beck, 1991-1992; *Physicians Desk Reference,* 1999). The fluoroquinolone group of antibiotics should be given 4 hours before or 2 hours after administration of antacids or sucralfate because these agents may interfere with the effectiveness of fluoroquinolone. Side effects include photosensitivity, rash, urticaria, seizures, monoclonus, or renal failure. Reduced levels may occur in patients taking nitrofurantoin, zinc, multiple vitamins, antacids, and sucralfate. Elevated levels may occur in patients taking cyclosporine, theophylline, or caffeine.

A frequent misperception among health care professionals is that the presence of bacteria or leukocytes in the urine of a patient with a chronic indwelling urinary catheter or foul-smelling or pustular drainage from a pressure ulcer requires antibiotic administration. Patients with either chronic condition commonly develop colonization of the urinary tract or ulcer site, respectively. The use of oral antibiotics in such cases is both ineffective and apt to promote resistance. Indications for the administration of parental antibiotics in such cases are presence of fever greater than 102°F rectally; elevation of the serum leukocyte count above 15,000 with a shift to granulocytosis; and other signs of systemic sepsis, including hypotension, change in mental status, central pallor, peripheral cyanosis, diaphoresis, and tachycardia (Beck, 1991-1992). Surrounding cellulitis or suspicion of osteomyelitis are additional indications for parental antibiotics in patients with necrotic pressure ulcers.

Acyclovir is an antiviral agent used to treat herpes zoster (shingles). Initially approved for the treatment of herpes type 2 infections, the dosage for zoster is at a much higher dose of 800 mg every 4 hours five times per day for 7 to 10 days. If given within 48 hours of the infection, it has been shown to reduce the duration and severity of symptoms. The dosage of the drug, the frequency of administration, or both should be lowered in patients with creatinine clearance below 25 ml per minute to prevent neurologic side effects such as confusion, dizziness, hallucinations, paresthesia, and lethargy (*Physicians Desk Reference,* 1999). Other side effects include skin rash, itching, myalgia, diarrhea, nausea, fever, headache, peripheral edema, lymphadenopathy, and leukopenia. The drug can be administered intravenously in severe cases associated with systemic involvement (ocular) or when associated with immune-deficiency states (*Physicians Desk Reference,* 1999). It has also been shown to significantly decrease the incidence of postherpetic neuralgia at 6 months follow-up in a metaanalysis of five randomized placebo-controlled trials. The patients' average age was 60 years. They were treated with 800 mg five times per day within 72 hours of onset of rash (Jackson et al., 1997). Famciclovir, an antiviral agent for acute zoster infection, has the advantage of less frequent dosing (three times per day) and a better side-effect profile. Dosage should also be reduced for renal insufficiency (*Physicians Desk Reference,* 1999).

Agents for Dizziness. It is common practice to prescribe meclizine for a patient who complains of "dizziness," especially in a hurried office visit. Older patients may be exhibiting one or a combination of three different syndromes in such cases, including "true" dizziness, presyncopal light-headedness, or disequilibrium. True dizziness implies a vertical or horizontal spinning of the surroundings that may or may not be associated with sensory or neurologic signs or symptoms. It can be secondary to a multitude of causes related to the inner ear or the central nervous system. Disequilibrium usually implies unsteadiness on the feet and usually on walking or turning. Disequilibrium may be secondary to a host of other disease processes as well. Presyncopal light-headedness implies a "feeling of being faint," usually on standing or sitting from the supine position and lasting 1 to 2 minutes in most cases. Various disease states and drugs previously mentioned in other sections may cause this syndrome. Appropriate evaluation of the type of dizziness as well as the associated signs and symptoms, time frame, and circumstance is necessary before prescribing meclizine for true dizziness because the treatment of the three syndromes is different. In addition, meclizine is an anticholinergic drug and should be used in the lowest dose possible, preferably 12.5 mg, to prevent side effects (Baloh, 1992).

Cardiac Drugs. There are only a few current indications for the use of digoxin, including systolic dysfunction of the myocardium and treatment of atrial arrhythmias. The drug is useful in such patients to improve cardiac function but does not increase survival. This drug should be avoided if possible in the elderly because it is excreted 90% unchanged in the urine and is highly dependent on creatinine clearance. Inappropriately high doses of digoxin may cause confusion, agitation, anxiety, nausea, vomiting, heart block, arrhythmias, and the visual perception of yellow or green colors. An early sign of digitalis toxicity is usually anorexia. In a study of 19 patients with moderate failure and left ventricular ejection fractions below 45%, the dose of digoxin was increased within the therapeutic range from 0.125 to 0.25 mg (low to moderate dose—mean levels of 0.8 to 1.5 ng/L) in patients with New York Heart Association class II or III heart failure. This dose adjustment did not significantly improve function further (Slatton et al., 1997). When used concomitantly with other cardiac drugs such as quinidine, verapamil, or amiodarone, the dosage should be monitored closely and reduced accordingly because of the potentiating effects of these drugs. Digoxin is contraindicated in certain cardiac disease states such as incomplete heart block, pericarditis, aortic stenosis, and hypertropic cardiomyopathy. The drug may also worsen myocardial ischemia with acute pulmonary edema (Luchi, Taffet, and Teasdale, 1991). A retrospective study of 416 women and 112 men in an academic hospital-based geriatric practice showed that 17% of the patients were taking digoxin. In addition to the indications for heart failure and atrial fibrillation, 9% of patients were on the drug for the inappropriate indication of coronary artery disease (Fishkind, Paris, and Aronow, 1997).

Quinidine is an old drug traditionally used to treat ventricular and atrial arrhythmias, including atrial fibrillation. A metaanalysis of controlled trials using quinidine to control normal heart rhythm after conversion indicated that its use increased mortality rate (Coplen et al., 1990). Common side effects of quinidine include ringing in the ears, diarrhea, flushing of the skin, bitter taste, nausea, stomach pain or cramping, headache, dizziness, light-headedness, blurred vision, skin rash, and wheezing. Rare side effects include confusion, fatigue, increased bleeding, and hemolytic anemia. Quinidine compared with sotalol was found to be significantly more effective (60% vs. 20%) in attempting to convert 50 patients with persistent atrial fibrillation to normal sinus rhythm. These patients were randomized to one of these two drug regimens over a 7-day period. At 6 months' follow-up, quinidine was still more effective (86% vs. 77%). However, patients on quinidine reported more proarrhythmic side effects (Hohnloser, van de Loo, and Baedeker, 1995). Another metaanalysis comparing amiodarone to flecainide involving 315 patients showed that 73% of patients on amiodarone vs. 48% on flecainide converted to normal sinus rhythm at 3 months, with 60% and 40%, respectively, still converted at 12 months (Zarembski et al., 1995).

Though flecainide and encainide are more recent and more potent antiarrhythmic agents, they have also been shown to increase mortality in patients with ventricular arrhythmias after acute myocardial infarction, with age being an independent risk factor (Akiyama et al., 1992). Procainamide has been shown to decrease short-term survival after cardiac arrest and resuscitation outside the hospital (Hallstrom et al., 1991). The side effects include nausea, vomiting, diarrhea, light-headedness, hypotension, edema, dizziness, and depression (*Physicians Desk Reference,* 1999). Procainamide can also cause a lupus syndrome. Because of the limited benefit-risk ratio for these drugs, they should be prescribed only under the close supervision and monitoring of a cardiologist.

Nitroglycerin preparations (nitrates), both orally and applied to the skin for treatment of ischemic heart disease and angina, may predispose the elderly patient to the development of light-headedness, postural hypotension, syncope, and falls, especially when used in an increasing dosage. Other common side effects include headache, faint or rapid heartbeat, nausea, and vomiting. Rare side effects include blurred vision, dry mouth, and skin rash occurring at the site of administration for topical preparations. Seizures may also occur in very high doses (Ishikawa et al., 1997). Patients who use the patch preparations should remove the patch for 4 to 6 hours per day to prevent the development of tolerance from the drug.

Hypolipidemic Agents

Hypocholesterolemic agents should be used with discretion in the elderly. A recent metaanalysis of 35 randomized trials of cholesterol-lowering treatments questions the value of intensive treatment of hypercholesterolemia. These agents are likely to benefit only people with significant risk factors for coronary heart disease, including smoking, hypertension, sedentary activity, previous stroke or myocardial infarction, and family history of risk factors (Smith et al., 1993). Two recent studies indicate that serum lipid levels (elevated cholesterol and low high-density lipoprotein [HDL] cholesterol) by themselves are poor predictors of coronary risk, coronary heart disease mortality, hospitalization for myocardial infarction, or unstable angina (Grover, Palmer, and Coupal, 1994; Krumholz et al., 1994). A recent metaanalysis of clinical trials involving cholesterol reduction has also failed to show any correlation with stroke risk (Hebert, Gaziano, and Hennekens, 1995). Serum cholesterol screening in healthy postmenopausal women has shown that serum cholesterol levels do not significantly change over the long term (7 to 10 years). Therefore a serum cholesterol performed every 5 to 10 years in elderly women without cardiovascular risk factors is sufficient (Hetland, Haarbo, and Christiansen, 1992). In addition, cholesterol-lowering agents used for patients with levels above 309 mg in the general population have not been shown to be cost-effective. In general, these agents cost $190,000 per extra year of life saved as opposed to population-based promotion of better eating habits at a cost of $20 per extra year of life saved (Kristiansen, Eggen, and Thelle, 1991).

Normal aging is accompanied by dulling of taste and smell sensations (Beck, 1991-1992). Certain conditions—anorexia secondary to dementia, depression, or malignancy;

visual or oral sensory deficits; living alone, with low income, lack of transportation, or living in an institutional setting (Beck, 1991-1992)—predispose older patients to the development of malnutritional states. Inappropriate dietary cholesterol restriction in these patients is unnecessary because it may worsen the process, leading to further anorexia, weight loss, and death. Liberalization of salt, carbohydrate, protein, and cholesterol restrictions for these patients may be one of the few quality-of-life measures that may make life worth living. Hypocholesterolemia (4 mmol/L) has been linked to increased mortality in the elderly. It is probably secondary to chronic inflammatory processes producing a catabolic state (Verdery and Goldberg, 1991). Restricted diets found in a majority of malnourished nursing home patients can contribute to the situation (Buckler, Kelber, and Goodwin, 1994).

For patients with cardiovascular risk factors and a higher than normal low-density lipoprotein (LDL) cholesterol level, the statin (HMG-CoA reductase inhibitors) drugs are very effective in lowering the LDL and total cholesterol. They also have the disadvantages of higher cost and the need for regular monitoring of liver function tests because of the development of rare hepatitis (Mach et al., 1995; Verdery and Goldberg, 1991). These agents should not be used in combination with cyclosporine, gemfibrozil, or niacin because the combination may cause rhabdomyolysis and renal failure (*Physicians Desk Reference,* 1999).

Nicotinic acid lowers total cholesterol to some extent but significantly elevates the HDL cholesterol (Vega and Grundy, 1994). Gemfibrozil reduces total cholesterol and elevates HDL cholesterol to a lesser extent than nicotinic acid and the statin drugs (Vega and Grundy, 1994). Niacin and gemfibrozil reduce serum triglyceride levels also. They should be used after an adequate trial of diet has failed, for patients who have a history of pancreatitis or recurrent abdominal pain resembling pancreatitis, and for patients with triglyceride levels greater than 2000 mg/dl (*Physicians Desk Reference,* 1999). Frequent bothersome side effects of niacin include pruritus, flushing, tingling, headache, and diarrhea, especially in high doses of several grams per day. Concomitant administration with aspirin can prevent cutaneous side effects (Whelan et al., 1992). Common side effects of gemfibrozil include dyspepsia, abdominal pain, and acute appendicitis. Less frequent side effects include diarrhea, nausea or vomiting, and fatigue. This agent should not be used concomitantly with anticoagulants because it may increase the risk of bleeding. Use of the drug may increase the severity of gallstones and can necessitate gallbladder surgery. Use of the drug in the presence of liver disease may increase levels of the drug and subsequently the chances of side effects (*Physicians Desk Reference,* 1999).

Clofibrate is a drug that causes modest reduction in cholesterol with a somewhat greater reduction in triglyceride levels. It is associated with potentially bothersome gastrointestinal side effects, including diarrhea and nausea. It is a relatively weak agent. It may potentiate the effect of anticoagulants when used concomitantly. Clofibrate also has been shown to increase the incidence of cholelithiasis and subsequent morbidity and mortality from surgery (*Physicians Desk Reference,* 1999).

Regular isotonic (walking, running, swimming, bicycling) exercise for 20 to 30 minutes three times per week is a very effective way of raising HDL cholesterol and can be effective in causing slow, progressive weight loss (Schuler et al., 1992). It also has been shown to significantly reduce mortality in postmenopausal women. The reduction was smallest in those performing moderate exercise (gardening, golfing, taking long walks) once per week (24%) and greatest in those performing it more than four times per week (38%) (Kushi et al., 1997). Moderate alcohol intake (one or more drinks per day) has been shown to be effective in elevating HDL cholesterol and reducing the subsequent risk of stroke, myocardial infarction, and total and cardiovascular mortality (Scherr et al., 1992). Alcohol has been shown to increase threefold the levels of estradiol, according to a study of 12 postmenopausal women on hormone replacement therapy (Ginsburg et al., 1996). The latter agent is thought to be one of the most potent lipid-lowering agents because it increases HDL, reduces LDL, and lowers total cholesterol (Scherr et al., 1992).

Recent studies indicate that estrogen is effective in retarding osteoporosis and reducing fracture risk at all bone sites (Fogelman, 1991; Daly et al., 1993; Robinson et al., 1994). Other positive effects of estrogen include less intimal thickening of the carotid arteries and less risk of stroke in postmenopausal women (Stampfer et al., 1991; Psaty et al., 1994; Manolio et al., 1993; Finucane et al., 1993). Other studies have shown a reduced risk of Alzheimer's disease at 5 years' follow-up (Tang et al., 1996), osteoarthritis of the hip in Caucasian women (Nevitt et al., 1996), and decreased incidence of myocardial infarction or death after angioplasty at 5.5 years' follow-up (O'Keefe et al., 1997). The effect on Alzheimer's disease is thought to be secondary to promoting the growth of cholinergic neurons and decreasing deposition of cerebral ameloid (Tang et al., 1996). In elderly women with a history of hysterectomy and in the presence of cardiovascular risk factors and an elevated total cholesterol, low HDL, and high LDL component, estrogen may offer a substantial advantage to the conventional cholesterol-lowering agents. In women without hysterectomies, estrogen should be used sequentially or in combination with progesterone to reduce the slight risk of endometrial cancer in patients taking unopposed estrogen (Voight et al., 1991). New formulations that combine estrogen and progesterone are currently in review by the FDA. Relative contraindications to estrogen use include fibrocystic disease and a history of migraine headaches. Absolute contraindications include a previous history or family history of breast cancer, previous pelvic cancer, and abnormal blood clotting (*Physicians Desk Reference,* 1999; Colditz et al., 1995). Recent studies are conflicting regarding the risk of breast cancer with estrogen use. One study showed a slight risk of breast cancer with consecutive use of estrogen (Daly et al., 1993). However, another study contradicts this association (Evans, Fleming, and Evans, 1995). Progesterone has recently been shown to reduce the risk of osteoporosis (Prince, 1991) and cardiovascular risk as well (Grodstein et al., 1996). The effect of estrogen for osteoporosis can be enhanced by the concomitant use of calcium in a dose of at least 1000 mg daily and vitamin D, 400 IU (Hazzard et al., 1994). The risk of epithelial ovarian cancer is not increased by the use of hormone replacement therapy (Hempling et al., 1997). There is a substantial risk of gallbladder disease in postmenopausal women and inflammation of the pancreas in women with high triglyceride (*Physicians Desk Reference,* 1999). Tamoxifen is a nonsteroidal antiestrogen useful for the treatment of node-negative breast cancer in women after total mastectomy, segmental mastectomy, axillary node dissection, or breast irradiation. It also may be used for male and female patients with metastatic breast cancer (*Physicians Desk Reference,* 1997). It was shown to significantly reduce the risk of myocardial infarction and also increase the risk of thromboembolic events in one study. Its positive effect on the heart is probably mediated by its effect on the lipid profile (McDonald et al., 1995).

Drugs for the Prevention of Osteoporosis

The question of whether to use hormone replacement therapy (estrogen and progesterone) in a woman involves the presence or absence of four factors: older age, osteoporosis risk factors, cardiovascular risk factors, and status of the uterus and ovaries. The effect of estrogen for the prevention of osteoporosis is thought to be dependent on a "window of opportunity" during which maximum effect can be achieved. The sooner hormone replacement therapy is started after the surgical or natural menopause, the greater the effect, with maximum effect achieved within 3 to 5 years afterward. The sole use of hormone replacement therapy for prevention of osteoporosis after age 62 is thought to be minimally effective, though specifics are unknown and current studies are ongoing. Said another way, the presence of osteoporosis risk factors in a postmenopausal woman may strengthen but by themselves have little impact on the argument to use hormone replacement therapy for osteoporosis unless cardiovascular risk factors are present. The major reason to use hormone replacement therapy during this age group is cardiovascular protection if cardiovascular risk factors are present. However, the use of hormone replacement therapy for prevention of cardiovascular risk is beneficial for the premenopausal woman as well, because the benefit has been shown to be achieved in the short term as well as long term. For the older woman with osteoporosis risk factors and no cardiovascular risk factors, modification of osteoporosis risk factors may be all that is necessary. This modification includes cessation of smoking and drinking, consumption of extra calcium and vitamin D, and regular exercise. For hormone replacement therapy, the presence of a uterus necessitates an understanding of the risk of endometrial cancer; the need for follow-up if prolonged, unexpected, or heavier than usual bleeding occurs; and the knowledge that the patient may have a regular period (Grady et al., 1992).

Other drugs that may be beneficial in the treatment of osteoporosis for the patient who has relative or absolute contraindications to hormone replacement therapy include calcitonin, sodium fluoride, and biphosphonates. Until recently calcitonin had to be given subcutaneously; a nasal spray is now available, although one disadvantage of the drug is its high cost. Sodium fluoride has been shown to increase bone formation, but it also increases risk of fracture because the bone that is formed is more brittle (Hazzard et al., 1994). It is still considered experimental. Etidronate, a biphosphonate, has been shown to be effective for the prevention of recurrent vertebral compression fractures in elderly women with osteoporosis when it is used cyclically in combination with calcium. Its disadvantages are cost and side effects, including, most commonly, diarrhea. Sodium alendronate, the first biphosphate, is approved for primary prevention of postmenopausal osteoporosis. It is useful especially as an alternative to estrogen for women who have relative or absolute contraindications. It has been shown to significantly decrease risk of vertebral and other fractures when used over a 3-year period. Common side effects include abdominal pain, musculoskeletal pain, acid reflux, dyspepsia, esophageal ulcer, vomiting, abdominal distention, and gastritis in 1% to 3% of patients (Liberman et al., 1995). Because of its gastrointestinal side effect profile, the drug should be taken in the morning with at least 8 ounces of water and at least 1 hour before other liquids or food (de Groen et al., 1996).

Drugs that Cause Anorexia

In the evaluation of causes of anorexia in the elderly, a review of the patient's drug list with prompt removal of the suspected offending agent is a simple but expedient method of resolving the problem. It is preferable to instituting a potentially unnecessary extensive workup to rule out organic causes such as malignancy, dementia, and depression. Drugs known to cause anorexia include digoxin, procainamide, thyroxine, theophylline, nitrofurantoin, and the SSRIs (Thompson and Morris, 1991).

Inappropriately high doses of thyroxine may also cause agitation, insomnia, unexpected weight loss, tachycardia, arrhythmias, and premature osteoporosis (*Physicians Desk Reference,* 1995). Dietary fiber or psyllium may interact with oral thyroxine and reduce the subsequent absorption and efficacy of the drug. In such cases hypothyroid patients may require unusually higher doses of thyroid to normalize the thyroid-stimulating hormone level (Liel, Harmon-Boehm, and Shany, 1996). Theophylline may also precipitate anxiety, arrhythmias, postural hypotension, nausea, insomnia, and even seizures (Hazzard et al., 1994). Because of these side effects, higher incidence of comorbid disease, and concomitant use of other drugs, theophylline is more difficult to use for older patients. The concomitant use of theophylline and fluoroquinolones can cause a severe adverse drug reaction secondary to doubling of the concentration of theophylline. This reaction may include seizures, agitation, confusion, nausea, and vomiting (Grasela and Dreis, 1992). For these reasons, if theophylline is to be used at all, a dose in the lower therapeutic range is appropriate (Hazzard et al., 1994). It is also prudent to use theophylline only for selected instances such as wheezing and asthma; the beta-agonist drugs, oral or inhaled, are the first line of treatment for chronic lung disease (Hazzard et al., 1994). Theophylline may be beneficial in the future for sleep-disordered breathing in patients with congestive heart failure and reduced left ventricular ejection fraction; a crossover study of 15 patients showed a significant reduction in the number of central apneas per hour as compared with placebo (Javaheri et al., 1996).

Drugs such as cotrimoxazole, tetracyclines, and nitrofurantoin should be avoided in the advanced elderly and patients with renal dysfunction. They should be used with caution in older patients in general because of their dependence on renal excretion (Sanderson, 1990). Chronic administration of tetracyclines may cause staining of the teeth and skin, photosensitivity of the skin, diarrhea, or stomach cramping. They also chelate with other drugs taken orally, including antacids, iron preparations, laxatives, and calcium supplements, and prevent absorption.

Drugs for Health Maintenance, General Prophylaxis, Minerals, Vitamins, and Antioxidants

Because of the greater risk of malnutrition secondary to multiple diseases, limited income, social isolation, or dental problems, patients who are 62 or older should be prescribed a general multiple vitamin. Recent advertisements on television and radio and in newspapers and periodicals encourage megadoses of specific vitamins, particularly A, C, and E. These vitamins are used primarily to prevent premature aging, especially with case-control studies indicating that vitamins A and C may reduce the incidence of heart disease and stroke (Riemersma et al., 1991; Gale et al., 1995). A popular theory of aging involves the production of free ionizing and chemical radical formation, causing damage to deoxyribonucleic acid and ribonucleic acid responsible for the production of proteins and enzymes and for cell function (Kristal and Yu, 1992). These vitamins may function as scavengers against free radicals or as antioxidants, preventing the aging process. However, other studies of these vitamins have shown unimpressive results. A trial compared 50 mg per day of vitamin E, 20 mg per day of beta carotene, a combination, and placebo in 22,269 male Finnish smokers without known coronary disease. Patients taking vitamin E showed no evidence of protection from the development of angina (Rapola et al., 1996). Another trial evaluated 1188 men and 532 women enrolled in a skin cancer prevention program using 50 mg per day of beta carotene or placebo for 4 years. At 8.2 years' follow-up, there was no difference in all causes of mortality including cardiovascular death (Greenberg et al., 1996). The effect of vitamin E alone on coronary atherosclerosis also has had mixed results. A randomized controlled trial in 2002 patients with angiography-proven disease using doses of 400 to 800 IU showed a dose-response effect, with significant reduction in cardiovascular deaths and nonfatal myocardial infarction but not overall mortality at 1.4 years' follow-up (Stephens et al., 1996).

Low folate level has also been implicated as a cause of coronary artery disease, according to a retrospective study of 5056 Canadian men and women (age 35 to 79) enrolled in a nutritional survey. The lowest serum quartile folate level was associated with a 69% increase (Morrison et al., 1996).

More disconcerting than these results is the association of beta carotene with cancer mortality. A trial of 18,000 current or former smokers and workers exposed to asbestos used a combination of 30 mg of beta carotene plus 25,000 IU of vitamin A compared with placebo. At 4 years follow-up, the intervention group had a significantly increased risk of lung cancer (Omenn et al., 1996).

Vitamins A, C, and E have been shown to increase cell-mediated immunity in the elderly (Penn et al., 1991). In addition, higher beta carotene and vitamin C levels have been correlated with better memory performance, according to a longitudinal study of 442 patients ages 65 to 94 (Perrig, Perrig, and Stahelin, 1997).

Although popular among the elderly, the use of specific vitamin and health food supplements should be discouraged until the results of numerous clinical trials definitely prove or disprove their effectiveness. Rather than a deficiency of vitamins, a more common problem among community-dwelling elderly is hypervitaminosis (Beck, 1991-1992). The fat-soluble vitamins A, D, E, and K accumulate in fat tissue with continued use, leading to vague and nonspecific but toxic symptoms that may be difficult to recognize. Specifically, megadoses of vitamin C can cause gastrointestinal irritability, a false-negative result on fecal occult testing, renal stones, and rebound scurvy. Megadoses of vitamin A can cause malaise, liver dysfunction, headache, hypercalcemia, and leukopenia (Beck, 1991-1992). Indications for specific vitamins include vitamin B_{12} for dementia, pernicious anemia, or malabsorption syndromes; vitamin C for pressure ulcers and for skin healing from incisions; vitamin D and calcium for osteomalacia and osteoporosis; vitamin K for bleeding problems; thiamine for chronic alcohol abuse; and folic acid supplementation for patients on phenytoin (phenytoin inhibits the production of folic acid) (Hazzard et al., 1994; Yao et al., 1992).

The need for supplemental iron therapy in elderly patients for nonspecific chronic anemia should be thoroughly investigated before prescription. The elderly, in general, tend to have a greater frequency of normal or increased tissue iron stores because of the high frequency of chronic diseases that cause iron-deficient erythropoiesis (Beck, 1991-1992). Side effects of oral iron therapy include constipation, black stools, hemosiderosis, and browning of the skin and teeth. The diagnosis of a microcytic hypochromic anemia related to iron deficiency in the elderly should always be distinguished from other common causes, such as malignancies and acute or chronic inflammatory diseases. Blood studies such as serum iron, ferritin level, transferrin level, and total iron-binding capacity can easily distinguish between that secondary to iron and other disease states (Damon, 1992).

Trace metals have shown interesting results. Zinc lozenges have been shown to resolve upper respiratory symptoms sooner than placebo in a randomized trial of 100 employees of the Cleveland Clinic (Mossad et al., 1996). A dose of 200 μg of selenium supplementation has been shown to reduce the total cancer incidence by 37% comparing it with placebo in a multicenter, randomized trial of 1312 patients followed for an average of 4.5 years (Clark et al., 1996).

Erythropoietin is one of the first of the new biotechnology drugs used to treat anemias of chronic disease. By stimulating the production of erythropoietin, it has been shown to increase mean hemoglobin levels and improve quality-of-life symptoms. It is indicated in patients with chronic renal failure and for rheumatoid arthritis. It also has been used to treat patients with chronic anemia secondary to human immunodeficiency virus (HIV) disease. It is a relatively safe drug, with little risk of anaphylactic reactions. There are no contraindications for use by the elderly. Because of its tendency to cause volume expansion, which could worsen blood control, its use should be monitored in patients with high blood pressure or chronic renal insufficiency (Damon, 1992). When using the drug, the patient should take an adequate substrate of iron supplementation for the production of red blood cells.

Aspirin in a dose of 81 mg has been shown to be significantly more effective than placebo in reducing the incidence of cerebral infarction, fatal myocardial infarction, subsequent risk of stroke, subsequent transient ischemic attack, and death in elderly patients with a history of previous transient ischemic attack. However, there was an associated, insignificant increase in hemorrhagic stroke (The SALT Collaborative Group, 1991). It has been shown to significantly reduce the risk of severe angina, myocardial infarction, and death at 6 and 12 months in elderly patients (age below 70) with non–Q-wave myocardial infarction or unstable angina (Wallentin, 1991). It also has been shown to be effective in significantly reducing cardiovascular and all-cause mortality, according to a survey of 2418 women with coronary artery disease at 3 years' follow-up. This risk reduction occurred in women over age 60, as well as those with hypertension, diabetes, and previous myocardial infarction (Harpaz et al., 1996). Because of its relative safety, a baby aspirin should be a part of every older patient's medication regimen unless contraindicated by active gastrointestinal bleeding, a history of bleeding diathesis, other blood disorder, or a history of allergy to aspirin. A dose of 75 mg is as effective as 325 mg, with significantly less chance of gastrointestinal bleeding. This dose may safely be used as prophylaxis in asymptomatic patients with a history of peptic ulcer disease as well. It has been shown to be equally as effective as warfarin in patients younger than 75 years of age with a history of nonrheumatic atrial fibrillation in preventing stroke. Exceptions include patients with risk factors such as a history of hypertension, previous thromboembolism, or heart failure (Stroke Prevention in Atrial Fibrillation Investigators, 1994). The 325-mg dose is also indicated in patients for prevention of a recurrent thrombotic stroke instead of the 75-mg prophylactic dose. Aspirin has also been shown in a case-control study to reduce the risk of colon cancer (Thun, Namboordiri, and Heath, 1991).

Low-dose heparin, in a dose of 5000 U twice daily, may be more effective than aspirin to prevent deep venous thrombosis and subsequent fatal or nonfatal pulmonary embolus and death in elderly patients who are temporarily immobile secondary to an acute illness or in patients with a history of previous deep venous thrombosis or pulmonary embolus, obesity, history of congestive heart failure, or chronic venous insufficiency (Beck, 1991-1992). This regimen is also recommended for general postoperative prophylaxis except for patients undergoing surgery for malignancies, repair of femoral or hip fracture, or lower extremity joint replacement. In these instances subcutaneous heparin used three times daily or preferably low-dose coumadin starting on the day of surgery and for up to 10 weeks after surgery is recommended because these patients are at greater risk for deep venous thrombosis and embolization. However, to prevent significant bleeding, the international normalized ratio should be maintained at the lowest therapeutic level to prevent complications.

Enoxaparin, a low-molecular-weight heparin, alleviates the need for blood monitoring of prothrombin time and is equally as effective for the prevention of deep vein thrombosis after hip replacement. Periodic complete blood counts, including platelet count, are recommended during the course of treatment (*Physicians Desk Reference,* 1999). Although it is traditionally used up to 10 days after surgery, another study has shown that 40 mg daily for up to 30 days can significantly prevent asymptomatic and symptomatic overall thromboembolism and proximal deep venous thrombi when compared with placebo (39% vs. 18%) (Bergqvist et al., 1996). A multicenter, randomized, double-blind trial compared adjusted-dose warfarin to enoxaparin. After 14 days' follow-up, 30 mg of enoxaparin given every 12 hours subcutaneously was significantly better than warfarin in preventing deep venous thrombosis (37% vs. 52%), with no difference in proximal venous thrombosis or bleeding between the two drugs (Leclerc et al., 1996). It also has been shown to be as effective in the home setting as intravenous heparin at 90 days' follow-up in treating patients with deep vein thrombosis, with the additional advantage of fewer hospital days (1.1 vs. 6.5) (Levine et al., 1996).

Whether to use warfarin or aspirin in an older patient is often a difficult question. A medical indication for the use of warfarin is a patient with a history of chronic atrial fibrillation secondary to rheumatic valvular heart disease to prevent embolic stroke (Hazzard et al., 1994). In addition, issues that should be factored into a decision include associated medical conditions, history of gastrointestinal disease, compliance, economic or psychosocial issues, cognitive dysfunction, or risk of falling. In each case the practitioner should weigh overall risk to expected benefit.

Associated medical conditions such as liver disease, malabsorption syndromes, and malignancy may predispose the patient to a greater risk of adverse drug reactions (disease-drug) when using warfarin because of its protein-binding properties. In such instances a reduction in the serum albumin may occur, which means less protein binding of the drug. Then a greater "free" portion of the drug is metabolically active, with a resultant increased chance of bleeding at the same dose. A patient with significant cognitive dysfunction may not be an ideal candidate because the patient may ultimately take too much in a single dose, which might predispose the patient to either increased risk of bleeding or insufficient amount to achieve the desired effect. The presence of other chronic medical conditions necessitating the use of other medications may increase the risk of drug-drug reactions as well.

The availability of a willing and able caregiver or interested party to administer the medication on a regular basis can resolve this issue. Pill administration vehicles may also be of benefit. In addition, communication and understanding of the need for regular monitoring of the bleeding time, the physician and laboratory costs involved, the availability of transportation, and the distance from the medical facility for the patient are essential components. The absence of any of these factors makes the use of warfarin impractical.

A patient at increased fall risk secondary to mobility problems, arthritis, neurologic disease, or specific drug therapy may be a less than optimal candidate for warfarin because of the increased risk of bleeding secondary to trauma. Patients taking warfarin after age 80 are at significantly increased risk of life-threatening and fatal bleeds (relative risk 4.5) compared with those under 50 (Fihn et al., 1996).

Patterned after the philosophy of the standard treatment of early myocardial infarction, thrombolytic agents (streptokinase and recombinant tissue plasminogen activator) have also been used in the last several years in various clinical trials in an attempt to prove their efficacy for early treatment of ischemic cerebrovascular accident. Because of the conflicting data on outcomes such as short-term complications (bleeding and death) and short- and long-term neurologic outcomes, their use is not recommended at this time (Miyawaki, 1997).

Ticlopidine hydrochloride is a platelet aggregation inhibitor. It is indicated for the prevention of thrombotic stroke in patients with a history of previous transient ischemic attacks who have not responded to aspirin therapy or are intolerant to aspirin (allergy or previous bleeding). In patients with reductions in creatinine clearance (50 to 80 ml/minute), there has been no significant difference in the clinical effects of the drug. The drug has the potential to cause neutropenia in less than 2% of patients. This problem is usually reversible but can be life-threatening in severe cases. Because of this, patients should have a neutrophil count initially before starting treatment and every 2 weeks for the first 3 months of therapy. Ticlopidine becomes 50% effective within 4 days of treatment and 60% to 70% effective in 10 to 11 days. It is contraindicated for patients who are hypersensitive to it and for patients with a history of hematopoietic disorders, severe liver impairment, or active intracranial or peptic ulcer (*Physicians Desk Reference,* 1999). Pentoxifylline is useful in treating intermittent claudication in patients with peripheral vascular disease by improving red blood cell flexibility, making it easier for these cells to pass through the microcirculation. This change translates clinically to greater pain-free walking distances (Cantwell-Gab, 1996).

Influenza vaccine should be given yearly to all elderly except patients with a history of egg allergy; 90% of deaths caused by influenza epidemics are people older than 64. It is usually given between October and December. If influenza develops in a long-term care institution, patients who have not been vaccinated or those allergic to the vaccine may be prophylactically treated with amantadine in a dose of 100 mg per day until the infection resolves. In high doses common side effects of the drug include confusion, irritability, headache, rash, lethargy, nausea, and fluid retention. The drug can also shorten the duration and severity of influenza A if started within 24 to 48 hours of onset of symptoms, but it is not effective against influenza type B (Beck, 1991-1992). Pneumonia vaccine should be administered to all elderly patients at least once. Some geriatricians advocate a repeat vaccination 6 years from the date of the last one for those at high risk of pneumococcal pneumonia, such as asplenic and chronic obstructive pulmonary disease patients (Beck, 1991-1992). Patients who have received the older 18 polyvalent strain do not need a repeat injection. Even though older patients have the greatest need for these vaccinations, studies indicate that they often develop an inadequate antibody response to them because of their blunted immune responses. Because the rate of pneumococcal vaccination is much lower than that of influenza vaccination in older adults, administration of both simultaneously can improve the rate of vaccination of the latter. There is little difference in side effects when they are given together rather than separately (Honkanen, Keistinen, and Knela, 1996).

Diphtheria tetanus prophylaxis is often ignored in the elderly, but recent studies indicate that only about 20% to 60% of the elderly have adequate antibody levels. Those especially at risk include diabetic patients with chronic foot ulcers and nursing home or homebound elderly with chronic pressure ulcers. Historically, many elderly were not exposed to childhood vaccinations, which were initiated after their youth. Any elderly patient who has not had vaccinations should receive three separate injections of diphtheria tetanus vaccination: initially, at 6 weeks, and at 1 year from the initial vaccine (Beck, 1991-1992; Holt, 1992; Gergen et al., 1995).

Elderly patients with a recent conversion (within 2 years) to positive tuberculin skin testing should be treated with isoniazid, 300 mg per day for 6 months, because studies indicate a high degree of protection (69%) against conversion from tuberculous infection to disease. Patients with a history of positive skin testing of unknown duration should not be treated with this drug because of the risk of morbidity and subsequent mortality for those patients who develop isoniazid-induced hepatitis. Exceptions to this rule include patients with diabetes mellitus, HIV disease, hematologic or reticuloendothelial malignancy, silicosis, previous gastrectomy, malnutrition, or scars of postprimary tuberculosis. Other exceptions include patients on 15 mg of steroids for more than 2 weeks, patients who have had close or household contact with an infected person, and those with scars of postprimary tuberculosis evidenced by chest radiograph (Hazzard et al., 1994). Patients on the drug should have liver function tests performed every 6 weeks initially to monitor for the development of this adverse reaction. The drug should be administered with B_6 (pyridoxine) because the drug interferes with the metabolism of this vitamin.

Steroids

Oral corticosteroid use in the older patient population should be a last resort after conventional therapy has failed and for specific indications because of the side effects that occur after prolonged use. These side effects include dependence, weight gain, masking of infection, fluid retention, worsening or precipitation of hypertension, diabetes, cataracts, and osteoporosis. Steroids serve no purpose for the uncomplicated treatment of osteoarthritis and should be reserved for severe cases of active rheumatoid arthritis.

Steroids may be very beneficial for the treatment of asthma resistant to conventional therapy, initial treatment of certain dermatoses, polymyalgia rheumatica (15 to 20 mg daily), and temporal arteritis (40 to 60 mg daily) (Beck, 1991-1992). Inhaled steroids are as effective as oral steroids for the treatment of chronic lung conditions without producing the systemic side effects of the oral route (Beck, 1991-1992). The use of these agents in patients with asthma is associated with a 50% reduction in hospitalization as opposed to beta agonists (Donahue et al., 1997). Oral prednisolone has also been shown to improve survival for up to 1 year in patients with severe alcoholic hepatitis as compared with placebo (Mathurin et al., 1996). Fludrocortisone acetate is an oral steroid specifically indicated for primary and secondary adrenocortical insufficiency of Addison's disease or for salt-losing adrenogenital syndrome. Although not specifically indicated, it also is used to treat refractory postural hypotension. It works by causing fluid retention, leading to an increase in intravascular volume (*Physicians Desk Reference,* 1997).

Laxatives

The chronic use of stimulant (cascara, bisacodyl, senna) laxatives should be discouraged in the elderly because of their tendency to produce a chemical deinnervation of the autonomic nerves as they detach from the mucosa of the large colon after many years of chronic use (Cefalu and Pike, 1981). This may subsequently lead to the development of a chronic nondilating megacolon syndrome, resulting in worsening constipation and even fecal impaction when the patient becomes immobile. Nonsystemic and bulk laxative agents (stool softener, psyllium) are the preferred agents of choice for the treatment of constipation. Prune juice serves an excellent purpose as a natural mild cathartic without long-term sequelae. Additional measures that should be used in conjunction with these agents include regular exercise; added fiber in the diet in the form of bran, fruits, and vegetables; and extra fluid intake (Beck, 1991-1992). An excellent laxative for the patient with gastrointestinal symptoms of hyperacidity is an inexpensive liquid magnesium containing antacid because these agents tend to cause diarrhea. Patients should also be advised that the frequency of regular bowel movements depends on a variety of factors, including associated medical conditions. What may be "abnormal" for one patient may be "normal" for another. In addition to discouraging chronic laxative use, drugs known to cause constipation should be identified and removed if possible. These drugs are most notably narcotics, anticholinergic agents, antispasmodics, antihistamines, major tranquilizers, tricyclic antidepressants, calcium channel blocking agents, iron salts, and diuretics (Cefalu and Pike, 1981).

Diabetic Agents

Chlorpropamide, a long-acting agent used for type 2 diabetes, is very potent and has been popular in the past. However, this agent has a half-life of 48 to 72 hours and an associated high risk of causing prolonged hypoglycemia, especially in patients with reduced appetite drive or cognitive dysfunction. It is generally considered an inappropriate drug for use in the elderly. It should be reserved for cases of diabetes complicated with diabetes insipidus (Willcox, Himmelstein, and Woolhandler, 1994). The newer hypoglycemic (sulfonylurea) agents, glipizide and glyburide, are shorter acting and considered more appropriate for the elderly. However, glyburide was shown to have the same risk of serious hypoglycemia as chlorpropamide, according to a Tennessee case-control study of Medicaid enrollees. Serious hypoglycemia was defined as a blood sugar of below 50 mg per dilution or that resulted in hospitalization, emergency room admission, or even death, associated with neuroglycopenic or autonomic symptoms, myocardial infarction, or stroke. Patients taking tolbutamide, tolazamide, and glipizide had lower risks of hypoglycemia than patients who took chlorpropamide and glyburide (Shorr et al., 1996). The main effect of glyburide and glipizide is to stimulate beta cells to release more insulin; they also have a peripheral effect. A major side effect as a result is the development of insulin resistance, hyperinsulinemia, and subsequent weight gain. These agents should be used with caution in elderly patients with reduced thirst and appetite drives secondary to dementia, depression, liver disease, or malnutrition because of the risk of serious hypoglycemia.

Newer agents such as metformin and acarbose work by different mechanisms. They may be used in combination with the sulfonylureas to potentiate their effect or alone in patients who have not responded to them or have only a minor response (*Physicians Desk Reference,* 1997). Metformin's principal action is on the liver to reduce glucose production. Major advantages include weight loss, lowering of insulin levels, and lipid levels. It also does not cause hypoglycemia by itself. It should not be used for patients with liver or renal disease or for patients with heart failure because it may cause lactic acidosis. Disadvantages are gastrointestinal side effects of nausea, flatulence, diarrhea, and nausea. Acarbose functions to delay carbohydrate absorption in the gut by interfering with dissacharide (complex sugar) metabolism. As a result, it causes a blunting of postprandial hyperglycemia and subsequent lowering of elevated glycosylated hemoglobin. It causes a major side effect of flatulence. To be effective, the drug should be given with food, and the dosage titrated up slowly.

Miscellaneous Drugs

Certain groups of drugs deserve special mention as being inappropriate and in some instances having no specific indications. Dipyridamole is an old drug that has been popular for the treatment of vascular problems by decreasing platelet "stickiness" and preventing stroke or myocardial infarction. It has not been shown to be superior to aspirin alone for the treatment of cerebral or coronary artery disease or in maintaining the patency of autologous grafts (Green and Miller, 1993). It is an inappropriate drug for use in the elderly (*Physicians Desk Reference,* 1995).

Muscle relaxers can cause sedation, lethargy, confusion, and cognitive dysfunction. They should be avoided in the elderly if possible (*Physicians Desk Reference,* 1999). The need for a "short-acting" muscle relaxer can best be served with a short-acting benzodiazepine such as lorazepam, 0.5 to 1 mg every 8 hours, used in a time-limited fashion.

Oxybutynin, an older drug with smooth muscle and anticholinergic properties, has traditionally been used to treat detrusa hyperreflexia associated with temporary or chronic urge incontinence in older patients. However, a recent study indicates that it is effective only in selective patients who have not responded to prompted voiding (Ouslander et al., 1995). Phenazopyridine is an old drug that may be useful to treat the uncomfortable symptoms of urinary tract infection initially (48 to 72 hours) until the antibiotic can become effective. It stains the urine a dark orange color (*The Complete Drug Reference,* 1992).

Quinine is another old drug that has been used traditionally for the treatment of nonspecific nocturnal leg cramps. A recent metaanalysis of five clinical trials using doses from 200 to 500 mg indicated that it reduces the frequency but not the severity or duration of leg cramps (Man-Sons-Hing and Wells, 1995). Hydroquinine hydrobromide in a dose of 300 mg per day has been shown to be significantly more effective than placebo for treatment of muscle cramps for 6 weeks, according to a clinical trial of 101 Danish patients (Jansen et al., 1997).

Elderly patients may present with intractable anorexia and weight loss, especially when associated with a worsening dementia process or cancer. Cyproheptadine is a serotonin and histamine-blocking agent that may be effective for these patients by stimulating central appetite centers (Beck, 1991-1992). However, patients, especially those with Alzheimer's disease, should be monitored closely for the development of anticholinergic side effects, including constipation, dry mouth, agitation, confusion, sedation, dizziness, restlessness, tremor, irritability, hypotension, difficulty with urination, and urinary retention.

Mitodrine, an alpha agonist, increases total peripheral vascular resistance. It has been proposed as a treatment for refractory (neurogenic) orthostatic hypotension. The drug has been shown to be significantly more effective than placebo in increasing standing and supine systolic blood pressure and in decreasing the symptoms of light-headedness but with more side effects at 2 weeks follow-up (Low et al., 1997).

Drugs for Sexual Potency

Alprostadil (prostaglandin E_1) has been approved for use in the United States for the treatment of erectile dysfunction. The drug is administered by intracavernous injection and causes erections by relaxing arteriolar and cavernous smooth muscle. The response is dose related. The drug also has been shown to improve sexual satisfaction as reported by either partner in up to 86% of injections. Side effects include penis pain in 11% of injections, priapism (erection for more than 6 hours), and prolonged erections (lasting 4 to 6 hours). The latter two side effects occurred in 5% and 1% of men, respectively, at 16 months follow-up. Study participants included those with vascular, neurogenic, and psychogenic causes of erectile dysfunction (Linet and Ogrinc, 1996).

Sildenafil citrate (Viagra) was approved by the FDA in 1998 for the treatment of erectile dysfunction. It has since revolutionized the treatment of male impotence and therefore has led to a sexual revolution. Sildenafil works by enhancing the effect of nitrous oxide, which is released in the corpus cavernosum during sexual stimulation, leading to an erection. Sildenafil is metabolized by the liver, and the dosage should be reduced in patients with hepatic cirrhosis. No dosage reduction is necessary for mild to moderate renal insufficiency (greater than 50 ml/minute creatinine clearance), but the dosage should be reduced in patients with severe renal insufficiency. Smaller starting dosages should also be used in healthy patients older than 65. Sildenafil is absolutely contraindicated in patients concurrently using nitroglycerin preparations; the combination can result in severe hypotension and cardiovascular death (*Physicians Desk Reference,* 1999). In more than 3000 patients age 19 to 87 with impotence for a mean duration of 5 years, it has been shown to be significantly more effective than placebo for organic, psychogenic, and mixed types of impotence. A study of men with diabetes indicated that sildenafil was significantly more effective than placebo (54% vs. 10%) in treating erectile dysfunction (Rendell et al., 1999).

The American College of Cardiology recently published an expert consensus document that lists patient categories for whom sildenafil is "potentially hazardous": (1) patients with stable coronary artery disease who are not using nitroglycerin preparations; (2) patients with congestive heart failure and borderline hypotension, (3) patients with hypertension using multiple antihypertensive regimens simultaneously; and (4) patients taking a long list of drugs that might prolong sildenafil's half-life (listed in publication). Dosage forms include 25-, 50-, and 100-mg tablets (*Physicians Desk Reference,* 1999).

Finasteride has been used in recent years for the treatment of initial symptomatic benign prostatic hyperplasia as a medical alternative to surgical treatment (transurethral resection of the prostate). It works by blocking the enzyme that converts testosterone to 5-alpha dihydrotestosterone. It has been shown to be effective in producing rapid regression of the size of the prostate, with 60% of treated patients experiencing a more than 10% improvement in urinary flow rate. Symptoms also improve in this group of patients by 30% or more. The drug should be used for at least 6 months. It should be used with caution because it can suppress serum prostatic antigen (PSA) levels in patients with prostate cancer. For this reason, a digital rectal examination should be performed initially and regularly while the patient is on the drug. Although not indicated for this purpose, PSA levels are used by clinicians to screen for the development of prostatic cancer while the patient is on the drug. A patient taking this drug with a PSA level above 10 ng/ml should be referred to a urologist for workup of prostate cancer, and a level of between 4 and 10 is advisable for the same (*Physicians Desk Reference,* 1997). Terazosin, an alpha blocker discussed previously, was compared with finasteride and placebo for the treatment of symptoms of benign prostatic hyperplasia in a 52-week multicenter trial of 1229 U.S. veterans. Symptom scores and urinary flow rates were significantly better with terazosin vs. placebo and finasteride alone but no different than using the combination together (Lepor, Williford, and Barry, 1996).

Cold and Over-the-counter Pain Medications

Older patients frequently seek advice about prescription and over-the-counter cold and cough medications. These agents usually have an antihistamine or decongestant component. In general, they should be avoided, especially in the presence of any medical illness that might contraindicate their use. Decongestants relieve nasal stuffiness, and antihistamines "dry up" bothersome watery secretions. Decongestants should be avoided for conditions such as anxiety and panic disorder, arrhythmias, and congestive heart failure. In addition, although studies in elderly patients are lacking, over-the-counter decongestant-antihistamine preparations have not been shown to improve symptoms in children (Hutton, Wilson, and Mellits, 1991). Patients with chronic nasal or allergic rhinitis or stuffiness should be instructed to use simple normal saline nasal spray three to four times daily to loosen secretions. If this remedy is insufficient and infection has been treated, topical steroid sprays combined with normal salt water sprays are available by prescription to relieve symptoms as a safer alternative.

Many older patients take over-the-counter analgesics for the relief of pain. These drugs often contain caffeine, which may be responsible for chronic symptoms of insomnia, especially if taken before bedtime (Brown et al., 1995). The most common categories of over-the-counter medications consumed by 1059 rural southwestern Pennsylvania elderly were analgesics (66.3%), followed by vitamin and mineral supplements (38.1%), antacids (27.9%), and laxatives (9.7%). The use of laxatives increased as that of analgesics decreased with increasing age (Stoehr et al., 1997).

Stimulants

Many dietary "natural" or "herbal" supplements used for weight loss, energy boosting, body building, or enhancement of performance contain ephedrine or related products. Frequent side effects of these agents include tachycardia, hypertension, coronary spasm, psychosis, seizures, and respiratory depression. Less frequent side effects include myocardial infarction, stroke, and death, according to a 1995 Texas Department of Health report of 500 toxic reactions (CDC, 1996). These effects can be magnified in the elderly, many of whom have preexisting hypertension or atherosclerotic cerebral or coronary disease.

Dexfenfluramine and fenfluramine were initially approved for appetite suppression and only for patients with moderate to severe obesity (at least 30% heavier than ideal body weight). Their use is associated with a significantly greater risk for pulmonary hypertension (odds ratio 6:3) according to a case-control study (Abenhaim et al., 1996). These drugs were withdrawn from the U.S. market in 1997 because of reports of serious heart valvular defects detected in users.

Chronic Pain Control

Chronic pain is often the rule rather than the exception in elderly patients burdened by multiple chronic diseases, especially secondary to arthritis and malignancy. For these patients the intensity and chronicity of perceived pain may produce or aggravate depressive symptoms. The latter can be a common symptom complex in older patients because of the loss of independence that occurs secondary to a myriad of problems: mobility problems; multiple sensory deficits in hearing, vision, taste, and smell; social isolation; institutionalization; and other losses including financial, family, friends, and personal possessions (Parmelee, Katz, and Lawton, 1991).

Relieving chronic pain in an elderly patient in a pharmacologically safe and effective manner requires that certain principles be followed: (1) avoid high-risk drug administration that may increase the risk of adverse drug reactions and side effects; (2) avoid prn medications for the relief of pain; (3) preferably use oral route of administration and reserve parental treatment for alimentary dysfunction; (4) dependence should not be a concern whereas tolerance is a minimal problem; (5) start with the simplest and safest drug available and switch to other categories as necessary; (6) always provide support for the patient in the form of counseling both informally from family, friends, and clergy and formally from social workers and psychologists as necessary; (7) never abandon the patient so that he or she feels alone or isolated; and (8) provide pharmacologic support for symptoms of depression (Rhymes, 1991; Patt, 1992).

Regarding specific drug therapy, acetaminophen given around the clock starting in a dose of 5 to 10 grains every 4 to 6 hours is often effective initially in providing pain relief secondary to arthritis. Patients with chronic pain and associated depressive symptoms often have associated insomnia and anorexia (Parmelee, Katz, and Lawton, 1991). In these cases 25 to 50 mg of amitriptyline may be effective because of its sedating side effects and because it stimulates appetite. Trazodone is an alternative antidepressant for the patient with Alzheimer's dementia that lacks the significant anticholinergic side effects of amitriptyline. The starting dose is 25 to 50 mg at bedtime. If acetaminophen alone is not effective, propoxyphene and acetaminophen, a narcotic antagonist, may be more effective without the side effect profile of NSAIDs or narcotics.

For patients with the chronic pain of bone metastasis from a terminal malignancy, NSAIDs are particularly useful, but increasing the dose provides a ceiling effect, at which the patient gets no further relief of pain (Rhymes, 1991). Steroids may also be effective for the relief of this type of pain (Rhymes, 1991). A narcotic such as codeine around the clock, with judicious use of laxatives, stool softeners, and a phenothiazine, may be the next step to relieving this type of pain. The phenothiazine may alleviate the side effect of the initial associated nausea and potentiate the effect of the narcotic. If this regimen is not effective, fentanyl patches with half-lives of 72 hours or morphine infusion pumps delivering a constant infusion with steady serum levels provide better relief (Stampfer et al., 1991; Psaty et al., 1994). Short-acting meperidine and meperidine-like preparations, given orally or parentally, with their short half-lives, have the disadvantage of allowing breakthrough pain and provide no added benefit over the use of morphine derivatives (Ishikawa et al., 1997). If used for acute pain, a dose of no more than 25 mg, in combination with an equal dose of a phenathiazine antiemetic (promethazine), may be effective. Higher doses may induce anticholinergic delirium.

Oncologic Drugs

Ondansetron and granisetron are agents useful for the treatment of nausea and vomiting secondary to cancer chemotherapeutic treatment. They function by selectively blocking the 5-hydroxytryptamine serotonin receptors. Dosage forms are available for both parental and oral use. As more potent agents, they are significantly more effective than traditional antiemetic agents. Principal side effects include headache, constipation, weakness, fatigue, abdominal pain, diarrhea, and dizziness (*Physicians Desk Reference*, 1997). According to one study, ondansetron was significantly more effective than placebo for treatment of postoperative nausea (Tramer et al., 1997).

Pamidronate is a bisphosphonate drug that inhibits the bone resorption that occurs as a result of some metastatic cancers. When used intravenously, it has been shown to be significantly more effective than placebo in reducing the frequency of nonvertebral fractures, hypercalcemia, bone surgery, and radiation therapy to bone. These results are from a randomized trial of 382 women with metastatic breast cancer and at least one lytic bone lesion (Hortobagyi et al., 1996).

Biotech Drugs

Interferon alfa shows promise as an adjuvant therapy for malignant melanoma according to a recent study of 280 patients followed after surgical removal of the primary lesion, with and without regional lymph node involvement. Patients treated for 48 weeks of high-dose interferon alpha-2b had higher 5-year relapse-free and overall survival than those not treated (37% vs. 26% and 36% vs. 37%, respectively) (Balch and Buzaid, 1996). It also has been shown to be significantly more effective than no treatment in eliminating serum markers and improving histology in patients with chronic hepatitis after 50 months of follow-up (Niederau et al., 1996). Interferon beta-1b has been shown to be significantly more effective than placebo in the treatment of patients with multiple sclerosis. Patients in the treatment group had fewer exacerbations of disease and less progression of disability than the placebo group at 2 years follow-up (Jacobs et al., 1996).

Drug Compliance

Compliance with drug regimens is a significant problem in the elderly more than in other age groups because of a host of factors: (1) multiplicity of diseases, requiring multiple

TABLE 5-2 Appropriate and Inappropriate Drug Therapy in the Elderly

Drug	Appropriate	Inappropriate	Special Consideration
Antiarrhythmic agents (quinidine, procainamide, flecainide)	Treatment of complicated arrhythmias	Treatment of routine arrhythmias	Use recommended for complicated cases under cardiologist supervision only
Antibiotics	Systemic symptoms of infected pressure ulcer or indwelling urinary catheter: fever, leucocytosis, hypotension, cellulitis, osteomyelitis, colored sputum	Surface exudate of pressure ulcers, bacteriuria and pyuria associated with indwelling urinary catheter; uncomplicated upper respiratory infection (viral)	May cause pseudomembranous colitis or promote resistance to antitiotics; adjust dose of penicillins, aminoglycosides, and fluoroquinolones consistent with creatinine clearance
Anticholinergic agents (antihistamines, tricyclic antidepressants, phenothiazine tranquilizers, narcotics)			Minimize or avoid use in patients with benign prostatic hyperplasia, glaucoma, chronic constipation, peripheral vascular disease, chronic bronchitis, Alzheimer's dementia
Antidizziness agents (meclizine)	"True" dizziness	Disequilibrium or presyncopal light-headedness	Use in low doses; anticholinergic effects may cause or worsen cognition
Antihypertensive Agents			
Alpha-blocker drugs	Hypertension	High doses may cause postural hypotension or syncope	Dual indication for hypertension and benign prostatic hyperplasia
Beta-blocker drugs	Shorter-acting selective agents; atenolol or metoprolol	Propranolol	For dual indications: angina and high blood pressure or atrial arrhythmias, after myocardial infarction or angina to reduce cardiovascular mortality
Calcium antagonists	Hypertension, angina, arrhythmias	Short-acting agents for hypertension, especially nifedipine	Cause vasodilation; side effects of flushing, pedal edema, constipation; verapamil useful in increasing pain-free

			walking distance in patients with intermittent claudication; increased mortality in patients taking short-acting agents for hypertension; increased risk of congestive heart failure or mortality in patients with left ventricular dysfunction; inhibit platelet function; increased risk for gastrointestinal hemorrhage; increased risk for transfusion postoperatively
Central-Acting Drugs			
Cold and OTC analgesic agents	See antihistamines and decongestants	See antihistamines and decongestants	Antihistamine-decongestant combination agents not found to be clinically effective in children
Antihistamines	For drying of excessive secretions	Alzheimer's patients	See anticholinergic drugs
Decongestants	For relief of nasal stuffiness	For patients with congestive heart failure, arrhythmias, anxiety disorders	
Analgesic agents	Pain relief	Patients with anxiety disorders or insomnia	Caffeine a frequent ingredient
Dementia Drugs			
Hydergine			Not significantly effective
Tacrine	For mild impairment (Alzheimer's type) for up to 30 weeks	Moderate to severe Alzheimer's disease	Monitor liver function tests monthly while on drug because of potential liver toxicity; side effects of nausea, diarrhea, and vomiting
Donepezil	For mild impairment (Alzheimer's type) for up to 30 weeks	Moderate to severe Alzheimer's disease	No need to monitor liver function tests; side effects of nausea, vomiting, and diarrhea
Pentoxifylline	Multiinfarct Dementia?		Slows cognitive deterioration but not memory loss

Table 5-2 Appropriate and Inappropriate Drug Therapy in the Elderly—cont'd

Drug	Appropriate	Inappropriate	Special Consideration
Vasodilators		Not effective	May cause postural hypotension
Digoxin	Congestive heart failure secondary to systolic dysfunction, atrial arrhythmias	Nonspecifically for other cardiac conditions	May cause anorexia, nausea, agitation, confusion; reduce dose according to creatinine clearance
Diuretics			
Loop	Treatment of fluid retention secondary to congestive heart failure or renal insufficiency; refractory and severe leg edema secondary to venous stasis or chronic venous insufficiency	Routine treatment of dependent edema or venous stasis secondary to chronic venous insufficiency, treatment of hypercalcemia; caution in using in advanced elderly or elderly with dementia or depression; treatment of uncomplicated hypertension	May cause contraction alkalosis, postural hypotension, hypokalemia, arrhythmias, and increased mortality; causes of hypercalciuria
Thiazide	Treatment of mild hypertension alone or in combination with other agents	Routine treatment of dependent edema or venous stasis secondary to chronic venous insufficiency; caution in using in advanced elderly or elderly with dementia or depression; doses greater than 50 mg ineffective for hypertension	May cause contraction alkalosis, postural hypotension, hypokalemia, arrhythmias, and increased mortality; prevents loss of calcium in urine; may have secondary benefit in retarding osteoporosis; may adversely affect lipid profile
Drugs for Diabetes			
Chlorpropamide		Long-acting (half-life 48-72 hours), potent	Use only in patients with diabetes mellitus and diabetes insipidus
Acarbose	Type 2 diabetes in combination with sulfonylureas or alone in patients who have not responded to them		Major side effects of flatulence, causes blunting of postprandial hyperglycemia and lowering of elevated glycosylated hemoglobin; given with food

Glipizide and glyburide	Type 2 diabetes	Cautious use in patients with reduced appetite drive: dementia; malnutrition; depression	Side effects of weight gain, hyperinsulinemia, and hypoglycemia
Metformin	Type 2 diabetes in combination with sulfonylureas or alone in patients who have not responded to them	Patients with liver or renal disease or congestive heart failure	Side effects of nausea, flatulence, diarrhea, and nausea; causes weight loss, lowering of insulin levels and lipid levels
Gastrointestinal Agents			
H_2 blocker drugs	Treatment or prevention of peptic ulcer disease or gastroesophageal reflux	Used prophylactically to prevent NSAID-induced gastric or duodenal bleeding; prophylaxis to prevent bleeding secondary to stress-induced gastritis in intensive care unit patients	Increased risk of aspiration pneumonia in bed-bound patients with swallowing abnormalities; indicated for prophylaxis against stress-induced gastritis for intensive care unit patients with a history of respiratory failure or bleeding disorders
Proton pump inhibitors (omeprazole, lansoprazole)	Severe or intractable gastrointestinal reflux disease	Treatment of uncomplicated peptic ulcer disease	Expensive
Smooth muscle relaxers (metoclopramide, cisapride)	Gastrointestinal reflux disease (for diabetic gastroparesis, prevention of nausea and vomiting postoperatively or secondary to chemotherapy, for implementation procedures for metoclopramide only)	Gastric emptying for gastrostomy patients	Less central nervous system sedation with cisapride Potential for extrapyramidal symptoms with metoclopramide
Sucralfate	Treatment of prevention of peptic ulcer disease	Used prophylactically to prevent NSAID-induced gastric or duodenal bleeding; prophylaxis to prevent bleeding secondary to stress-induced gastritis in intensive care unit patients	Increased risk of aspiration pneumonia in bed-bound patients with swallowing abnormalities, indicated for prophylaxis against stress-induced gastritis for intensive care unit patients with a history of respiratory failure or bleeding disorders

TABLE 5-2 Appropriate and Inappropriate Drug Therapy in the Elderly—cont'd

Drug	Appropriate	Inappropriate	Special Consideration
Hypolipidemic Agents			
Hypocholesterolemic drugs	For patients with significant history of or cardiovascular risk factors	Population-based treatment of hypercholesterolemia to prevent cardiovascular mortality	HMG-CoA reductase agents used with niacin, gemfibrozil, or cyclosporine may cause rhabdomyolysis and renal failure; need to monitor liver function tests when using HMG-CoA reductase (statin) agents; HMG-CoA agents more expensive; probucol can worsen cardiac conduction abnormalities; clofibrate may increase the incidence of cholelithiasis, subsequent morbidity and mortality from surgery; gemfibrozil and clofibrate may increase risk of bleeding when used with anticoagulants
Hypotriglyceridemic drugs	For patients in whom diet has failed, for triglyceride levels between 1000 and 2000 mg/dl, pancreatitis, recurrent abdominal pain resembling pancreatitis		See hypocholesterolemic drugs
Meperidine	Acute pain in low doses (25 mg)	Chronic pain	Short half-life
Miscellaneous Drugs			
Dipyridamole			Not shown to be superior to aspirin for vascular disease or for autologous grafts
Muscle relaxers		May cause sedation, lethargy, cognitive dysfunction, postural hypotension, falls	

Oxybutynin			Effective only in selected patients who have not responded to prompted voiding
Quinine	Metaanalysis indicates it reduces the frequency but not the duration or severity of leg cramps		
NSAIDs	PRN use, lowest possible dose, for acute flares of arthritis for 5-7 days	Indomethacin, chronic use of NSAIDs, active bleeding	May cause or worsen hypertension, congestive heart failure, renal insufficiency, or hepatitis; high doses associated with acute confusion and cognitive dysfunction, especially indomethacin; monitor hemogram and renal function with chronic use; acetaminophen as effective for osteoarthritis
Psychotropic Drugs			
Antidepressants	Treatment of depressive symptoms	Nonspecific treatment of insomnia or agitation, amitriptyline in most cases	SSRIs can worsen appetite, insomnia, anxiety, and weight loss in frail elderly or patients with dementia or depression; high doses of tricyclic agents can cause or worsen cognitive dysfunction, precipitate postural hypotension and falls; properly document need for drug; reduce dose of drug when possible
Hypnotics	Occasional use for sleep	Regular use for sleep	Can cause sedation, cognitive dysfunction, falls; possible association with increased length of stay, hospital costs, and severity of illness

HMG-CoA, 3-hydroxy-3-methylgutaryl coenzyme A; *NSAIDs,* nonsteroidal antiinflammatory drugs; *PRN,* as needed; *SSRIs,* selective serotonin reuptake inhibitors.

TABLE 5-2 Appropriate and Inappropriate Drug Therapy in the Elderly—cont'd

Drug	Appropriate	Inappropriate	Special Consideration
Psychotropic Drugs—cont'd			
Major (phenothiazine) tranquilizers	Psychotic behavior, hallucinations or delusions that are troublesome for patient; aggressive, hostile, combative behavior in dementia patients	Nonspecific diagnosis of dementia	May cause or worsen cognitive dysfunction, functional decline, postural hypotension, and falls; Parkinsonian side effects and risk of tardive dyskinesia; reduce dose and discontinue drug when possible; properly document need for drug
Minor (benzodiazepine) tranquilizers	Anxiety that is troublesome for patients	Nonspecific use for sleep	Reduce dose and discontinue when possible; avoid PRN use; properly document need for drug
Barbiturates	Seizure disorder	Nonspecific treatment of insomnia or anxiety	Monitor drug levels, properly document need for drug; may cause or worsen cognitive dysfunction, postural hypotension, and falls
Sexual Potency and Prostate			
Finasteride	Initial symptomatic benign prostatic hyperplasia	Patients with diagnosed or suspected prostate cancer	Should be used for at least 6 months; use with caution because it can suppress PSA levels in patients with prostate cancer
Steroids	Polymyalgia rheumatics (15-20 mg/daily); temporal arteritis (40-60 mg/daily); acute flares of rheumatoid arthritis, acute attacks of asthma resistant to conventional therapy; moderate to severe chronic lung disease; allergic rhinitis; initial treatment of certain dermatoses	Initial treatment of asthma; osteoarthritis	Side effects of weight gain; fluid retention; dependence; worsening or precipitation of hypertension or diabetes, cataracts, or osteoporosis

Fludrocortisone acetate	Replacement therapy for Addison's disease or adrenogenital syndrome	Not officially indicated for treatment of refractory postural hypotension	
Prostaglandin	Erectile dysfunction secondary to vascular, neurogenic, or psychogenic causes	General use to increase sexual potency	Side effects of penis pain, priapism, and prolonged erections
Stimulants			
Dexfenfluramine and fenfluramine		Cause pulmonary fibrosis and valvular heart defects	Withdrawn for use because of serious side effects
Theophylline	Acute wheezing or a diagnosis of asthma	Routine treatment of chronic obstructive lung disease	Can cause postural hypotension, nausea, anorexia, weight loss, arrhythmias, anxiety, insomnia
Vitamins and Prophylaxis			
Aspirin (81 mg)	Daily for all patients	Active gastrointestinal bleeding or history of bleeding diathesis or other blood disorders; allergy to aspirin	
Aspirin (325 mg)	For patients with a history of previous stroke	Active gastrointestinal bleeding or history of bleeding diathesis or other blood disorders; allergy to aspirin	
Heparin	Prophylaxis for transiently immobile patients with a history of deep venous thrombosis or pulmonary embolus; obesity, history of congestive heart failure, or chronic venous insufficiency		
Enoxaparin	Prevention of deep vein thrombosis and pulmonary embolism in patients postoperative hip or knee replacement; home follow-up treatment for deep venous thrombosis	General postsurgical prophylaxis	Shown to be as effective as warfarin in preventing deep venous thrombosis; when used for home treatment of deep venous thrombosis, associated with decreased hospital stay

PSA, Prostate-specific antigen.

TABLE 5-2 Appropriate and Inappropriate Drug Therapy in the Elderly—cont'd

Drug	Appropriate	Inappropriate	Special Consideration
Vitamins and Prophylaxis—cont'd			
Warfarin	For deep venous thrombosis and pulmonary embolism prevention in patients after surgery for cancer, hip fracture, knee or hip replacement; prophylaxis for patients with chronic atrial fibrillation and rheumatic heart disease	General postsurgical prophylaxis; patients at risk for falls, with cognitive dysfunction or dementia, liver disease, or malnutrition	Maintain INR 1.2-1.5 normal to prevent excess bleeding tendency; increased bleeding in patients over age 80; use with caution in patients with liver disease and malnutrition; avoid use of NSAIDs and aspirin concomitantly because of increased risk of bleeding
Iron supplement	Proven iron deficiency	Nonspecific treatment of microcytic hypochromic anemia	
Zinc	Lozenges shown to be effective for reduction in severity and duration of upper respiratory symptoms; wound healing in event of pressure ulcers		Not yet approved by FDA
Selenium	Shown to be effective in reduction in incidence of cancer		
Vitamin (antioxidant) A, C, E	For deficiency states only	For prophylaxis against premature aging	Effective in increasing cell-mediated immunity; controversial regarding benefits for cancer and heart disease prevention
Vitamin (multiple)	For all patients		

INR, International normalized ratio; *FDA*, Food and Drug Administration.

medications, often obtained through multiple pharmacies, all of which may cause confusion for the patient; (2) cognitive dysfunction associated with memory loss and subsequent failure to take medication appropriately, leading to exacerbation of disease or toxicity states; (3) restricted income and inability to pay for medication, leading to exacerbation of disease; (4) difficulty in complying with office or hospital visits because of mobility problems for the patient or transportation problems in obtaining medication from the pharmacist promptly or at all in some cases; (5) visual problems that may increase the frequency of inappropriate medication or dose, leading to adverse drug reactions; and (6) medical diseases that may interfere with fine and gross coordination of the upper extremities for medication administration, such as stroke, Parkinson's disease, cervical stenosis, dementia, and arthritis.

Drug compliance for the older patient can be enhanced in the following general ways: (1) educating the patient or family about the purpose of the medication and potential side effects; (2) educating the patient or family about the disease process and signs or symptoms of worsening disease; (3) asking the patient or family to bring all prescription and over-the-counter medications to each clinic or hospital visit for reevaluation; (4) assigning key family members or friends who may be of assistance in helping the patient secure needed medication from the pharmacy or clinic in a timely fashion; (5) asking family, friends, or nursing personnel when available to assist in or monitor medication administration for the elderly patient with visual, coordination, or cognitive problems; (6) using pill administration boxes that can be refilled weekly by the patient, family, friends, or nursing personnel; and (7) referring to social service agencies, home health agencies, senior citizen centers, and volunteer agencies to assist in securing financial and transportation assistance as applicable.

Specific drug compliance can be increased for the elderly patient by encouraging the prescriber to: (1) prescribe medication administered no more than once or twice daily; (2) administer one drug to treat two conditions when possible; (3) start with one third to one half the normal starting dose to decrease the risk of adverse drug reactions; (4) maximize the dose of one drug to treat a specific condition before adding a second agent to reduce the risk of adverse drug reactions; and (5) use the cheapest drug possible (Beck, 1991-1992).

Summary

Basic principles of drug therapy for the elderly include an understanding of normal changes that occur during the aging process: reduced immune defenses, blunting and reduction of receptor sites, loss of physiologic reserve, and physiologic and structural changes in organ systems. These systems include the skin, gastrointestinal tract, liver, kidney, and brain. Advancing age is associated with the development of chronic disease, multiple diseases, and the need to take more over-the-counter and prescription medications. All of these factors increase the risk of adverse drug reactions. The high incidence of sensory deficits, cognitive dysfunction, mobility problems, transportation difficulty, socioeconomic concerns, and arthritis necessitate extreme caution and attention to compliance issues as well. All of these points make the topic of drug therapy in the elderly much different than drug therapy in the general adult population.

Resources

Center Watch, Inc.
Clinical Trials Listing Service
581 Boylston Street, Suite 200
Boston, MA 02116
http://www.centerwatch.com

Rx List Internet Drug Index
http://www.rxlist.com

References

Abenhaim L et al: Appetite-suppressant drugs and the risk of primary pulmonary hypertension, *N Engl J Med* 335:609-616, 1996.

Akiyama T et al: Effects of advancing age on the efficacy and side effects of antiarrhythmic drugs in post-myocardial infarction patients with ventricular arrhythmias, *J Am Geriatr Soc* 40:666-672, 1992.

Australia/New Zealand Heart Failure Research Collaborative Group. Randomised, placebo-controlled trial of carvedilol in patients with congestive heart failure due to ischemic heart disease, *Lancet* 349:375-380, 1997.

Bagger JP et al: Effect of verapamil in intermittent claudication: a randomized, double-blind, placebo-controlled, cross-over study after individual dose-response assessment, *Circulation* 95:411-414, 1997.

Balch CM, Buzaid AC: Finally, a successful adjuvant therapy for high-risk melanoma, *J Clin Oncol* 14:1-3, 1996.

Baloh RW: Dizziness in older people, *J Am Geriatr Soc* 40:713-721, 1992.

Beck JC: *Geriatric review syllabus: a core curriculum in geriatric medicine.* New York, 1991-1992, American Geriatrics Society.

Berggren D et al: Postoperative confusion after anesthesia in elderly patients with femoral neck fractures, *Anesth Analg* 66:497-504, 1987.

Bergqvist D et al: Low-molecular-weight heparin (Enoxaparin) as prophylaxis against venous thromboembolism after total hip replacement, *N Engl J Med* 335:696-700, 1996.

Bixler EO et al: Next-day memory impairment with Triazolam use, *Lancet* 337:827-831, 1991.

Bjorck S et al: Renal protective effect of enalapril in diabetic nephropathy, *Br Med J* 304:339-343, 1992.

Black RS et al: Pentoxifylline in cerebrovascular dementia, *J Am Geriatr Soc* 40:237-244, 1992.

Bradley JD et al: Comparison of an antiinflammatory dose of ibuprofen, an analgesic dose of ibuprofen, and acetaminophen in the treatment of patients with osteoarthritis of the knee, *N Engl J Med* 325:87-91, 1991.

Braunwald E: Ace inhibitors: a cornerstone of the treatment of heart failure, *N Engl J Med* 325:351-353, 1991.

Brown SL et al: Occult caffeine as a source of sleep problems in an older population, *J Am Geriatr Soc* 43:860-864, 1995.

Buckler DA, Kelber ST, Goodwin JS: The use of dietary restrictions in malnourished nursing home patients, *J Am Geriatr Soc* 42:1100-1102, 1994.

Buring JE, Glynn RJ, Hennekens CH: Calcium channel blockers and myocardial infarction: a hypothesis formulated but not yet tested, *JAMA* 274:654-655, 1995.

Cahill L et al: Beta-adrenergic activation and memory for emotional events, *Nature* 371:702-704, 1994.

Calkins E, Ford AB, Katz PR: *Practice of geriatrics,* ed 2, Philadelphia, 1992, WB Saunders.

Cantwell-Gab K: Identifying chronic peripheral arterial disease, *Am J Nurs* 96:44, 1996.

Cefalu CA, Pike J: Fecal impaction: a practical approach to the problem, *Geriatrics* 36(5):143-145, 1981.

Centers for Disease Control and Prevention: Adverse events associated with ephedrine-containing products: Texas, December 1993–September 1995, *MMWR* 45:689-693, 1996.

Clark LC et al: Effects of selenium supplementation for cancer prevention in patients with carcinoma of the skin: a randomized controlled trial, *JAMA* 276(24):1957-1963, 1996.

Coates ML, Rembold CM, Farr BM: Does pseudoephedrine increase blood pressure in patients with controlled hypertension? *J Fam Pract* 40:22-26, 1995.

Cohn JN et al: A comparison of enalapril with hydralazine-isosorbide dinitrate in the treatment of chronic congestive heart failure, *N Engl J Med* 325:303-310, 1991.

Colditz GA et al: The use of estrogens and progestins and the risk of breast cancer in postmenopausal women, *N Engl J Med* 332:1589-1593, 1995.

Colenda CC: Drug treatment of behavior problems in elderly patients with dementia, *part I, Drug Therapy* 15-20, 1991.

Cook DJ et al: Risk factors for gastrointestinal bleeding in critically ill patients, *N Engl J Med* 10(330):377-381, 1994.

Cooper JW: Probable adverse drug reactions in a rural geriatric nursing home population: a four-year study, *J Am Geriatr Soc* 44:194-197, 1996.

Coplen SE et al: Efficacy and safety of quinidine therapy for maintenance of sinus rhythm after cardioversion, *Circulation* 82:1106-1116, 1990.

Culter AF et al: Accuracy of invasive and non-invasive tests to diagnose *Helicobacter pylori* infection, *Gastroenterology* 109:136-141, 1995.

Cummings SR et al: Risk factors for hip fracture in white women, *N Engl J Med* 23(332):767-773, 1995.

Curb JD et al: Effect of diuretic-based antihypertensive treatment on cardiovascular disease risk in older diabetic patients with isolated systolic hypertension, *JAMA* 276:1886-1892, 1996.

Daly E et al: Measuring the impact of menopausal symptoms on quality of life, *Br Med J* 307:836-840, 1993.

Damon LE: Anemias of chromic disease in the aged: diagnosis and treatment, *Geriatrics* 47:47-57, 1992.

De Groen PC et al: Esophagitis associated with the use of alendronate, *N Engl J Med* 335:1016-1021, 1996.

Donahue JG et al: Inhaled steroids and the risk of hospitalization for asthma, *JAMA* 277:887-891, 1997.

Doucet J et al: Drug-drug interactions related to hospital admissions in older adults: a prospective study of 1000 patients, *J Am Geriatr Soc* 44:944-948, 1996.

Evans MP, Fleming KC, Evans FM: Hormone replacement therapy: management of common problems, *Mayo Clin Proc* 70:800-805, 1995.

Figulla HR et al: Diltiazem improves cardiac function and exercise capacity in patients with idiopathic dilated cardiomyopathy: results of the diltiazem in dilated cardiomyopathy trial, *Circulation* 94:346-352, 1996.

Fihn SD et al: The risk for and severity of bleeding complications in elderly patients treated with warfarin, *Ann Intern Med* 124:970-979, 1996.

Finucane FF et al: Decreased risk of stroke among postmenopausal hormone users: results from a national cohort, *Arch Intern Med* 153:73-79, 1993.

Fishkind D, Paris BE, Aronow WS: Use of digoxin, diuretics, beta blockers, angiotensin-converting enzyme inhibitors, and calcium channel blockers in older patients in an academic hospital-based geriatrics practice, *J Am Geriatr Soc* 45:809-812, 1997.

Fogelman L: Viewpoint: oestrogen, the prevention of bone loss and osteoporosis, *Br J Rheumatol* 30:276-281, 1991.

Frierson RL, Wey JJ, Tabler JB: Psychostimulants for depression in the medically ill, *Am Fam Physician* 43:163-170, 1991.

Furberg CD, Psaty BM, Meyer JV: Nifedipine: dose-related increase in mortality in patients with coronary heart disease, *Circulation* 92:1326-1331, 1995.

Gale CR et al: Vitamin C and risk of death from stroke and coronary heart disease in cohort of elderly people, *Br Med J* 310:1563-1566, 1995.

Garcia Rodriquez LA et al: The role of non-steroidal antiinflammatory drugs in acute liver injury, *Br Med J* 305:865-868, 1992.

Gergen PJ et al: A population-based serologic survey of immunity to tetanus in the United States, *N Engl J Med* 332:761-766, 1995.

Ginsburg ES et al: Effects of alcohol ingestion on estrogens in postmenopausal women, *JAMA* 276:1747-1751, 1996.

Gottlieb SS et al: Renal response to Indomethacin in congestive heart failure secondary to ischemic or idiopathic dilated cardiomyopathy, *Am J Cardiol* 70:890-893, 1992.

Grady D et al: Hormone therapy to prevent disease and prolong life in postmenopausal women, *Ann Intern Med* 117:1016-1032, 1992.

Graham DY et al: Effect of treatment of *Helicobacter pylori* infection on the long-term recurrence rate of gastric or duodenal ulcer, *Ann Intern Med* 116:705-708, 1992.

Graham DY et al: Epidemiology of *Helicobacter pylori* in an asymptomatic population in the United States: effects of age, race, and socioeconomic status, *Gastroenterology* 100:1495-1501, 1991.

Grasela TH, Dreis MW: An evaluation of the quinolone-theophylline interaction using the Food and Drug Administration spontaneous reporting system, *Arch Intern Med* 152:617-621, 1992.

Green D, Miller V: Role of dipyridamole in the therapy of vascular disease, *Geriatrics* 48:46, 1993.

Greenberg ER et al: Mortality associated with low plasma concentration of beta carotene and the effect of oral supplementation, *JAMA* 275:699-703, 1996.

Greenblatt DJ et al: Sensitivity to triazolam in the elderly, *N Engl J Med* 324:1691-1698, 1991.

Griffin MR et al: Nonsteroidal antiinflammatory drug use and the increased risk for peptic ulcer disease in elderly persons, *Ann Intern Med* 114:257-262, 1991.

Grisso JA et al: Risk factors for falls as a cause of hip fracture in women, *N Engl J Med* 324:1326-1331, 1991.

Grodstein F et al: Postmenopausal estrogen and progestin use and the risk of cardiovascular disease, *N Engl J Med* 335:453-461, 1996.

Grover SA, Palmer CS, Coupal L: Serum lipid screening to identify high-risk individuals for coronary death, *Arch Intern Med* 154:679-684, 1994.

Gurwitz JH et al: Initiation of antihypertensive treatment during nonsteroidal antiinflammatory drug therapy, *JAMA* 272:781-786, 1994.

Gurwitz JH, Noonan JD, Soumerai SB: Reducing the use of H_2-receptor antagonists in the long-term care setting, *J Am Geriatr Soc* 40:359-364, 1992.

Guthrie R: Terazosin in the treatment of hypertension and symptomatic benign prostatic hyperplasia: a primary care trial, *J Fam Pract* 39:129-133, 1994.

Hallstrom AP et al: An antiarrhythmic drug experience in 941 patients resuscitated from an initial cardiac arrest between 1970 and 1985, *Am J Cardiol* 68:1025-1031, 1991.

Hannedouche T et al: Randomized controlled trial of enalapril and B blockers in nondiabetic chronic renal failure, *Br Med J* 309:833-837, 1994.

Harpaz D et al: Effect of aspirin on mortality in women with symptomatic or silent myocardial ischemia, *Am J Cardiol* 78:1215-1219, 1996.

Hazzard WR et al: *Principles of geriatric medicine and gerontology,* ed 3, New York, 1994, McGraw-Hill.

Hebert PR, Gaziano JM, Hennekens CH: An overview of trials of cholesterol lowering and risk of stroke, *Arch Intern Med* 155:50-55, 1995.

Heidrich FE, Stergachis A, Gross KM: Diuretic drug use and the risk for hip fracture, *Ann Intern Med* 115:1-6, 1991.

Hempling RE et al: Hormone replacement therapy as a risk factor for epithelial ovarian cancer: results of a case-control study, *Obstet Gynecol* 89:1012-1016, 1997.

Henry D et al: Variability in risk of gastrointestinal complications with individual nonsteroidal antiinflammatory drugs: results of a collaborative meta-analysis, *Br Med J* 312:1563-1566, 1996.

Henry D et al: Meta-analysis workshop in upper gastrointestinal hemorrhage. *Gastroenterology* 100(5):1481-1482, 1991.

Hentschel E et al: Effect of ranitidine and amoxicillin plus metronidazole on the eradication of *Helicobacter pylori* and the recurrence of duodenal ulcer, *N Engl J Med* 328:308-312, 1993.

Hetland ML, Haarbo J, Christiansen C: One measurement of serum total cholesterol is enough to predict future levels in healthy postmenopausal women, *Am J Med* 92:25-28, 1992.

Hohnloser S, van de Loo A, Baedeker F: Efficacy and proarrhythmic hazards of pharmacologic cardioversion of atrial fibrillation: prospective comparison of sotalol versus quinidine, *J Am Coll Cardiol* 26:852-858, 1995.

Hollenberg NK, Moore TJ: Age and the renal blood supply: renal vascular responses to angiotensin converting enzyme inhibition in healthy humans, *J Am Geriatr Soc* 42:805-808, 1994.

Holt DM: Recommendations, usage and efficacy of immunizations for the elderly, *Nurse Pract* 17:51-59, 1992.

Honkanen PO, Keistinen T, Knela SL: Reactions following administration of influenza vaccine alone or with pneumococcal vaccine to the elderly, *Arch Intern Med* 156:205-208, 1996.

Hortobagyi GN et al: Efficacy of pamidronate in reducing skeletal complications in patients with breast cancer and lytic bone metastases, *N Engl J Med* 335:1785-1791, 1996.

Hutton N, Wilson MH, Mellits ED: Effectiveness of an antihistamine-decongestant combination for young children with the common cold: a randomized, controlled clinical trial, *J Pediatr* 118:125-130, 1991.

Ishikawa K et al: Short-acting nifedipine and diltiazem do not reduce the incidence of cardiac events in patients with healed myocardial infarction, *Circulation* 95:2368-2373, 1997.

ISIS-4 Collaborative Group: ISIS-4: a randomized factorial trial assessing early oral captopril, oral mononitrate, and intravenous magnesium sulphate in 58,050 patients with suspected acute myocardial infarction, *Lancet* 345:669-685, 1995.

Jackson JL et al: The effect of treating herpes zoster with oral acyclovir in preventing postherpetic neuralgia: a meta-analysis, *Arch Intern Med* 157:909-912, 1997.

Jacobs LD et al: Intramuscular interferon beta-Ia for disease progression in relapsing multiple sclerosis, *Ann Neurol* 39:285-294, 1996.

Jansen PH et al: Randomised controlled trial of hydroquinine in muscle cramps, *Lancet* 349:528-532, 1997.

Javaheri S et al: Effect of theophylline on sleep-disordered breathing in heart failure, *N Engl J Med* 335:562-567, 1996.

Jick SS, Dean AD, Jick H: Antidepressants and suicide, *Br Med J* 310:215-218, 1995.

Jones AC, Berman P, Doherty M: Nonsteroidal antiinflammatory drug usage and requirement in elderly acute hospital admissions, *Br J Rheumatol* 31:45-48, 1992.

Kalish SC et al: Antipsychotic prescribing patterns and the treatment of extrapyramidal symptoms in older people, *J Am Geriatr Soc* 43:967-973, 1995.

Kapur S, Mieczkowski J, Mann JJ: Antidepressant medications and the relative risk of suicide attempt and suicide, *JAMA* 268:3441-3445, 1992.

Knapp MJ et al: A 30-week randomized controlled trial of high-dose tacrine in patients with Alzheimer's disease, *JAMA* 271:992-998, 1994.

Kristal BS, Yu BP: An emerging hypothesis: synergistic induction of aging by free radical and Maillard reactions. *J Gerontol Biol Sci Med Sci* 47:B107-B114, 1992.

Kristiansen IS, Eggen AE, Thelle DS: Cost-effectiveness of incremental programmes for lowering serum cholesterol concentration: is individual intervention worthwhile? *Br Med J* 302:1119-1122, 1991.

Krumholz HM et al: Lack of association between cholesterol and coronary heart disease: mortality and morbidity and all-cause mortality in persons older than 70 years, *JAMA* 272:1335-1340, 1994.

Kushi LH et al: Physical activity and mortality in postmenopausal women, *JAMA* 277:1287-1292, 1997.

Lam RW et al: Multicenter, placebo-controlled study of fluoxetine in seasonal affective disorder, *Am J Psychiatry* 152:1765-1770, 1995.

Langman MJ et al: Risks of bleeding peptic ulcer associated with individual nonsteroidal antiinflammatory drugs, *Lancet* 343:1075-1078, 1994.

Leclerc JR et al: Prevention of venous thromboembolism after knee arthroplasty, *Ann Intern Med* 124:619-626, 1996.

Lees AJ: Comparison of therapeutic effects and mortality data of levodopa and levodopa combined with seligiline in patients with early, mild Parkinson's disease, *Br Med J* 311:1602-1607, 1995.

Lepor H, Williford WO, Barry MJ: The efficacy of terazosin, finasteride, or both in benign prostatic hyperplasia, *N Engl J Med* 335:533-539, 1996.

Lesage J: Polypharmacy in geriatric patients, *Nurs Clin North Am* 26:273-289, 1991.

Lesar TS, Briceland L, Stein DC: Factors related to errors in medication prescribing., *JAMA* 277:312-317, 1997.

Lessem JN, Weber MA: Antihypertensive treatment with a dual-acting beta-blocker in the elderly, *J Hypertens* 11:S29-S36, 1993.

Levine JS: Misoprostol and nonsteroidal antiinflammatory drugs: a tale of effects, outcomes, and costs, *Ann Intern Med* 123:309-310, 1995.

Levine M et al: A comparison of low-molecular-weight heparin administered primarily at home with unfractionated heparin administered in the hospital for proximal deep-vein thrombosis, *N Engl J Med* 334:677-681, 1996.

Lewis EJ et al: The effect of angiotensin-converting-enzyme inhibition on diabetic nephropathy, *N Engl J Med* 329:1456-1462, 1993.

Liberman UA et al: Effect of oral alendronate on bone mineral density and the incidence of fractures in postmenopausal osteoporosis, *N Engl J Med* 333:1437-1443, 1995.

Lichstein E et al: Relation between beta-adrenergic blocker use, various correlates of left ventricular function and the chance of developing congestive heart failure, *J Am Coll Cardiol* 16:1327-1332, 1990.

Liel Y, Harmon-Boehm I, Shany S: Evidence for a clinically important adverse effect of fiber-enriched diet on the bioavailability of levothyroxine in adult hypothyroid patients, *J Clin Endocrinol Metab* 81:857-859, 1996.

Lindley CM et al: Inappropriate medication is a major cause of adverse drug reactions in elderly patients, *Age Ageing,* 21:294-300, 1992.

Linet OI, Ogrinc FC: Efficacy and safety of intracavernosal alprostadil in men with erectile dysfunction, *N Engl J Med* 334:873-877, 1996.

Low PA et al: Efficacy of midodrine versus placebo in neurogenic orthostatic hypotension: a randomized, double-blind multicenter study, *JAMA* 277:1046-1051, 1997.

Luchi RJ, Taffet GE, Teasdale TA: Congestive heart failure in the elderly, *J Am Geriatr Soc* 39:810-825, 1991.

Mach JR et al: Serum anticholinergic activity in hospitalized older persons with delirium: a preliminary study, *J Am Geriatr Soc* 43:491-495, 1995.

Maltby N et al: Efficacy of tacrine and lecithin in mild to moderate Alzheimer's disease: double blind trial, *Br Med J* 308:879-883, 1994.

Mangano DT et al: Effect of atenolol on mortality and cardiovascular morbidity after noncardiac surgery, *N Engl J Med* 335:1713-1720, 1996.

Manolio TA et al: Associations of postmenopausal estrogen use with cardiovascular disease and stroke risk factors in older women, *Circulation* 88:2163-2171, 1993.

Man-Sons-Hing M, Wells G: Meta-analysis of efficacy of quinine for treatment of nocturnal leg cramps in elderly people, *Br Med J* 310:13-17, 1995.

Mathurin P et al: Survival and prognostic factors in patients with severe alcoholic hepatitis treated with prednisolone, *Gastroenterology* 110:1847-1853, 1996.

McDonald CC et al: Cardiac and vascular morbidity in women receiving adjuvant tamoxifen for breast cancer in a randomised trial, *Br Med J* 311:977-980, 1995.

Miyawaki E: Thrombolysis for stroke: some concern, some hope—an editorial, *Journal Watch* 16(6):51-52, 1997.

Monane M et al: The impact of thiazide diuretics on the initiation of lipid-reducing agents in older people: a population-based analysis, *J Am Geriatr Soc* 45:71-75, 1997.

Morrison HI et al: Serum folate and risk of fatal coronary heart disease, *JAMA* 275:1893-1896, 1996.

Mossad SB et al: Zinc gluconate lozenges for treating the common cold: a randomized, placebo-controlled study, *Ann Intern Med* 125:81-88, July 15, 1996.

Nevitt MC et al: Association of estrogen replacement therapy with the risk of osteoarthritis of the hip in elderly white women, *Arch Intern Med* 156:2073-2080, 1996.

Newbern VB: Cautionary tales on using beta blockers, *Geriatr Nurs* 12(3):119-122, 1991.

Niederau C et al: Long-term follow-up of HbeAG-positive patients treated with interferon alfa for chronic hepatitis B, *N Engl J Med* 334:1422-1427, 1996.

O'Keefe JH Jr et al: Estrogen replacement therapy after coronary angioplasty in women, *J Am Coll Cardiol* 29:1-5, 1997.

Oldroyd KG et al: Effects of early captopril administration on infarct expansion, left ventricular remodeling and exercise capacity after acute myocardial infarction, *Am J Cardiol* 68:713-718, 1991.

Omenn GS et al: Effects of a combination of beta carotene and vitamin A on lung cancer and cardiovascular disease, *N Engl J Med* 334:1150-1155, 1996.

O'Riordan TG, Tobin A, O'Morain C: *Helicobacter pylori* infection in elderly dyspeptic patients, *Age Ageing* 20:189-192, 1991.

Ouslander JG et al: Does oxybutynin add to the effectiveness of prompted voiding for urinary incontinence among nursing home residents? a placebo-controlled trial, *J Am Geriatr Soc* 43:610-617, 1995.

Packer M et al: Double-blind, placebo-controlled study of the effects of carvedilol in patients with moderate to severe heart failure: the precise trial, *Circulation* 94:2793-2799, 1996.

Packer M et al: Effect of amlodipine on morbidity and mortality in severe chronic heart failure, *N Engl J Med* 335:1107-1114, 1996b.

Pahor M et al: Risk of gastrointestinal haemorrhage with calcium antagonists in hypertensive persons over 67 years old, *Lancet* 347:1061-1065, 1996.

Park KC, Forman DE, Wei JY: Utility of beta-blockade treatment for older postinfarction patients, *J Am Geriatr Soc* 43:751-755, 1995.

Parmelee PA, Katz IR, Lawton MP: The relation of pain to depression among institutionalized aged, *J Gerontol B Psychol Sci Soc Sci* 46:15-21, 1991.

Patt RB: PCA: prescribing analgesia for home management of severe pain, *Geriatrics* 47:69-84, 1992.

Penn ND et al: The effects of dietary supplementation with vitamins A, C, and E on cell-mediated immune functions in elderly, long-stay patients, *Age Ageing,* 20:169-174, 1991.

Perrig WJ, Perrig P, Stahelin HB: The relation between antioxidants and memory performance in the old and very old, *J Am Geriatr Soc* 45:718-724, 1997.

Pestotnik SL et al: Adverse drug events in hospitalized patients: excessive length of stay, extra costs, and attributable mortality, *JAMA* 277:301-306, 1997.

Peura DA: *Helicobacter pylori:* a diagnostic dilemma and a dilemma of diagnosis, *Gastroenterology* 109:313-315, 1995.

Physicians Desk Reference. Montvale, NJ, 1995, 1997, 1999, Medical Economics.

Pinkowish MD: Practical briefings: clinical news you can put into practice now, *Patient Care* 6-21, 1995.

Prince RL: Prevention of postmenopausal osteoporosis: a comparative study of exercise, calcium supplementation, and hormone replacement therapy, *N Engl J Med* 325:1189-1195, 1991.

Psaty BM et al: The risk of myocardial infarction associated with the combined use of estrogens and progestins in postmenopausal women, *Arch Intern Med* 154:1333-1339, 1994.

Rapola JM et al: Effect of vitamin E and beta-carotene on the incidence of angina pectoris: a randomized, double-blind, controlled trial, *JAMA* 275:693-698, 1996.

Ray WA, Griffin MR, Malcolm E: Cyclic antidepressants and the risk of hip fracture, *Arch Intern Med* 151:754-756, 1991.

Rendell MS et al: Sildenafil for treatment of erectile dysfunction in men with diabetes, *JAMA* 281:421-426, 1999.

Rhymes JA: Clinical management of the terminally ill, *Geriatrics,* 46:57-67, 1991.

Riemersma RA et al: Risk of angina pectoris and plasma concentrations of vitamins A, C, and E and carotene, *Lancet* 337:1-5, 1991.

Rogers SL, Friedhoff LT: The efficacy and safety of donepezil in patients with Alzheimer's disease: results of a U.S. multicentre, randomized, double-blind, placebo-controlled trial. The Donepezil Study Group, *Dementia* 7(6):293-303, 1996.

Rovner BW et al: Research and reviews: the prevalence and management of dementia and other psychiatric disorders in nursing homes, *Int Psychogeriatrics* 2(13):22, 1990.

Rummans TA et al: Learning and memory impairment in older, detoxified, benzodiazepine-dependent patients, *Mayo Clin Proc* 68:731-737, 1993.

The SALT Collaborative Group: Swedish aspirin low-dose trial (SALT) of 75 mg aspirin as secondary prophylaxis after cerebrovascular ischemic events, *Lancet* 338:1345-1349, 1991.

Saltz BL: Tardive dyskinesia in the elderly patient, *Hosp Pract (Off Ed)* 27:167-184, 1992.

Saltz BL et al: Prospective study of tardive dyskinesia incidence in the elderly, *JAMA* 266:2402-2406, 1991.

Sanderson P: Antibiotics and the elderly, *Practitioner* 234:1064-1066, 1990.

Scherr PA et al: Light to moderate alcohol consumption and mortality in the elderly, *J Am Geriatr Soc* 40:651-657, 1992.

Schuler G et al: Regular physical exercise and low-fat diet; effects on progression of coronary artery disease, *Circulation* 86:1-11, 1992.

Shankel SW et al: Acute renal failure and glomerulopathy caused by nonsteroidal antiinflammatory drugs, *Arch Intern Med* 152:986-990, 1992.

Sheikh J: The pharmacological treatment of depression in older patients. Paper presented at annual meeting, American Geriatrics Society, New Orleans, 6 October 1995.

SHEP Cooperative Research Group: Prevention of stroke by antihypertensive drug treatment in older persons with isolated systolic hypertension: final results of the systolic hypertension in the elderly program (SHEP), *JAMA* 265:3255-3264, 1991.

Shorr RI et al: Individual sulfonylureas and serious hypoglycemia in older people, *J Am Geriatr Soc* 44:751-755, 1996.

Slataper R et al: Comparative effects of different antihypertensive treatments on progression of diabetic renal disease, *Arch Intern Med* 153:973-980, 1993.

Slatton ML et al: Does digoxin provide additional hemodynamic and autonomic benefit at higher doses in patients with mild to moderate heart failure and normal sinus rhythm? *J Am Coll Cardiol* 29:1206-1213, 1997.

Smith GD et al: Cholesterol lowering and mortality: the importance of considering initial level of risk, *BMJ* 306:1367-1373, 1993.

Soumerai SB et al: Adverse outcomes of underuse of beta-blockers in elderly survivors of acute myocardial infarction, *JAMA* 277:115-121, 1997.

Stampfer MJ et al: Postmenopausal estrogen therapy and cardiovascular disease: ten year follow-up from the nurses' health study, *N Engl J Med* 325:756-762, 1991.

Stephens NG et al: Randomised controlled trial of vitamin E in patients with coronary disease: Cambridge Heart Antioxidant Study (CHAOS), *Lancet* 347:781-786, 1996.

Stewart WF et al: Risk of Alzheimer's disease and duration of NSAID use, *Neurology* 48:626-632, 1997.

Stoehr GP et al: Over-the-counter medication use in an older rural community: the MoVIES Project, *J Am Geriatr Soc* 45:158-165, 1997.

Stroke Prevention in Atrial Fibrillation Investigators: Warfarin versus aspirin for prevention of thromboembolism in atrial fibrillation: stroke prevention in atrial fibrillation II study, *Lancet* 343:687-691, 1994.

Taha AS et al: Famotidine for the prevention of gastric and duodenal ulcers caused by nonsteroidal antiinflammatory drugs, *N Engl J Med* 334:1435-1439, 1996.

Tang M et al: Effect of oestrogen during menopause on risk and age at onset of Alzheimer's disease, *Lancet* 348:429-432, 1996.

Tariot PN et al: Lack of carbamazepine toxicity in frail nursing home patients: a controlled study, *J Am Geriatr Soc* 43:1026-1029, 1995.

Tariot PN et al: Carbamazepine treatment of agitation in nursing home patients with dementia: a preliminary study, *J Am Geriatr Soc* 42:1160-1166, 1994.

Thiessen BQ et al: Increased prescribing of antidepressants subsequent to beta-blocker therapy, *Arch Intern Med* 150:2286-2290, 1990.

Thompson MP, Morris LK: Unexplained weight loss in the ambulatory elderly, *J Am Geriatr Soc* 39:497-500, 1991.

Thun MJ, Namboodiri MM, Heath CM Jr: Aspirin use and reduced risk of fatal colon cancer, *N Engl J Med* 325:1593-1596, 1991.

Tramer MR et al: A quantitative systematic review of ondansetron in treatment of established postoperative nausea and vomiting, *Br Med J* 314:1088-1093, 1997.

US Department of Health and Human Services: *Core curriculum on tuberculosis: what the clinician should know,* ed 3, Washington, DC, 1994, USDHHS.

Vega GL, Grundy SM: Lipoprotein responses to treatment with lovastatin, gemfibrozil, and nicotinic acid in normolipidemic patients with hypoalphalipoproteinemia, *Arch Intern Med* 154:73-82, 1994.

Verdery RB, Goldberg AP: Hypocholesterolemia as a predictor of death: a prospective study of 224 nursing home residents, *J Gerontol A Biol Sci Med Sci* 46:84-90, 1991.

Voight LF et al: Progesterone supplementation of exogenous estrogens and risk of endometrial cancer, *Lancet* 338:274-277, 1991.

Wallentin LC: Aspirin (75 mg/day) after an episode of unstable coronary artery disease: long-term effects on the risk for myocardial infarction, occurrence of severe angina and the need for revascularization, *J Am Coll Cardiol* 18:1587-1593, 1991.

Warram JH et al: Excess mortality associated with diuretic therapy in diabetes mellitus, *Arch Intern Med* 151:1350-1566, 1991.

Weinberger MH: Hypertension in the elderly, *Hosp Pract* 27:103-120, 1992.

Whelan AM et al: The effect of aspirin on niacin-induced cutaneous reactions, *J Fam Pract* 34:165-168, 1992.

Willcox SM, Himmelstein DU, Woolhandler S: Inappropriate drug prescribing for the community-dwelling elderly, *JAMA* 272(4):292-295, 1994.

Winter M: *Basic clinical pharmaco-kinetics,* ed 2, Vancouver, Wash, 1988, Applied Therapeutics.

Wooley D: Peripheral vascular disease. In Ham RJ, Sloane PD, editors: *Primary care geriatrics: a case-based approach,* ed 2, St Louis, 1992, Mosby.

Yao Y et al: Prevalence of vitamin B_{12} deficiency among geriatric outpatients, *J Fam Pract* 35:524-528, 1992.

Yassa R, Nair NP: A 10 year follow-up study of tardive dyskinesia, *Acta Psychiatr Scand* 86:262-266, 1992.

Zarembski DG et al: Treatment of resistant atrial fibrillation, *Arch Intern Med* 155:1885-1891, 1995.

Zisselman MH et al: Sedative-hypnotic use and increased hospital stay and costs in older people, *J Am Geriatr Soc* 44:1371-1374, 1996.

Zuccala G et al: Use of calcium antagonists and need for perioperative transfusion in older patients with hip fracture: observational study, *Br Med J* 314:643-644, 1997.

6

Aging Skin

The skin of an old person serves as a window through which the body reveals much of its internal pathology. As part of comprehensive health care, providers should be encouraged to be attentive to the skin of their older patients.

People age at different rates, depending on a host of factors. Many older adults view skin problems as a normal consequence of the aging process and thus hesitate to mention them to their provider, even when they cause considerable discomfort or anxiety (Kaminer and Gilchrest, 1994). This reticence must be considered and addressed by providers. In a study of 68 noninstitutionalized volunteers ages 50 to 91, none of whom had ever consulted a dermatologist, two thirds had medical concerns about their skin. Of those age 70 to 80, 83% complained of cutaneous problems. On examination, all subjects had at least one abnormal skin finding, and almost two thirds had a clinically significant cutaneous abnormality. These abnormal findings did not include what are referred to as the normal intrinsic changes of aging or the chronic exposure to sun (photoaging) that occurs as a result of a long life. The investigators indicated that this high prevalence of previously unrecognized symptomatic skin disease is virtually identical to that recorded for the 65- to 74-year-old cohort in the most recent federal Health and Nutrition Examination Survey of more than 20,000 Americans. This sends an overdue message to providers that asking the older person about skin problems and changes in pigmentation, particularly in areas that are covered by clothing, is essential. This point cannot be overemphasized. Asking these questions may assist in a diagnosis and or prevent an exacerbation of another disease. This chapter's purpose is to provide practitioners with a guide to assess and treat the integument of an older person.

Normal Skin and Age-related Changes

The human skin is composed of three layers: epidermis, dermis, and subcutaneous. These layers are a protective barrier between the body and the environment. The epidermis is the outer visible covering that reveals the physical changes of aging. The dermis and subcutaneous layer contain blood vessels and glands that provide pigmentation,

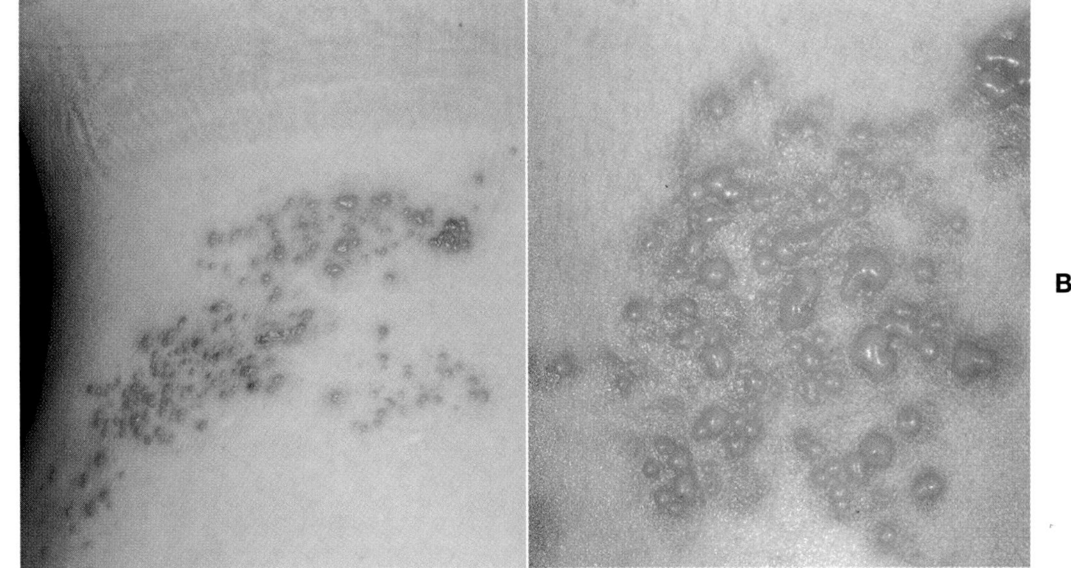

Figure 6-1 Herpes zoster. A, A common presentation with involvement of a single thoracic dermatome. B, A group of vesicles that vary in size. Vesicles of herpes simplex are a uniform size. (From Habif TP: *Clinical dermatology: a color guide to diagnosis and therapy,* ed 3, St Louis, 1996, Mosby.)

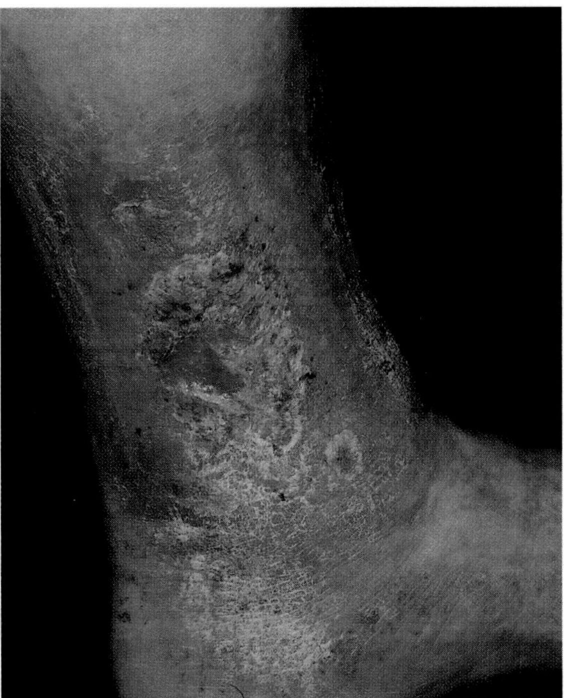

Figure 6-2 Venous stasis ulcer. (From Habif TP: *Clinical dermatology: a color guide to diagnosis and therapy,* ed 3, St Louis, 1996, Mosby.)

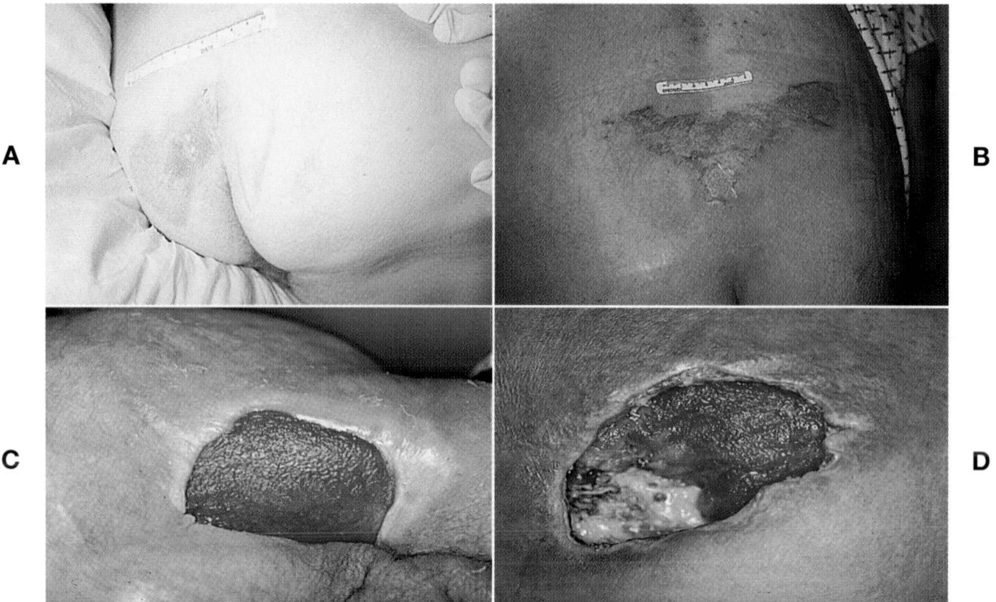

Figure 6-3 A, Stage I pressure ulcer. B, Stage II pressure ulcer. C, Stage III pressure ulcer. D, Stage IV pressure ulcer. (Courtesy Laurel Wiersema-Bryant, RN, MSN, Clinical Nurse Specialist, Barnes Hospital, St Louis. In Potter PA, Perry AG: *Basic nursing: a critical thinking approach,* ed 4, St Louis, 1999, Mosby.)

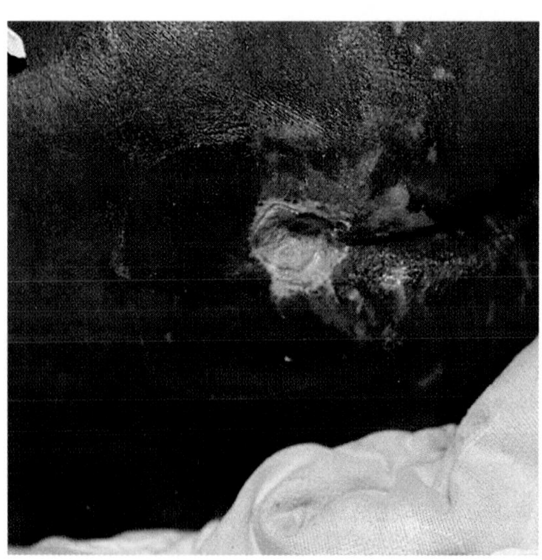

Figure 6-4 Pressure ulcer with tissue necrosis. (From Potter PA, Perry AG: *Basic nursing: a critical thinking approach,* ed 4, St Louis, 1999, Mosby.)

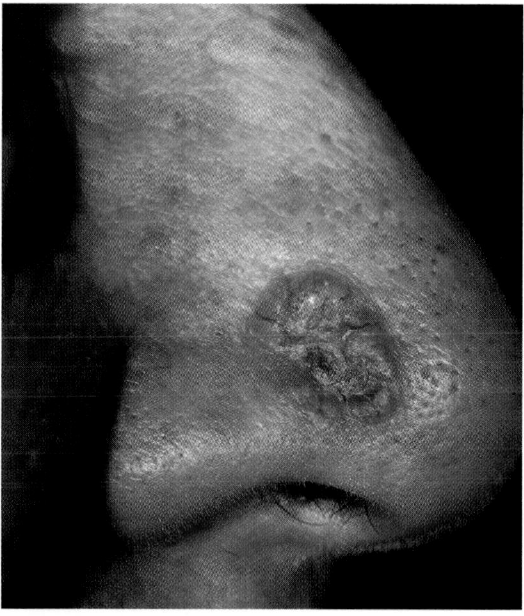

Figure 6-5 Basal cell carcinoma. (From Habif TP: *Clinical dermatology: a color guide to diagnosis and therapy,* ed 3, St Louis, 1996, Mosby.)

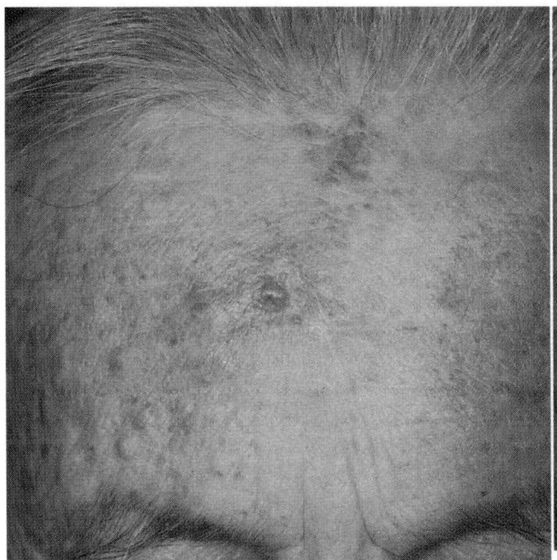

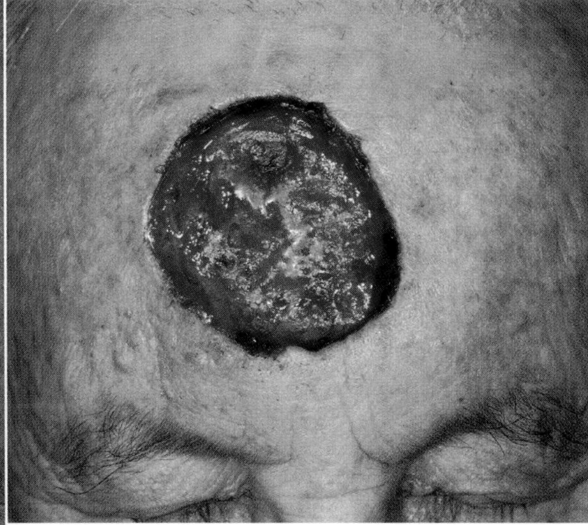

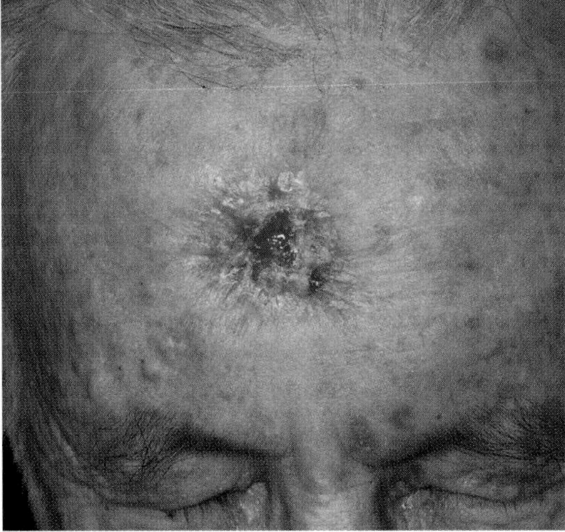

Figure 6-6 Basal cell carcinoma before (**A**), immediately after surgery (**B**), and 6 weeks after surgery using Mohs' micrographic surgical technique (**C**). (From Habif TP: *Clinical dermatology: a color guide to diagnosis and therapy,* ed 3, St Louis, 1996, Mosby.)

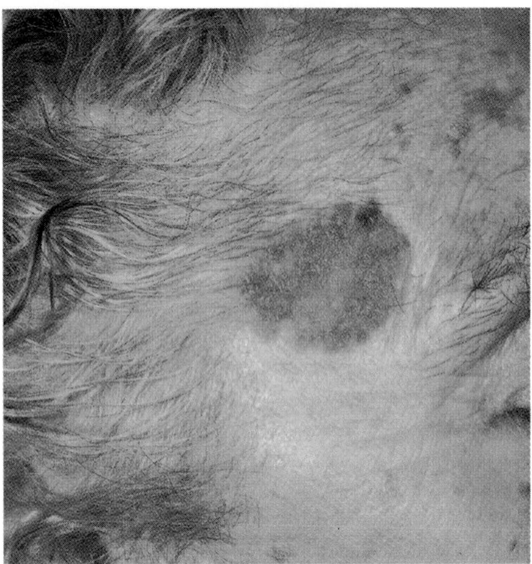

Figure 6-7 Seborrheic keratosis. (From Habif TP: *Clinical dermatology: a color guide to diagnosis and therapy,* ed 3, St Louis, 1996, Mosby.)

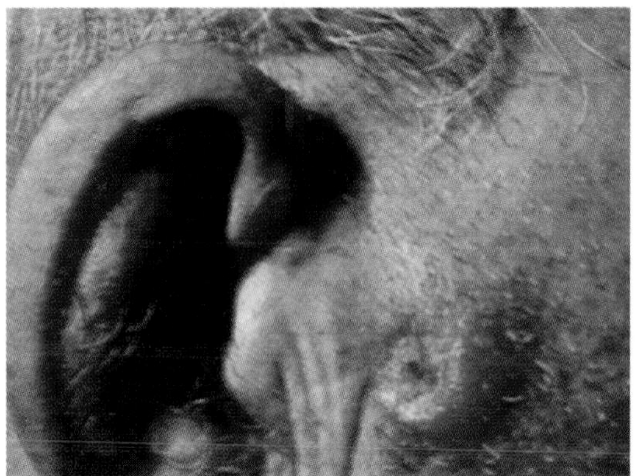

Figure 6-8 Squamous cell carcinoma. (Courtesy Gary Monheit, MD, University of Alabama at Birmingham School of Medicine.)

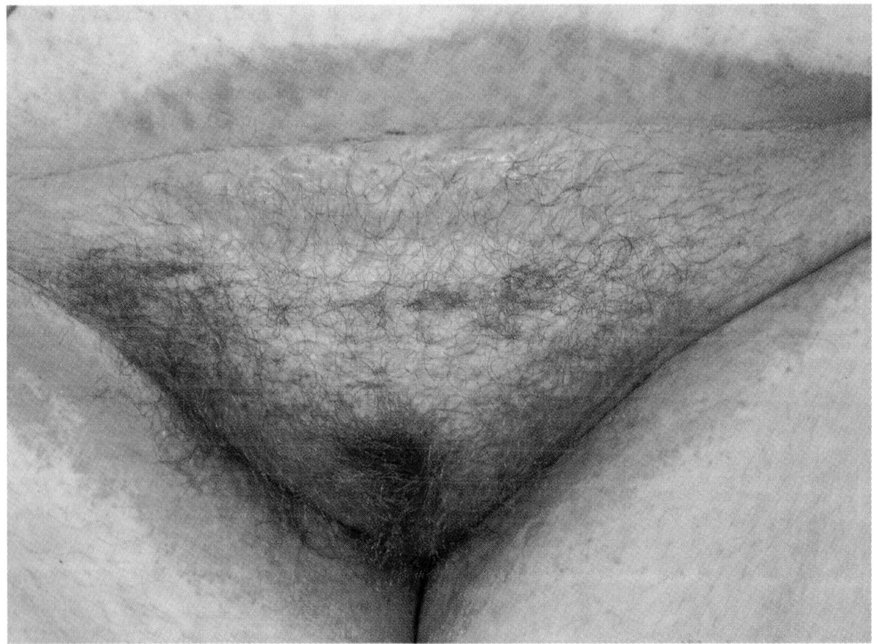

Figure 6-9 Candida intertrigo. (From Habif TP: *Clinical dermatology: a color guide to diagnosis and therapy,* ed 3, St Louis, 1996, Mosby.)

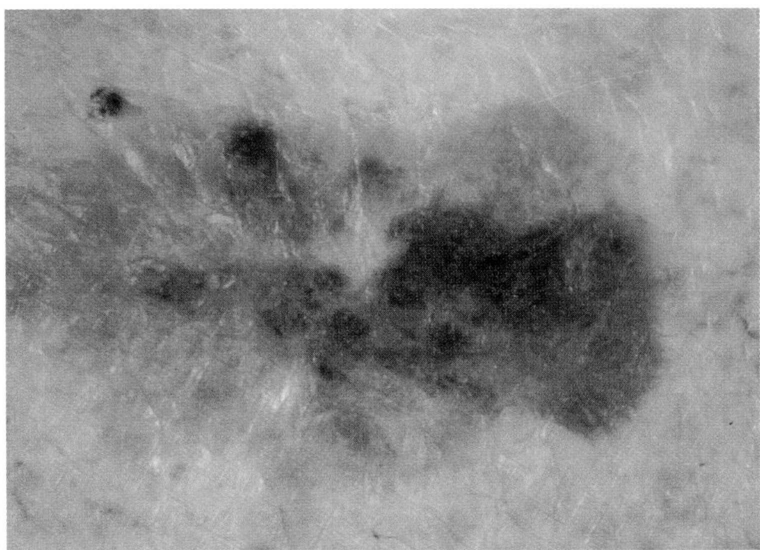

Figure 6-10 Lentigo malignant melanoma. (From Habif TP: *Clinical dermatology: a color guide to diagnosis and therapy,* ed 3, St Louis, 1996, Mosby.)

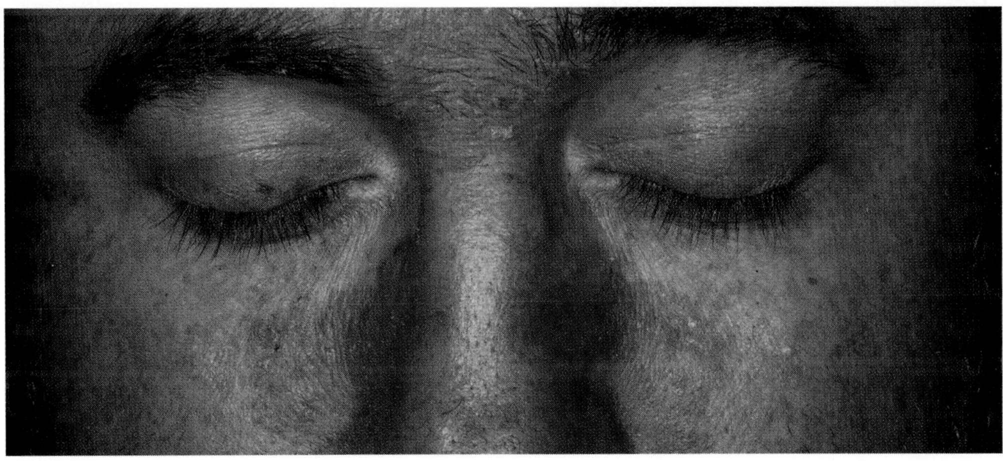

Figure 6-11 Seborrheic dermatitis. (From Habif TP: *Clinical dermatology: a color guide to diagnosis and therapy,* ed 3, St Louis, 1996, Mosby.)

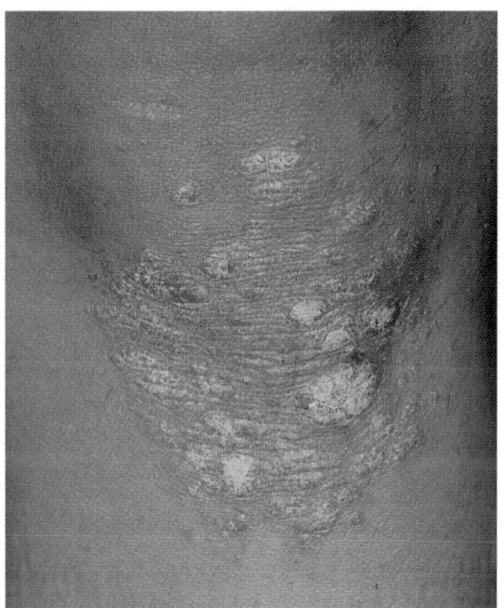

Figure 6-12 Psoriasis. (From Habif TP: *Clinical dermatology: a color guide to diagnosis and therapy,* ed 3, St Louis, 1996, Mosby.)

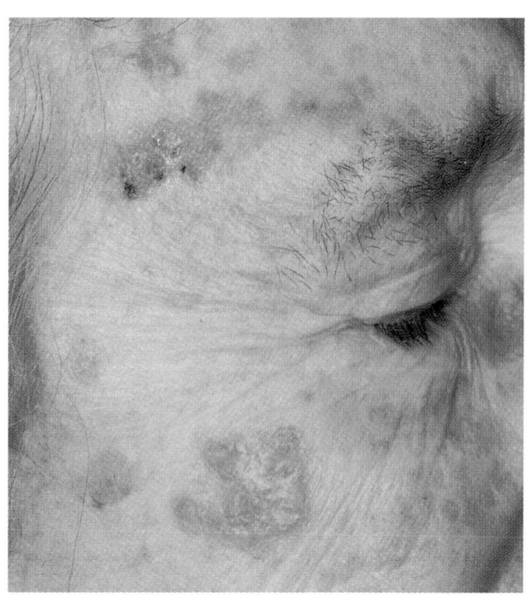

Figure 6-13 Actinic keratosis. (From Habif TP: *Clinical dermatology: a color guide to diagnosis and therapy,* ed 3, St Louis, 1996, Mosby.)

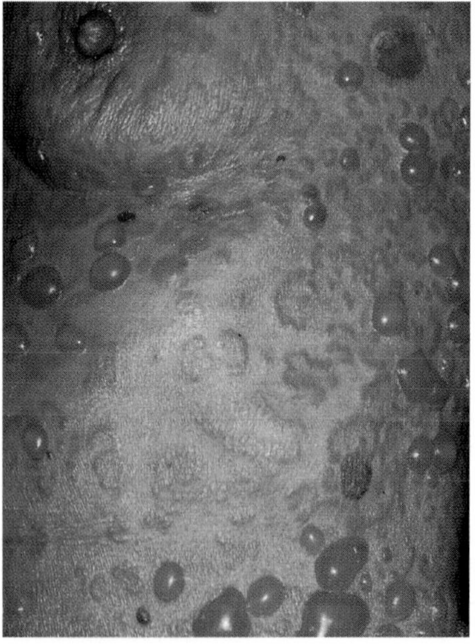

Figure 6-14 Bullous pemphigoid. Generalized eruption with tense blisters arising from an edematous, erythematous annular base. (From Habif TP: *Clinical dermatology: a color guide to diagnosis and therapy,* ed 3, St Louis, 1996, Mosby.)

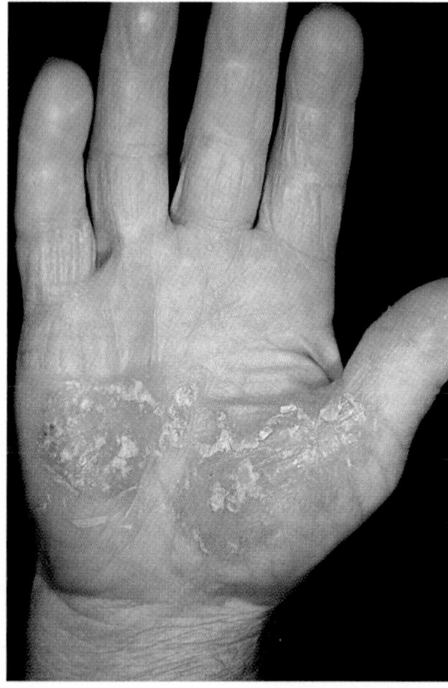

Figure 6-15 Subacute eczematous inflammation. Acute vesicular eczema has evolved into subacute eczema with redness and scaling. (From Habif TP: *Clinical dermatology: a color guide to diagnosis and therapy,* ed 3, St Louis, 1996, Mosby.)

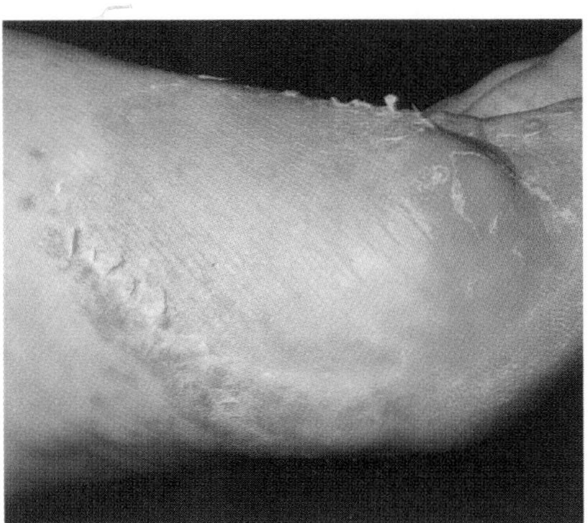

Figure 6-16 Tinea infection. Active border, which contains vesicles that indicate acute inflammation. (From Habif TP: *Clinical dermatology: a color guide to diagnosis and therapy,* ed 3, St Louis, 1996, Mosby.)

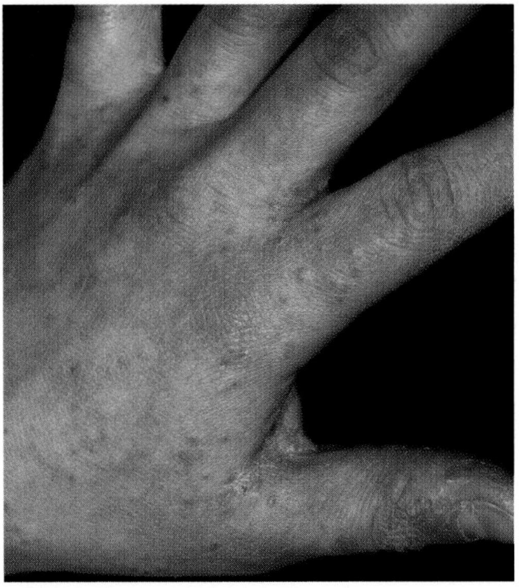

Figure 6-17 Scabies. Tiny vesicles and papules in the finger webs and back of the hand. (From Habif TP: *Clinical dermatology: a color guide to diagnosis and therapy,* ed 3, St Louis, 1996, Mosby.)

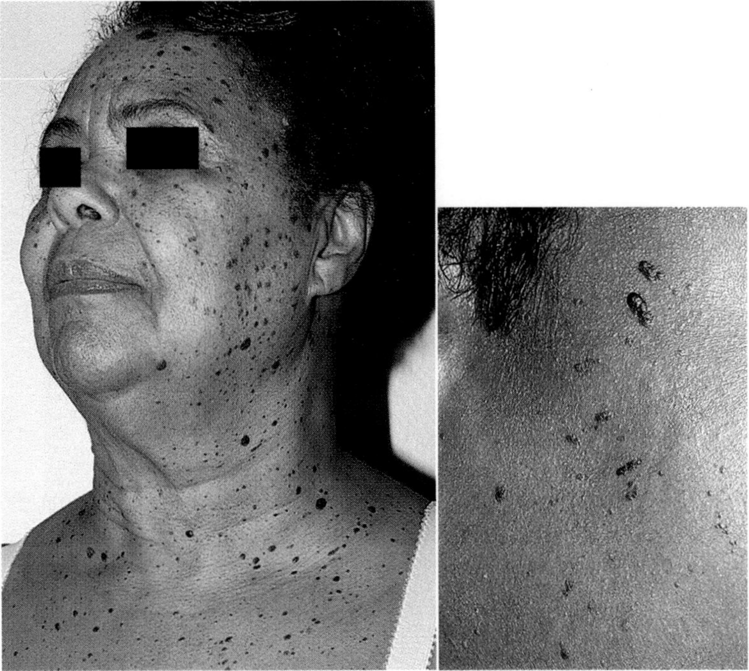

Figure 6-18 Dermatosis papulosa nigra. (From Johnson BL, Moy RL, White GM: *Ethnic skin: medical and surgical,* St Louis, 1998, Mosby.)

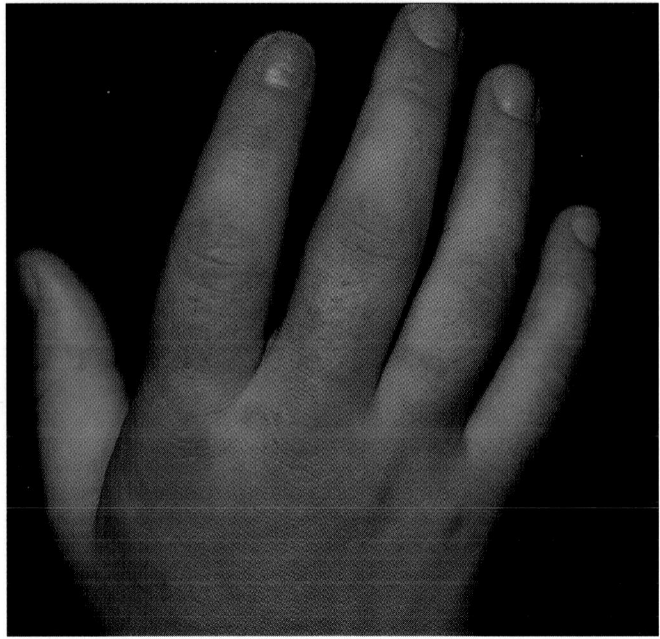

Figure 6-19 Erysipeloid. Approximately 3 days after animal or fish contact, a dull red erythema appears at the inoculation site and extends centrifugally. (From Habif TP: *Clinical dermatology: a color guide to diagnosis and therapy,* ed 3, St Louis, 1996, Mosby.)

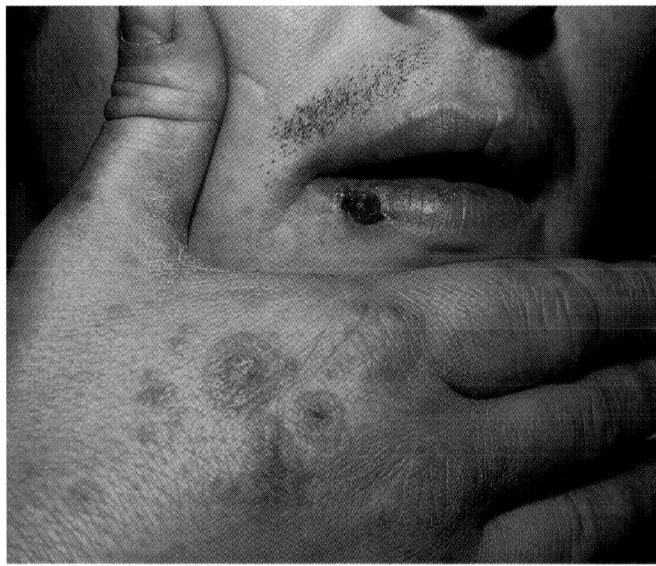

Figure 6-20 Erythema multiforme. An episode may be precipitated by herpes simplex infection. (From Habif TP: *Clinical dermatology: a color guide to diagnosis and therapy,* ed 3, St Louis, 1996, Mosby.)

TABLE 6-1 Functions of the Skin

Skin Function	Mechanism
Protection	Intact skin covering creates a physical barrier against bacteria, minor physical trauma, and foreign substances
Synthesis of keratin	Keratinocytes are produced in the basal layer, develop, and then move to the surface of the skin
Excretion of wastes	Sweat, sodium chloride, urea, and lactic acid are excreted through the skin
Blood pressure regulation	Skin blood vessels can constrict, which promotes venous return and increases the cardiac output and blood pressure
Fluid regulation	Skin keeps fluids contained in the body
Temperature regulation	Skin blood vessels can (1) dilate to promote heat loss or to prevent tissue freezing (radiation), (2) constrict to conserve heat, or (3) regulate temperature by conduction, convection, and evaporation
Tissue repair	Skin replaces damaged skin cells and forms scar tissue
Production of vitamin D	In the presence of ultraviolet light, a precursor of vitamin D is converted to vitamin D in the skin
Sensory perception	Special sensors in the skin respond to touch, pain, heat, cold, pressure, vibration, tickling, itching, wetness, oiliness, and stickiness
Expression of emotional feelings	Surface of the skin can respond to emotions through sweating, pallor, or flushing

From Burke MM and Walsh MB: *Gerontologic nursing: wholistic care of the older adult,* ed 2, St Louis, 1997, Mosby.

insulation, and protection of the underlying organs (Burke and Walsh, 1997). Table 6-1 outlines the multiple functions of the skin.

Changes in appearance and function over time are termed *intrinsic aging.* In most people, the majority of unwanted changes are due not to aging alone but to a combination of aging and chronic environmental damage, largely sun exposure. The epidermis, dermis, subcutaneous fat, and appendages all change during the life of a person. Table 6-2 shows the age-related changes that occur with intrinsic aging.

Epidermis

The epidermis, the most evident and superficial compartment, serves as the major interface with the external environment. Made up largely of keratinocytes, which are the major barrier cells to chemical and microbial insults, the epidermis undergoes periodic turnover (characteristically 28 days) to shed old insulted cells and replace them. This turnover time is reduced by 50% between the third and eighth decades. This change can affect wound healing and causes drying of the epidermis (Lavken and Sun, 1982). Vitamin D synthesis is a major function of the epidermis and keratinocytes, and it is significantly decreased in aged skin. This problem can be easily addressed if pursued by providers.

Melanocytes and Langerhans' cells comprise the other epidermal cell type. Melanin determines skin color and tanning capacity and is the skin's major protection against

TABLE 6-2 Skin Changes Associated with Intrinsic Aging

Compartment	Component	Change	Biologic Consequence
Epidermis	Keratinocytes	Decreased proliferative potential	↓ Wound healing, ↓ vitamin D production
	Melanocytes	Decreased 10%-20% per decade	↓ Photoprotection, white hairs
	Langerhans' cells	Decreased as much as 40%	↓ Delayed hypersensitivity reactions
	Basement membrane	Decreased surface area	↓ Epidermal-dermal adhesion, ↑ blistering
Dermis	Fibroblasts	Decreased collagen/elastin	↓ Tensile strength, ↓ elasticity
	Blood vessels	Decreased	↓ Thermoregulation, ↓ response to injury
	Mast cells	Decreased	↓ Immediate hypersensitivity reactions
	Neural elements	Decreased by one third	↓ Sensation, ↑ pain threshold
Subcutis	Fat	Decreased	↓ Mechanical protection and insulation
Appendages	Eccrine glands	Decreased number and output	↓ Thermoregulation
	Apocrine glands	Decreased number and output	Unknown
	Sebaceous glands	Increased size, decreased output	Unknown
	Hair	Decreased number and growth rate	Cosmetic

From Hazzard WR et al: Principles of geriatric medicine and gerontology, ed 3, New York, 1994, McGraw-Hill.

damaging solar radiation. The number of enzymatically active melanocytes decreases by 10% to 20% each decade in both sun-protected and sun-exposed skin. Photosensitivity increases as the number of melanocytes declines. Loss of melanocytes results in graying hair and, coupled with a reduced capillary blood supply, fading normal skin color.

Langerhans' cells are derived from the bone marrow and are distributed diffusely throughout the epidermis. Their dendritic and immunocompetent capacities contribute to antigen recognition and presentation. In the aged skin Langerhans' cells are reduced by about 40%. This loss is believed to account for the observed age-associated decrease in delayed hypersensitivity. In sun-exposed skin, there is a greater loss of Langerhans' cells. Organisms have a greater chance of invading the body through the skin (Kaminer and Gilchrest, 1994).

Dermis

Age-related changes in the dermis are numerous. The dermis, largely connective tissue, is inhabited by blood vessels, lymphatics, and multiple cellular components. It is involved in thermoregulation and the inflammatory response, as well as delivery of nutrients and oxygen to the skin. A 20% loss in dermal thickness occurs with aging, which often leads to the paper-thin or transparent skin appearance in older adults. In addition, the remaining dermis is relatively acellular and avascular, which interferes with its temperature-regulating capacity. This change predisposes older people to hypothermia and heat stroke during temperature extremes. With the decreased vascular supply (50% decrease in mast cells), there is a diminished response to cutaneous hypersensitivity reactions. These muted inflammatory reactions often fail to alert the physician or the patient to the need for intervention and therapy. These changes delay wound healing, which may be further compromised many times by the multiple chronic illnesses of an older adult.

Subcutaneous Layer

The subcutaneous layer is composed of loose connective tissue, fat cells, and glands. Its main functions are to provide heat, insulation, and caloric reserves and to act as a shock absorber (Sparks, 1997). Atrophy in this layer results in a reduction of many of these functions and primarily affects the face, extremities, hands, and soles of the feet. Because of the loss of the shock absorber quality of the subcutaneous tissue, skin becomes more susceptible to trauma, particularly the soles of the feet. This change increases the trauma of walking and magnifies the many foot problems experienced by older people (Hogstel, 1989).

The cutaneous appendages are composed of eccrine, apocrine, and pilosebaceous units, which are hair follicles and sebaceous glands. The eccrine, or sweat, glands decrease with age, and apocrine glands in humans cause the characteristic odor associated with sweating. Sebaceous glands are found everywhere on the body with the exception of the palms, soles, and proximal nail folds. They secret sebum, a lipid-rich substance that decreases by 40% to 60% in the older adult. The function of sebum and its clinical implications are as yet unknown (Kaminer and Gilchrest, 1994).

Aging is associated with a gradual decrease in the number of hair follicles, as well as a decrease in their growth rate. The hair of older people is sparse and thin, and it fails to grow with the same rapidity of a younger person. Loss of hair color and graying are also common because of the decrease in melanocytes. The nails thicken, develop longitudinal lines, and also have a decreased growth rate (Sparks, 1997).

Environmental Effects on Skin

Environmental damage to the skin is largely due to sun exposure. Photoaging describes many of these preventable changes. Each individual is affected differently by the sun, and varied chemical changes within the skin take place.

Photoaging

Photoaging consists of those changes in cutaneous appearance and function that are a direct result of repeated sun exposure superimposed on intrinsic aging. Although many providers and patients perceive no difference between them, photoaging and chronologic aging are two distinct entities. This point must be made clear, since it is estimated that more than 90% of cosmetically undesirable skin changes in older people are due to photoaging, and more than 90% of skin cancer arises in chronically sun-exposed (photoaged) vs. sun-protected skin. Photoaged skin appears wrinkled and leathery, yellowing, and coarse, with telangiectasia, atrophy, easy bruising, and various premalignant neoplasms, as well as basal and squamous cell carcinomas (Kurban and Kurban, 1993).

The skin of older patients must be carefully assessed, and its protective aspects guarded. Although many of the intrinsic changes associated with aging cannot be diminished, many of their negative implications can be prevented if properly assessed by the provider. The changes associated with photoaging, particularly the high incidence of basal and squamous cell carcinomas, can be prevented. Many older people do not refer to their skin as problematic because they have come to accept their age and never critically see change. The provider needs to be conscious of this first organ that is seen.

More than 60% of older people are estimated to have a skin problem. The common manifestations of skin disorders in the elderly follow.

Common Skin Disorders

As a person ages, neoplasms and infections are more prevalent. The disorders reviewed here address those found most commonly in the elderly population, but they are not exclusive to them.

Benign Neoplasms

Seborrheic keratoses are commonly found on sun-exposed skin. They appear as waxy, warty, greasy papules that have a "stuck-on" appearance. The color may vary from a flesh color to a darker brown. These lesions are most commonly found on the trunk, scalp, neck, extremities, and face. Size varies from a few millimeters up to 5 cm. The etiology is not well known; however, a hereditary component is common in up to 50% of cases. Dermatosis papulosa nigra is a subtype of seborrhea found most commonly in older adults of African heritage. They appear on the face as dark papules that are sometimes pedunculated.

Treatment is usually light cautery or curettage. Another option is liquid nitrogen. Appearing most often in the older adult, usually beginning in the early 50s, seborrheic keratoses are benign and removed for cosmetic purposes.

Acrochordons or skin tags are papillomas that are benign. They appear most often in the middle-aged and elderly and are commonly found on the neck, axillae, and trunk. Treatment is usually scalpel removal or electrocautery.

Keratoacanthomas appear as nodules that enlarge rapidly. They have a keratin center, and the outline is smooth. Treatment is sometimes not necessary as they may resolve on their own. They are often confused with squamous cell carcinoma. Although benign, treatment is based on diagnosis of a well-differentiated squamous cell carcinoma. Removal is performed by scalpel, curettage, or cautery.

Premalignant Conditions

Actinickeratoses appear as raised, rough lesions that may range in color from a light tan to dark brown, well-defined patches. Mild to moderate erythema may also be present. If the practitioner is doubtful of the assessment, a skin biopsy is appropriate because the lesions may develop into squamous cell carcinoma. The location is the sun-exposed areas of the skin. Thus, treatment and prevention involve avoidance of sun and use of sunscreen with a high sun protection factor (SPF).

Treatment is cryotherapy with liquid nitrogen or curettage; 5-fluorouracil (5-FU) is also used in varying percentages, 1% to 2% for facial lesions and up to 5% for truncal lesions. Initially, erythema and burning occur, leading to ulceration in 2 to 4 weeks. Finally, vesiculation leads to ulceration and reepithelialization. This process takes up to 2 months, and the use of cream is stopped on ulceration. If no results are seen with 5-FU alone, combination therapy with tretinoin cream is used on more resistant cases.

Bowen's disease is a chronic, scaly, erythematous plaque with well-defined margins. These plaques can occur in mucous membranes or anywhere else on the body. Often the patient's history includes arsenic exposure as a youth. Close monitoring is mandated because multiple lesions are associated with an increased incidence of internal malignancies. Treatment is with liquid nitrogen or curettage and cautery. Radiotherapy has been used; however, full-tumor doses are required.

Malignant Skin Conditions

Malignant skin conditions, for example, basal and squamous cell carcinomas, are common to the geriatric population. Factors such as sunlight, UV exposure, radiation, and carcinogenic chemicals predispose individuals to such conditions (Box 6-1).

Basal cell carcinoma (BCC) develops from the basal layer of the epidermis. It usually has a pearly appearance and is characterized as a firm nodule with rolled edges and an umbilicated center.

It occurs most often in those with freckled, fair, or ruddy skin and is the most common of all cancers, including skin cancer. Occasionally, BCC is confused with malignant melanoma.

Box 6-1

Risk Factors for Skin Cancer

Overexposure to frost, wind, and UV radiation from the sun
Occupational exposure to radiation
Chemical carcinogen exposure
Genetic predisposition
Thermal burn scars
Chronic trauma and irritation to an area
X-ray therapy
Skin that is fair, ruddy, freckled, light hair or eyes; skin that burns easily
Precancerous skin lesions
Age over 50
Indoor occupation with blasts of outdoor recreation
History of severe sunburn before age 18

From Mayfield P: Skin. In Hogstel MO, editor: *Clinical manual of gerontological nursing*, St Louis, 1992, Mosby.

The warning signs for BCC are as follows:

A sore that lasts for 3 weeks or more
An irritated, reddened area that may be itchy or painful
A smooth growth with an elevated, shiny border
A pearly or translucent nodule resembling a mole
A white or yellow lesion that resembles scar tissue (Mayfield, 1992)

Before treatment for BCC, histologic confirmation is done. The biopsy techniques can be shave, punch, or excisional, depending on tumor size, tissue involvement, and location. Treatment of BCC is dependent on the carcinoma's size, level of invasion, and patient history. Curettage and cauterization are used to treat small tumors. The procedure is usually repeated to ensure complete removal. Cryotherapy is also used as an effective treatment for small tumors. Other treatment methods include complete excision and Mohs' cryosurgery for recurrent and high-risk BCC. If surgery is not an option, a common circumstance in the elderly, radiotherapy is an option. Another alternative is topical 5-FU, which is used only on superficial lesions, especially when they present as numerous tumors. Unfortunately, there is a high recurrence, warranting close follow-up. All BCC patients should be monitored for recurrence or new lesions for 5 years.

Like BCC, squamous cell carcinoma (SCC) usually presents on sun-damaged skin. It is the second most common skin cancer in white adults. It develops from the squamous epithelium and affects areas of chronic inflammation or chronic ulceration, such as the lower extremities. Venous stasis ulcers, systemic lupus erythematosus, and lupus vulgaris are often associated with SCC lesions. Initially the area affected becomes erythematous and indurated, causing the overlying layer to become hyperkeratotic or scaly, leading to ulceration. Unlike the translucent BCC nodule, SCC lesions present as opaque nodules. The carcinoma may appear as a red nodule with a rough, scaly nodule. Sometimes, an ulcerated nodular mass occurs. Risk factors for SCC are a high occurrence of actinic keratoses, which are considered to be a premalignant form of SCC. Other factors include exposure to chemicals such as coal, pitch, asphalt, tar, soot, and creosote, all carcinogenic. There is a risk of metastases, depending on the tumor etiology. Lesions found on mucocutaneous junctions are most likely to metastasize (Abrams et al., 1995).

Like BCC, SCC is treated initially by punch or incisional biopsy methods to confirm the diagnosis. Once it is confirmed, surgical excision involving at least 5 mm beyond the tumor's edges is used. Other methods include cryotherapy for small tumors and radiotherapy for poorly defined tumors.

Malignant melanoma is a malignant neoplasm of pigmented cells called melanocytes. There are different types of melanoma nodules. The etiology is unclear: however, sun exposure is thought to be a major contributing factor, especially a blistering sunburn before age 18. This trauma is believed to damage the Langerhans' cells, affecting the cells' immune response. Malignant melanomas often occur in preexisting moles; a smaller portion of melanomas are seen in new moles. Thus any change in existing moles or the appearance of a new mole, especially after age 40, warrants careful examination (Box 6-2).

Lentigo maligna (Hutchinson's freckle) presents as a pigmented macular lesion, usually less than 1 cm in diameter. It has an irregular border and is found on sun-exposed areas of the skin (face, neck, hands). One lesion may have areas varying in color among

Box 6-2

Assessment Tool to Identify Moles at Risk of Developing into Malignant Conditions

The ABCD Rule

A. Asymmetry: One half does not match the other half
B. Border irregularity: Ragged, notched, or blurred edges
C. Color: Not uniform in color, with differing shades of color such as brown, black, or a mottling of red, white or blue
D. Diameter: A diameter greater than 6 mm or an increase in size

Data from McGovern M, Kwaiser-Kuhn J: Skin assessment of the elderly client, *Journal of Gerontological Nursing* 18(4):39-43, 1992.

brown, black, red, and white. Over time, lentigo maligna enlarges, and pigmentation becomes irregular. Approximately 5% to 7% of melanomas are lentigo maligna. It is referred to as a freckle because it presents in those over age 60 as a tan flat lesion that gradually changes in size and color.

Treatment of lentigo maligna often involves a wide local incision, including a skin flap or skin graft. As with all melanoma patients, careful and routine follow-up is essential to detect any other areas of suspicion (bleeding moles, pigmentation changes).

Superficial spreading melanoma is the most common type of melanoma, accounting for approximately 65% to 75% of all melanomas. This melanoma spreads horizontally and peaks in middle age. It occurs on any area of the body and usually presents as a pigmented plaque with varying pigmentation and an irregular border. They are common to other melanomas because it is usually asymptomatic. If bleeding or pruritus is seen, the lesion is likely to be in an advanced stage. Treatment is discussed under nodular melanoma.

Nodular melanoma accounts for 20% of all melanomas. It occurs in a multitude of patients and is found on any body site. Presentation is usually a vertically growing lesion with dark pigmentation. It can be seen as amelanotic (pink); however, this is rare.

Treatment for superficial spreading and nodular melanoma involves an excisional or incisional biopsy for histologic interpretation. On diagnosis, referral to an experienced physician is needed for proper management. Further treatment involves excision with 1- to 3-cm margins, depending on the histologic diagnosis. Lymphadenectomy for prophylactic purposes has shown little, if any, benefit. Other treatment options include an isolated limb perfusion with chemotherapy or immunotherapy (interleukins, interferons). Table 6-3 describes the prognosis for melanomas of various depths.

Kaposi's sarcoma presents as an indolent tumor in the elderly of European origin, most often those of Jewish or Italian ancestry. It is also common in patients with acquired immunodeficiency syndrome (AIDS); however, the AIDS-related tumor is the lymphadenopathic form and is associated with a poor prognosis. Appearance is usually a dark blue or purple macula that gradually becomes a nodule or ulcer. Upon histologic examination, these cells are of endothelial origin, proliferating vessels, and connective tissue. Treatment is usually either simple excision or radiotherapy, if symptomatic. Among the elderly, this tumor often grows slowly and is benign.

TABLE 6-3 Prognosis for Patients with Melanoma

Melanoma Depth	Prognosis
<0.85 mm	Highly curable; 99% of patients disease free at 8 yr
0.85-1.69 mm	Low metastatic risk; 93% of patients disease free at 8 yr
1.7-3.64 mm	Moderate metastatic risk; 67% of patients disease free at 8 yr
>3.65 mm	High metastatic risk; 35% of patients disease free at 8 yr

Benign Skin Conditions

Pruritus

A common complaint among the elderly is itching. A thorough examination for skin lesions should be performed. In addition, systemic disorders involving the liver or kidneys and diagnoses such as leukemia, iron-deficiency anemia, lymphoma, and polycythemia rubra vera may cause severe itching. A review of the drugs the patient takes may reveal side effects of itching. Although underlying conditions are often not the cause of the pruritus, a research study has shown that almost half the patients presenting with a chief complaint of pruritus did have an underlying condition (Kaminer and Gilchrest, 1994). Another fact to consider is that the dry, scaly skin common to the elder is very itchy.

Treatment for the patient who does not have an obvious skin lesion involves screening, such as a complete blood count, erythrocyte sedimentation rate, electrolyte and urea levels, and liver function tests. Tests for the presence of glucose in the urine and, if warranted, guaiac stools, should be performed. If symptoms are unresponsive to treatment, abrupt in onset, and severe, thorough examination and evaluation is necessary.

Xerosis

Dry skin is most common in the winter months, usually when humidity decreases indoors secondary to heating. Also, exposure to outdoor cold and windy conditions contributes to xerosis. The skin appears scaly, and the areas most involved are the hands, lower legs, and forearms. The process begins when the stratum corneum barrier is compromised by fissure or excoriations that expose this layer to environmental irritants.

Treatment includes home humidification and avoidance of strong soaps, rubbing alcohol, and detergents. Bathing should be kept to a minimum, with mild soap. Avoidance of irritating materials such as wool should also be practiced. Emollients or creams containing lactic acid or urea can be used frequently and liberally, especially following bathing. Petrolatum jelly is an excellent inexpensive option. If a patient's skin is eczematous, a topical corticosteroid ointment with an occlusive dressing is helpful once or twice a day.

Infectious Diseases

Infections in the skin occur more often as a person ages. Aging produces a slower healing process, compromised circulation, edematous extremities, and the overall decline of the skin's immune function. Thus bacterial infections have a greater tendency to develop. Skin infections can be bacterial, fungal, viral, yeast, or parasitic in origin.

Bacterial

Staphylococcal Scalded Skin Syndrome (SSSS). Lyell's syndrome or SSSS is a severe, extensive bullous condition caused by a staphylococcal infection of the skin. The epithelium lifts off in sheets, leaving a large denuded area. It is common in young children and immunocompromised adults. Staphylococci are cultured from the skin or blood. It often leads to septicemia and ultimately death. A differential diagnosis of toxic epidermal necrolysis (TEN) should also be considered. Both diagnoses are life-threatening, and hospitalization is necessary. Differentiation is done by skin biopsy or scraping. The difference is that SSSS presents with cleavage in the epidermis and TEN presents with subepidermal blisters. Patients with SSSS are immediately treated with penicillinase-resistant antistaphylococcal antibiotics. Treatment also includes fluid and electrolyte replacement, topical silver sulfadiazine cream for prevention of cutaneous infection, and systemic antibiotics. Both SSSS and TEN have a poor prognosis. This disorder is further discussed in the section on drug-induced skin reactions.

Erysipelas. Erysipelas is an infection of the skin caused by group A or group C hemolytic streptococci that enter the skin by wounds, insect bites, or minor cuts. Erysipelas presents as an area of erythema and swelling, with lesions having well-defined margins that may spread. Hemorrhage may occur in the elderly, in addition to the vesicles or bullae that can be seen. Development of malaise, lethargy, and lymphadenopathy is not uncommon. Treatment consists of oral erythromycin 250 to 500 mg four times a day for 14 days. If erysipelas is seen on the face, treatment with IV antibiotics is needed because spreading continues for the first 24 to 48 hours and sinus involvement is possible.

Cellulitis. A common occurrence in the elderly, cellulitis is a deep skin infection usually caused by group A streptococci. Gram-negative organisms have been seen. It presents usually as a complication of an open wound or a venous ulcer. Cellulitis may also appear in intact skin, usually a lower extremity that is edematous; however, sites such as the parotid gland have also become involved. The area appears erythematous, warm, tender, and swollen. Lymph involvement is possible. Treatment with oral erythromycin or penicillin 250 to 500 mg four times a day for 14 days is the treatment of choice. Continue to assess the patient for response to therapy.

Fungal

The elderly commonly have fungal infections of the skin, which may be partially related to the decreased immunologic response of the skin as people age. The word *tinea* refers to a fungal class, dermatophytes, that are present in the dead outer layer of the nail beds or stratum corneum (Kaminer and Gilchrest, 1994).

Tinea Pedis. Tinea pedis or athlete's foot is an infection caused by dermatophytes *Trichophyton mentagrophytes* and *T. rubrum*. It usually begins between the toes and spreads to the toenails and plantar surfaces. Patients often complain of itching and scaly skin. Maceration of the interdigital spaces is common. There is a potential for cellulitis development, so careful examination is needed. Diagnosis is done by scrape biopsy and visualizing under a microscope with potassium hydroxide (KOH) solution, which reveals green fungal hyphae.

Treatment is with miconazole or clotrimazole 1% to 2% creams. Several months of application may be needed to prevent recurrence (Kaminer and Gilchrest, 1994). Nail beds are treated with griseofulvin, which can cause gastrointestinal (GI) upset, leukopenia, vertigo, and headaches. Foot care should include full drying of the interdigital spaces, proper footwear, and medicated powder or cotton between the toes for moisture absorption.

Tinea Unguium. This infection is seen on the toenails and occasionally the fingernails and is caused by *T. rubrum* or *T. mentagrophytes*. Nails may appear thickened and enlarged, impeding shoe wearing. Treatment is with griseofulvin 500 to 1000 mg/day for 6 to 9 months for fingernails and 12 to 18 months for toenails. Recurrence is common, especially within the first year. Management such as nail trimming and clipping by podiatry is also recommended.

Tinea Cruris. This is a cutaneous skin infection of the groin commonly seen in the elderly. Patients who are obese, wear nonbreathable clothing, and are immobile are at risk. A common complaint is itching, and examination reveals an erythematous scaly area with well-defined margins. Common complications include maceration, lichenification, and secondary bacterial or candidal infections. Diagnosis is confirmed by KOH smear. Treatment two or three times a day with miconazole cream 2% or clotrimazole 1% to the affected area is recommended. Good hygiene to the area and moisture prevention are important.

Yeast

Candidiasis. The definition of candidiasis is an infection caused by yeast. *Candida albicans,* the responsible microorganism, grows in warm, moist areas, usually the groin, axilla, and below the breasts. This infection is common among those receiving antibiotic therapy, the immunocompromised older adult, and patients with diabetes. Sites such as the vagina, mouth, and bowel may carry this organism asymptomatically, creating sources of reinfection. The three types of *Candida* infections follow.

Candidal Vulvovaginitis. This infection presents as a milky vaginal discharge, with examination revealing vulvar erythema and edema. Patients often complain of vaginal itching. It may also be due to the presence of glycosuria, and testing is encouraged.

Oral Candidiasis. Oral candidiasis or thrush appears on the tongue as white creamy plaques. It is often seen in patients following prolonged use of inhaled glucocorticoids. It can be prevented by gargling with water after treatment or using a spacer connected to the inhaler. It is also seen in those with poorly fitting dentures, those with deep skin folds in that area, and those who are saliva and food retainers. For local irritation to the skin, nystatin or miconazole cream three times a day for a week is helpful.

Intertrigo. This infection is caused by yeast and is seen between two skin folds. It is most frequently between the buttocks, the thighs, or the scrotum and the thigh. Intertrigo appears as a moist, reddened rash that may have some flaky, itchy areas at the creases. Itching is a common complaint. It occurs most commonly in individuals who do not practice adequate personal hygiene, are obese, or wear tight-fitting clothing that does not provide adequate ventilation (Bentz et al, 1996).

Treatment for intertrigo is antifungal creams applied to clean dry skin. Nystatin cream does not work effectively against dermatophytes and thus is not useful for treatment. If inflammation is present, a low-dose corticosteroid cream may be used.

Viral

Herpes Zoster. Herpes zoster is an acute vesicular eruption caused by an infection of the varicella-zoster virus. Shingles or herpes zoster can occur at any age but is most common in those ages 50 to 70. In the elderly postherpetic neuralgia is more common, and the severity and duration are more severe. Pain in the infected area usually precedes the outbreak by 48 hours or more.

The presentation is usually an outbreak of an itchy, annoying-to-painful rash. The lesions are grouped, red vesicles distributed unilaterally along the neural pathway, usually on the trunk. Regional lymph glands may be tender and swollen (Berger, Sanford, and Odon, 1997). The papules turn into vesicles and may become hemorrhagic. This process is painful. Over the next couple of weeks, the vesicles dry, and scarring or hyperpigmentation may occur. An underlying lymphoma or immune disease should be suspected if the vesicles spread outside the dermatome area. Herpes zoster may appear in the eyes again because of nerve root involvement affecting the ophthalmic portion of the trigeminal nerve. An ophthalmologic consult is appropriate; conjunctivitis, iridocyclitis, and keratitis may occur. If the nose tip has a lesion, the nasociliary and ophthalmic nerves are involved. Diagnosis is done by cytologic smear with the appearance of multinucleate giant cells.

Treatment is a high dose of oral acyclovir, 800 mg five times a day for 7 days, to accelerate healing and reduce acute pain. Patients with reduced renal function must be monitored closely, and all patients should be advised to maintain good hydration. Although decreased, the risk of postherpetic neuralgia, a dermatomal pain syndrome, is still possible and occurs in approximately 10% of patients (Burke and Walsh, 1997). Pain medication such as acetaminophen (Tylenol) around the clock is usually sufficient in the elderly; opiate usage should be avoided because of medication errors and potential side effects (Abrams, Beers, and Berkow, 1995). Treatment for the vesicles is Burow's solution, an aluminum acetate solution diluted 1:20 or 1:40 for external use (Abrams, Beers, and Berkow, 1995), or a topical cream with capsaicin, which alleviates pain (Burke and Walsh, 1997). Usually after 2 to 3 weeks, the patient has completely recovered and returned to normal function.

Parasitic

Scabies. Scabies is an eruption caused by a mite, the *Sarcoptes scabiei* var hominis, specifically. The female mite deposits eggs beneath the skin, and they hatch into larvae in days. Transmission is skin-to-skin contact, especially among those living together (families, nursing homes, shelters). It is important to inquire about other household members and animal contact in the history.

The chief complaint is usually unrelenting pruritus, usually at night. The skin is excoriated, and the telltale sign of the burrow mark is from the mite. It appears as a linear ridge, and the mite is usually at one end, where a vesicle is also located. Areas commonly affected include the interdigital webs, umbilicus, wrists (especially the flexor aspect), genitalia, buttocks, and areola. Erythematous nodules or papules in these areas are also common. Among the elderly scabies is sometimes confused with eczema or exfoliative dermatitis because of the presence of crusted lesions. Evaluation for erythroderma or a generalized lymphadenopathy should be done, especially if scabies goes undetected for a prolonged period.

Examination of the mite under a microscope is possible by removing the mite with a scalpel. However, it is often difficult to locate one, especially if the area is widespread. Presumptive diagnosis is often the best option.

Treatment with permethrin 5% cream is the first-line choice. Lindane (Kwell) wasformerly the choice for treatment; however, resistance and neurotoxicity have downgraded it to an alternative treatment. It is important to apply the cream to the entire body, from neck down. Thorough application is important, and assistance is recommended. This treatment kills the mite and ova, but the burrow and its sensitization remain until the skin naturally sheds. Reapplication 1 to 2 weeks apart may be needed. Treatment of all household members is recommended. Prevention of reinfestation by washing bed linens and underwear in hot water is usually effective.

Pediculosis (Lice). Lice affect different areas: the body, the head, or the genitals. The problem is caused by different organisms. It is often seen among the elderly who practice poor hygiene or live in an overcrowded environment. Grandparents with school-age grandchildren may also be affected by outbreaks in schools. Lice are wingless, dorsoventrally flattened, blood-sucking insects.

Pediculosis capitis, head lice, can be transmitted by hairbrushes, hair accessories, and close contact. Scalp itching is seen usually in conjunction with secondary eczematous and impetiginization. Small, gray-white ova (nits) are present on examination. The occipital portion of the scalp and sometimes the postauricular area are affected.

Pediculosis corporis (body lice) are responsible for generalized itching. Bacterial infections, eczematous changes, and excoriated areas are often a consequence of body lice. The seams of the patient's clothing can be inspected for nits.

Pediculosis pubis is caused by the crab louse and is sexually transmitted. Transmission by towels or clothing is possible but unlikely. Inspection of the pubic hair is necessary. However, the eyelashes, leg hairs, axillae, and chest hairs may also be involved.

Treatment for head lice is a permethrin 1% cream rinse applied to the hair, left on for 10 minutes, and rinsed. Lindane shampoo is effective, but its neurotoxicity has called for stricter guidelines for use by pregnant women and younger populations. Treatment, like that for scabies, involves all household members and washing all bed linens, hair utensils, and accessories in warm water.

Body lice are treated by dry cleaning the patient's clothing or washing them in hot water. Using a hot iron on clothing seams will kill any nits. Use of a medicated powder with malathion 1% on the clothing may help. Malathion lotion 0.5% may also be effective, but it does have an unpleasant odor. If eyelashes are involved, treatment with petrolatum jelly will suffocate any lice. Physostigmine ophthalmic ointment 0.25% to lashes four times a day for 3 days also helps.

Pubic lice are treated like head lice, and any sexual partners should also be treated. Patient and family education is important, especially for prevention measures.

Dermatitis. Also referred to as eczema or eczematous dermatitis, atopic dermatitis and contact dermatitis are superficial inflammations of the skin secondary to allergen exposure, irritant exposure, or a genetic predisposition. The patient presents with pruritus, edema, and erythema. If vesiculation, oozing, or crusting is present, the process has been longstanding.

Atopic dermatitis is thought to have a genetic component as an important factor. Many patients also have family members with asthma, hay fever, or atopic dermatitis. Contributing factors include stressful events; extremes in temperature or humidity; and allergies to cosmetics, rubber, and *Rhus* plant (e.g., poison ivy, oak). Age is not a diagnosing factor; however, in older adults, it may be more severe and generalized than in younger patients (Burke and Walsh, 1997). It presents with extreme itching, lichenification, and eczematous changes. The neck, wrists, postauricular area, and popliteal and antecubital areas are often involved. Patch testing is sometimes done to identify the precipitating irritant. A variant, termed *nummular dermatitis* or *discoid eczema*, presents as itchy, scaly, coin-shaped lesions, usually on the posterior trunk, buttocks, and limbs. The lesions may become purulent after oozing and crusting. The precipitating cause is unknown.

Contact Dermatitis. Contact dermatitis can be a challenging diagnosis to make. The area may be chronically irritated (dishpan hands) and appear vesiculated or pustular. In the elderly a common diagnosis is dermatitis of unknown origin. Complaints of pruritus, excoriation, and dry, scaling skin are common. The location of the affected area may lead to the responsible irritant. It is caused by an irritant that penetrates and disrupts the stratum corneum, causing an inflammatory reaction within the underlying epidermis. Common irritants include acids, detergents, and solvents. Lichen simplex chronicus or neurodermatitis is a possible diagnosis. This is a localized pruritic area characterized by extreme itching. The area appears well circumscribed or lichenified, with scaling and papulation. It is common in the elderly, especially women. The usual sites include the occipital area, wrists, thighs, and lower limbs. Improvement is seen when itching ceases.

Management is multifaceted. Elimination of all irritants is vital. If the lesion is wet, dry it. If dry, hydrate it, and if it is inflamed, apply corticosteroid cream. Drying can be accomplished with Burow's solution compresses. For chronic cases, patients must avoid drying detergents, frequent showers, and irritants. Use of topical steroids of moderate to strong potency may control symptoms. Use of an Unna's boot, especially on affected limbs, is helpful in breaking the itch-scratch cycle.

Stasis dermatitis is inflammation secondary to venous hypertension, usually in the lower limbs. Edema, venous stasis skin changes, and dilation of superficial venules around the ankles are seen. It is affected by edema, contact dermatitis secondary to medicated preparations such as neomycin, and scratching. The etiology is unknown.

Management that includes controlling the edema with elastic stockings, elevation, and hydrocortisone 1% may alleviate some symptoms.

Seborrheic Dermatitis. Seborrheic dermatitis is an inflammatory benign disease with an unknown cause. A relationship to the yeast *Pityrosporum ovale* has not been confirmed. It is common in the adult population and difficult to cure because of its chronic and recurrent nature. It appears as scaly, erythematous patches that are slightly papular. It is often asymptomatic, but itching may occur. The scalp is often involved, and dandruff must be ruled out as a possibility. Other areas commonly affected include the postauricular and beard areas, nasolabial folds, eyelids, and eyebrows. Blepharitis or conjunctivitis may occur with eyelid involvement. It is associated with Parkinson's disease, phenylketonuria, zinc deficiency, and epilepsy.

Treatment consists of applying ketoconazole (Nizoral) cream topically to the affected areas. It is also available in a shampoo. For milder cases, daily use of a dandruff shampoo with 1% selenium or 2% pyrithione zinc may be effective, with weekly use of Nizoral shampoo. Maintenance therapy may be needed once or twice a week indefinitely. This treatment often becomes costly, and for maintenance use an over-the-counter dandruff shampoo is adequate. For the erythema a topical steroid may be used; however, a spray or gel may be best for hairy areas. Eyelid involvement is treated with baby shampoo applied to the affected area with a cotton swab. Patient education includes reassurance that it is not contagious; however, the chronicity of this disease must be stressed.

Exfoliative Dermatitis. Exfoliative dermatitis or erythroderma is a generalized, severe dermatitis, most often the result of eczema, psoriasis, a drug reaction, or an undetected malignancy. Erythroderma occurs quickly and has a thick, scaly appearance. The exfoliation process creates cutaneous heat loss, which may lead to rigors. In addition, examine the patient for lymphadenopathy. Shedding of hair and nails is seen in extreme cases.

The treatment depends on the severity of the disease. Hospital admittance is necessary for severe cases because of the extensive heat, fluid, and protein loss. Topical use of an emollient cream is recommended. Prednisone (40 to 60 mg a day) is used when it is first diagnosed and then gradually tapered.

Scaling Diseases

Psoriasis

Psoriasis is a skin disorder that presents with plaques that have a shiny, silver-tinted, scaly appearance. A family history is usually positive, as it is transmitted genetically. Also, inquire about use of beta-blockers, which are known to exacerbate psoriasis. Psoriasis is seen usually in the third and eighth decades of life and more commonly in Caucasians than in African-Americans. Psoriasis may appear throughout the body but is most commonly seen on bony areas (knees, elbows, scalp, buttocks). It may also affect the palms, soles, and nails; nail pitting is a common nail abnormality in chronic cases (Bentz, 1996).

In the older adult look for signs of psoriatic arthritis such as fusiform swelling and tenderness of the distal interphalangeal joint. The rheumatoid factor is negative, although other forms of arthritis may develop. Other sequelae include exfoliative dermatitis and pustular psoriasis.

Treatment includes assessment of the patient's mobility and ability to comply with instructions. Coal tar ointments work well, but they stain, have a distinct odor, and are difficult to work with because of their gluelike texture. Anthralin is a cream or paste that is used on thick, scaly plaques. It comes in varying strengths (0.1% to 1%) and is applied to the plaque for a limited time (20 minutes to overnight), depending on strength. In conjunction with these methods, corticosteroids are effective, especially under an occlusive dressing. If plaques appear on the skin, a tar-based shampoo can be used. For more resistant, widespread cases, phototherapy is effective, as is natural sunlight with proper precautions. Other alternatives include photochemotherapy, which involves a photoactive drug (methoxsalen). Finally, methotrexate is helpful in pustular and exfoliative psoriasis. Low doses of 2.5 to 5 mg a week are common doses for the elderly. Dermatology evaluation is recommended, as is monitoring of hepatic and renal function for agents such as methotrexate.

Bullous Disorders

Bullous Pemphigoid

Bullous pemphigoid presents as a localized or generalized bullous eruption. It appears often in the elderly on either normal or erythematous skin. Approximately half of the cases have involvement of the mucous membranes. It is a chronic condition that affects men and women equally. On histologic examination, subepidermal bullae are seen with complement (C3) present after immunofluorescent staining and immunoglobulin (IgG) on the dermal-epidermal border. If the disease is active, the bullous pemphigoid antigen may be present in some patients.

Treatment for bullous pemphigoid differs, depending on its presentation. For a mild, localized infection, treatment is high-dose topical corticosteroids. More generalized cases may require hospitalization and systemic administration of prednisone. Elderly patients should be closely followed for complications such as upper GI bleeding, fluid retention, hypertension, and confusion. Tapering of the steroid therapy begins once the lesions have resolved. It may take several months of systemic therapy for patients to achieve total remission.

Pemphigus Vulgaris

This disorder is uncommon and occurs most often in middle age; however, many patients are 60 or older. Pemphigus vulgaris presents as intraepidermal bullae on the skin or mucous membranes. The bullae easily rupture and can lead to erosions on the abdomen, extremities, and mucous membranes. A common complaint is a painful mouth lesion, which is common in the early stages of the disease. If the disease progresses, widespread blistering and the risk of sepsis and secondary infection may occur. The diagnosis may be difficult to make and confused with bullous pemphigoid, benign mucous membrane pemphigoid, toxic epidermal necrolysis, a drug-induced reaction, or erythema multiforme.

Hospitalization is necessary if it is widespread, and prednisone is used to control the disease. For milder cases prednisone is used and warrants close follow-up in the elderly patient. Once the skin lesions have cleared, the prednisone is tapered, and topical or intralesional corticosteroid therapy is used on resistant lesions. Management is similar to bullous pemphigoid, and close monitoring of the elderly patient for steroid complications is again stressed.

Drug-Induced Eruptions

Drug-induced eruptions usually present as a pruritic, symmetric, maculopapular rash, 1 to 10 days following the initiation of a new medication (Abrams, 1995). The rash may last up to 14 days after the drug is stopped. The most common culprits are penicillins, sulfonamides, gold, phenylbutazone, and gentamicin. Over-the-counter (OTC) and new hygiene products may also cause a reaction. Treatment precautions include a careful review of all medications (prescribed, OTC, herbal remedies), a detailed history of possible environmental factors, and any medication changes.

Erythema Multiforme

Erythema multiforme presents as symmetric, edematous, erythematous lesions of the skin or mucous membranes. It is an inflammatory eruption, and the lesions may have a bullous appearance. It is thought to be caused by a hypersensitivity reaction to a drug or infection; commonly herpes simplex. Many cases do not fit this classic profile and appear with an unknown etiology (Abrams, 1995). Disease severity varies from lesions with a red circumference and a cyanotic middle to clusters on the extremities to widespread erosion with bullae on the mucous membranes (Stevens-Johnson syndrome). Corneal ulceration may occur in severe cases.

Treatment involves removal of all susceptible agents. If the disease is severe, hospitalization is needed. Localized areas are treated symptomatically, and the use of systemic corticosteroids is debatable and not routine.

Toxic Epidermal Necrolysis

Also known as Lyell's syndrome, TEN is a severe condition that presents with lethargy, general malaise, skin erythema, and tenderness, which quickly progress to blistering and erosion of the skin. One third of the cases are caused by drugs such as a nonsteroidal antiinflammatory drug, barbiturate, antibiotic, or hydantoin (Abrams, 1995). This disorder is life threatening and has a high mortality rate. The classic sign of this disease is the shearing off of the overlying epidermis when force is applied laterally, which is termed Nikolsky's sign.

Treatment for TEN includes hospitalization on a burn unit and use of a biologic dressing. An ophthalmologist is recommended for management of eye care.

Treatment of all patients involves patient education. If the patient resides in a long-term care facility, the staff must be updated on current trends and the rationale for such treatment.

Primary and Secondary Skin Lesions

Skin lesions are divided into primary and secondary lesions, although some experts would include a third special category. The classification is flexible, with overlap, and should serve only as a guide.

Primary (Elementary) Lesions

A primary lesion is the first grossly recognizable or most characteristic structural change of skin disease:

- Flat lesions
  - Macule: Flat, circumscribed change in color, ordinarily less than 2 cm in diameter
    - Hypopigmentation
    - Hyperpigmentation
    - Transient or permanent (telangiectasia) vascular dilation
  - Patch: Larger flat, circumscribed color change
- Solid lesions
  - Papule: Circumscribed elevation no more than 1 cm in diameter

Nodule: Circumscribed larger (greater than 1 cm) and deeper elevation
Tumor: Circumscribed elevation larger and deeper than a nodule; also refers to neoplastic elevations of any size
Plaque: Elevation greater than 1 cm with relatively large surface area compared with height (often confluent papules)
Wheal (hive): Distinctive elevation, usually white to pink, due to localized transient tissue edema
Fluid-filled lesions (blisters)
Vesicle: Sharply circumscribed collection of free fluid no more than 0.5 cm in diameter
Bulla: Large vesicle (greater than 0.5 cm)
Pus-filled lesions
Pustule: Circumscribed elevation containing free pus
Folliculitis: Pustule of a hair follicle
Abscess: Localized deeper and larger accumulation of pus
Furuncle: Abscess of hair follicle
Carbuncle: Coalescent furuncles
Purpura: Discoloration of skin or mucous membrane due to intracutaneous or subcutaneous bleeding
Petechia: Purpura less than 3 mm in diameter
Ecchymosis (bruise): Large area of purpura (borders indistinct)
Hematoma: Large area of purpura producing swelling
Comedo (pl. comedones): Sebum and keratin that occlude pilosebaceous ostium
Open comedo: "Blackhead," darkened sebum and keratin that shows at pilosebaceous ostium
Closed comedo: "Whitehead," undarkened sebum and keratin in pilosebaceous apparatus that does not show at narrow ostium
Burrow: Tunnel or channel in stratum corneum of variable size and shape containing a parasite, such as scabies, creeping eruption

Secondary Lesions

Secondary lesions evolve from primary lesions, either naturally or from adventitious events such as scratching, secondary infection, and treatment:

Pus-filled lesions
Pustule: Circumscribed elevation containing free pus
Abscess: Localized deeper and larger accumulation of pus
Crust (scab): Dried exudate (blood, serum, pus)
Scale: Accumulation of loose, horny fragments of stratum corneum
Scar (cicatrix): Permanent fibrotic skin change following damage to dermis
Localized loss of substance from surface downward
Erosion: Superficial denudation of part or all of epidermis
Excoriation: Superficial loss of skin (often linear or punctate) because of scratching or picking
Fissure: Linear cleavage in the skin
Ulcer: Localized loss of substance extending into dermis and sometimes subcutaneous tissue

Atrophy: Loss of or lack of full development of tissue
Epidermal: Thin, translucent epidermis with fine wrinkling (cigarette paper); may actually reflect histologic changes in papillary dermis
Dermal: Depression of the skin without changes in color or surface markings
Maceration: Changes secondary to prolonged wetting of skin
Lichenification: A lichenlike thickening of the skin, with accentuation of skin markings resulting from chronic rubbing

Summary

Many older people view skin problems as a normal part of the aging process. They often hesitate to mention skin problems to their health care provider. It is important for the provider to ask the older person about changes in pigmentation or any skin problems so that assessments can be made and any necessary treatment can take place.

Resources

American Society for Dermatologic Surgery
http://www.asds-net.org/scfactsheet.html

Skin Cancer Zone
http://www.melanoma.com

Dermatology Journals and Publications
http://tray.dermatology.uiowa.edu

References

Abrams WB, Beers MH, Berkow R, editors: *The Merck manual of geriatrics,* ed 2, Whitehouse Station, NJ, 1995, Merck Research Laboratories.

Bentz MA et al: Selected topics in dermatology for the primary care physician, *Compr Ther* 22(3):135-143, 1996.

Berger T, Sanford MG, Odon R: Skin and appendages. In Tierney LM, McPhee SJ, Papadakis MA, editors: *Current medical diagnoses and treatment 1997,* ed 36, Norwalk, Conn, Appleton & Lange.

Burke MM, Walsh MB: *Gerontologic nursing: Wholistic care of the older adult,* ed 2, St Louis, 1997, Mosby.

Hogstel M: The integumentary system. In Burggraf V, Stanley M, editors: *Nursing the elderly: a care plan approach,* Philadelphia, 1989, JB Lippincott.

Kaminer MS, Gilchrest BA: Aging of the Skin. In Hazzard RW et al, editors: *Principles of geriatric medicine and gerontology,* ed 3, New York, 1994, McGraw-Hill.

Kurban RS, Kurban AK: Common skin disorders of aging: diagnosis and treatment, *Geriatrics* 48(4):30-42, 1993.

Lavken RM, Sun TT: Heterogeneity in epidermal basal keratinocytes: morphological and functional correlations, *Science* 2(15):1239, 1982.

Mayfield P: Skin. In Hogstel MO, editor: *Clinical manual of gerontological nursing,* St Louis, 1992, Mosby.

Sparks SM: Integument. In Burke MM, Walsh MB, editors: *Gerontologic nursing: wholistic care of the older adult,* ed 2, St Louis, 1997, Mosby.

7

Respiratory System

Age-related Changes

There is a gradual age-related decline in pulmonary function beginning at about age 40. The elastic recoil of the lungs decreases, owing to changes in elastin and collagen. The lung weight is decreased by approximately one fifth, the bronchi harden, and the bronchial epithelium and mucous glands degenerate. The alveolar ducts and bronchioles enlarge, with an accompanying decrease in the depth of the alveolar sacs. The alveoli decrease in number, and the cilia become less active. With inhalation, the lung bases of the elderly do not inflate well, and secretions are not expelled. There is a greater resistance to airflow, owing to narrowing of the bronchioles. The vital capacity decreases, and the residual volume increases because of loss of elastic recoil. Additional age-related respiratory system changes in the elderly include the following:

- The thoracic muscles of inspiration and expiration grow weaker, leading to incomplete lung expansion and decreased elastic recoil.
- Pulmonary function test changes are reduced respiratory function, reduced vital capacity, reduced breathing capacity, and increased residual lung volume.
- Poor ciliary function, reduced cough reflex, and decreased T-cell immunity develop.
- The number of functioning alveoli decreases.
- The number of beta receptors decreases.
- Concerning the arterial blood gases (ABGs), Pao_2 decreases with age; Pao_2 corrected for age equals 109 minus 0.43 times (patient's age); Pao_2 in an 80-year-old is 75 mm Hg.
- $Paco_2$ and pH may be outside the normal range, and the response to change may be blunted.
- There is decreased oxygen uptake by cells.
- The incidence of sleep apnea and sleep disorders increases.
- The anteroposterior chest diameter increases, the thoracic transverse measurement decreases, and kyphosis ensues.
- Costal cartilage calcifies, and the ribs become less mobile.

The clinical implications of the age-related changes are as follows (Witta, 1997):

1. Barrel-shaped chest or senile emphysema
2. Bibasilar crackles at baseline; increased risk for respiratory muscle fatigue
3. Increased risk for pneumonia and aspiration; increased risk for reactivation of tuberculosis
4. Decreased reserve (Patients are more prone to disease.)
5. Decreased response to beta agonists
6. Possible normal hypercapnia (Therefore oxygen should be titrated cautiously to prevent impairment of hypercapnia-driven respiration.)
7. Delayed symptoms of hypoxemia and hypercapnia
8. Decreased response to exercise, stress, and disease
9. Increased risk for nocturnal hypoxemia

The elderly population may present with a number of clinical entities in the primary care setting.

Chronic Cough

Cough is the host defense mechanism to clear the airway of secretions and inhaled particles. A chronic cough is one that lasts at least 3 weeks. In adults, chronic bronchitis due to cigarette smoking or inhaled irritants and postnasal drip from chronic sinusitis or allergic rhinitis may be contributors. Additional illnesses causing chronic cough include viral infections, bacterial infections, asthma, gastroesophageal reflux disease (GERD), foreign body aspiration, tuberculosis (TB), medications such as beta blockers or angiotensin converting enzyme (ACE) inhibitors, and psychogenic factors. Worrisome causes of chronic cough include mediastinal masses and chronic lymphadenopathy.

Conditions

Chronic bronchitis: A dry hacking cough is present and is worse in the morning.

Postnasal drip: 41% of patients with a chronic cough complain of a clear nasal discharge, nasal congestion, and frequent throat clearing (Uphold and Graham, 1994).

Asthma: Individuals have cough at bedtime or after exercise, laughing, or exposure to cold air. Cough is seasonal in occurrence with a strong family history. Cough may be nonproductive or productive but not purulent. Associated symptoms may include wheezing and intercostal retraction; but cough may be the sole manifestation.

GERD: Individuals describe a history of heartburn, dysphagia, or a sour taste in the mouth, which may be relieved by sitting up.

Viral infections: Symptoms often occur in the winter, with a nonproductive cough, rhinitis, and nasal congestion.

Bacterial infections: Cough may be productive or purulent, accompanied by fever, respiratory distress, or both.

Aspiration of a foreign body: The cough may persist for weeks or months, and there is a fixed, localized wheezing on auscultation that suggests a distinct affected area.

TB: Initially individuals describe minimal production of yellow-green mucus on arising, but with progressive disease the cough becomes more productive. Associated symptoms include fever, night sweats, dyspnea, and hemoptysis.

Tumor: Characteristics of the cough depend on the location of the primary tumor.

Psychogenic factors: The cough disappears during sleep, it is worse when attention is brought to it, it is worse under stress, and it lacks associated symptoms.

Bronchitis

Bronchitis is an inflammatory condition of the tracheobronchial tree characterized by hyperemic, edematous bronchi, heightened bronchial secretions, impaired mucociliary activity, and destruction of the epithelium. Bronchitis may be acute or chronic in nature and may result from infections with rhinoviruses, pneumococci, *Mycoplasma*, *Chlamydia*, or *Moraxella catarrhalis*. There may be a secondary bacterial infection resulting from *Streptococcus pneumoniae* or *Haemophilus influenzae*.

History

Onset and duration of symptoms
Associated symptoms: fever, pharyngitis, dyspnea, chest pain
Other household members with infectious illness
Past medical history of respiratory illnesses
Past and current smoking history
Quality and nature of sputum production
Drug or environmental allergies
Current medications, including over-the-counter (OTC)

Symptoms

Cough is the hallmark symptom
Fever (unless infected with rhinovirus or coronavirus)
Chest pain
Bronchospasm with wheezing (uncommon in nonsmokers)

Focused Physical Examination

The physical examination should include vital signs; a mental status examination; an eyes, ears, nose, and throat (EENT) examination; a lymph node examination; and a heart and lung examination.

Pay particular attention to fever, edematous turbinates or pharynx, enlarged lymph nodes, wheezing, and tachycardia.

Differential Diagnoses

Acute bronchitis and pneumonia are extremely difficult to differentiate. Patients with pneumonia often have high fevers, rigors, pleuritic chest pain, rusty or bloody sputum, focal crackles, and x-ray abnormalities. However, the elderly may present atypically, without evidence of high fever or with less severe constitutional symptoms.

Pneumonia
Tuberculosis
Pneumocystis carinii pneumonia
Asthma
Exposure to airborne irritants
Congestive heart failure
Drug-related: beta blockers, ACE inhibitors, acetylsalicylic acid (ASA), nonsteroidal antiinflammatory drugs (NSAIDs), particularly naproxen
Foreign body obstruction
Paroxysmal nocturnal dyspnea as a complication of chronic sinusitis
Allergic rhinitis
GERD: glottic dysfunction
Cerumen: impacted in external canal (Barker, Burton, and Zieve, 1995)
Tumors
Psychogenic

Diagnostic Tests

Bronchitis is a diagnosis of exclusion. A complete blood cell count (CBC) with differential, sputum culture, and chest x-ray examination are necessary only if the patient has worsening symptoms despite management. Consider a purified protein derivative (PPD) test if the patient is at risk for tuberculosis.

Treatment

Therapeutics

Because most cases are viral in origin, antibiotics are generally not needed. Increase fluids and rest and discontinue cigarettes. Cough suppressants, antihistamines, and sedatives should be used sparingly, based on the severity of symptoms. Expectorants have not proven helpful.

Clearance of secretions should be promoted with postural drainage and therapeutic doses of bronchodilators (e.g., albuterol [Proventil] metered-dose inhaler, 90 µg per puff, 2 puffs every 4 to 6 hours, with an onset of action in 5 to 15 minutes, peak effect in 60 to 90 minutes, and duration of 3 to 6 hours).

If a bacterial infection complicates the viral infection, treat with *one* of the following:

Erythromycin 250 mg to 500 mg four times a day for 10 days ***or***
Trimethoprim sulfamethoxazole (TMP/SMX) twice a day for 10 days ***or***
Doxycycline 100 mg twice a day for 10 days

In patients with coexisting chronic obstructive pulmonary disease (COPD), treat with antibiotics when there is a change in the color, consistency, and amount of sputum production.

Education

Teach the patient to avoid individuals with upper respiratory infections. Increase fluid intake and rest. Monitor temperature daily. Notify health care provider if symptoms do not improve within 3 days. Take medications as instructed.

Follow-up

If symptoms last longer than 14 days, begin antibiotic therapy for a 10-day course. If there is no improvement within an additional 2 weeks, consider referral to a specialist. Chronic cough resolves completely within 1 month in half of those patients who are motivated by an acute illness to discontinue cigarettes permanently (Barker, Burton, and Zieve, 1995).

Chronic Obstructive Pulmonary Disease

COPD is a complex syndrome of airway obstruction or airflow limitation. There are two components of COPD: emphysema and chronic bronchitis.

Emphysema is a pathologic diagnosis based on a permanent, abnormal dilation and obstruction of alveolar ducts and air spaces distal to the terminal bronchioles. Emphysema is characterized by airway obstruction, hyperinflation, loss of elastic recoil, and destruction of alveolar-capillary interface, which impairs gas exchange.

Chronic bronchitis is a clinical diagnosis based on the presence of cough and sputum production that occurs on most days of a 3-month period during 2 consecutive years. It is characterized by thickened bronchial walls; hyperplasia and hypertrophied mucous glands; and mucosal inflammation in the bronchial walls, large central airways, and, later, smaller airways.

Sequelae of emphysema or chronic bronchitis may be chronic hypoxemia, which causes pulmonary hypertension, and cor pulmonale, conditions associated with poor survival if untreated (Barker, Burton, and Zieve, 1995).

History

Onset and duration of symptoms

Occupational and environmental exposures to dusts (e.g., grain, wood, cotton, mineral, or polyurethane) and chemical fumes

Cigarette smoking (number of packs times number of years equals pack-year smoking history)

Number of attempts to quit smoking and duration of cigarette-free time

Shortness of breath (Ask if individual has trouble keeping up with peers doing routine activities such as walking, sports, or work activities. More advanced dyspnea is roughly quantified by distance walked or flights of stairs walked before stopping.)

Quantity and characteristics of sputum production
Drug or environmental allergies
Current medications, including OTC

Alpha$_1$ antitrypsin deficiency (α_1-antitrypsin) is an uncommon genetic disorder, found in about 1 in 2500 whites, in which the circulating levels of antiproteases are less than 10% of normal. A DNA-base substitution causes an amino acid substitution that prevents secretion of antiproteases from liver cells. Serum levels are less than 15% of normal, which leads to development of premature emphysema in deficient individuals. Although affected people present for medical care with severe emphysema in the third and fourth decades, many individuals with α_1-antitrypsin deficiency have normal or only mildly abnormal lung function if they do not smoke (Barker, Burton, and Zieve, 1995).

Symptoms

Chronic cough
Wheezing
Weight changes
Recurrent respiratory infections
Progressive exertional dyspnea
Lack of libido
Tachypnea
Sputum production
Fatigue
Insomnia
Limitation of activities of daily living from shortness of breath

Focused Physical Examination

Check vital signs. Be alert for fever, tachypnea, tachycardia, and irregular pulse.
Check for increase in resting chest anteroposterior diameter, flattening of the angle of the clavicle and trapezius, widening of the xiphocostal angle, and increase in the intercostal spaces.
Check for diminished muscle mass in the thighs and legs.
The characteristic seating posture is leaning forward with both hands on the knees to elevate the shoulders.
Note purse-lipped breathing and prolonged time of expiration.
Note cyanosis and clubbing of the nails.
Note tobacco staining of the fingers.
Chest percussion reveals increased resonance and a low diaphragm.
Auscultation shows diminished transmission of breath sounds and early inspiratory crackles.
Wheezing may be elicited with forced expiration.

Systemic findings include neck vein distention, peripheral edema, hepatomegaly, tricuspid regurgitation, and a ventricular heave.

Differential Diagnoses

Emphysema
Chronic bronchitis
Congestive heart failure
Asthma
Pneumonia
Lung cancer
Tuberculosis

Diagnostic Tests

Chest x-ray film is abnormal only in advanced disease. There is hyperinflation with flattening of the diaphragm, increased retrosternal air space on the lateral view, narrow cardiac silhouette, and a paucity and tapering of peripheral blood vessels. The electrocardiogram (ECG) shows a vertical or indeterminate heart axis and low voltage. Enlarged P waves, right axis deviation, or right ventricular hypertrophy is present with cor pulmonale (Barker, Burton, and Zieve, 1995).

Administer a PPD and obtain CBC with differential and chemistries, in particular, liver function tests (LFTs). Consider Gram stain and culture of sputum if infection is suspected.

Spirometry

As a general rule, forced expiratory volume at 1 second (FEV_1) measurements greater than 2 liters indicate mild obstruction; 1 to 2 L, moderate obstruction; and less than 1 L, severe obstruction.

Bronchodilator Testing

Bronchodilator testing can reveal reversible bronchospasm, and the postbronchodilator measure of FEV_1 is the best overall predictor of life expectancy in COPD (Barker, Burton, and Zieve, 1995).

Carbon Monoxide Diffusing Capacity Test

The carbon monoxide diffusing capacity test is a test to evaluate the amount of functioning pulmonary capillary bed in contact with functioning alveoli. It is helpful in distinguishing emphysema from asthma. Cigarette smokers without emphysema have mild reductions in diffusing capacity because of the accumulation of carbon monoxide in the blood, which is only partially reversible with smoking cessation. A diffusing capacity below 70% of the predicted value is present with emphysema but may also be found with interstitial fibrosis and pulmonary vascular diseases. In chronic asthmatic bronchitis the diffusing capacity tends to be preserved.

Consider ABGs and pulse oximetry as conditions warrant.

Treatment

Therapeutics

The recommended stepped-treatment approach to COPD is to start with anticholinergic agents, then beta-adrenergic agents, followed by theophylline and corticosteroids. Response to treatment is judged by symptomatic improvement and spirometry.

Drug treatment should use the minimum number of agents and the least frequent dosing schedule possible, starting with the agents having the greatest benefit and least toxicity (Barker, Burton, and Zieve, 1995). See Table 7-1.

TABLE 7-1 Pharmacologic Therapy for Chronic Obstructive Pulmonary Disease

Name of Drug	Dosage	Side Effects	Other Clinical Pearls
Inhaled Anticholinergic			
Ipratropium (Atrovent)	2 puffs t.i.d. to 6 puffs q.i.d.	Mouth irritation and cough	Side effects may be decreased by use of a spacer.
Beta-adrenergic Agonists			
Albuterol (Proventil)	2-4 puffs 2-4 times daily	Hypokalemia and occasional tachycardia or tremor	Supplemental potassium may be needed. Avoid over-the-counter inhalers, as many contain epinephrine.
Theophylline	200 mg q12 hr; actual dose based on drug levels	Tremors, potential for drug-drug interactions	Thought to be the most useful drug for the prevention of nocturnal symptoms.
Oral Corticosteroids			
Prednisone	40 mg daily for 2 weeks	Weight gain, appetite increase, increased risk of infection, fluid and electrolyte imbalance	An improvement in spirometry of 15% indicates a positive response. Taper to lowest possible dose.
Inhaled Steroids			
Triamcinolone (Azmacort)	2 puffs t.i.d. to q.i.d.	Oral candidiasis; rinse mouth well and use spacer	Benefit is mainly in nonsmokers or those with asthmatic bronchitis.

Oxygen Therapy. Oxygen therapy prolongs survival and improves physical and psychologic functioning in hypoxemic patients with COPD. Indications for continuous oxygen therapy include the following:

Pao_2 55 mm Hg or O_2 saturation 88% while in usual state of health *or*
Pao_2 60 mm Hg or O_2 saturation 89% with evidence of chronic hypoxemia, such as erythrocytosis, ankle edema, venous engorgement, or psychologic impairment

Oxygen should be prescribed at the lowest level necessary to maintain an arterial oxygen saturation at or above 90%, usually 1 to 4 L/min via nasal cannula for a minimum duration of 18 hr/day. Portable liquid oxygen systems allow mobility out of the home and should be used whenever possible. Stress the danger of smoking in the presence of oxygen.

Education

Educate the patient regarding the disease process, prevention of disease progression, treatment of complications, drug treatment to maximize lung function, and rehabilitation to optimize activity levels. The patient should be given realistic expectations about the long-term progressive course of the disease, tempered by the understanding that temporary worsenings are treatable. Achievement of maximum social and physical functioning may be assisted by simple measures such as special parking areas for the disabled, use of wheelchairs and motorized carts in shopping malls, and portable oxygen and oxygen supplementation during air travel. Patients and their families should understand that the dyspnea that occurs with exertion is not harmful to the lung and that, with the appropriate pacing of activities, a certain level of dyspnea is actually desirable to achieve and maintain functioning (Barker, Burton, and Zieve, 1995). Inquiries about sexual functioning should be encouraged. Education of the patient's bed partner about proper techniques and the use of prophylactic bronchodilators and oxygen can establish more normal sexual functioning, even with severe disease. Discuss with the patient and family issues surrounding advance directives and mechanical ventilation as treatments for acute respiratory failure. Educate the patient about smoking cessation, to include cigarettes, cigars, marijuana, and cocaine. Avoid respiratory irritants. Pneumococcal vaccination is recommended every 6 years. Influenza vaccination is recommended annually. Amantadine prophylaxis for unimmunized individuals during an influenza epidemic can prevent or attenuate this potentially fatal infection. Instruct the patient to contact health care providers at the onset of upper respiratory tract infection symptoms. Encourage the patient to become involved in a pulmonary rehabilitation program and support group.

If a bacterial infection ensues, treat it with *one* of the following:

Erythromycin 250 mg to 500 mg four times a day for 10 days *or*
TMP/SMX twice a day for 10 days *or*
Doxycycline 100 mg twice a day for 10 days

Follow-up

After an acute exacerbation, follow up by phone in 24 to 48 hours. After beginning oral theophylline, follow up for drug level 2 weeks after the initiation of therapy. Follow stable patients every 3 to 6 months. Instruct patients to consult with their health care provider immediately with the signs and symptoms of respiratory infection or distress.

Pneumonia

Pneumonia is a lower respiratory tract infection accompanied by systemic symptoms and evidence of consolidation on chest x-ray film. Bronchitis and pneumonia represent a continuum of lower respiratory infection. Aspirated pathogens, including bacteria, *Mycoplasma*, and viruses, invade the bronchial epithelium, causing inflammation, edema, and leukocyte infiltration. X-ray examination findings depend on the extent of involvement of adjacent lung parenchyma. It may take 24 hours or longer to visualize x-ray film changes that support clinical findings. Patients seen early and those with emphysema may fail to show any infiltrate or may show a patchy infiltrate on their chest films despite considerable inflammation. Thus the clinical distinction between acute bronchitis and acute pneumonia is often an arbitrary radiologic distinction (French, 1995).

Pneumonia is increasingly common among elderly patients and those with coexisting illnesses. Patients over age 65 are at increased risk for mortality from bacteremic pneumococcal disease.

The most commonly cultured organisms in people 65 and older are *S. pneumoniae, H. influenzae,* and other gram-negative bacilli. In the absence of laboratory analysis and documentation of a causative organism, consideration should be given to where the patient lives. If the patient is living at home, consider the most common pathogens in community-acquired pneumonia. Expand your suspicions about causative organisms if the patient resides in a long-term care facility or was recently hospitalized (French, 1995).

History

History of previous pneumonia
Frequency of upper respiratory infections (URIs)
Fever
Shortness of breath
Quality and nature of sputum production
Cough
Constitutional symptoms
Wheezing
Rhinorrhea
Weight changes
Rigors
Nausea or diarrhea
Smoking history
TB history and recent exposure
Travel history (especially recent travel)
Comorbid illness (e.g., diabetes, hypertension, cancer or chronic illnesses such as rheumatoid arthritis or lupus, asthma, COPD, emphysema)
Alcohol intake

Drug and environmental allergies
Current medications, including OTC

Symptoms

Bacterial pneumonias are commonly preceded by a virallike prodrome of headache, myalgias, and malaise. Also, there may be some of the following:

Abrupt onset of shaking chills
Fever
Pleuritic chest pain
Cough productive of purulent or rusty sputum

Nonbacterial pneumonias (atypical pneumonia) are distinguished by a prodrome of headache and myalgia before the respiratory symptoms. The onset is a flulike illness. See Table 7-2.

Fever
Headache
Sore throat
Myalgia and malaise
Nonproductive hacking cough at onset or several days later
Substernal chest pain
Dyspnea and respiratory distress

When caring for the elderly, a clinician must be alert for subtle changes in behavior. Two common indicators of illness in this age group are tachycardia and tachypnea. People who live at home are more likely to present with classic symptoms, whereas residents of long-term care facilities may exhibit mental status changes, falls, anorexia, and new behavioral problems. Early recognition of subtle changes in this population, leading to early interventions, decreases morbidity and mortality.

Focused Physical Examination

Check vital signs.
Consider weight if patient has coexisting illness.
Inspect and observe respiratory rate, ability to speak in sentences, use of pursed-lip breathing, jugular venous distention (JVD), use of accessory muscles, positioning to relieve shortness of breath, cyanosis, tachypnea, grunting, nasal flaring, and mental status changes.
Auscultation: Crackles may be an age-related change.

Crackles that do not clear with cough are suggestive of pneumonia of either type. Signs of consolidation (bronchial breath sounds, dullness to percussion, and egophony) are more common in bacterial pneumonia.

In early stages of pneumonia the examination may be normal, despite an infiltrate on x-ray film. However, crackles and rhonchi may indicate pneumonia before the appearance of an infiltrate.

TABLE 7-2 Pneumonia-Producing Organisms

Organism	Symptoms	Statistics of Interest
Pneumococcus: may occur in previously healthy adults or after URI.	Presents abruptly High fever Shaking chills Productive cough of purulent or rusty sputum Headache Prostration Pleuritic chest pain	Bacteremia occurs in 15%-30% of cases.
H. influenzae: predilection for elderly or patients with COPD or preexisting illnesses but may affect healthy persons. Often occurs after a period of influenza.	Symptoms are similar to other bacterial pneumonias	
Staphylococcus: often occurs in patients with specific risk factors: nursing home residents, alcohol abusers, or individuals with chronic disease. Also occurs after an influenza epidemic.	Symptoms are similar to other bacterial pneumonias	
M. catarrhalis: consider in individuals with chronic illness or underlying COPD.	Symptoms are mild, no myalgias, chills, pleuritic chest pain or extreme prostration	
Gram-negative bacilli: rare in previously healthy adults. High risk: old age, nursing home residents, immobilization, lack of independence for some portion of ADLs, incontinence, stroke, severe underlying illness, alcohol abusers, malnutrition.		There is a high risk for complications. There is a 20%-30% mortality rate.
M. pneumoniae: close contact is necessary for transmission. Epidemics have occurred in cramped housing areas and in the military.	Symptoms: Mild and course is self-limited. There is an insidious onset, with hacking cough, fever, malaise, headache.	Only 3%-10% of all community-acquired pneumonias are from this organism. In individuals age 30-60, symptoms may last up to 6 weeks despite treatment.
Chlamydia pneumonia	Symptoms are similar to *M. pneumoniae*	

From Uphold CR, Graham MV: *Clinical guidelines in adult health,* Gainesville, Fla, 1994, Barmarrae.

Table 7-2 Pneumonia-Producing Organisms—cont'd

Organism	Symptoms	Statistics of Interest
Legionella pneumonia	Symptoms are more severe than other atypical pneumonias. Unique characteristics include hyponatremia, neurologic symptoms of confusion, headache, nausea, diarrhea, hematuria, and elevated serum transaminase.	There is a 10%-30% mortality rate.
Viruses are not a common cause of pneumonia in adults except in the immunocompromised.	Symptoms are fever, chills, dry hacking cough, and pharyngitis.	
RSV is increasingly being recognized as a cause of pneumonia in adults. CMV and herpes simplex viruses in immunocompromised patients cause pneumonias that are treatable.	Patients with viral pneumonias have more prolonged prodromal illness, milder symptoms and less elevated white blood cells than patients with bacterial pneumonias. Chest x-rays films do not reveal lobar infiltrates with pleural effusions as in bacterial pneumonias.	
Pneumocystis	Symptoms are insidious onset of fever, cough, and dyspnea in an immunocompromised patient.	

Palpation and percussion may show tactile fremitus and dullness over the area of consolidation.

Diagnostic Tests

In a patient with classic symptomatology, diagnostic studies serve only to confirm the diagnosis. In an elderly patient with an atypical presentation, a broader workup may be required to determine an etiology and therefore better focus case management. An appropriate diagnostic workup should be focused and cost-effective.

Chest x-ray examination is helpful in the differential diagnosis of cough, shortness of breath, or chest pain. It may also be helpful in revealing other underlying conditions such as cardiomegaly, lung abscess, TB, obstruction, tumor, and multilobar involvement

(French, 1995). Although the x-ray is essential for the firm diagnosis of pneumonia, a normal x-ray does not necessarily rule out pneumonia, and subsequent films may actually reveal a progression of pulmonary infiltrates. One reason for this change may be that the elderly tend to be dehydrated at the time of presentation, and rehydration causes the infiltrate to appear (French, 1995). There may be a 24-hour lag time between the clinical presentation and x-ray changes.

Sputum microbiology and chest x-ray film are appropriate.

Consider pulse oximetry if available. Consider blood gases if O_2 saturation is less than 90. The O_2 saturation and ABGs should be used to assist in determining the severity of illness. Severe hypoxemia is an indicator of poor outcome and may require admission to an intensive care unit. The spirometry change is that FEV_1 is decreased.

The ECG shows atrial changes.

A blood chemistry 20 (Chem 20) and a CBC with differential are appropriate if the patient is older than 60 or has coexisting illnesses. In a classic scenario the CBC reveals a marked leukocytosis with a left shift; this phenomenon can be absent or delayed in the elderly patient.

Consider PPD. Consider sputum acid-fast bacilli (AFB) each morning for three mornings if history indicates.

Do blood cultures if bacteremia is suspected.

Treatment

Hospitalization vs. outpatient management is based on a number of factors, including physical parameters, social support, insurance issues, and the ease of treatment for the probable causative organism.

Hospitalization should be strongly considered for patients with the risk factors in Box 7-1, especially if there are multiple risk factors present.

Therapeutics

Provide antipyretics for general comfort. Consider guaifenesin for tenacious secretions; avoid dextromethorphan, which suppresses cough reflex.

Outpatient treatment for patients 60 years or older is based on the presumptive diagnosis from the signs and symptoms exhibited. The most common pathogens include *S. pneumoniae,* respiratory viruses, *H. influenzae,* aerobic gram-negative bacilli, *Staphylococcus aureus, M. catarrhalis, Legionella, Mycobacterium tuberculosis,* and endemic fungi.

Antimicrobial therapy in the elderly should provide broad-spectrum activity. Initiate therapy with a third-generation cephalosporin or with multiple antibiotics. Before the results of microbiologic analysis, ceftriaxone (Rocephin), 250 to 500 mg intramuscularly, allows the clinician to treat the patient in the office setting, the long-term care facility, or the hospital. Other choices for treatment include second-generation cephalosporins, TMP/SMX, beta-lactam or beta lactamase inhibitors, and macrolides. Fluoroquinolones such as sparfloxacin (Zagam) and levofloxacin (Levaquin) may occasionally cause skin rashes or gastrointestinal disturbances. Central nervous system toxicity, including dizziness, insomnia, confusion, hallucinations, and seizures, can occur, particularly in elderly patients. Tendinitis or tendon rupture has occurred with sparfloxacin, as it has

Box 7-1

Risk Factors for Mortality or a Complicated Course of Pneumonia

Age Over 65 Years

Presence of coexisting illnesses such as chronic structural disease of the lung, postsplenectomy state, chronic alcohol abuse or malnutrition or appears toxic.

Physical Findings

Respiratory rate in excess of 30 breaths/minute and/or hemoptysis
Diastolic blood pressure ≤60 mm Hg or a systolic blood pressure 90 mm Hg
Temperature >38.3° C (101° F)
Presence of extrapulmonary sites of disease, presence of septic arthritis, meningitis

Laboratory Findings

White blood cell count $<4 \times 10^9$/L or $>30 \times 10^9$/L or an absolute neutrophil count below 1×10^9/L
Pao_2 <60 mm Hg or $Paco_2$ of 50 mm Hg while breathing room air
Serum creatinine of >1.2 mg/dl or a blood urea nitrogen >20 mg/dl
Chest x-ray: more than 1 lobe involvement, presence of a cavity, rapid radiographic spreading, and presence of pleural effusion
Other evidence of sepsis or organ dysfunction: metabolic acidosis, increased prothrombin time, and increased partial thromboplastin time, decreased platelets, or the presence of fibrin split products >1:40

Modified from American Thoracic Society: Guidelines for the initial management of adults with community acquired-pneumonia: diagnosis, assessment of severity, and initial antimicrobial therapy, *Am Rev of Respir Dis* 148:1418-1426, 1993.

with other fluoroquinolones, and will probably occur with levofloxacin as well. All fluoroquinolones have been associated with cartilage damage in high doses in animal studies (Abramowicz, 1997).

Issues to consider in selecting an antimicrobial agent are cost-benefit ratio, dosage schedule, patient tolerability, and site of administration (i.e., home or long-term care facility) (French, 1995).

When microbes have been identified, treat *H. influenzae, Staphylococcus* species, *M. catarrhalis,* and gram-negative bacilli with *one* of the following:

Augmentin 250 to 500 mg every 8 hours for 10 days ***for everything except gram-negative bacilli or***
Ceftin 250 to 500 mg every 12 hours for 10 days for all organisms ***or***
TMP/SMX twice a day for 7 to 14 days ***or***
Ciprofloxacin 200 mg twice daily for 10 days for gram-negative organisms

Treat *S. pneumoniae* with *one* of the following:

Procaine penicillin 300,000 U intramuscularly for the first dose ***then***
Penicillin VK 250 to 500 mg four times a day for 7 to 10 days ***or***
Erythromycin 250 to 500 mg three or four times a day for 7 to 10 days

Treat *Mycoplasma* and *Chlamydia* species with *one* of the following:

Doxycycline 100 mg twice daily for 10 to 14 days ***or***
Erythromycin 250 to 500 mg three or four times daily

For *Legionella* species, hospitalize and administer *one* of the following:

Erythromycin intravenously ***or***
Doxycycline 100 mg twice daily for 14 days ***or***
Ciprofloxacin 200 mg twice daily for 10 to 14 days

Treat *Pneumocystis carinii* with TMP/SMX twice a day for 21 days.
Treat viral infections with symptomatic treatments.

Education

Stop smoking.
Take deep breaths: 10 each hour.
Increase hydration and nutritional intake.
Educate about the importance of antibiotic therapy. The patient should finish all medication.
Instruct the patient about what to do for missed doses.
Avoid other individuals with upper respiratory infections.
Patient and family members should practice good handwashing techniques.
Instruct the patient to schedule activities with rest periods.
Establish practice mechanisms to ensure that elderly patients receive pneumococcal vaccines every 6 years and influenza vaccine yearly.

Follow-up

A telephone contact with the patient within 24 hours of the initial visit provides a check on antibiotic compliance, side effects, and the status of symptoms. This contact also reassures ill patients that the health care provider is available if their condition worsens. A follow-up visit to the office 3 to 4 days later can assess response to therapy. Symptoms of pneumococcal pneumonia in the uncompromised patient abate dramatically within 48 to 72 hours of initiation of penicillin therapy. If substantial response has not occurred, consider switching to erythromycin or hospitalizing the patient.

Early follow-up chest x-ray films are mandatory in patients who fail to show clinical improvement by 5 to 7 days of therapy or who have a later relapse. Old age, COPD, and alcoholism may delay radiologic clearing for an additional 2 to 6 weeks (Barker, Burton, and Zieve, 1995).

Asthma

According to the National Heart, Lung, and Blood Institute of the National Institutes of Health, the following is the current, accepted, working diagnosis of asthma:

Asthma is a chronic, inflammatory disorder of the airways in which many cells and cellular elements play a role. In part, mast cells, eosinophils, T-lymphocytes, macrophages, neutrophils, and epithelial cells are involved. In susceptible individuals, this inflammation causes recurrent episodes of wheezing, breathlessness, chest tightness, and coughing, particularly at bedtime or in the early morning. These episodes are usually associated with widespread, but variable airflow obstruction that is often reversible, either spontaneously or with therapy. The inflammation also causes an associated increase in the existing bronchial hyperresponsiveness to a variety of stimuli (Richman, 1997).

Individuals older than 55 have the highest rate of asthma-related deaths. The prevalence, severity, and death rate have increased in the past decade, particularly in blacks and Hispanics. There are an estimated 15 million patients with asthma (Richman, 1997).

History

Determine if symptoms worsen in association with the following specific factors:

Airborne chemicals or dust
Animals with fur or feathers
Changes in weather
Exercise
House dust mites in mattresses, upholstered furniture, and carpets
Menses
Mold
Nighttime
Pollen
Smoke: tobacco or wood
Strong emotional expression: laughing or crying hard
Viral infection
Medications: ASA, ACE inhibitors, NSAIDs, beta blockers

Ask about the following factors:

Family history
Impact of disease
Previous therapies and responses
Drug and environmental allergies
Current medications, including OTC

Symptoms

Cough, especially nocturnal
Recurrent wheeze
Recurrent dyspnea
Chest tightness

Occupational asthma should be considered in all patients with adult-onset asthma and in patients with asthma that worsens in adulthood. Roughly 200 chemicals have been implicated in occupational asthma (Table 7-3).

The total duration of exposure, duration of symptoms, and the severity of symptoms at the time of diagnosis are important determinants of outcome. Early diagnosis and early withdrawal from exposures to offending chemicals are the keys to recovery.

TABLE 7-3 Examples of Occupational Hazards Implicated in Asthma

Chemical	Occupation
Grain dust	Grain store workers
Henna	Hairdressers
Coffee beans	Coffee roasters
Penicillin	Pharmacists and health care workers
Oil mists	Tool setters
Cobalt dust	Metal grinders
Flour	Bakers

From Richman E: Asthma diagnosis and management: new severity classifications and therapy alternatives, *Clin Rev* 7(8):76-112, 1997.

Focused Physical Examination

Check vital signs.
Observe general appearance, noting distress or decreased responsiveness.
Note accessory muscle use, retraction, posture, nasal flaring, diaphoresis, and cyanosis.
Examine skin for eczema and atopy.
EENT examination: nasal discharge, allergic shiners, nasal polyps, postnasal drip, frontal tenderness.
Pulmonary examination: note adventitious sounds, particularly prolonged expiratory phase and wheezing. Unilateral wheezing suggests an aspirated foreign body.

Differential Diagnoses

Obstructed airway, foreign body, tumor, or anatomic changes
Chronic bronchitis or emphysema
Pneumonia
Pulmonary infiltrates with eosinophilia
Congestive heart failure
Allergic reaction
Laryngeal dysfunction
Cough secondary to drugs
Vocal cord dysfunction

Diagnostic Tests

Consider chest x-ray film or CBC with differential if infection is suspected. Consider pulse oximetry or ABGs as the patient's condition warrants. Perform peak expiratory flow with a peak flowmeter. Consider spirometry evaluation. In patients with persistent asthma, despite taking appropriate daily medication, identify allergen exposure, assess sensitivity to seasonal allergies with a thorough history, and assess sensitivity to perennial indoor allergens with skin or in vitro testing.

Treatment

Therapeutics

According to the Second Expert Panel, the goals of asthma therapy are (Richman, 1997):

- Prevent chronic and troublesome symptoms, such as coughing or breathlessness at night, in the morning, or after exertion
- Maintain nearly normal pulmonary function
- Maintain normal activity levels (including exercise)
- Prevent recurrent exacerbations and minimize the need for emergency care and hospitalization (Table 7-4)
- Provide optimal pharmacotherapy with minimal or no adverse effects
- Meeting patient's and family's expectations of, and satisfaction with, asthma care

The goals can be met by the following measures:

- Prescribing daily antiinflammatory therapy to provide the most effective control
- Following the stepped-care approach by initiating therapy at higher levels and stepping down as stability is achieved (Table 7-5)

TABLE 7-4 Management of Asthma Exacerbations/Severity

Assess Severity
Measure PEFR: A value <50% of personal best or of the predicted value suggests a severe exacerbation. Note signs and symptoms: degree of cough, breathlessness, wheeze, and chest tightness correlate imperfectly with severe exacerbation. Accessory muscle use and suprasternal retractions suggest severe exacerbation.

Initial Treatment
Inhaled short-acting β_2-agonist: up to three treatments of 2-4 puffs by metered-dose inhaler at 20-minute intervals or single nebulizer treatment

Good Response	Incomplete Response	Poor Response
Mild Exacerbation PEFR >80% predicted or personal best. No wheezing or shortness of breath. Response to β_2-agonist sustained for 4 hours. • May continue β_2-agonist every 3-4 hours for 24-48 hours • For patients on inhaled glucocorticoid, double dose for 7-10 days	**Moderate Exacerbation** PEFR 50% to 80% predicted or personal best. Persistent wheezing and shortness of breath. • Add oral glucocorticoid • Continue β_2-agonist	**Severe Exacerbation** PEFR <50% predicted or personal best. Marked wheezing and shortness of breath. • Add oral glucocorticoid • Repeat β_2-agonist immediately • If distress is severe and nonresponsive, consider calling ambulance or 911

From Richman E: Asthma diagnosis and management: new severity classifications and therapy alternatives, *Clinician Rev* 7(8):76-112, 1997.
PEFR, Peak expiratory flow rate.

Table 7-5 Classification and Stepped Care in Asthma Therapy

Step	Daily Medication for Long-Term Control	Medication for Quick Relief
Step 4: Severe Persistent Symptoms: Continual Limited physical activity Frequent exacerbations Frequent nocturnal symptoms Pulmonary function: FEV_1/PEFR is no greater than 60% of predicted PEFR variability exceeds 30%	Antiinflammatory agent (high-dose inhaled glucocorticoid) **and** long-acting bronchodilator (inhaled or oral β_2-agonist or theophylline) **and** oral glucocorticoid	Short-acting inhaled β_2-agonist. Daily use or increasing use indicates need for additional long-term therapy.
Step 3: Moderate Persistent Symptoms: Daily Daily use of inhaled short-acting β_2-agonist Exacerbations affect activity Exacerbations at least twice weekly and may last for days Nocturnal symptoms more frequent than once weekly Pulmonary function: FEV_1/PEFR exceeds 60% but is less than 80% of predicted PEFR exceeds 30% variability	Antiinflammatory agent (medium-dose inhaled glucocorticoid) **and/or** medium-dose inhaled glucocorticoid plus long-acting bronchodilator	Short-acting inhaled β_2-agonist. Daily use or increasing use indicates need for additional long-term therapy.
Step 2: Mild Persistent Symptoms: more frequent than twice weekly but less than once a day Exacerbations may affect activity Nocturnal symptoms more frequent than twice monthly Pulmonary function: FEV_1/PEFR is at least 80% of predicted PEFR variability is between 20%-30%	**One daily medication:** antiinflammatory agent (low-dose inhaled glucocorticoid, cromolyn, or nedocromil) **or** sustained-release theophylline	Short-acting inhaled β_2-agonist. Daily use or increasing use indicates need for additional long-term therapy.
Step 1: Mild Intermittent Symptoms: no more frequent than twice weekly Asymptomatic and with normal PEFR between exacerbations Exacerbations brief (hours to days) Intensity of exacerbations varies Nocturnal symptoms no more frequent than twice monthly Pulmonary function: FEV_1/PEFR is at least 80% of predicted PEFR variability is less than 20%	**No daily medication**	Short-acting inhaled β_2-agonist. Use more than twice weekly may indicate need to initiate long-term therapy.

From Richman E: Asthma diagnosis and management: new severity classifications and therapy alternatives, *Clinician Rev* 7(8):76-112, 1997.

FEV_1, Forced expiratory volume (in one second), *PEFR*, peak expiratory flow rate.

- Performing office-based assessment at intervals ranging from 1 to 6 months
- Considering referral to an asthma specialist when control of asthma cannot be maintained or the patient requires step 4 care

Pharmacologic Therapy. The most effective medications continue to be those with antiinflammatory actions, inhaled steroids, mast cell stabilizers, and leukotriene modifiers. The next step includes medications that provide relief from acute symptoms, such as short-acting beta adrenergics, anticholinergics, and systemic glucocorticoids.

Asthma treatment is based on a stepped approach. Guidelines for treatment should be initiated at higher levels or steps rather than higher doses of medications (Murphy, 1997).

Antiinflammatory drugs
  Corticosteroids
  Beclomethasone (Beclovent, Vanceril metered-dose inhaler [MDI]) 2 puffs four times a day or 4 puffs twice a day
  Flunisolide (Aerobid MDI) 2 to 4 puffs twice a day
  Triamcinolone acetonide (Azmacort MDI) 2 puffs three or four times a day or 4 puffs twice a day
  Fluticasone (Flovent MDI) 2 to 4 puffs twice a day
  Prednisone or prednisolone tablets for acute treatment, up to 80 mg per day for 7 to 14 days; for chronic treatment, up to 40 mg every other day
  Cromolyn (Intal MDI) 2 to 4 puffs four times a day
Bronchodilators
  B_2 Adrenergics
    Albuterol (Proventil, Ventolin MDI) 2 puffs every 4 to 6 hours as needed
    Ipratropium plus albuterol (Combivent MDI) 2 puffs four times a day
  Long acting:
    Salmeterol (Serevent MDI) 2 puffs every 12 hours
Anticholinergics
  Ipratropium (Atrovent MDI) 2 puffs four times a day
Leukotriene Receptor Antagonist
  Zafirlukast (Accolate tablet) 20 mg twice a day 1 hour before or 2 hours after meals
5-Lipoxygenase Inhibitor
  Zileuton (Zyflo tablet) 600 mg four times a day

Management of upper respiratory tract symptoms is an integral component of asthma management. Coexisting rhinitis, sinusitis, and GERD require treatment.

Education

Patient education is key in the management of chronic asthma and acute exacerbations. Education is a partnership between patients and clinicians.

The asthma education program should include five components:

1. Basic asthma facts: Review pathophysiology.
2. Roles of asthma medications: See previous instructions.
3. Skills for use of inhaler, spacer, and peak flowmeter.
4. Office spirometry should be performed at the initial assessment and diagnosis of asthma, then after the patient's condition has stabilized following initiation of therapy, and at least every 1 to 2 years thereafter.

5. Peak expiratory flow rates (PEFR) should be recorded by patients two to four times daily for 2 to 3 weeks during initial medication therapy. Average the morning and afternoon scores, after removing the two high results and two low results. These values show the patient's personal best before medication (morning value) and after medication therapy (afternoon value). After maximum medical therapy has occurred and the patient's medical condition has stabilized, have patient perform PEFRs in the early afternoon. Patients should contact their health care provider if the PEFR falls to less than 80% of their personal best.

Because predicted values vary across racial and ethnic populations, the personal best PEFR is a better choice for individual monitoring than population-based normative values.

Environmental Control and Avoidance Measures

Avoid exposure to tobacco smoke and allergens to which the patient is sensitive.

Avoid pets. If pets cannot be removed from the home, have designated pet-free living areas. Close bedroom doors, use air filters, and remove carpets or upholstery from pet-free areas.

Avoid exertion when pollution levels are high.

Avoid foods and beverages containing sulfites, including wine.

Avoid nonselective beta blockers in patients with cardiovascular disease, ophthalmologic indications, migraines, or stage fright.

Mattresses and pillows should be encased in allergen-free cases. Sheets and blankets should be washed weekly in water hotter than 140° F.

Consider allergy testing and immunotherapy when the connection between symptoms and exposure to allergens is unavoidable. Skin or in vitro testing may also be considered when patients are perennially exposed to indoor allergens.

When and How to Take Rescue Steps. Provide written signs and symptoms, in appropriate language, of acute exacerbations and treatment plan changes (such as when to use short-acting bronchodilators). Educate patients to recognize symptoms and changes in symptom patterns that herald a diminution of asthma control and the need for stepping up the therapy.

Follow-up

For acute exacerbations requiring a nebulizer or corticosteroids, see the patient within 24 hours and then reevaluate in 3 to 5 days. After the exacerbation has resolved completely, schedule follow-up visits every 1 to 3 months.

For patients on theophylline, obtain serum drug levels after 2 weeks of initiating therapy and every 4 to 6 months thereafter.

Schedule a yearly influenza vaccine (if the patient is not allergic to eggs).

Consider pneumococcal vaccine every 6 years.

Influenza

Influenza is an infection of the respiratory tract caused by the influenza virus. There are three types of virus, labeled A, B, and C. The proteins that coat the flu virus change constantly, making it difficult for the immune system to recognize and fight new strains. The virus is mainly spread by airborne transmission vs. direct contact, as in the common cold. Therefore people with lung disease, the elderly, or those with weakened immunity are prone to severe and possibly fatal complications from the flu.

During flu epidemics, up to 40% of people in a given community may develop flu symptoms during the time span of a few weeks. Flu season is usually November through February. Illness is severe for 3 to 14 days, and convalescence lasts for 1 to 4 weeks.

History

There is an abrupt onset of systemic symptoms.
Headache and myalgias that involve the back, arms, legs, and occasionally the eyes are the predominant symptom.
Fever may rise up to 106° F for 3 days and may persist for 5 to 7 days.
Respiratory symptoms such as cough, nasal discharge, hoarseness, and sore throat appear as systemic symptoms wane.
Cough and weakness usually subside after 2 weeks but may persist longer.
Drug or environmental allergies.
Current medications, including OTC.

Symptoms

Sudden onset of fevers, chills, muscle aches, malaise, cough, and sore throat
Symptoms usually self-limiting

Focused Physical Examination

Check vital signs: appears constitutionally ill; flushed face, hot skin, watery red eyes, clear nasal discharge, tender cervical lymph nodes, and occasionally localized crackles in the chest.
There is anorexia, nausea, vomiting, diarrhea.
White cell count and differential count usually demonstrate mild neutropenia and relative lymphocytosis because of absolute granulocytopenia.

Differential Diagnoses

Common cold
Pneumonia
Allergic rhinitis
Sinusitis
Streptococcal pharyngitis
Otitis media

Diagnostic Tests

Consider CBC if bacterial infection is suspected. Generally, diagnostic tests are not indicated.

Treatment

Therapeutics

Treatment is entirely symptomatic. Give acetaminophen or NSAIDs for aches and fever. Use combination products with decongestants, such as pseudoephedrine or phenylephrine, for congestion, cough, and nasal discharge. Do not use nasal sprays longer than 3 days to decrease the chance of rebound nasal congestion. Other medications that can be used are antihistamines such as diphenhydramine, chlorpheniramine, or clemastine or cough suppressants such as dextromethorphan.

Two antivirals that may be helpful in treating symptoms of influenza A infection **when started within 48 hours** are amantadine (Symmetrel) and rimantadine (Flumadine). These drugs attenuate clinical disease in all patients with influenza A by reducing fever by 50% and by shortening the duration of illness by 1 or 2 days. Side effects include insomnia, nervousness, dizziness, and difficulty in concentrating and may occur in about 7% of adults. Dose is 100 mg twice a day for 7 days. In frail, elderly patients and patients with an elevated creatinine clearance, 100 mg daily should be given.

Education

Advise patients that if they develop dyspnea, hemoptysis, wheezing, purulent sputum, fever persisting more than 7 days, dark urine, or severe muscle pain or tenderness, prompt medical attention is needed.

Encourage bedrest. Return to full activity should be delayed until symptoms are gone.

Supportive measures, including increased nutrition, are important, and symptoms should be managed as previously discussed with combination products.

Influenza Vaccine

For maximum protection, patients should receive the vaccine between the beginning of October and mid-November. However, the vaccine should be administered at any time there are symptoms in the community. People age 65 and older should also receive the pneumococcal vaccine every 6 years. Both vaccines may be given at the same time without increasing the risk of vaccine side effects. Elderly people and certain patients with chronic disease may develop lower postvaccination titers and remain susceptible to infection. Vaccinated individuals develop antibody titers that are protective against illnesses caused by strains similar to those in the vaccine. Related variants may emerge during outbreak periods.

Individuals who are allergic to eggs should never be vaccinated. Individuals who have an acute illness with fever should not be vaccinated until the illness has subsided.

Follow-up

Because this illness is usually self-limited, follow-up is dictated by persistent symptoms beyond 7 to 10 days or if signs and symptoms of bacterial infection ensue.

Common Cold

The common cold is a minor infection of the nose and throat that causes symptoms that last from a few days to a few weeks. There are five different families of viruses that cause colds. Rhinoviruses are the etiologic agent in 25% to 30% of colds, with seasonal peaks in the early fall and mid to late spring. Nearly 100 strains of rhinovirus have been found to date. Coronaviruses account for another 10% to 15% of annual colds, with a seasonal peak in midwinter. Multiple cases occur in family, work, and school settings. The virus is commonly spread via hand-to-hand contact and infrequently via droplet infection. Infectious material can survive on the hand for as long as 4 hours. Adults average two to four colds per year.

History

Presence of facial, ear, throat, or chest pain
Number and seasonal patterns of colds for the previous year
Exposure to others with similar symptoms
Drug or environmental allergies
Current medications, including OTC

Symptoms

Symptoms develop 1 to 3 days after the virus enters the body. Illness is characterized by one or more of the following symptoms:

General malaise
Low-grade or no fever
Nasal discharge, obstruction, or congestion
Sneezing, coughing, sore throat, and hoarseness
Conjunctivae may be watery and inflamed

Patients can readily make the correct diagnosis of the common cold. The challenge for health care providers is to identify patients with complicating secondary bacterial sinusitis and otitis media, for whom antimicrobials will be beneficial.

Focused Physical Examination

Check vital signs. Physical examination should include the pharynx, nasal cavity, ears, and sinuses.

Watery red eyes and clear nasal discharge may be the only objective signs unless bacterial infection complicates the clinical picture.

Differential Diagnoses

Influenza
Pneumonia
Allergic rhinitis
Sinusitis
Streptococcal pharyngitis
Otitis media

Diagnostic Tests

Consider CBC with differential if bacterial infection is suspected. Generally, diagnostic tests are not indicated.

Treatment

Therapeutics

Treatment is entirely symptomatic. Give acetaminophen or NSAIDs for aches and fever. Use combination products with decongestants, such as pseudoephedrine or phenylephrine, for congestion, cough, and nasal discharge. However, caution is recommended when using decongestants in hypertensive patients. Do not use nasal sprays for more than 3 days to decrease the chance of rebound nasal congestion. Other medications that can be used are antihistamines such as diphenhydramine, chlorpheniramine, and clemastine, and cough suppressants such as dextromethorphan. Advise patients about the side effects of all these drugs.

Education

Supportive measures are important, including increased nutrition and symptom management as described previously with combination products. Because transmission of colds occurs chiefly by physical contact, it is reasonable to counsel patients, and those around them, that transmission can be minimized by handwashing, reduced finger-to-nose contact, and reduced exposure to the cold sufferer.

The prophylactic and therapeutic properties of large doses of vitamin C have been examined in a number of trials, and no consistent beneficial effect has been found.

Follow-up

Because this illness is usually self-limited, follow-up is dictated by persistent symptoms beyond 7 to 10 days or if signs and symptoms of bacterial infection ensue.

Sinusitis

Sinusitis is inflammation of the mucosal lining of the paranasal sinuses, which leads to stasis, obstruction, and subsequent infection. Factors that may induce a response include allergens and environmental irritants such as nicotine or other air pollutants. The sinuses are air-filled bony cavities that produce and drain up to 2 pints of mucus every day. Self-cleaning occurs by movement of the mucus, propelled by cilia, through the ostia, which are located behind the turbinates. Acute sinusitis is a bacterial infection of one or more paranasal sinuses, which occurs when the normal drainage is impaired because of blockage of one or more ostia. Up to 10% of cases of acute sinusitis are extensions of dental abscess. Nursing home or homebound patients with nasogastric tubes occasionally have occult sinusitis as a cause of persistent fever (Barker, Burton, and Zieve, 1995).

Sinusitis is subdivided by duration into acute sinusitis, with symptoms lasting up to 3 weeks; subacute sinusitis, with symptoms lasting from 3 weeks to 3 months; and chronic sinusitis, with symptoms occurring longer than 3 months. Allergy is the most common underlying cause of chronic sinusitis. Colds are the most common cause of acute sinusitis.

History

Recent URI
Allergies
Recent swimming or diving
History of nasal polyps
Dental abscess
Adenoidal hypertrophy
Foreign body
Immune deficiency

Symptoms

Acute Sinusitis

Dull pain over maxillary sinuses that becomes throbbing pain in later stages
Fever
Congestion
Green nasal discharge
Postnasal drip
Cough
Fatigue
Congested ears or nose unresponsive to oral decongestants
Headache
Toothache
Facial fullness
Coughing, dependency, and percussion over the involved sinus exacerbate the pain
Early morning periorbital swelling

Chronic Sinusitis

Nasal discharge, nasal congestion, or cough lasting more than 30 days
Hallmark sign: dull ache or pressure across midface or headache
Thick postnasal drip
Popping ears, eye pain, halitosis, and fatigue

Focused Physical Examination

Check vital signs.
Examination should include the pharynx, nose, and ears. Transillumination of the sinuses can be attempted but is often unreliable.
Examine teeth and gingiva for caries and inflammation; tap maxillary teeth with tongue blade because 5% to 10% of maxillary sinusitis is caused by dental root infection.
Auscultate heart and lungs.

Differential Diagnoses

Dental abscess
Cluster headache
Migraine headache
Allergic rhinitis
Vasomotor rhinitis
Nasal polyp
Tumor
Uncomplicated upper respiratory infection

Diagnostic Tests

Radiologic examination of the sinuses is not necessary in patients with typical signs and symptoms.

Acute sinusitis can be treated without culture. Nasopharyngeal swabs are usually contaminated with normal flora and are of no use.

Consider CBC with differential if patient exhibits constitutional signs.

Treatment

Therapeutics

Of acute infections, 60% are caused by *S. pneumoniae* and *H. influenzae*. *S. aureus* causes fewer than 5% and tends to be associated with pansinusitis and general toxicity:

Ampicillin or amoxicillin 250 to 500 mg four times a day for 14 days ***or***
TMP/SMX two tablets twice daily for 14 days ***or***

Augmentin 500 mg every 12 hours for 14 days, dose based on patient's creatinine clearance, if known, ***or***
Cefuroxime 250 to 500 mg twice a day for 14 days

For treatment of chronic sinusitis, the same antimicrobial therapy is used. However, extend therapy for a total of 3 to 4 weeks:

Topical decongestants (e.g., phenylephrine 0.25% or 0.5%) 1 to 2 sprays every 3 to 4 hours for 2 to 4 days
Oral decongestants (e.g., pseudoephedrine 30 to 60 mg) every 4 to 6 hours
Topical corticosteroids (beclomethasone) 1 to 2 sprays each nostril twice daily
Guaifenesin (Robitussin 100 mg/5 ml) 10 to 20 ml every 4 hours
Nasal sinus irrigation daily with saline solution

Pain relief is important, and codeine may be required.

Education

Instruct patient to return for further evaluation if symptoms are not improved within 48 hours. Increase fluids. Steam inhalation and warm compresses may relieve pressure. Avoid allergens and excessively dry heat. Avoid swimming and diving during acute sinusitis. Avoid the use of antihistamines, which slow the movements of secretions out of the sinuses. Encourage smoking cessation. Avoid air travel during acute phase.

Follow-up

Patients whose symptoms worsen during the first 48 hours of vigorous ambulatory therapy should be referred to an EENT specialist.

Tender periorbital swelling, associated with proptosis (downward or outward displacement of the eyes) and chemosis (scleral edema), represent orbital cellulitis and require immediate referral to an EENT specialist.

Allergic Rhinitis

Allergic rhinitis, the most common of all allergic disorders, is inflammation of the mucous membranes of the nose, usually accompanied by edema of the nasal mucosa and nasal discharge. It is estimated that 17% of Americans suffer from acute and chronic conditions generally considered to be allergic in origin. Allergic rhinitis alone accounts for 7% of common allergic conditions in the general population. The majority of office visits to health care providers are for conditions known to be mediated by antibodies of the immunoglobulin E (IgE) class or for conditions that resemble IgE-mediated allergy. The most common form of allergic rhinitis is seasonal and caused by ragweed pollen. The perennial form of allergic rhinitis occurs year round and is usually related to house dust mites, mold, cockroaches, and animal dander. This form of rhinitis is more difficult to diagnose and treat. The onset of symptoms is most common between the ages of 10 and 20 and rarely begins before age 4 or after age 40.

Atrophic or geriatric rhinitis is a perennial nonallergic rhinitis resulting from progressive degeneration and atrophy of nasal mucous membranes and bones of the nose.

History

Age of onset of symptoms
Recent use of nasal decongestants
History of allergies
History of nasal polyps or deviated septum
Seasonal versus perennial symptoms

Symptoms

Triad of symptoms: nasal congestion, sneezing, and clear rhinorrhea
Cough, sore throat, pruritic, edematous eyelids
Obstructed airflow

Focused Physical Examination

Check vital signs.
Palpate lymph nodes.
Assess allergic shiners or dark discoloration beneath both eyes.
Verify that nasal mucosa is pale and boggy, with thin, clear secretions. Turbinates are enlarged, and the edematous membranes may be difficult to differentiate from nasal polyps, which may resemble peeled green grapes in the nasal cavity.
There is cobblestone appearance of conjunctiva due to concurrent allergic conjunctivitis.
There is transverse nasal crease due to chronic upward wiping of the nose.
Tonsils and adenoids are enlarged.
Speech is nasal speech or breathing is through the mouth.
Examine heart and lungs.

Differential Diagnoses

Upper respiratory infection
Sinusitis
Otitis media
Foreign body if blockage is unilateral
Deviated septum if blockage is unilateral
Nasal polyps
Hypothyroidism
Pregnancy
Drug related: oral contraceptives, hormonal replacement therapy

Diagnostic Tests

Diagnosis and treatment are based on history and physical examination.
Consider CBC with differential if the patient exhibits signs and symptoms of infection.

Treatment

Therapeutics

Antihistamines or H_1-receptor antagonists are the primary sources of symptomatic relief. It may be necessary to try several antihistamines before an effective one is found. Also, it may be necessary to switch medications occasionally to avoid tolerance:

Diphenhydramine (Benadryl) 12.5 to 50 mg three or four times a day (dose based on symptom relief versus somnolence) ***or***
Clemastine (Tavist) 1 to 2 tablets twice daily ***or***
Chlorpheniramine (Chlor-Trimeton) 4 mg four times a day ***or***
Hydroxyzine (Atarax, Vistaril) 10 to 25 mg three or four times a day ***or***
Brompheniramine (Dimetane) 4 mg four times a day ***or***
Loratadine (Claritin) 10 mg daily

Many of these medications come in combination preparations:

Topical decongestants (phenylephrine 0.25 or 0.5%) 1 or 2 sprays every 3 to 4 hours for 2 to 4 days
Oral decongestants (pseudoephedrine 30 to 60 mg) every 4 to 6 hours
Topical corticosteroids
- Beclomethasone 1 to 2 sprays each nostril twice daily
- Mometasone furoate (Nasonex) 2 sprays each nostril once daily
- Guaifenesin (Robitussin 100 mg/5 ml) 10 to 20 ml every 4 hours
- Nasal sinus irrigation daily with saline solution

Environmental Control and Avoidance Measures

Avoid exposure to tobacco smoke and allergens to which patients are sensitive.
Avoid pets. If pets cannot be removed from the home, have designated pet-free living areas. Close bedroom doors, use air filters, and remove carpets or upholstery from pet-free areas.
Avoid exertion when pollution levels are high.
Avoid foods and beverages containing known allergy triggers.
Mattresses and pillows should be encased in allergen-free cases. Sheets and blankets should be washed weekly in water hotter than 140° F.

Consider allergy testing and immunotherapy when the connection between symptoms and exposure to allergens is unavoidable. Skin testing or in vitro testing may also be considered when patients are perennially exposed to indoor allergens.

Reduce humidity in the home.

Stay inside with closed doors and windows while running the air conditioner during times of peak pollen exposure.

Follow-up

Consider referral to an EENT specialist or allergist if symptoms are not well controlled with adequate trial of environmental control and medications.

Hemoptysis

Hemoptysis is expectoration of both blood-tinged and grossly bloody sputum. Inflammation of the tracheobronchial mucosa is the causative factor in many cases of hemoptysis. Minor mucosal erosion can occur from upper respiratory infections, bronchitis, bronchiectasis, tuberculosis, and endobronchial inflammation due to sarcoidosis. Bronchogenic cancer may injure the mucosa, whereas metastatic lung cancer rarely results in hemoptysis. Lung tumors account for approximately 20% of the cases of hemoptysis. In addition, there may be injury to the pulmonary vasculature via necrotizing pneumonia (e.g., *Klebsiella*), lung abscesses, aspergillomas, and pulmonary infarction secondary to embolization. Hemoptysis may also occur because of elevations in the pulmonary capillary pressure as in pulmonary edema, multiple sclerosis, Wegener's syndrome, Goodpasture's syndrome, and arteriovenous malformations. Patients with mitral stenosis and pulmonary vascular congestion are prone to hemoptysis with any source of lung irritation. Additional causes may be bleeding disorders, excessive coagulant therapy, or chest trauma (Table 7-6).

Conditions

Bronchitis and bronchiectasis: occasionally blood-tinged sputum; patient usually has chronic cough and dyspnea, which may be worse in the morning.

Lung tumors: occur most frequently in persons over 40 and in smokers; there is a change in the cough pattern; chest ache may be an accompanying symptom.

Pneumonia: sputum appears red-brown or red-green and is mixed with pus; there may be fever, pleuritic chest pain, or malaise.

TABLE 7-6 Differentiation

	pH	Color	Characteristics
Blood-streaked sputum			Common and may occur in nonthreatening conditions
Hemoptysis	Alkaline	Bright red and frothy	Blood is mixed with sputum
Hematemesis	Acid	Darker brown	Blood may be mixed with food particles

Pulmonary infarction secondary to pulmonary embolus: sudden onset of pleuritic chest pain in conjunction with hemoptysis; patient has diaphoresis and syncope, dyspnea, and anxiety. Frequently, the patient has a history of calf pain, deep venous thrombosis, or phlebitis.

Pulmonary edema: pink frothy sputum, diaphoresis, tachypnea, tachycardia, anxiety; JVD, hepatomegaly, or ankle edema may be present.

History and Symptoms

Question patient about the onset of hemoptysis:

Question if this is a first-time episode or a recurrent problem. Explicitly determine if the bleeding is coming from the lungs or from expectorated blood from the nasopharynx.

Describe color, consistency, and characteristics of sputum.

Quantify the amount of bleeding.

Inquire about associated symptoms: weight loss, fatigue, persistent cough, dyspnea, wheezing, fever, night sweats, or excessive bruising.

What is the past medical history, particularly regarding lung, cardiac, hematologic, or immunologic disorders?

Inquire about recent respiratory infection or exposure to TB, environmental exposures (e.g., asbestos), use of anticoagulants, history of chest trauma, cigarette smoking, family history of hemoptysis, last chest x-ray or PPD, drug or environmental allergies, and current medications, including OTC.

Focused Physical Examination

Check vital signs, particularly noting fever or tachypnea.

Observe skin for ecchymoses and telangiectasias and nails for clubbing.

Examine nose and pharynx for signs of bleeding. Differentiate hemoptysis from epistaxis.

Inspect neck for JVD, and check for lymphadenopathy.

Perform a complete lung and cardiovascular examination.

Assess for ankle edema.

Differential Diagnoses

Bronchitis or bronchiectasis

Lung tumors

Pneumonia

Pulmonary infarction secondary to pulmonary embolus

Pulmonary edema

Diagnostic Tests

Perform chest x-ray examination.
Consider Gram stain for suspected infection.
Consider AFB for suspected TB.
Consider cytology for suspected malignancy.
Consider PPD.
Consider ventilation-perfusion (V/Q) scan or angiography when pulmonary embolus is suspected.
Consider bronchoscopy for patients who smoke and are over 40 or who have an abnormal chest x-ray and recurrent hemoptysis.
Consider prothrombin time, partial thromboplastin time, and platelet count studies.

Treatment

Therapeutics

Treat any underlying illness or infection. Encourage judicious use of mild cough suppressants.

Patients with blood-tinged or blood-streaked sputum who have an upper respiratory infection or bronchitis that does not resolve in 2 to 3 days should be reevaluated or referred to a specialist.

Education

Explain that blood is irritating to the tracheobronchial tree and mucus should be expectorated, not swallowed.

Have patient record the number of episodes of hemoptysis and collect the blood that is expectorated.

Have patient return to the clinic or emergency room if the amount of blood increases or becomes filled with clots or if the patient develops respiratory distress, diaphoresis, chest pain, or tachypnea.

Follow-up

Because hemoptysis is usually self-limited, follow-up is indicated with persistence or recurrence of symptoms or with suspicion of neoplastic process or coagulopathy.

Tuberculosis

Tuberculosis is a necrotizing bacterial infection most commonly affecting the lungs. Primary or initial infection occurs by inhalation of the etiologic agent, *Mycobacterium tuberculosis,* which is dispersed as microdroplet nuclei by a person who is positive for tuberculosis. Of primary tuberculosis infections, 90% to 95% remain in a latent or dormant infection stage. It is estimated that 10 to 15 million Americans have latent TB infections.

Active TB may develop during periods of stress, when the body is going through change or fighting off a disease such as human immunodeficiency virus (HIV) or diabetes, with use of corticosteroids, during adolescence, and during old age.

Apical areas of the lungs are the most common sites for TB, but TB is a systemic disease that may result in pleural effusion, disseminated TB, or infections in the lymphatic or genitourinary systems.

From 1985 to 1991, annually reported TB cases increased by 18% because of a variety of issues, including an increase in diagnosis of HIV disease, deterioration of the medical infrastructure, an increase in adverse social and economic conditions, and an increase in foreign-born individuals who have emigrated and have TB infection (U.S. Department of Health and Human Services, 1994).

In the United States the highest incidence of TB, except for people with HIV disease, is in people over age 65.

Efforts to control the spread of TB have been confounded by the emergence of strains of TB that are resistant to multiple drugs. In April 1991 as many as one third of all positive TB cultures in New York City were resistant to one or more anti-TB drugs (U.S. Department of Health and Human Services, 1994).

Tuberculosis control in the United States depends on screening populations at high risk and providing preventive therapy to those who are most likely to develop active disease (Box 7-2).

History

Onset and duration of symptoms
Exposure to TB at home, school, social occasions
Previous history of TB infection
Review of risk factors (e.g., chronic disease)

Box 7-2

Individuals at High Risk for Tuberculosis

- Racial or ethnic minority populations as defined locally.
- Foreign-born individuals, especially children, who arrive from countries with a high incidence of TB (African, Asian, and Latin American nations). In 1995, 63% of new cases of TB were in individuals from the following countries: Haiti, India, Mexico, Philippines, People's Republic of China, and Vietnam.
- Domestic or occupational contacts of infectious TB cases.
- Alcoholic and injection drug users.
- Residents and staff of acute and long-term facilities (hospitals, nursing homes, correctional and mental health institutions).
- Individuals with chronic disease such as HIV, diabetes, ESRD, hematologic disease, history of intestinal bypass or gastrectomy, chronic malabsorption syndromes, silicosis, cancer of the upper gastrointestinal tract or oropharynx, prolonged steroid use and immunosuppressive therapy, and being 10% or more *below* the ideal body weight.

From U.S. Department of Health and Human Services: *The clinician's handbook of preventive services,* McLean, Va., 1994, International Medical.
TB, Tuberculosis; *ESRD,* end-stage renal disease.

Review of dates of TB skin tests and chest x-ray examination
Recent travel to countries where TB is prevalent
Drug or environmental allergies
Current medications, including OTC

Symptoms

Symptoms vary but may include the following:

Increasing fatigue
Malaise
Anorexia
Weight loss
Periodic fever
Night sweats
Hemoptysis
Productive, prolonged cough lasting longer than 3 weeks

Focused Physical Examination

Note the patient's vital signs. The physical examination often may be entirely negative, even with obvious evidence of pulmonary disease on the chest x-ray film. The following positive findings, when present, may be of considerable help in supporting the diagnosis:

Crackles localized to the upper posterior chest or auscultatory evidence of pulmonary cavitation (bronchovesicular breath sounds and whispered pectoriloquy)
Evidence of pleural effusion
Supraclavicular and infraclavicular retraction
Lymphadenopathy
Skin pallor
Evidence of weight loss and fever

Differential Diagnoses

Malignancy
Silicosis
COPD
Asthma
Bronchiectasis
Pneumonia

Diagnostic Tests

The incubation period is 2 to 10 weeks from the time of exposure to the development of a positive reaction to a TB test.

The response to PPD may wane with age and be restored with repeat testing. Because of this booster effect, patients (particularly those over 55) who undergo repeated testing may be falsely classified as new converters and unnecessarily treated with isoniazid. Some authorities advise initial screening of adults in institutional and hospital settings with a two-step PPD testing procedure. If the first Mantoux test is negative, a second should be performed in 1 to 2 weeks. Reaction to the booster test usually indicates old—not new—TB infection. The Centers for Disease Control and Prevention also recommends this two-step procedure for the initial screening of residents and employees of long-term care facilities such as nursing homes, adult foster care homes, and board and care homes (U.S. Department of Health and Human Services, 1994) (Figure 7-1).

The Mantoux test should be read 48 to 72 hours after placement by palpating the margin of induration and measuring the diameter transverse to the long axis of the forearm. It may be helpful to outline the margin of induration with a ballpoint pen. Erythema surrounding the induration should not be considered in evaluating test results. Providers should always record the actual millimeters of induration. Simply recording positive or negative is not precise enough and may lead to improper treatment.

Absence of tuberculin reaction does not exclude a diagnosis of TB infection, especially when symptoms suggest active disease. Induration of less than 5 mm may occur early in the course of TB infection or in individuals with altered immune function. Anergy testing with at least two other delayed-type hypersensitivity skin tests (i.e., *Candida,* mumps, or tetanus toxoid) should be used in conjunction with PPD testing in adults with decreased cell-mediated immune function (including those with HIV infection).

Adverse reactions to TB skin testing are very uncommon. Reactions described include pain, fever, ulceration, vesiculation, and regional adenopathy. Because of the potential for adverse reactions, it is not advisable to retest patients who have a documented history of a positive Mantoux test.

Although bacillus Calmette-Guérin (BCG) vaccine can cause false-positive Mantoux reactions, this response decreases with time and rarely causes reactions 15 mm or greater. In general, BCG-vaccinated individuals with positive Mantoux tests should be considered to have true infection with TB and given appropriate follow-up care (Table 7-7).

Administer chest x-ray examination

Take sputum culture. A positive culture is essential to confirm the diagnosis. Three sputum samples should be examined for AFB smear and culture. Culture results may take from 3 to 6 weeks.

Administer baseline laboratory tests: liver function tests (LFTs) and CBC with differential.

Determine baseline drug susceptibility of the first isolate. Repeat drug susceptibility testing in patients whose isolates do not convert to negative within 3 months.

Urinalysis should be obtained routinely; if sterile pyuria is found, it is suggestive of renal TB, and cultures should be sent.

If clinical features suggest infection outside the lung, smears and cultures of other body fluids such as cerebrospinal fluid are appropriate.

ADMINISTERING

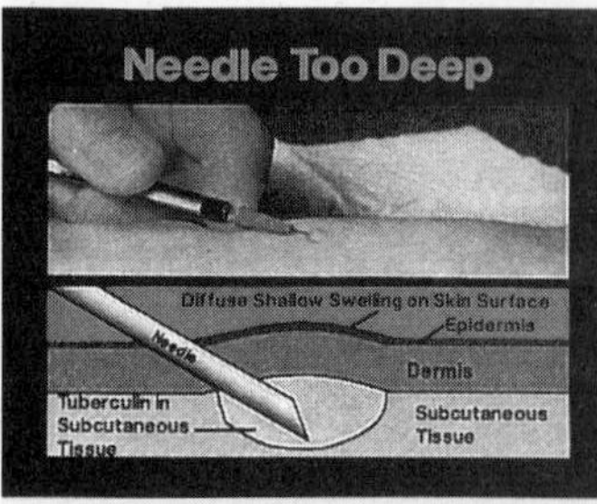

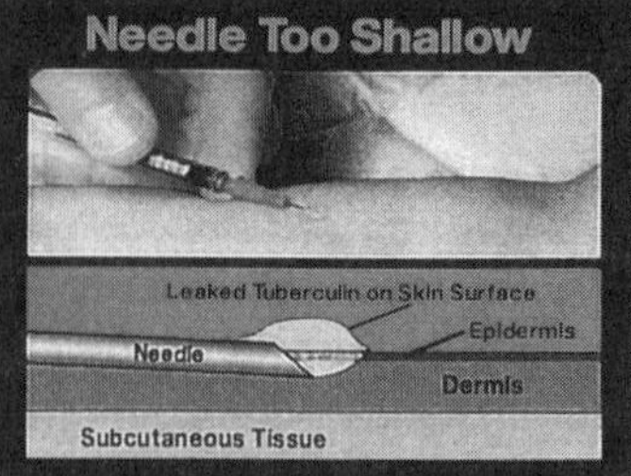

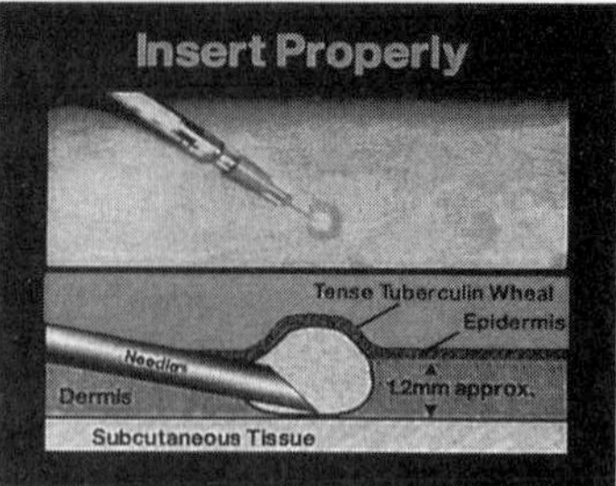

READING

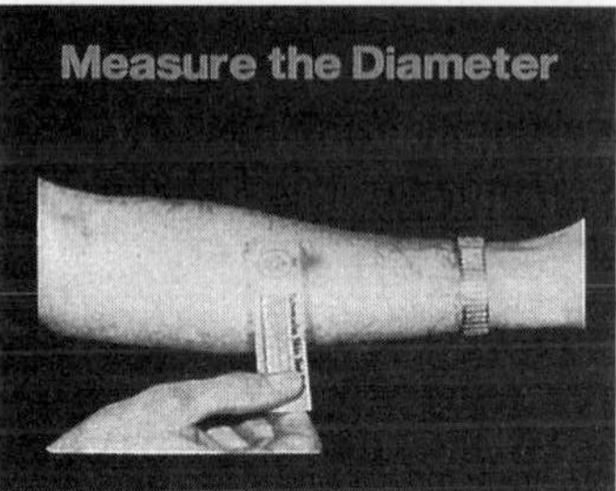

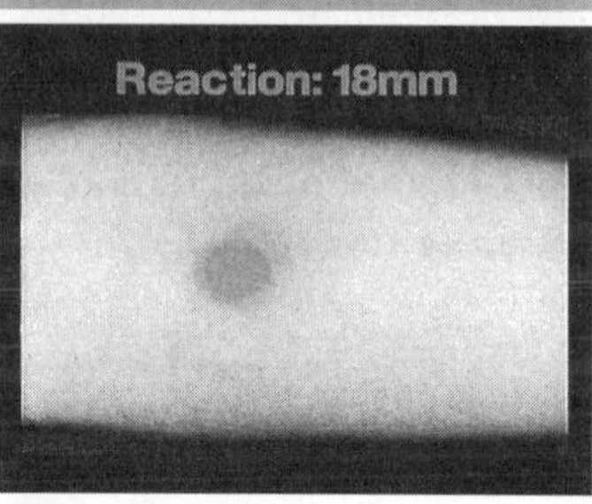

Give 0.1 cc of 5 Tuberculin Units PPD intradermally.

All tests should be read between 48-72 hours. If more than 72 hours has elapsed and there is not an easily palpable positive reaction, repeat the test on the other arm and read at 48-72 hours.

Measure induration - not erythema.

Measure and report results in millimeters of induration.

All persons with positive reactions should be evaluated for preventive therapy, once TB disease has been ruled out.

5 or more millimeters induration is considered positive for the highest risk groups, such as:

- Persons with HIV infection;
- Persons who have had close contact with an infectious tuberculosis case;
- Persons who have chest radiographs consistent with old, healed tuberculosis;
- Intravenous drug users whose HIV status is unknown.

10 or more millimeters induration is considered positive for other high risk groups, such as:

- Foreign-born persons from high prevalence areas (such as Asia, Africa, and Latin America);
- Intravenous drug users known to be HIV seronegative;
- Medically-underserved low income populations, including high-risk racial or ethnic minority populations (especially blacks, Hispanics, and Native Americans);
- Residents of long-term care facilities (such as correctional institutions, nursing homes, mental institutions);
- Persons with medical conditions which have been reported to increase the risk of tuberculosis such as silicosis, being 10 percent or more below ideal body weight, chronic renal failure, diabetes mellitus, high dose corticosteroid and other immunosuppressive therapy, some hematologic disorders (such as leukemias and lymphomas), and other malignancies;
- Locally identified high risk populations;
- Children who are in one of the high risk groups listed above; and
- Health care workers who provide services to any of the high risk groups.

15 or more millimeters induration is considered positive for persons with no risk factors for tuberculosis.

Negative Reactions *- For each of the categories, reactions below the cutting point are considered negative.*

CDC

U.S. DEPARTMENT OF HEALTH & HUMAN SERVICES
Public Health Service
Centers for Disease Control and Prevention
National Center for Prevention Services
Division of TB Elimination
Atlanta, Georgia 30333

Please use this wall chart in conjunction with the CDC skin test video

Figure 7-1 The Mantoux Tuberculin Skin Test. (Courtesy U.S. Department of Health and Human Services, Public Health Service, Centers for Disease Control and Prevention, National Center for Prevention Services, Division of TB Elimination, Atlanta, Ga.)

TABLE 7-7 Criteria for Determining Need for Preventive Therapy with Positive PPD

Category	<35	≥35
With risk factor	Treat all ages if reaction to 5 TU PPD is ≥10 mm (or ≥5 mm and recent TB contact, HIV infected or has radiographic evidence of old TB)	
Without risk factor High-incidence group*	Treat if PPD is ≥10 mm	Do not treat
Without risk factor Low-incidence group	Treat if PPD is ≥15 mm	Do not treat

From U.S. Department of Health and Human Services: *The clinician's handbook of preventive services,* McLean, Va, International Medical, 1994.

*High-incidence groups include foreign-born persons, medically underserved low-income populations, and residents of long-term care facilities.

Treatment

Therapeutics

Option 1 is to administer daily isoniazid, rifampin, and pyrazinamide for 8 weeks, followed by 16 weeks of isoniazid and rifampin daily or two to three times per week. *All regimens administered two to three times per week should be monitored by directly **observed** treatment for the duration of therapy:*

Isoniazid: 5 mg/kg up to 300 mg for everyday dosing ***or***
15 mg/kg up to 900 mg for two to three times weekly dosing
Rifampin: 10 mg/kg up to 600 mg for all dosing schedules
Pyrazinamide: 15 to 30 mg/kg up to 2 g for daily dosing ***or***
50 to 70 mg/kg up to 3 g for two to three times weekly dosing

In areas where resistance to isoniazid is documented, add ethambutol or streptomycin for at least 6 months, as well as 3 months beyond culture conversion:

Ethambutol: 15 to 25 mg/kg for daily dosing ***or***
25 to 30 mg/kg up to 2.5 g for two to three times weekly dosing
Streptomycin: 15 to 20 mg/kg up to 1 g intramuscular for daily dosing ***or***
25 to 30 mg/kg up to 1 g for two to three times weekly dosing

Option 2 is to administer daily isoniazid, rifampin, pyrazinamide, and streptomycin or ethambutol for 2 weeks, followed by twice weekly administration of the same drugs for 6 weeks by directly observed treatment. Subsequent administration is twice weekly with isoniazid and rifampin for 16 weeks by directly observed treatment.

Option 3 is directly observed treatment three times per week with isoniazid, rifampin, pyrazinamide, and ethambutol or streptomycin for 6 months (Uphold and Graham, 1994).

*Consult a TB medical expert if the patient continues to remain symptomatic or if the smear **or** culture remains positive after 3 months.*

Education

Teach patient the possible side effects of medications, including the following:

Peripheral neuritis from isoniazid
Multiple drug interactions
Orange urine and tears that may stain contact lenses with rifampin
Possible eighth cranial nerve damage with streptomycin: have hearing tested
Hyperuricemia with pyrazinamide
Optic neuritis with ethambutol: have vision, especially color sensitivity, tested

All antitubercular medications have possible liver damage as a side effect. *No alcohol is allowed.*

Teach proper disposal of secretions and tissues, as well as the mode of transmission, and reinforce the need to cover mouth with coughing.

Have patients take pyridoxine (vitamin B_6) 25 mg daily while on isoniazid.

Patients are usually back to their usual state of health in 1 to 2 months.

Follow-up

The patient's role in successful treatment of TB, daily self-administration of drugs for a period of 6 to 9 months and return for regular follow-up schedules, is crucial. After treatment has been initiated, the patient should be seen or contacted at least once per month, chiefly to ensure drug compliance and to monitor for drug side effects.

Sputum cultures should be obtained monthly for the first 3 months. At 3 months and between 6 and 12 months, chest x-ray films should be obtained.

Sputum cultures should be negative after 3 months of therapy, although occasionally nonculturable acid-fast organisms can be seen on smear for longer periods. A test-of-cure culture should be done on all patients at 5 or 6 months.

At the cessation of traditional chemotherapy regimen (9 months), prolonged follow-up is not necessary. After short-course (6 months) chemotherapy, it is recommended that follow-up be continued for another 12 months to detect relapses by symptoms and sputum culture.

Summary

Age-related changes in the respiratory system are significant, as are the number of potential acute and chronic diseases of the lungs and airways. The practitioner must be able to distinguish between acute, self-limiting, life-threatening, and chronic lung diseases and to treat each appropriately to minimize discomfort and loss of function. It is important to know the risk factors for lung disease so that prevention and appropriate screening can be started early. This point is important whether the concern is COPD, cancer of the lung, or infectious concerns such as TB, a resurgent and significant threat.

Resources

American Lung Association
www.lungusa.org

New York Online Access to Health (NOAH)
COPD Website
http://www.noah.cuny.edu

National Coalition for Adult Immunization
http://www.nfid.org/ncai

References

Abramowicz M, editor: Sparfloxacin and levofloxacin, *Med Lett Drugs Ther* 39:41-43, 1997.

American Lung Association: *Guidelines for the prevention and treatment of influenza and the common cold for the general public,* Atlanta, 1997, the Association.

American Thoracic Society: Guidelines for the initial management of adults with community-acquired pneumonia: diagnosis, assessment of severity, and initial antimicrobial therapy, *American Review of Respiratory Disease* 148:1418-1426, 1993.

Barker LR, Burton JR, Zieve PD: *Ambulatory medicine,* ed 4, Baltimore, 1995, Williams & Wilkins.

Burke MM, Walsh MB: *Gerontologic nursing: wholistic care of the older adult,* ed 2, St Louis, 1997, Mosby.

Fischbach F: *A manual of laboratory & diagnostic tests,* ed 4, Philadelphia, 1992, JB Lippincott.

French M: Pneumonia in the elderly, *Adv Nurse Pract* 3:40-44, 1995.

Miller CA: *Nursing care of older adults: theory and practice,* ed 2, Philadelphia, 1995, JB Lippincott.

Richman E: Asthma diagnosis and management: new severity classifications and therapy alternatives, *Clin Rev* 7:76-112, 1997.

Stanley M, Beare PG: *Gerontological nursing,* Philadelphia, 1995, FA Davis.

Uphold CR, Graham MV: *Clinical guidelines in adult health,* Gainesville, Fla, 1994, Barmarrae.

US Department of Health and Human Services: *The clinician's handbook of preventive services,* McLean, Va, 1994, International Medical.

US Department of Health and Human Services: *Core curriculum on tuberculosis: what every clinician should know,* ed 3, Atlanta, 1999, Centers for Disease Control and Prevention.

Witta KM: COPD in the elderly: controlling symptoms and improving quality of life, *Adv Nurse Pract* 5:18-27, 72, 1997.

8

The Aging Cardiovascular System

Epidemiology

Eight of every 10 people 65 or older have at least one chronic medical problem, but 60% of those over 65 are without any functional or physical limitations from their conditions. However, when there is illness or disability in the elderly population, cardiovascular disease is still the most frequent cause. Congestive heart failure is the most common medical problem necessitating hospitalization in the elderly. More than half of the patients hospitalized annually for acute myocardial infarctions are more than 65 years old. Finally, coronary artery disease causes 70% to 80% of the deaths in the over-65 age group (Duncan and Vittone, 1996). Therefore proper diagnosis and treatment of cardiovascular diseases can help to both maintain the health of the large number of functionally independent elderly and reduce morbidity and mortality in the elderly in acute and chronic care settings.

Changes in the cardiovascular system occur with aging. Some of these changes can be considered natural in an aging organism. Others occur with the onset of a disease process in the cardiovascular system itself. Still other changes are the result of coexisting medical conditions. There are anatomic changes in the blood vessels, the heart itself, the heart valves, and the conducting systems, as well as physiologic or functional changes.

Age-related Changes in the Vasculature

With aging, there is gradual buildup of atherosclerotic plaque in the vascular tree throughout the body. The plaques are complex aggregates of necrotic cells, mostly smooth muscle cells, connective tissue such as collagen and elastin, and lipid deposits. There is often deposition of calcium in and around these plaques. The result is a hardened, irregular vessel wall and a narrowing of the lumen of the vessel, with obstruction or partial obstruction of blood flow. Commonly referred to as "hardening of the arteries," this process probably begins in late adolescence and advances with aging. During the Korean War, autopsies done on soldiers who were war casualties revealed that atherosclerotic changes had already begun in some as young as 18 years old. Of course, other factors influence the rate at which atherosclerosis progresses. Known risk factors for development of atherosclerosis are listed in Box 8-1.

Other changes in the vascular tree occur as a natural consequence of aging, and these changes take place regardless of the presence or rate of atherosclerosis. The cells of the arterial walls become more and more irregular in size and shape with aging. Their usual orderly layering becomes deranged, with the orientation of the cells one to another irregular and disorderly. The subendothelial layer thickens because of increased connective tissue production and increased calcium and lipid deposition. In the medial layer there are thickened smooth muscle layers. The smooth muscle cells have more protein and calcium deposition. The surrounding elastin or connective tissue is prone to fragmentation. The loss of the integrity of elastin means poor elasticity in the vessel wall. In the intimal layer there is similar fragmentation of elastin and increased collagen content. The intimal surface becomes irregular, leaving more pits and crevices for lipids to deposit. All of these changes result in thicker, less distensible, less pliable arterial walls. With any atherosclerotic change, the stiffening is even worse. These aged arteries cannot distend when blood flow increases, effectively increasing the peripheral "resistance" to flow. An aorta affected by these aging changes has decreased compliance or resistance to the systolic ejection, affecting the percentage of the blood volume pumped by the left ventricle during systole that actually is ejected into the peripheral circulation (ejection fraction). At some point, when circulatory demand increases, these stiff, noncompliant blood vessels cannot expand to accommodate the demand, leading to higher pressures within the arterial tree.

In the coronary arteries these aging changes tend to affect the proximal part of the artery first and the left coronary artery before the right, with autopsy studies consistently finding changes as young as middle adulthood, whereas changes in the right are noted in the 50s (Wei, 1992).

Changes also occur in the function of the blood vessel walls. With aging the usual constriction response of the vascular smooth muscle to alpha-adrenergic stimulation is unchanged. However, the usual relaxation response of the vascular smooth muscle to beta-adrenergic stimulation declines with age, another factor in the aged blood vessel's decreased ability to relax. This response to alpha-adrenergic input without corresponding response to beta-adrenergic input may be part of the etiology of isolated systolic

Box 8-1

Risk Factors for the Development of Atherosclerosis

- Cigarette smoking
- Diabetes
- Hypertension
- Hyperlipidemia
- Obesity
- Genetic factors

hypertension in the elderly, in addition to the increase in the level of plasma catecholamines in the elderly (Applegate, 1989).

Changes in the Heart Muscle

The age-related changes in the myocardium include enlargement of the cardiac muscle cells, the myocytes. Inside the cell there are lipid and lipofuscin deposits, the tubules dilate, and there is decreased mitochondrial activity, resulting in abnormal products of oxidation, such as malonaldehyde, which irreversibly denatures deoxyribonucleic acid. This leads to a bigger cell, with impaired cellular functions, that does not get replaced by replication when there is cell death. At age 75 a body has only 10% as many sinus node cells as it had at age 20, according to one study (Wei, 1992). This change may account for the increased incidence of sinus node disease, such as SSS or supraventricular tachyarrhythmias, in the elderly.

Around the myocytes, as in the blood vessel walls, there is increased deposition of elastic tissue, fat, and collagen; and multiple foci of fibrosis and calcification may occur. The result is a stiff, inelastic, noncompliant myocardium. There may also be deposition of amyloid, especially in the left ventricle. The left ventricle thickens slightly, but in general the overall size of the left ventricle remains the same with aging changes alone. Within the myocardium capillaries are obliterated because of the deposition of lipids, connective tissue, and calcium. Therefore the myocardium can actually be relatively ischemic, with inadequate blood flow, because of this small-vessel disease, even with the major coronary arteries open. Small-vessel ischemic disease occurs with increased frequency in patients with diabetes.

These changes have a functional consequence for the myocardium. The stiffer the myocardial wall becomes, the more time is required for this stiff heart muscle to relax, and the relaxation phase requires more energy and uses more oxygen. The first result is that decreased relaxation of the myocardial wall impedes diastolic filling and therefore effectively reduces cardiac output. With severe impairment to diastolic filling, there is reduced forward flow or cardiac output. The result can be left-sided congestive heart failure (CHF), leading to pulmonary vascular congestion and systemic congestion and edema. Second, with increased myocardial oxygen demand, there can be a relative hypoxia or ischemia in the heart muscle, even with the major coronary arteries undiseased. Compounding this effect is the fact that, as people age, there is a decrease in the arterial oxygen tension. It decreases by 4 mm Hg per decade, from an average of 90 mm Hg at age 30 to 75 mm Hg at age 80 (Wei, 1992).

Changes in the Heart Valves and Conducting System

Again, the aging changes in the heart valves and the conductive system are largely deposition of calcium; an increase in connective tissue, with fragments of degenerated connective tissue and cells remaining or deposited within the normal tissue; and fibrosis. In the heart valves calcium deposition has the largest effect. Calcium deposits below the mitral valve, in the space between the posterior leaflet of the mitral valve and the adjacent myocardial wall, effectively decrease the motion of the valve leaflets and prevent complete opening of the valve. Calcium deposits in the mitral annulus likewise decrease excursion of the valve leaflets. The physiologic result is mitral stenosis, decreased left ventricular filling, and eventual left atrial strain and enlargement. There is a twelvefold increase in atrial fibrillation with submitral calcium deposits, and frequently there are associated conduction defects (Duncan and Vittone, 1996).

In the conducting system, similar aging changes occur, with predictable effects. In addition, there is a loss of conducting cells. As described earlier, there may be a 90% loss of the number of cells in the sinus node by age 75. The atrioventricular (AV) node and bundle of His show a decrease in the number of both cells and conducting fibers. From the AV node the bundle of His emerges as a main bundle, then branches into the left and right bundles. Proximally there are fewer fascicles connecting the main bundle with the left bundle. There are also fewer distal conducting fibers. Predictably, conduction disorders such as left or right bundle branch blocks and AV node blockade have increased incidence with aging. Box 8-2 lists the structural and functional changes in the aging heart (Duncan and Vittone, 1996).

Changes in Cardiovascular Physiology

The structural changes described translate into specific cardiovascular problems, such as hypertension, decreased cardiac output, CHF, valvular dysfunction, and cardiac arrhythmias or conduction disturbances. Other changes in cardiovascular physiology compound these problems. Already mentioned is the decreased arterial oxygen tension, which can aggravate any vascular problem and make elderly patients with circulatory compromise (coronary artery or peripheral artery insufficiency) have more severe symptoms than they would, based on their anatomic vascular disease alone. The elderly also have an increased resting heart rate, perhaps related in part to an increased level of catecholamines. Nonetheless, when increased heart rate or contractility is needed, in the case of physiologic stress, there is a decrease in responsiveness to beta-adrenergic stimulation. Thus maximum heart rate and ability to increase the ejection fraction are less.

The elderly are also much more sensitive to small changes in plasma volume. The natural changes of aging in the kidneys, coupled with changes in the function of the renin-angiotensin axis, actually make the elderly person more susceptible to dehydration. There is a decreased thirst drive. Vasopressin secretion is decreased in response to decreased plasma volume. There is also decreased renin production, therefore decreased angiotensin, and, ultimately, decreased aldosterone production. In addition, when plasma volume is decreased, the elderly person may be more symptomatic because compensatory mechanisms such as the baroreceptor reflex are also less responsive. Thus the elderly person with small decreases in plasma volume might be light-headed, dizzy, or even syncopal.

One study found a substantial drop in arterial blood pressure in elderly patients after a meal. There have been significant increases in this group in postprandial symptoms, including syncope, angina, and myocardial infarction (MI). The mechanism of postprandial hypotension is thought to be the diversion of blood flow to the gut, resulting in a relatively reduced intravascular volume elsewhere in the vascular tree. Other relatively mild hemodynamic changes occur with defecation, urination, and postural change. The incidence of symptomatology associated with such mild hemodynamic changes is negligible in the young but significant in the elderly. There is a significant increase in the frequency of falls in the elderly, and although falls are often multifactorial, no doubt a

Box 8-2

Age-Related Changes in Cardiovascular Structure and Function

Structure

- Myocardial
  - Increased myocardial mass
  - Increased LV wall thickness
  - Increased deposition of collagen
- Valvular
  - Increased thickness of aortic and mitral leaflets
  - Increased circumference of all four valves
  - Calcification of mitral annulus
- Arterial
  - Increased intimal thickness
  - Increased collagen content

Function

- Heart rate
  - Decreased heart rate at rest
  - Decreased maximal heart rate during exercise
  - Decreased heart rate variability
  - Decreased sinus node intrinsic rate
- LV systolic
  - Unchanged cardiac output
  - Increased stroke volume index
- LV diastolic
  - Decreased LV compliance
  - Increased early diastolic LV filling
- Myofibril
  - Unchanged peak contractile force
  - Increased duration of contraction
  - Decreased Ca^{++} uptake by sarcoplasmic reticulum
  - Decreased β-adrenergic-mediated contractile augmentation
- Vascular
  - Decreased compliance
  - Increased pulsed-wave velocity

LV, Left ventricular.
From Duncan A, Vittone JM: Cardiovascular disease in elderly patients, *Mayo Clin Proc* 71:184-196, 1996.

number are related to events such as those described, which can cause small but eventful hemodynamic changes in the elderly. Add to that diuretic therapy for hypertension or CHF, and the elderly person is at even more risk.

As an illustration of the impact of aging changes in the elderly heart and vascular system, imagine the elderly person facing a physiologic stress such as surgery, acute illness, or perhaps pneumonia. In either instance the elderly heart now needs to increase its cardiac output to generate a greater circulatory flow to vital organs. First, the left ventricular early (passive) diastolic filling is less because of a stiffened, less compliant ventricle. Less volume is delivered to the aorta in systole. Therefore an increase in systolic contraction may be required. The left ventricle is slightly thickened, but unless there has been an MI or there is ischemia, contractile strength should be preserved. Yet the maximum increase possible in ejection fraction is lower in the elderly. Increased heart rate can compensate for decreased filling volume, but the maximum heart rate attainable is lower in the elderly. In addition, because of aging changes in the arterial tree, the peripheral resistance is higher. There is increased afterload for the systolic contraction to overcome. The blood volume that is delivered to the peripheral circulation is therefore less, despite the increased demand. Add to that any decrease in plasma volume, and the situation is compounded. Beta-adrenergic stimulation is present, but the aging heart responds less to this stimulus. If aging coronary arteries are also affected by atherosclerotic changes, there may be ischemia and increased risk for MI. All of this, plus decreased arterial oxygen tension and decreased efficiency of oxygen extraction, can make an elderly cardiovascular system unable to deliver increased cardiac output on demand.

Age-related changes in the cardiovascular system are a combination of changes natural to aging, cardiovascular disease present, and comorbid conditions that affect the cardiovascular system. Overall, the natural history of heart disease is that it increases with aging. The manifestations of heart disease, the treatments, and the outcomes may all differ in the elderly person, compared with the younger person. Yet elderly people can improve their cardiovascular function with exercise. With regular cardiovascular exercise such as a gradual program of brisk walking for 30 minutes at least three times a week, exercise tolerance improves through increased arterial oxygen tension but chiefly through increased efficiency of oxygen uptake and extraction (air to blood to tissue). As a result, resting heart rate and blood pressure fall. Body fat percentage can be decreased, and muscle strength and joint flexibility can be increased, resulting in better mobility, balance, and gait. Therefore the aging cardiovascular system, like the aging musculoskeletal system, can still be conditioned.

Cardiac Examination of the Elderly Patient

The cardiac examination of the elderly person contains the same elements as that of any other patient. However, as cardiac disease increases with age, there may be findings encountered infrequently in the young. First, measure the blood pressure and the heart rate, and assess the heart rhythm for regularity and ectopic beats. For blood pressure measurement of all patients, even more pertinently in the elderly, the cuff should be inflated initially to 200 mm Hg or just over. Failure to do this may result in a falsely low reading. Another method is to palpate the brachial artery as the cuff is inflated. Inflate the cuff at least 20 mm Hg above the point at which the artery ceases to be palpable (the palpable systolic blood pressure). Deflate the cuff slowly. If Korotkoff's sounds are heard immediately as deflation begins, chances are that the cuff was not inflated to a high enough pressure, and the patient's systolic pressure could be higher than measured. (This caution applies even if the cuff was initially inflated to 200 mm Hg or above.) Repeat the measurement on the other arm, and inflate to a higher level. In evaluating elderly patients for hypertension, it is prudent to take a series of blood pressure readings and to measure blood pressure while the patient is both sitting and standing.

Orthostatic Hypotension

The increased incidence of orthostatic hypotension in the elderly is due to a number of normal aging structural and physiologic changes that have been discussed. Older people have a lower resting heart rate and are less able to increase cardiac output with demand. They have lower plasma renin activity, a decreased vasopressin response to thirst, and decreased renal conservation of salt with decreased volume. Thus they may have a relatively decreased intravascular volume. As a result, blood pressure may fall significantly with change from a lying or sitting posture to a standing position, a phenomenon called orthostatic blood pressure change. If that change causes abnormally low blood pressure or symptoms such as light-headedness, dizziness, or syncope, the diagnosis is orthostatic or postural hypotension. The blood pressure criterion for a diagnosis of orthostatic hypotension is a drop of more than 20 mm Hg in systolic pressure or a drop of more than 10 mm Hg in diastolic pressure, on change of position. Orthostatic hypotension can be a result of volume depletion, as in fluid or blood loss, or it can be from other causes, such as autonomic nervous system dysfunction. Alternately, a rise in pulse of more than 20 beats per minute on change of position can be considered a sign more specific for volume depletion. The presence of symptomatic orthostatic hypotension can have important therapeutic implications for the elderly.

Auscultation of the Heart

Bruits

Listen for carotid bruits. Asymptomatic carotid bruits are indicative of diffuse atherosclerotic disease. Asymptomatic carotid bruits can be predictors of increased stroke risk, but the incidence of stroke in these patients is contralateral as often as ipsilateral. Totally occluded carotid arteries are silent and do not produce a bruit (Schneiderman, 1993).

Heart Sounds

Listen for the heart sounds and physiologic splitting of the second heart sound, S_2. It should be split in inspiration because of delayed pulmonic closure that occurs from increased filling of the right heart. It should be heard best at the left sternal border. As one listens toward the apex, the splitting should disappear; the pulmonic component of S_2 should be so faint as to be inaudible there. There can be a reversed split, called a paradoxic split (i.e., a splitting or two-component sound in expiration, and no split in inspiration). It accompanies left ventricular conduction delay as in left bundle branch block (LBBB). Pacemaker patients have paradoxic splitting, as pacemakers activate the right heart before the left. The delay in the closing of the aortic valve makes the second heart sound a one-component sound in inspiration because both pulmonic closure and aortic closure are delayed. In right bundle branch block, the pulmonic valve closure is delayed in both inspiration and expiration, so the second heart sound is constantly split. See Table 8-1 for the normal occurrence of heart sounds.

Although a fourth heart sound is common in the elderly patient, a third heart sound represents disease. A third heart sound is common in CHF, but it is not found exclusively in CHF. In CHF rapid passive (early) diastolic filling is associated with a gallop if there is increased end-systolic volume. If the systolic ejection fraction is lower than normal, there is increased residual volume in the left ventricle after systole. In other words, the ventricle does not empty well with systole. The flow of blood into that residual pool of blood is one of the conditions that causes an S_3 gallop.

TABLE 8-1 Relative Differences of Heart Sounds

	Cause	End-piece	Location	Pitch	Respirations	Position	Variables
S_1	Closure of tricuspid and mitral valves	Diaphragm	Entire precordium (apex)	High	Softer on inspiration	Any position	Increased with excitement, exercise, amyl nitrate, epinephrine, and atropine
S_2	Closure of pulmonary and aortic valves	Diaphragm	A_2 at 2nd RICS; P_2 at 2nd LICS	High	Fusion of A_2P_2 on expiration; physiologic split on inspiration	Sitting or supine	Increased in thin chest walls and with exercise

	Aortic	Pulmonic	Second Pulmonic	Mitral	Tricuspid
Pitch	$S_1 < S_2$	$S_1 < S_2$	$S_1 < S_2$	$S_1 < S_2$	$S_1 < S_2$
Loudness	$S_1 < S_2$	$S_1 < S_2$	$S_1 < S_2$*	$S_1 > S_2$†	$S_1 > S_2$
Duration	$S_1 > S_2$	$S_1 > S_2$	$S_1 > S_2$	$S_1 > S_2$	$S_1 > S_2$
S_2 split	>inhale	>inhale	>inhale	>inhale‡	>inhale
	<exhale	<exhale	<exhale	<exhale	<exhale
A_2	Loudest	Loud	Decreased		
P_2	Decreased	Louder	Loudest		

Modified from Seidel HM: *Mosby's guide to physical examination,* St Louis, 1999, Mosby.

*S_1 is relatively louder in second pulmonic area than in aortic area.

†S_1 may be louder in mitral area than in tricuspid area.

‡S_2 split may not be audible in mitral area if P_2 is inaudible.

Murmurs

Perhaps the most common murmur heard in the elderly heart is the murmur of aortic sclerosis, a calcified valve with an irregular orifice that causes turbulent flow but without a hemodynamically significant decrease in the dimensions of the valve orifice. It is a systolic murmur that can be heard in the second intercostal spaces, radiating to the neck over both carotids; depending on intensity, it may radiate to the base or the apex. The presence or absence of symptoms or evident hemodynamic compromise helps to make the important distinction between benign aortic sclerosis and aortic valve stenosis.

Usually in aortic stenosis, palpable carotid upstrokes are diminished (pulsus parvus et tardus), but there may be a palpable systolic thrill over the carotids. Delayed aortic closure can result in paradoxic splitting of the second heart sound. There is usually low-normal blood pressure (BP) with a narrowed pulse pressure (systolic BP not much higher than diastolic), but in elderly patients noncompliant arteries may result in normal or even hypertensive blood pressures, even in the face of significant aortic stenosis. In tight stenosis the reduced flow through the valve may result in a softer murmur than in benign aortic sclerosis. More important than these signs may be symptoms. Any elderly person with an aortic outflow murmur and symptoms suggestive of angina or CHF needs evaluation of the aortic valve by echocardiogram.

Respiratory Examination

On a lung examination of an elderly patient, crackles at the lung bases are not an infrequent finding. Crackles often reflect mild fibrotic pulmonary changes that can be a part of the natural aging process. They may not represent congestion, as in CHF. In fact, CHF in the elderly can present with no crackles or rales at all, but with "cardiac asthma," a wheezing that mimics bronchospastic disease, or simply with persistent cough. Severe pulmonary vascular congestion might present with cough productive of rusty, blood-tinged sputum. The significance of crackles heard on the examination of the lungs of the older patient must be determined by other related findings such as jugular venous distention, edema, or productive cough.

Abdominal Examination

Palpating the abdomen for silent, asymptomatic abdominal aortic aneurysms has diagnostic sensitivity in thin persons but not in the obese (Schneiderman, 1993).

Peripheral Vascular Examination

Check pulses: femoral, popliteal, dorsalis pedis, and posterior tibial. Note asymmetry. Note skin lesions, dryness, hair loss, duskiness, and edema. Absence of pulses without symptoms and with intact skin that is appropriately warm, with good capillary filling, is usually no cause for alarm. Try to elicit any history that suggests claudication with exercise. In that case, and certainly if there is ulceration of the skin, arterial Doppler studies and vascular surgery evaluation should be considered.

Hypertension in the Older Person

Definition

Hypertension is defined as systolic blood pressure (SBP) of 140 mm Hg or greater, diastolic blood pressure (DBP) of 90 mm Hg or greater, or taking antihypertensive medication (NIH, 1997). The objective of identifying and treating high blood pressure is to reduce the risk of cardiovascular disease and associated morbidity and mortality. Table 8-2 provides a classification of blood pressure for adults.

Epidemiology

It is not surprising, given the changes in the arterial tree that occur with aging, compounded by the progression of atherosclerosis, that stiffened, noncompliant arteries in elderly people result in increased peripheral resistance or hypertension. Studies done to ascertain the prevalence of hypertension in the elderly give greatly varying estimates, from 10% to 50%. Generally the prevalence increases with age, with more hypertension found, for example, in those in the 80- to 90-year-old age group than in those a decade younger. The prevalence of hypertension in elderly black patients is consistently higher than that in elderly white patients (Applegate, 1989).

In the Framingham Heart Study, the presence of hypertension resulted in a twofold increase in CHF in men and a threefold increase in CHF in women. The type of CHF to

TABLE 8-2 Classification of Blood Pressure for Adults Age 18 and Older*

Category	Systolic (mm Hg)		Diastolic (mm Hg)
Optimal†	<120	and	<80
Normal	<130	and	<85
High-normal	130-139	or	85-89
Hypertension‡			
Stage 1	140-159	or	90-99
Stage 2	160-179	or	100-109
Stage 3	≥180	or	≥110

From National Institutes of Health: *The sixth report of the Joint National Committee on prevention, detection, evaluation, and treatment of high blood pressure,* Bethesda, Md, 1997, International Medical.

*Not taking antihypertensive drugs and not acutely ill. When systolic and diastolic blood pressures fall into different categories, the higher category should be selected to classify the individual's blood pressure status. For example, 160/92 mm Hg should be classified as stage 2 hypertension, and 174/120 mm Hg should be classified as stage 3 hypertension. Isolated systolic hypertension is defined as SBP of 140 mm Hg or greater and DBP below 90 mm Hg and staged appropriately (e.g., 170/82 mm Hg is defined as stage 2 isolated systolic hypertension). In addition to classifying stages of hypertension on the basis of average blood pressure levels, clinicians should specify presence or absence of target organ disease and additional risk factors. This specificity is important for risk classification and treatment.

†Optimal blood pressure with respect to cardiovascular risk is below 120/80 mm Hg. However, unusually low readings should be evaluated for clinical significance.

‡Based on the average of two of more readings taken at each of two or more visits after an initial screening.

which long-standing hypertension predisposes is diastolic failure. A hypertrophic left ventricle is most likely to have poor ventricular relaxation and reduced compliance. On the contrary, coronary artery disease (CAD) and ischemia of the heart muscle are more likely to result in CHF from systolic dysfunction.

Isolated Systolic Hypertension

In the elderly diastolic and systolic hypertension can certainly be found together, but there is an increase in the incidence of isolated systolic hypertension (i.e., elevated systolic blood pressures) with normal diastolic pressures. Isolated systolic hypertension, which is peculiar to the elderly, is actually more of a predictor for some cardiovascular morbidities than is diastolic hypertension and therefore must be treated. The presence of isolated systolic hypertension in those older than 65 has more predictive value for future stroke, MI, and CHF than the presence of diastolic hypertension (Kannel, 1989; Kannel, Dawber, and McGee, 1980).

Because of the increased arterial stiffness, or decreased compliance, there is probably an exaggerated rise in hypertension in the elderly in all situations that result in transient BP elevations, such as stress and anxiety, increased heart rate, or increased stroke volume with exercise. As a result, it is unwise to make a diagnosis of hypertension based on one reading. Unless BPs require urgent intervention, such as systolic readings above 200 or diastolic readings above 115, it is preferable to have the patient get a series of readings before instituting treatment. Without this precaution, hypertension in the elderly may be overdiagnosed, with significant side effects when patients are treated who are really usually normotensive.

Pseudohypertension

Occasionally a phenomenon called pseudohypertension is encountered. When the elderly have a brachial artery with walls so thickened, calcified, and sclerosed that the artery is essentially noncompressible by the standard BP cuff, an inaccurately high BP may result. To rule out pseudohypertension, first palpate the pulsating brachial artery. Then inflate the cuff and listen for Korotkoff's sounds. When these sounds disappear, palpate the arm for the brachial artery again. If the pulseless artery can still be palpated, this indicates a stiff, noncompressible artery, and an elevated systolic reading under these circumstances may represent pseudohypertension. This procedure is known as Osler's maneuver. Pseudohypertension is actually rare. If needed, an accurate reading in this circumstance would require an intraarterial line.

Evaluation of Hypertension

History

A medical history should include the following (NIH, 1997):

- Known duration and levels of elevated BP
- Patient history or symptoms of CAD, heart failure, cerebrovascular disease, periph-

eral vascular disease, renal disease, diabetes, dyslipidemia, other comorbid conditions, gout, or sexual dysfunction

- Family history of high BP, premature CAD, stroke, diabetes, dyslipidemia, or renal disease
- Symptoms suggesting causes of hypertension
- History of recent changes in weight, leisure time physical activity, and smoking or other tobacco use
- Dietary assessment, including intake of sodium, alcohol, saturated fat, and caffeine
- History of all prescribed and over-the-counter medications, herbal remedies, and illicit drugs, some of which may raise BP or interfere with the effectiveness of antihypertensive drugs
- Results and adverse effects of previous antihypertensive therapy
- Psychosocial and environmental factors (e.g., family situation, employment status, and working conditions) that may influence hypertension control

Physical Examination

The initial physical examination should include the following (NIH, 1997):

- Two or more BP measurements separated by 2 minutes with the patient either supine or seated and after standing for at least 2 minutes
- Verification in the contralateral arm (if values are different, the higher value should be used)
- Measurement of height, weight, and waist circumference
- Funduscopic examination for hypertensive retinopathy (i.e., arteriolar narrowing, focal arteriolar constrictions, arteriovenous crossing changes, hemorrhages and exudates, disk edema)
- Examination of the neck for carotid bruits, distended veins, or an enlarged thyroid gland
- Examination of the heart for abnormalities in rate and rhythm, increased size, precordial heave, clicks, murmurs, and third and fourth heart sounds
- Examination of the lungs for rales and evidence of bronchospasm
- Examination of the abdomen for bruits, enlarged kidneys, masses, and abdominal aortic pulsation
- Examination of the extremities for diminished or absent arterial pulsations, bruits, and edema
- Neurologic assessment

Laboratory Assessment

Routine laboratory tests recommended before initiating therapy are tests to determine the presence of target organ damage and other risk factors. These routine and optional tests as recommended in the sixth report of the Joint National Committee on Blood Pressure (NIH, 1997) are listed in Table 8-3.

TABLE 8-3 Tests and Procedures in Evaluating Hypertension

Routine	Optional
Urinalysis	Creatinine clearance
CBC	Microalbuminuria
Electrolytes	24-hour urinary protein
Renal function tests	Blood calcium
Glucose	Uric acid
Total cholesterol and HDL	Fasting triglycerides/LDL
12-lead electrocardiogram	Glycosylated hemoglobin
	TSH
	Echocardiography

From National Institutes of Health: *The sixth report of the Joint National Committee on prevention, detection, evaluation, and treatment of high blood pressure,* Bethesda, Md, 1997, International Medical.
CBC, Complete blood count; *HDL,* high-density lipoprotein; *LDL,* low-density lipoprotein; *TSH,* thyroid-stimulating hormone.

Treatment

Fortunately, treatment of hypertension can make a difference in the outcome. In studies of people over age 60, treatment of hypertension, including isolated systolic hypertension, has shown a reduction in strokes of up to 32% in some series. Although the number of nonfatal MIs did not decrease, the number of fatal MIs and the number of deaths from CHF did decrease. In fact, the number of cardiac deaths from all causes was decreased by 38% in elderly persons whose hypertension was treated (Applegate, 1989).

The decision to treat is based on risk stratification (NIH, 1997). Box 8-3 lists the components of cardiovascular risk stratification in patients with hypertension. Use this information and refer to Table 8-4 for treatment guidelines.

Initial therapy in mildly elevated BP should consist of lifestyle modification: diet, exercise, and attention to reversible risk factors. Box 8-4 lists lifestyle modifications for hypertension prevention and management.

Pharmacologic Treatment

If pharmacologic treatment is required, a number of agents are available: diuretics, angiotensin-converting enzyme (ACE) inhibitors, beta blockers, adrenergic inhibitors, and calcium channel blockers. See Tables 8-5 and 8-6 for information regarding oral antihypertensive drugs.

Diuretics. The physiologic mechanisms that leave elderly patients with relatively lower plasma volumes and at risk for dehydration have been discussed. As a rule, it is prudent to try to avoid diuretics in elderly patients for these reasons. Diuretics lower both SBPs and DBPs, but in addition to the risk for volume depletion or dehydration, diuretics also affect potassium, glucose, and lipid metabolism. However, hypokalemia can be critical, and patients who are also taking digoxin must be closely monitored to avoid arrhythmia. Administration of potassium supplements necessitates close monitoring of potassium levels for hyperkalemia. The risk of hyperkalemia is increased if the patient is

Box 8-3

Components of Cardiovascular Risk Stratification in Patients with Hypertension

Major Risk Factors

Smoking
Dyslipidemia
Diabetes mellitus
Age older than 60 years
Sex (men and postmenopausal women)
Family history of cardiovascular disease: women under age 65 or men under age 55

Target Organ Damage/Clinical Cardiovascular Disease

Heart diseases
- Left ventricular hypertrophy
- Angina/prior myocardial infarction
- Prior coronary revascularization
- Heart failure

Stroke or transient ischemic attack
Nephropathy
Peripheral arterial disease
Retinopathy

From National Institutes of Health: *The sixth report of the Joint National Committee on prevention, detection, evaluation, and treatment of high blood pressure,* Bethesda, Md, 1997, International Medical.

TABLE 8-4 Risk Stratification and Treatment*

Blood Pressure Stages (mm Hg)	Risk Group A (No Risk Factors No TOD/CCD)†	Risk Group B (At Least 1 Risk Factor, Not Including Diabetes; No TOD/CCD)	Risk Group C (TOD/CCD and/or Diabetes, with or without Other Risk Factors)
High-normal (130-139/85-89)	Lifestyle modification	Lifestyle modification	Drug therapy‡
Stage 1 (140-159/90-99)	Lifestyle modification (up to 12 months)	Lifestyle modification† (up to 6 months)	Drug therapy
Stages 2 and 3 (≥160/≥100)	Drug therapy	Drug therapy	Drug therapy

For example, a patient with diabetes and a blood pressure of 142/94 mm Hg plus left ventricular hypertrophy should be classified as having stage 1 hypertension with target organ disease (left ventricular hypertrophy) and with another major risk factor (diabetes). This patient would be categorized as Stage 1, Risk Group C, and recommended for immediate initiation of pharmacologic treatment.

From National Institutes of Health: *The sixth report of the Joint National Committee on prevention, detection, evaluation, and treatment of high blood pressure,* Bethesda, Md, 1997, International Medical.

*Lifestyle modification should be adjunctive therapy for all patients recommended for pharmacologic therapy.

TOD/CCD, Target organ disease/clinical cardiovascular disease.

†For patients with multiple risk factors, clinicians should consider drugs as initial therapy plus lifestyle modifications.

‡For those with heart failure, renal insufficiency, or diabetes.

Box 8-4

Lifestyle Modifications for Hypertension Prevention and Management

- Lose weight if overweight.
- Limit alcohol intake to no more than 1 oz (30 ml) ethanol (e.g., 24 oz [72 ml] beer, 10 oz [300 ml] wine, or 2 oz [60 ml] 100-proof whiskey) per day or 0.5 oz (15 ml) ethanol per day for women and lighter-weight people.
- Increase aerobic physical activity (30 to 45 minutes most days of the week).
- Reduce sodium intake to no more than 100 mmol/day (2.4 g sodium or 6 g sodium chloride).
- Maintain adequate intake of dietary potassium (approximately 90 mmol/day).
- Maintain adequate intake of dietary calcium and magnesium for general health.
- Stop smoking and reduce intake of dietary saturated fat and cholesterol for overall cardiovascular health.

From National Institutes of Health: *The sixth report of the Joint National Committee on prevention, detection, evaluation, and blood pressure,* Bethesda, Md, 1997, International Medical.

on ACE inhibitors, which conserve potassium. Loop diuretics such as furosemide (Lasix) and bumetanide (Bumex) are in general more effective in treating edema and CHF but give less even BP control. They are generally not good choices as single-agent antihypertensives because of their short duration of action. Because of their rapid onset of action and rapid progression to peak action, some elderly patients experience urge or functional incontinence with these agents. They may frequently delay or deliberately omit these medications if they have a social engagement. Compliance must always be considered in choosing a medication.

Angiotensin-converting Enzyme Inhibitors. An alternative to diuretics may be ACE inhibitors in some patients. The ACE inhibitors decrease sodium and water retention by interfering with the conversion of angiotensin I to angiotensin II, a step in the overall production of aldosterone. However, the elderly with hypertension are more likely to be "low renin" hypertensives; i.e., they have low serum renin values. Their hypertension is less likely a volume-dependent hypertension. Therefore ACE inhibitors may be less effective in this type of patient. Some elderly patients have side effects from ACE inhibitors, such as rash, loss of taste, increase in blood urea nitrogen (BUN) and creatinine, persistent cough, and angioedema. If ACE inhibitors are chosen, start with the smallest therapeutic dose. The initial dose, especially if the patient is already on diuretics or has hyponatremia, can cause marked hypotension within the first 3 hours of dosing. If the patient has renal insufficiency and is already on a diuretic, use reduced doses of both the diuretic and the ACE inhibitor, and follow renal functions and serum potassium carefully. Avoid potassium-sparing diuretics with ACE inhibitors, or monitor serum potassium regularly.

The angiotensin II receptor blocker losartan (Cozaar) likewise reduces sodium and water retention. Similar cautions apply.

Beta Blockers. This class may be less effective in the elderly, again because there is decreased renin activity with aging. In addition, there is decreased response to beta-adrenergic stimulus. Therefore the elevation of BP in an elderly person is less likely to involve either of these two mechanisms, or, at least, these mechanisms are less likely to

Text continued on p. 222

Table 8-5 Oral Antihypertensive Drugs*

Drug	Trade Name	Usual Dose Range, Total mg/day* (Frequency per Day)	Selected Side Effects and Comments*
Diuretics (partial list)			Short-term: increases cholesterol and glucose levels; biochemical abnormalities: decreases potassium, sodium, and magnesium levels, increases uric acid and calcium levels; rare: blood dyscrasias, photosensitivity, pancreatitis, hyponatremia
Chlorthalidone (G)†	Hygroton	12.5-50 (1)	
Hydrochlorothiazide (G)	Hydrodiuril, Microzide, Esidrix	12.5-50 (1)	
Indapamide	Lozol	1.25-5 (1)	(Less or no hypercholesterolemia)
Metolazone	Mykrox	0.5-1.0 (1)	
	Zaroxolyn	2.5-10 (1)	
Loop Diuretics			
Bumetanide (G)	Bumex	0.5-4 (2-3)	(Short duration of action, no hypercalcemia)
Ethacrynic acid	Edecrin	25-100 (2-3)	(Only nonsulfonamide diuretic, ototoxicity)
Furosemide (G)	Lasix	40-240 (2-3)	(Short duration of action, no hypercalcemia)
Torsemide	Demadex	5-100 (1-2)	

From National Institutes of Health: *The sixth report of the Joint National Committee on prevention, detection, evaluation, and treatment of high blood pressure,* Bethesda, Md, 1997, International Medical.

*These dosages may vary from those listed in the *Physician's Desk Reference* (51st edition), which may be consulted for additional information. The listing of side effects is not all-inclusive, and side effects are for the class of drugs except where noted for individual drugs (in parentheses); clinicians are urged to refer to the package insert for a more detailed listing.

†(G) indicates generic available.

‡Also acts centrally.

||Has intrinsic sympathomimetic activity.

§Cardioselective.

Continued

TABLE 8-5 Oral Antihypertensive Drugs*—cont'd

Drug	Trade Name	Usual Dose Range, Total mg/day* (Frequency per Day)	Selected Side Effects and Comments*
Diuretics (partial list)—cont'd			
Potassium-Sparing Agents			Hyperkalemia
Amiloride hydrochloride (G)	Midamor	5-10 (1)	
Spironolactone (G)	Aldactone	25-100 (1)	(Gynecomastia)
Triamterene (G)	Dyrenium	25-100 (1)	
Adrenergic Inhibitors			
Peripheral Agents			
Guanadrel	Hylorel	10-75 (2)	(Postural hypotension, diarrhea)
Guanethidine monosulfate	Ismelin	10-150 (1)	(Postural hypotension, diarrhea)
Reserpine (G)‡	Serpasil	0.05-0.25 (1)	(Nasal congestion, sedation, depression, activation of peptic ulcer)
Central Alpha-Agonists			Sedation, dry mouth, bradycardia, withdrawal hypertension
Clonidine hydrochloride (G)	Catapres	0.2-1.2 (2-3)	(More withdrawal)
Guanabenz acetate (G)	Wytensin	8-32 (2)	
Guanfacine hydrochloride (G)	Tenex	1-3 (1)	(Less withdrawal)
Methyldopa (G)	Aldomet	500-3,000 (2)	(Hepatic and "autoimmune" disorders)
Alpha-Blockers			Postural hypotension
Doxazosin mesylate	Cardura	1-16 (1)	
Prazosin hydrochloride (G)	Minipress	2-30 (2-3)	
Terazosin hydrochloride	Hytrin	1-20 (1)	
Beta-Blockers			Bronchospasm, bradycardia, heart failure, may mask insulin-induced hypoglycemia; less serious: impaired peripheral

			circulation, insomnia, fatigue, decreased exercise tolerance, hypertriglyceridemia (except agents with intrinsic sympathomimetic activity)
Acebutolol‖	Sectral	200-800 (1)	
Atenolol (G)§	Tenormin	25-100 (1-2)	
Betaxolol§	Kerlone	5-20 (1)	
Bisoprolol fumarate§	Zebeta	2.5-10 (1)	
Carteolol hydrochloride‖	Cartrol	2.5-10 (1)	
Metoprolol tartrate (G)§	Lopressor	50-300 (2)	
Metoprolol succinate§	Toprol-XL	50-300 (1)	
Nadolol (G)	Corgard	40-320 (1)	
Penbutolol sulfate‖	Levatol	10-20 (1)	
Pindolol (G)‖	Visken	10-60 (2)	
Propranolol hydrochloride (G)	Inderal	40-480 (2)	
	Inderal LA	40-480 (1)	
Timolol maleate (G)	Blocadren	20-60 (2)	
Combined Alpha- and Beta-Blockers			Postural hypotension, bronchospasm
Carvedilol	Coreg	12.5-50 (2)	
Labetalol hydrochloride (G)	Normodyne, Trandate	200-1,200 (2)	
Direct Vasodilators			Headaches, fluid retention, tachycardia
Hydralazine hydrochloride (G)	Apresoline	50-300 (2)	(Lupus syndrome)
Minoxidil (G)	Loniten	5-100 (1)	(Hirsutism)
Calcium Antagonists			
Nondihydropyridines			Conduction defects, worsening of systolic dysfunction, gingival hyperplasia
Diltiazem hydrochloride	Cardizem SR	120-360 (2)	(Nausea, headache)
	Cardizem CD	120-360 (1)	
	Dilacor XR, Tiazac		

Continued

TABLE 8-5 Oral Antihypertensive Drugs*—cont'd

Drug	Trade Name	Usual Dose Range, Total mg/day* (Frequency per Day)	Selected Side Effects and Comments*
Calcium Antagonists—cont'd			
Nondihydropyridines—cont'd			
Mibefradil dihydrochloride (T-channel calcium antagonist)	Posicor	50-100 (1)	(No worsening of systolic dysfunction; contraindicated with terfenadine [Seldane], astemizole [Hismanal], and cisapride [Propulsid])
Verapamil hydrochloride	Isoptin SR, Calan SR	90-480 (2)	(Constipation)
	Verelan, Covera HS	120-480 (1)	
Dihydropyridines			Edema of the ankle, flushing, headache, gingival hypertrophy
Amlodipine besylate	Norvasc	2.5-10 (1)	
Felodipine	Plendil	2.5-20 (1)	
Isradipine	DynaCirc	5-20 (2)	
	DynaCirc CR	5-20 (1)	
Nicardipine	Cardene SR	60-90 (2)	
Nifedipine	Procardia XL, Adalat CC	30-120 (1)	
Nisoldipine	Sular	20-60 (1)	
ACE Inhibitors			Common: cough; rare: angioedema, hyperkalemia, rash, loss of taste, leukopenia
Benazepril hydrochloride	Lotensin	5-40 (1-2)	
Captopril (G)	Capoten	25-150 (2-3)	
Enalapril maleate	Vasotec	5-40 (1-2)	
Fosinopril sodium	Monopril	10-40 (1-2)	
Lisinopril	Prinivil, Zestril	5-40 (1)	
Moexipril	Univasc	7.5-15 (2)	
Quinapril hydrochloride	Accupril	5-80 (1-2)	
Ramipril	Altace	1.25-20 (1-2)	
Trandolapril	Mavik	1-4 (1)	
Angiotensin II Receptor Blockers			Angioedema (very rare), hyperkalemia
Losartan potassium	Cozaar	25-100 (1-2)	
Valsartan	Diovan	80-320 (1)	
Irbesartan	Avapro	150-300 (1)	

TABLE 8-6 Combination Drugs for Hypertension

Drug	Trade Name
Beta-Adrenergic Blockers and Diuretics	
Atenolol, 50 or 100 mg/chlorthalidone, 25 mg	Tenoretic
Bisoprolol fumarate, 2.5, 5, or 10 mg/hydrochlorothiazide, 6.25 mg	Ziac*
Metoprolol tartrate, 50 or 100 mg/hydrochlorothiazide, 25 or 50 mg	Lopressor HCT
Nadolol, 40 or 80 mg/bendroflumethiazide, 5 mg	Corzide
Propranolol hydrochloride, 40 or 80 mg/hydrochlorothiazide, 25 mg	Inderide
Propranolol hydrochloride (extended release), 80, 120, or 160 mg/hydrochlorothiazide, 50 mg	Inderide LA
Timolol maleate, 10 mg/hydrochlorothiazide, 25 mg	Timolide
ACE Inhibitors and Diuretics	
Benazepril hydrochloride, 5, 10, or 20 mg/hydrochlorothiazide, 6.25, 12.5, or 25 mg	Lotensin HCT
Captopril, 25 or 50 mg/hydrochlorothiazide, 15 or 25 mg	Capozide*
Enalapril maleate, 5 or 10 mg/hydrochlorothiazide, 12.5 or 25 mg	Vaseretic
Lisinopril, 10 or 20 mg/hydrochlorothiazide, 12.5 or 25 mg	Prinzide, Zestoretic
Angiotensin II Receptor Antagonists and Diuretics	
Losartan potassium, 50 mg/hydrochlorothiazide, 12.5 mg	Hyzaar
Calcium Antagonists and ACE Inhibitors	
Amlodipine besylate, 2.5 or 5 mg/benazepril hydrochloride, 10 or 20 mg	Lotrel
Diltiazem hydrochloride, 180 mg/enalapril maleate, 5 mg	Teczem
Verapamil hydrochloride (extended release), 180 or 240 mg/trandolapril, 1, 2, or 4 mg	Tarka
Felodipine, 5 mg/enalapril maleate, 5 mg	Lexxel
Other Combinations	
Triamterene, 37.5, 50, or 75 mg/hydrochlorothiazide, 25 or 50 mg	Dyazide, Maxide
Spironolactone, 25 or 50 mg/hydrochlorothiazide, 25 or 50 mg	Aldactazide
Amiloride hydrochloride, 5 mg/hydrochlorothiazide, 50 mg	Moduretic
Guanethidine monosulfate, 10 mg/hydrochlorothiazide, 25 mg	Esimil
Hydralazine hydrochloride, 25, 50, or 100 mg/hydrochlorothiazide, 25 or 50 mg	Apresazide
Methyldopa, 250 or 500 mg/hydrochlorothiazide, 15, 25, 30, or 50 mg	Aldoril
Reserpine, 0.125 mg/hydrochlorothiazide, 25 or 50 mg	Hydropres
Reserpine, 0.10 mg/hydralazine hydrochloride, 25 mg/hydrochlorothiazide, 15 mg	Ser-Ap-Es
Clonidine hydrochloride, 0.1, 0.2, or 0.3 mg/chlorthalidone, 15 mg	Combipres
Methyldopa, 250 mg/chlorothiazide, 150 or 250 mg	Aldochlor
Reserpine, 0.125 or 0.25 mg/chlorthalidone, 25 or 50 mg	Demi-Regroton
Reserpine, 0.125 or 0.25 mg/chlorothiazide, 250 or 500 mg	Diupres
Prazosin hydrochloride, 1, 2, or 5 mg/polythiazide, 0.5 mg	Minizide

From National Institutes of Health: *The sixth report of the Joint National Committee on prevention, detection, evaluation, and treatment of high blood pressure,* Bethesda, Md, 1997, International Medical.

ACE, Angiotensin-converting enzyme.

*Approved for initial therapy.

be the major mechanism at work. The important role of beta blockade in the treatment of angina and CAD is discussed later. However, as antihypertensives in the elderly, they may be less efficacious. In addition, side effects such as lethargy, depression, aggravation of the peripheral vascular disease, and sleep disturbance may be exaggerated in the elderly. The high incidence of CHF in the elderly is also reason for caution. But recent studies of patients treated with beta blockers for CAD have shown that even patients with CHF have been able to tolerate beta blockers in many cases. This tolerance is definitely to their advantage in CAD. By decreasing heart rate and contractility, the beta blockers decrease the myocardial oxygen demand. Beta blockers have been shown to be effective in preventing both extension of the infarct after acute MI and repeat MI. However, for patients with CHF who need an antihypertensive and have no history of MI, it is probably desirable to try other antihypertensives first. Nitrates and calcium channel blockers can still be used if CAD is suspected or if there are anginal symptoms.

Adrenergic Inhibitors. Centrally acting adrenergic inhibitors decrease sympathetic output from the brain and central nervous system to the peripheral vascular system. Decreased sympathetic stimulation results in decreased vasoconstriction, smooth muscle in the vessel walls relaxes, and peripheral resistance falls. Alpha methyldopa (Aldomet), clonidine (Catapres), guanabenz (Wytensin), guanadrel sulfate (Hylorel), and guanfacine hydrochloride (Tenex) are some of the products available. These agents work in various ways on the alpha-adrenergic system. They may stimulate these receptors as false transmitters, effectively blocking the reception of the true neurotransmitters that would, in turn, trigger the release of adrenergic agents such as norepinephrine from neuronal storage sites. They may stimulate alpha-adrenergic inhibitory receptors. Some may even prevent norepinephrine reuptake by the nerve once it is released from the neuronal stores. The net result is decreased tissue concentration of norepinephrine and other sympathetic stimulants.

More peripherally acting alpha blockers such as prazosin (Minipress) and terazosin (Hytrin) stimulate alpha-adrenergic receptors, acting as false transmitters in the postsynaptic or peripheral site. These medications avoid the sedation or drowsiness of the more centrally acting drugs, but orthostatic hypotension is still a potential problem. Also, the profound drop in BP that can occur with first exposure to these drugs makes it prudent to give the first dose to the patient at bedtime; should a profound drop in pressure occur, the patient is in the supine position. Labetalol (Normodyne, Trandate) has some beta-blockade properties but is primarily alpha blockade.

Centrally or peripherally, alpha blockade is generally an effective approach to treatment of hypertension in the elderly. Although the elderly have reduced responsiveness to beta-adrenergic stimuli, they have normal alpha-adrenergic responsiveness and increased circulating norepinephrine levels.

Calcium Channel Blockers. Calcium channel blockers are usually a good choice for BP control in the elderly. As a class, they are vasodilators. They have effectiveness in vasodilation of the coronary artery bed and therefore are effective antianginals. Thus when hypertension and CAD coexist, calcium channel blockers are an excellent therapeutic choice. The different products available do have different properties, as far as negative inotropism and effect on AV node conduction are concerned. Verapamil, diltiazem (Cardizem), and nifedipine do depress left ventricular contractility, probably in that order, and have to be used carefully or avoided in CHF on account of systolic dysfunction. Nifedipine is prone to provoking reflex tachycardia, as some of the others can also do to a lesser extent. Verapamil and diltiazem depress AV node conduction and may be used for that purpose to control ventricular rate in supraventricular tachyarrhythmias such as atrial fibrillation. They are usually used in conjunction with digitalis in this setting but can be effective alone, particularly diltiazem. However, they may have an adverse effect in the presence of conduction defects or any degree of heart block. Amlodipine (Norvasc) has the advantage of little or no effect on left ventricular contractility or on AV node conduction. In treating hypertension, amlodipine may require 2 to 3 weeks before its maximum effect is shown, and it may provoke reflex tachycardia. As a class, calcium channel blockers can cause edema, and orthostatic hypotension can be a problem.

Adverse Effects of Antihypertensive Therapy

The elderly are more likely to suffer side effects, both from prescribed medications and from the effects of reduced intraarterial pressures. In general, however, reducing the peripheral vascular resistance is compensated for by an increase in cardiac output. The heart is able to circulate a larger blood volume when the force against which it must work (i.e., the peripheral vascular resistance) is lower. That seems to be the case with blood flow to vital organs when high BP is treated. There may be a level of BP below which compensatory increase in cardiac output is compromised; i.e., there can be a BP that is too low for optimum perfusion of vital organs, especially if that pressure is low because of volume depletion. The perfect BP that is under good control but not too low may be a delicate balance that is difficult to achieve. One easy indication to follow may be renal function, BUN, and creatinine, which tend to rise when renal perfusion is compromised. On first encountering the elderly person with hypertension, administer a medication regimen that gradually reduces the BP to desired levels. Abrupt, large drops in pressure may cause symptoms such as light-headedness and dizziness, have an adverse effect on gait and balance, put the patient at risk for falls, and contribute to confusion. When BP has been elevated for a time, the cerebral autoregulatory mechanisms have been reset regarding what is normal cerebral blood flow. However, when BP is lowered slowly and gradually, these autoregulatory mechanisms can reset appropriately (Applegate, 1989). As with any medication in the older person, "start low, and go slow" with dosing. Figure 8-1 is an algorithm for the treatment of hypertension.

Coronary Artery Disease

Epidemiology

Estimates vary of the incidence of CAD in the elderly, but in all series the numbers are high. In one study estimates are that 15% of men and 9% of women over age 70 have CAD, and that figure increases to 20% of both men and women by age 80. Of those with CAD, 40% of patients in their 80s are estimated to be symptomatic, and 70% or more of those in their 90s have at least one coronary artery totally occluded (Duncan and Vittone, 1996). These figures are at the low end of the estimates. Other studies have estimated that 30% to 40% of people over age 60 have significant CAD Still another study reports that at least 60% of those over age 65 have at least one coronary artery with critical narrowing (i.e., more than 75% stenosis). One study estimates that 10% to 12% of the chronic disease limitations in the elderly are due to CAD. Mortality rates from acute MIs are down in the elderly, but more patients are suffering the complications of chronic coronary

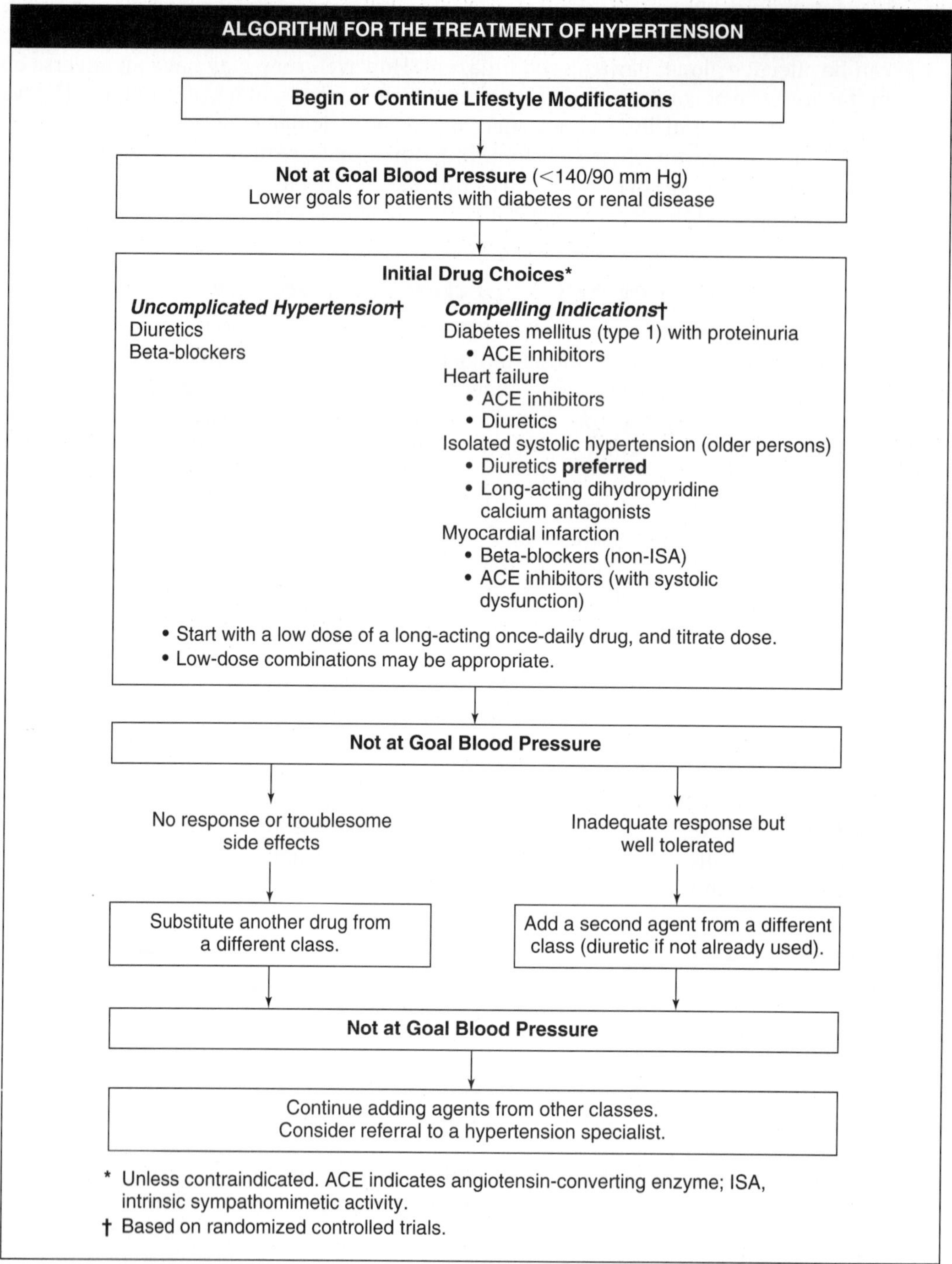

ALGORITHM FOR THE TREATMENT OF HYPERTENSION
Begin or Continue Lifestyle Modifications
Not at Goal Blood Pressure (<140/90 mm Hg)
Lower goals for patients with diabetes or renal disease
Initial Drug Choices*
Uncomplicated Hypertension†
Diuretics
Beta-blockers
Compelling Indications†
Diabetes mellitus (type 1) with proteinuria
• ACE inhibitors
Heart failure
• ACE inhibitors
• Diuretics
Isolated systolic hypertension (older persons)
• Diuretics preferred
• Long-acting dihydropyridine calcium antagonists
Myocardial infarction
• Beta-blockers (non-ISA)
• ACE inhibitors (with systolic dysfunction)
• Start with a low dose of a long-acting once-daily drug, and titrate dose.
• Low-dose combinations may be appropriate.
Not at Goal Blood Pressure
No response or troublesome side effects
Inadequate response but well tolerated
Substitute another drug from a different class.
Add a second agent from a different class (diuretic if not already used).
Not at Goal Blood Pressure
Continue adding agents from other classes.
Consider referral to a hypertension specialist.
* Unless contraindicated. ACE indicates angiotensin-converting enzyme; ISA, intrinsic sympathomimetic activity.
† Based on randomized controlled trials.

Figure 8-1 Algorithm for the treatment of hypertension. (Modified from National Institutes of Health: The sixth report of the Joint National Committee on prevention, detection, evaluation, and treatment of high blood pressure, Bethesda, Md, 1997, International Medical.)

Box 8-5
Risk Factors for the Development of Coronary Artery Disease

- Cigarette smoking
- Diabetes
- Hypertension
- Elevated cholesterol and serum lipids
- Obesity
- Sedentary lifestyle
- Male sex
- Family history

insufficiency (i.e., CHF, systolic and diastolic) due to myocardial ischemia (Senni and Redfield, 1997; Stemmer and Aronow, 1997). The risk factors for the development of CAD are listed in Box 8-5.

Atypical Presentation of Coronary Artery Disease in the Elderly

The diagnosis of CAD in the elderly may present a challenge. Like so many other syndromes, presentation of CAD in the elderly may be atypical. Typical angina is less likely to be the presenting symptom. Precordial chest pain, pressure, or heaviness that might radiate to the neck, jaw, or shoulder or down the left arm is often completely absent in the elderly patient. Dyspnea is the most common presenting symptom of CAD in the elderly. This presentation can make recognition of early symptoms difficult, as there is often concomitant respiratory disease in the elderly, and symptoms may be attributed to it. Sometimes CAD in the elderly is completely silent.

If patients do present with chest pain, pressure, or heaviness, it, too, may have an atypical pattern. In the elderly the complaint of pain radiating to both shoulders and arms has been a symptom that can confound the diagnosis. When the elderly do present with symptoms that suggest new-onset angina, whatever the presentation, there is a higher likelihood, compared with younger persons, that CAD will be confirmed. Therefore it pays to have a lower threshold of suspicion in the elderly, and CAD should be considered when any elderly patient complains of dyspnea.

Although referral to a cardiologist is definitely indicated, there is strong evidence to support admitting for an inpatient evaluation the elderly patient with convincing symptoms of new-onset angina. In fact, it is justifiable to consider new-onset angina in this age group as “unstable” angina. Certain other findings predict a very high likelihood that symptoms represent significant coronary artery stenosis: if the patient is male and over 60 or if the patient if female and over 70, if there are transient hemodynamic changes during the pain, if there are transient electrocardiogram (ECG) changes associated with the pain, if there are ST segment elevations or depressions equal to or greater than 1 mm, or if there are marked symmetric T wave inversions in multiple precordial leads (Fauci et al., 1994). Such findings can help make the decision as to whether the patient needs coronary artery catheterization in the diagnostic workup.

Confirming the Diagnosis

To confirm the suspicion of CAD, noninvasive stress testing is usually the first step. A range of tests are available. The treadmill stress test may not be useful for many elderly patients because physical limitations from conditions such as arthritis may prevent effective exercise. Even those without such limitations may not be able to accomplish a meaningful exercise stress test. Resting heart rate and maximum achievable heart rate with exercise both decline with aging. Many elderly are not able to reach the 85% maximum predicted heart rate that is the target for interpreting the exercise stress test. For those who can exercise but have baseline ECG abnormalities that would make it difficult to interpret the recordings made during exercise, such as LBBB or ST segment abnormalities, radionucleotide scanning combined with exercise can be used. The rest and stress thallium test uses an injection of thallium to trace or scan perfusion of the heart muscle at rest, during exercise, and after exercise. The radioactive thallium is distributed evenly in the blood, and scanning can then give a pictorial estimate of relative volumes of blood flowing through the heart muscle in different locations. Less thallium activity in an area of heart muscle means less blood flow there. When an area of heart muscle shows decreased blood flow during exercise, this means that the coronary artery supplying that area is not able to increase blood flow or perfusion to meet the increased oxygen demands of exercise. Thus that area of heart muscle would likely be ischemic with exercise. If the flow increases again with rest, the coronary artery supplying that area is not completely obstructed and, with decreased demand, is able to meet the perfusion needs of that segment of muscle. This segment is in jeopardy of ischemic injury or infarction. Coronary angiography would be indicated to directly visualize the coronary artery in question and determine the degree of stenosis. Any area that is underperfused with rest and exercise and does not reperfuse after exercise is termed a "fixed defect"; the muscle is already permanently damaged by ischemia. If the area also moves abnormally, i.e., is hypokinetic, that fact further suggests prior permanent damage by MI. If there has been no clinical history of MI, this patient most likely has had a subclinical, unrecognized, or silent MI. The presence of evidence of prior silent MI, coupled with new symptoms compatible with angina, may be indication enough for coronary angiography to evaluate the degree of CAD.

If an elderly person cannot exercise at all, radionucleotide scanning of the myocardium can still be done by using dipyridamole (Persantine), dobutamine, or adenosine injections to create a physiologic stress on the heart. These nonexercise thallium scans are valuable and almost noninvasive. However, the agents used to induce the physiologic stress can have side effects. For instance, dipyridamole may cause bronchospasm and aggravate any concomitant pulmonary disease, and it is contraindicated in patients with active pulmonary disease.

Echocardiography with Doppler flow studies is an excellent tool for diagnosing valvular disease; evaluating chamber size; and evaluating left ventricular function, systolic and diastolic. Presence of wall motion abnormality on echocardiogram can also indicate ischemic or scarred myocardium. Exercise echocardiography can be even more specific in demonstrating heart muscle that functions inadequately with exercise, most likely because of ischemia or prior infarct.

Patients found to have significant abnormalities on exercise or nonexercise stress testing are most likely recommended for cardiac catheterization if their overall medical condition and prognosis are good. Knowing the exact anatomy of the coronaries, whether there is diffuse or single-vessel disease, whether the left main coronary artery is diseased, and the extent of stenosis in each vessel is the only way of verifying whether coronary artery bypass grafting is indicated in the patient who is healthy enough to be a surgical candidate. Yet in the elderly, multivessel disease is statistically more common than left main CAD alone. The presence of other concomitant illnesses such as severe CHF might make the patient an unacceptable operative risk. Other concomitant conditions such as advanced dementia may make it ethically impossible to pursue major surgery, or surgery may be contraindicated because of overall poor condition or poor prognosis. Nonetheless, even in some patients who are definitely not surgical candidates, by choice or because of overall condition and prognosis, cardiac catheterization can be beneficial by identifying patients with single-vessel disease or other anatomic patterns that are amenable to percutaneous transluminal coronary angioplasty.

Therapy for Coronary Artery Disease

For the elderly patient with CAD who is not going to undergo coronary artery bypass grafting, the therapy for angina is medication. Medications used in the elderly are the same as in other age groups: nitrates, beta blockers, and calcium channel blockers. These medications and their side effect potential in the elderly have been discussed under the subject of hypertension. In summary, the elderly are more likely to be compromised by the postural hypotension, atrioventricular blockade, and negative inotropism that some of these agents cause. Doses of each are lower in the elderly in general, but doses still must be titrated to achieve elimination of anginal symptoms, which is the standard for treatment success. It is important to maximize control of concomitant conditions such as hypertension and CHF because decompensation of control of either condition aggravates angina, and a previously well-controlled angina patient may become symptomatic again.

Nitrates

Nitrates are available in many forms and routes of administration. They act primarily as coronary vasodilators by improving myocardial blood flow and decreasing preload. Nitrates are well tolerated and effective, but chronic use can induce tolerance. The degree of tolerance can be limited by prescribing a regimen that includes a minimum 8 to 10 hours without nitrates. Available longer-acting nitrates include isosorbide dinitrate 10 to 40 mg orally twice a day, isosorbide mononitrate 10 to 40 mg orally twice a day or 60 to 120 mg once a day in a sustained-release preparation, oral sustained-release nitroglycerin preparations 6.25 to 12.5 mg two to four times daily, and transdermal nitroglycerin patches that deliver nitroglycerin at a predetermined rate. Side effects of nitrates include headache, nausea, dizziness, and hypotension (Massie and Amidon, 1997).

Therapy for Acute Myocardial Infarction

The elderly patient who is actually having an acute MI, like the elderly patient with angina, may present atypically. Most have some chest discomfort, but there is again likely

Box 8-6

Complications of Acute Myocardial Infarction

- Stroke
- Atrial arrhythmias
- Conduction disturbances
- Congestive heart failure

to be dyspnea more than pain or pressure. Elderly patients are less likely to become diaphoretic. Instead, the presenting symptoms of acute MI in the elderly may be acute confusion, syncope, and stroke, if not sudden death. Interestingly, in the elderly, the common early complication of acute MI is stroke, and a common complication of acute stroke is acute MI (Duncan and Vittone, 1996). There is greater in-hospital and long-term mortality from acute MI in the elderly than in the younger age group. The mortality in those over age 70 is four times greater than the average. Complications that are more frequent in the elderly patient with a new acute MI are listed in Box 8-6.

The increase in CHF is due to increased incidence of prior infarction, cardiomyopathy, hypertensive cardiac hypertrophy, and increased frequency of multivessel CAD, meaning more and larger areas of heart muscle already compromised by ischemia. Incidence of papillary muscle rupture is also increased, causing acute mitral valve dysfunction and secondary CHF, and the incidence of myocardial wall rupture is also increased. The incidence of postinfarction pericarditis is not increased in the elderly patient. There is also no increased frequency of ventricular tachycardia (V-Tach) (Duncan and Vittone, 1996).

Emergency Treatment of Acute Myocardial Infarction

Initial therapy of the patient should include an immediate aspirin 160 to 325 mg, administration of sublingual nitrates (NTG SL 1/150 every 5 minutes × three), and immediate transfer to an emergency room or acute care setting. If available, administration of oxygen (carefully noting any history of chronic obstructive pulmonary disease [COPD]), pain relief with morphine as required, and use of nitrates unless the systolic BP is below 90 or the heart rate is below 50 or higher than 100 are indicated. Once the patient is in an acute setting, intravenous (IV) heparin is started, as well as thrombolytic therapy if the history and ECG meet the criteria. Currently thrombolytic therapy, using streptokinase, urokinase, or tissue plasminogen activator, is reserved for those with symptoms compatible with acute MI and ST segment elevation more than 1 mm or LBBB on ECG (Ryan et al., 1996). This same regimen, except, of course, for thrombolytics, should be used for the patient presenting with anginal symptoms for whom acute MI is possible and must be ruled out. Oxygenation should be monitored by pulse oximetry and subsequent arterial blood gas measurements if there is significant history of lung disease. If pain is not relieved, narcotics should be administered, starting with 2 to 5 mg of IV morphine if not otherwise contraindicated (e.g., by allergy). If pain persists, the patient is a candidate for IV nitroglycerin drip, for which the starting dose is usually 5 μg per minute, titrated upward to a maximum of 75 to 100 μg per minute, as required to control pain. The patient presenting with symptoms compatible with angina, in whom suspicion of acute MI is high, should also be heparinized, hospitalized on a telemetry unit, and evaluated by a cardiologist (Fauci et al., 1994).

After the acute perimyocardial infarction period, long-term management should include aspirin therapy, beta-blocker therapy with or without other antianginals (nitrates and calcium channel blockers), and ACE inhibitors. Nonmedical management of cardiac risk factors is equally important. Treatment goals should include maintenance of ideal weight, control of hyperlipidemia, and, if necessary and appropriate, estrogen replacement therapy. Diet should be the American Heart Association step 2 diet for most. It contains less than 7% saturated fat and 200 mg per day of cholesterol minimally. Target for total low-dose lipoproteins should be below 130. Smoking cessation is essential to success. Patients who are functionally able should be in a formal rehabilitation program, which should include working up to a goal of 20 minutes of exercise at least three times per week. Such programs have shown positive benefit in the elderly but have been underused (Duncan and Vittone, 1996; Ryan, et al., 1996).

Coronary Artery Bypass Grafting in the Elderly

Coronary artery bypass grafting (CABG) in elderly patients can be appropriate for long-term treatment of CAD. If the patient is a good surgical candidate and in the course of evaluation and treatment of angina or acute MI is found to meet the indications for surgery, it should never be avoided or eliminated because of advanced age alone.

Not unexpectedly, the operative mortality for CABG does go up with age, and it increases when the procedure is done as an emergency. Nonetheless, elderly people who undergo successful CABG do better than those with medical or even angioplasty treatment in terms of prolonged survival, relief of symptoms, and restoration of an active lifestyle. They have fewer cardiac events, including acute MI and cardiovascular deaths. CABG gives more symptom-free time, therefore enhancing quality of life. This is not to say that CABG in the elderly can be approached cavalierly. Indeed, the decision must be approached with great caution. In addition to a greater operative risk of mortality, elderly surgical patients have greater morbidity; they stay in the hospital longer, up to 38% longer for the over-80 age group, and with up to 21% higher costs (Stemmer and Aronow, 1997).

In younger patients newer approaches to avoid CABG include coronary artery stents. In the elderly the rate of clinical success has been lower with coronary artery stents, and the event-free survival time has been shorter (Duncan and Vittone, 1996).

Common Arrhythmias in the Elderly

Changes in the conducting system of the heart lead to an increased incidence of arrhythmias and other conduction abnormalities in the elderly. Degeneration and fibrosis occur throughout the conduction system, in the sinus node, in the AV node, and in the bundle of His. As a result, there is a high prevalence of SSS and other atrial arrhythmias in the elderly. There is increased incidence also of AV node block of all degrees, of LBBB, and of RBBB. However, the internodal tracts do not lose as many muscle cells with aging and do not accumulate as much fibrous tissue as the sinus and AV nodes (Wei, 1992). Thus when there is LBBB, there is usually accompanying CAD. Likewise, when left anterior hemiblock (LAHB) and RBBB coexist, the combination almost always implies some structural heart disease, such as coronary artery insufficiency or ischemia or previous MI (Duncan and Vittone, 1996). This degree and type of conduction system disease would be unlikely on account of aging changes in the heart alone. Atrial fibrillation, SSS, and AV node blockade such as second-degree or third-degree (complete) heart block can occur solely as a consequence of an aging conductive system.

Atrial Fibrillation

The incidence of atrial fibrillation in the elderly is approximately 4%. In those over age 70, that incidence increases to 11%, and for those over age 84, the incidence is 17%. Increased mortality is most often due to increased incidence of stroke. Other complications of atrial fibrillation include systemic emboli, with embolic infarction in the extremities, or loss of vision from thromboemboli to the ophthalmic branches of the carotid arteries. See Box 8-7 for factors that predispose older people to atrial fibrillation.

Because the patient is elderly, do not discount acute alcohol excess as part of the differential diagnosis for the etiology of new-onset atrial fibrillation! Alcohol can be indicated in both acute and long-term atrial fibrillation, acute from alcohol's toxic effect and long-term from alcoholic cardiomyopathy.

Drugs, particularly stimulants, can also contribute to atrial fibrillation. Drugs that can cause or contribute to atrial fibrillation include caffeine, nicotine, and cough and cold

Box 8-7

Factors That Predispose Older Persons to Atrial Fibrillation

- Dilation of the atrium
- Sinus node disease (due to muscle cell loss, loss of nodal fibers, fibrosis, deposition of fatty tissue and amyloid in the sinus node)
- Calcification of the mitral valve
- Acute myocardial ischemia or infarct
- Inflammatory or infiltrative diseases that affect the myocardium (e.g., myocarditis from autoimmune disease such as lupus, rheumatoid arthritis)
- Pericarditis
- Cardiac surgery
- Pulmonary diseases
- Hypoxia
- Acute pulmonary embolism
- Hypokalemia
- Hypomagnesemia
- Hypocalcemia
- Hypoglycemia
- Hypothermia
- Alcohol
- Drugs

remedies such as decongestants, which are sympathetic stimulants, as well as local anesthetics such as lidocaine (Xylocaine), which are often combined with epinephrine for injection. Some drugs with anticholinergic side effects predispose to tachycardia, palpitations, and tachyarrhythmias as well.

Diagnosis of Atrial Fibrillation

Atrial fibrillation as diagnosed on the ECG shows a wavy baseline with no, or only occasional, deflections that resemble P waves and with irregular ventricular contractions. The ventricular rate is rapid, usually in the 100 to 160 range. The primary goal for treatment of atrial fibrillation is to control the ventricular rate. A usual goal is a ventricular rate of 90 or below. Some elderly patients have atrial fibrillation with a controlled ventricular rate, with no treatment, which indicates that intrinsic AV node disease is already present. With the usual rapid rate, the stiffened, less compliant ventricle, which may not be able to stretch for optimum filling, has even more decreased filling. There is less time for diastolic filling at a faster rate. In addition, the phase of diastolic filling, the atrial contraction, is completely missing. Less diastolic filling means less end-diastolic volume. The systolic function of the left ventricle may be normal, with the heart ejecting the normal 45% to 50% of the end-diastolic volume (i.e., a normal ejection fraction). However, the volume is smaller, so even with a normal ejection fraction, the volume of blood actually pumped into the circulation is smaller (i.e., the cardiac output is smaller). The difference may be enough to result in hypotension and decreased perfusion to the vital organs. There may be CHF and pulmonary vascular congestion, with dyspnea and hypoxia resulting. Acute atrial fibrillation can result in hemodynamic instability based on rapid ventricular rate alone.

Even the patient with AV node disease whose rate with atrial fibrillation is not rapid can be compromised because of the lack of atrial contraction. The atrial contraction is the last phase of diastolic filling. The stiffened ventricle that does not fill well during the passive, or stretch, phase of filling, may need the atrial contraction to achieve an effective filling volume. Without the atrial contraction, cardiac output can decrease, even without a rapid rate. The elderly are much more likely to be dependent on this atrial contraction to achieve adequate ventricular filling during diastole. Therefore the ultimate goal is to restore normal sinus rhythm, but rate control must be achieved first. At the same time, giving the patient oxygen after checking pulse oximetry or arterial blood gases, establishing IV access, and other supportive measures are indicated as well. It is wise to presume that acute new-onset atrial fibrillation could be a sign of myocardial ischemia or MI. Therefore treating any chest pain or discomfort with nitrates is indicated while monitoring vital signs. Telemetry should also be instituted.

Diagnostic Testing in New-onset Atrial Fibrillation

Appropriate diagnostic laboratory studies to rule out MI (creatinine phosphokinase, isoenzymes, cardiac troponin levels) should be ordered. A complete blood count (CBC) to rule out severe anemia, chemistry profiles to look for metabolic disorders, and thyroid function studies to rule out hyperthyroidism should be ordered. When the patient is stable enough, a chest x-ray film to rule out an acute pulmonary process should be done, as well as an echocardiogram to look for intraatrial thrombi, pericardial effusion, valvular disease, and abnormality in chamber size or contractility. In the case of intraatrial thrombus or valvular vegetation, some prefer the transesophageal echocardiogram for greater accuracy.

Rate Control in Atrial Fibrillation

The usual first drug used to control a rapid ventricular rate in atrial fibrillation is digoxin. Digoxin slows conduction across the AV node by increasing AV node refractory time. Therefore the number of beats that are successfully conducted from the rapidly fibrillating atrium, through the AV node, and into the ventricle are fewer, and the ventricle slows down. As a result of a slower ventricular rate and therefore increased time for diastolic ventricular filling, and with the addition of the positive inotropic effect of digoxin on the strength of systolic contractions, cardiac output increases. Often hemodynamic instability is corrected just by slowing the ventricular rate. Generally, a rate of 90 or less is the target. The usual dosage of digoxin is 1 mg total over 24 hours, or less, if the rate slows sufficiently. Some give digoxin initially in a dose of 0.5 mg IV, followed by 0.25 mg IV another one to two times, approximately 6 hours apart. If rate is controlled, a daily dose of oral digoxin at 0.125 to 0.25 mg can be started. If the rate is still a problem after a total of 1 mg of digoxin, the practice in the past has been to continue to give additional IV doses at intervals of 6 to 12 hours until the rate was controlled. Of course, this practice increased the possibility that patients would develop signs of digoxin toxicity, including nausea and vomiting and ventricular ectopy.

With the availability of calcium channel blockers, some of which have the property of slowing AV node conduction, especially verapamil and diltiazem, there is now an adjunct to digoxin for rate control in atrial tachyarrhythmias. Diltiazem is usually chosen because it has less negative inotropic effect (i.e., less depression of ventricular contractility) than verapamil. Therefore diltiazem is better tolerated in the CHF patient and in the patient who has acute CHF because of arrhythmia. Also, diltiazem, unlike verapamil, does not aggravate COPD or bronchospastic disease. In the acute setting it is prudent to use the short-acting form of diltiazem, starting at 30 mg orally three times a day. All patients treated for rate control with atrial fibrillation should be on cardiac monitoring or telemetry. It is always possible that, after multiple doses of digoxin along with verapamil or diltiazem, the patient could develop excessive AV node blockade, varying degrees of heart block, or severe bradycardia, when serum levels of these drugs equilibrate. Digoxin toxicity can contribute to dangerous ventricular arrhythmias. Digoxin does not itself convert atrial fibrillation to normal sinus rhythm. However, what frequently happens when it does result in a slowing of rate and AV node blockade is spontaneous conversion by the heart back to a normal sinus rhythm.

Beta blockers can also be used for rate control of supraventricular tachyarrhythmias. Although less useful in atrial fibrillation, they can be effective in paroxysmal atrial tachycardia or in patients with short bursts, but not sustained, supraventricular tachyarrhythmia. In hyperthyroidism associated with atrial fibrillation, beta blockers may be very effective. Of course, beta blockers are contraindicated in patients with asthma and COPD and can aggravate CHF with their negative inotropy, and even those that are in theory selective for cardiac beta receptors may still show some negative effects on lung function.

On the rare occasion that drugs do not work to control the rapid rate in atrial fibrillation, pacing with electrical destruction of the sinus node, called ablation of the sinus node, is a last-choice, last-chance option. Afterwards, a pacemaker must be inserted permanently.

Once the rate is controlled, if conversion to sinus rhythm has not occurred spontaneously, other medications can be added to attempt conversion. Quinidine is most commonly added. Other drugs that can convert atrial fibrillation to sinus rhythm are procainamide, flecainide, and amiodarone. None of these drugs lacks potential for serious side effects, which may limit their usefulness in the elderly. At times they can be temporary. After conversion occurs and is maintained for a period of 3 or 4 months, it may be possible to taper the drug. Unfortunately, recurrence of atrial fibrillation once the patient is off antiarrhythmic drugs is more frequent in the elderly. Additional factors that seem to affect the likelihood that a patient will or will not remain in sinus rhythm once converted are left atrial size and mitral valve disease. If the left atrium is significantly dilated on echocardiogram, the success rate at maintaining sinus rhythm without antiarrhythmics, and perhaps even with them, is poor.

Atrial Flutter

A variation on atrial fibrillation is atrial flutter. The hallmark of atrial flutter is a regular rhythm. The atria are beating at a rapid but regular rate. Usually the rate is not as rapid as in atrial fibrillation. The rate is slow enough and regular enough that some of the beats are regularly conducted across the AV node and capture the ventricles in a regular fashion. The result is that the atria may contract at a ratio of 2:1, 3:1, 4:1, or any ratio of atrial to ventricular contractions. In the case of a 3:1 atrial flutter, an ECG shows P waves in a sawtooth pattern, with every third P wave successfully conducting and resulting in a ventricular contraction and a QRS complex. The degree of block may not be constant. Portions of a rhythm strip from a patient in atrial flutter may show a 3:1 block, another part of the strip may show a 4:1 block, and still another part of the strip may show 2:1 or 6:1 blockade. Each portion shows a regular pattern for a time, until the ratio changes. The treatment of rapid atrial flutter is the same as that for rapid atrial fibrillation. In either case, if the ventricular rate is already 90 or less without treatment, treatment for rate control is not necessary and could cause excessive bradycardia. A rate that is controlled without medication treatment indicates intrinsic AV node disease in the patient. In this case, attention can be turned immediately to determining the underlying cause of the arrhythmia, if possible.

Anticoagulation in Atrial Fibrillation

It is estimated that atrial fibrillation is responsible for as much as 85% of the systemic emboli originating in the heart. Of those emboli, two thirds travel to the brain and cause a stroke. Of all nonhemorrhagic strokes, 15% to 20% are believed due to atrial fibrillation (Reardon and Camm, 1996). Instead of a clot that forms in the venous circulation, it may be a clot that forms in the right atrium with atrial fibrillation that is responsible for at least some of the pulmonary emboli that occur. The risk for stroke can be dramatically reduced by chronic anticoagulation with warfarin; there has been a reduction of up to 86% of stroke risk for atrial fibrillation in the patient with nonrheumatic heart disease in one series. Aspirin therapy alone did not show any benefit at low doses; although some benefit with one whole aspirin a day, 325 mg, was shown in one series, it was obtained only in those under age 75. Aspirin at a low dose, 81 mg a day, has been shown effective as a stroke preventive, and many in clinical practice recommend increasing that dose to 325 mg a day for those who have already had one stroke, but these benefits were seen in patients who were not in chronic atrial fibrillation.

To anticoagulate with warfarin or not is a difficult decision to make in some patients. Obviously, the risk of hemorrhagic events with warfarin is increased. In some situations warfarin is definitely contraindicated. Patients whose stroke was hemorrhagic should not be anticoagulated. Patients with hypertension should be well controlled before they are anticoagulated to reduce the risk of hemorrhagic stroke. Patients with any active bleeding, with allergy to warfarin, or with recent central nervous system or eye surgery should not be given warfarin. Patients may need to have laboratory tests to monitor the prolongation of prothrombin time, often weekly initially and then sometimes as frequently as every 3 to 4 weeks chronically. If access to regular laboratory monitoring at appropriate intervals is not available, the patient should not be put on warfarin. If the patient is unreliable about following instructions and following up with appointments and there is no remedy for this behavior, the patient should not be put on warfarin. If the patient has bleeding dyscrasias, including thrombocytopenia, warfarin should not be used. Relative contraindications to warfarin include high risk for injury from falls, significant dementia, history of gastrointestinal bleeding, or presence of known pathology in any system that predisposes to bleeding. Age alone should not be considered a contraindication to warfarin therapy. For anticoagulation in chronic atrial fibrillation, the therapeutic range of the international normalized ratio (INR) is from 2 to 3. With the elderly the goal should be to keep the INR at the low end of the therapeutic range, if possible. Surprisingly, if properly monitored, warfarin therapy is not associated with an increased rate of spontaneous bleeding except in the central nervous system, where intracranial bleeding in patients over 75 on warfarin occurred at 1.8% in one series. If a patient does bleed from other sites on warfarin, there is most likely trauma or another underlying reason. If the patient does not have excessively prolonged prothrombin times, hematuria, hemoptysis, or gastrointestinal bleeding in a patient on warfarin should prompt an investigation for genitourinary, pulmonary, or gastrointestinal pathology. Excessively prolonged prothrombin times associated with abnormal bleeding can be corrected with parenteral vitamin K or, in emergent cases, with infusions of fresh frozen plasma. There is no doubt that, barring contraindications, patients in chronic atrial fibrillation should be anticoagulated to prevent morbidity and mortality from stroke. It is important to educate the patient and caregiver regarding dietary vitamin K intake while the patient is on warfarin.

Cardioversion to Achieve Normal Sinus Rhythm

Patients who achieve rate control but remain in atrial fibrillation have such significantly increased risks for stroke and other thromboembolic events that converting them back to normal sinus rhythm is desirable. However, it is not always possible. There are risks to chronic anticoagulation, but most patients who are cardioverted electrically or medically must remain on antiarrhythmic drugs chronically, and these drugs likewise have risks.

In which group is outcome better in terms of lifestyle, illness burden, function, and survival? That question has not yet been answered. However, the elderly do seem more likely to miss their "atrial kick" and suffer reduced cardiac output and, as a result, reduced function. What about electrical cardioversion for the elderly, then?

Electrocardioversion carries a small risk of thromboembolism from the procedure itself. Therefore if the patient has been in atrial fibrillation for more than 1 to 2 days, it is customary to anticoagulate the patient for about 3 weeks before to the electrocardioversion and to continue it for about 3 weeks afterwards. Another risk to the procedure, particularly in elderly patients and in those with known sinus node disease, is that the patient can go into sinus arrest as a result of the cardioversion. This event is usually followed by bradycardia and then a return to normal sinus rhythm. However, when sinus node disease is known, it may be prudent to use temporary pacing before cardioversion. The long-term success of cardioversion depends on the age of the patient and the duration of the atrial fibrillation. Cardioversion is most successful if done within 3 months of onset. In one series of patients cardioverted early after onset, 70% remained in sinus rhythm after 1 year. Other factors affecting the success of cardioversion are the presence of mitral valve disease, the cardiac functional class of the patient, and left ventricular size. A left atrial dimension of 45 mm or greater is a negative predictor for success. In another series of patients, because of multiple factors, only 30% were still in sinus rhythm at 3 months and only 25% at 1 year, and half of these required antiarrhythmic drugs to maintain sinus rhythm. If there is a clear precipitating cause such as pneumonia or heavy alcohol intake, conversion to and remaining in sinus rhythm are much more successful. Otherwise, the elderly are overall less likely to have successful conversion to sinus rhythm. The elderly are also less likely to maintain sinus rhythm, and they are more likely to be among those requiring antiarrhythmic drugs to maintain sinus rhythm. Therefore the decision to attempt cardioversion, medically or electrically, must be weighed carefully.

Sick Sinus Syndrome

Another common arrhythmia in the elderly is sick sinus syndrome (SSS), also called sinus node dysfunction (SND). Again, idiopathic degeneration of the sinus node occurs with aging. Ischemia can also affect sinus node function. SND occurs in 4% to 45% of patients after CABG. In this setting it is usually temporary, and less than 1% of CABG patients have SND that lasts long term and requires pacing. However, when this occurs, it is usually in patients over age 64. In fact, in all settings, SSS or SND is primarily a problem of the elderly.

SSS occurs because of abnormal sinus node pulse formation and abnormal sinoatrial conduction. It is characterized by intermittent episodes of both bradycardia and tachyarrhythmia. There may be sinus pauses and sinus arrest. The patients have symptoms according to whether the bradycardia episodes or the tachycardia episodes predominate in their presentation. Symptoms may be fatigue or palpitations. Light-headedness and syncope can occur with both bradycardia and tachycardia episodes. There can be sudden death as well. Ambulatory heart monitoring is a helpful tool in evaluating sinus node dysfunction. If symptoms are not frequent enough to demonstrate on 24-hour Holter monitoring, prolonged event monitoring for up to 1 week may be necessary. Patients can trigger the recordings when there is an event, call in, and have the recording transmitted by telephone.

Patients with symptomatic or sustained tachyarrhythmias can be treated medically. Beta blockers are effective for short, unsustained bursts of supraventricular ectopy from which patients are symptomatic. Beta blockers are also effective in most episodic paroxysmal atrial tachycardia. For episodes of atrial fibrillation, digoxin is often the choice, but verapamil or diltiazem can be used as first-line therapy or as an adjunct to digoxin, just as in atrial fibrillation of any etiology. However, patients documented to have recurrent, "in and out" atrial fibrillation should be anticoagulated.

The bradycardia associated with SSS is treated only if it is symptomatic (i.e., if it causes light-headedness, dizziness, syncope, or fatigue or is associated with chest discomfort or dyspnea). Sometimes in the elderly with a lot of comorbidity, it is difficult to assess whether nonspecific symptoms are due to a relative bradycardia or to other chronic illnesses and disabilities. In this case, monitoring that shows sinus pauses greater than 3 seconds and a heart rate less than 40 should probably lower the threshold for pacemaker insertion. In SSS, the bradycardia may not be symptomatic enough to require pacing. However, an attempt to treat the tachyarrhythmias with medication may worsen the bradycardia to the degree that the patient becomes more symptomatic, and pacemaker implantation is then necessary.

Pacemakers

Pacemakers may be atrial, ventricular, or dual chamber. The mode of pacing does not seem to affect survival in SSS. In fact, pacing at all may not improve survival in SSS. In one series of 50 patients, 5-year mortality was 50% and not significantly influenced by pacemaker implantation. Causes of death are mostly CHF, acute MI, and stroke in SSS patients (Duncan and Vittone, 1996). However, in cases of heart block from AV node disease (i.e., AV node block), pacing and the mode of pacing do seem to affect survival. Patients with AV node blockade do better with dual-chamber pacemakers. There seems to be a hemodynamic benefit to having the atria and then the ventricles fire in physiologic synchrony. For patients with either atrial or dual-chamber pacing, there is a lower incidence of atrial fibrillation. The advantages of that are obvious.

Ventricular Arrhythmias

In the elderly the most common ventricular arrhythmias, premature ventricular contractions (PVCs), increase in frequency with age. There are also increased numbers of "premalignant" PVCs, i.e., PVCs with characteristics that portend the possibility of ventricular tachycardia, a life-threatening arrhythmia often responsible for sudden death phenomena. Premalignant characteristics are PVCs that are multifocal or multiform, that occur in pairs (couplets), that fall on the previous T wave (R on T), or that occur with a frequency greater than 5 per minute. As for every age group, treating these PVCs, benign or premalignant in their characteristics, does not decrease mortality but does improve quality of life if the patient is symptomatic from them. Some of the drugs used to treat ventricular ectopy are themselves associated with increased mortality. For a person whose left ventricular function is good, the first approach to treatment should be a trial of a cardioselective beta blocker. Ventricular tachycardia (V-Tach) is defined as a run of PVCs, three or more in a row, at a rate or interval equivalent to 100 per minute or more. The usual rate is 120 to 180 beats per minute. Episodes of V-Tach may last from just seconds, to minutes, to hours. Patients may report transient light-headedness or dizziness, weakness, nausea, or faintness, with or without chest discomfort or palpitations, from a few seconds of V-Tach. Many patients lose consciousness from V-Tach sustained beyond a few seconds because of the very poor perfusion capability of a heart whose ventricles are contracting so rapidly that there is literally no time for filling. Many patients have acute pulmonary vascular congestion to further complicate their hemodynamics. Finally, most patients with sustained V-Tach have some underlying structural heart disease, either cardiomyopathy or CAD causing myocardial ischemia.

Antiarrhythmic drugs used to treat ventricular tachyarrhythmias include quinidine, beta blockers, encainide, flecainide, and amiodarone. The problem with many of the drugs used to treat ventricular arrhythmias is their potential for serious side effects, often including the promotion of ventricular arrhythmias themselves. Acute treatment of sustained ventricular tachycardia is IV lidocaine, sometimes in conjunction with electric shock therapy. Long-term therapy in some patients may include implantable electric "defibrillators." When a patient has had life-threatening arrhythmias of any type, electrophysiologic studies are often used to induce the arrhythmia and study its electrophysiology (i.e., its point of origin and the conduction pathways involved). They can help to determine the appropriate therapy (i.e., which drugs vs. the need for pacemaker placement or defibrillator implantation). They can also be used to check the effectiveness of drug therapy by testing to see if the arrhythmia is still inducible when the patient is on the optimum dosage and regimen of a particular drug.

Valvular Disease

Aortic Stenosis

In the elderly the most common valvular disorder is aortic stenosis. The orifice of the aortic valve is narrowed, and the opening and closing movements of the aortic valve leaflets are inhibited, further decreasing the flow of blood through the valve. These changes occur largely from degenerative changes and calcium deposition in the valve tissue. Aortic stenosis most often becomes a hemodynamically significant problem for patients in their 80s and 90s. In one series of patients undergoing aortic valve replacement, only 18% of those under age 70 had aortic stenosis purely on the basis of aging and degenerative changes, whereas 48% of those over age 70 had purely "senile" aortic stenosis. The others had histories of rheumatic heart disease or congenitally bicuspid valves, where the valve orifice is occluded by the tendency of the valve leaflets to fuse together over time.

Diagnosis is aided by the characteristic aortic systolic ejection type of murmur. The murmur is harsh, crescendo-decrescendo, but peaking late in systole. It is heard best in the second right intercostal space and radiates up over both carotids and to the base of the heart. If the murmur is loud enough, it may be heard at the apex as well. If aortic valve closure is sufficiently delayed, there may be paradoxic splitting of the second heart sound, splitting on expiration and closing to one sound on inspiration. There may also be present a short early diastolic puff or blow compatible with aortic insufficiency. So many elderly patients have some calcium deposition in the aortic valve leaflets, causing turbulent, noisy flow through the valve and loud systolic murmurs, that it can be difficult to differentiate this benign aortic "sclerosis" from significant aortic valve outflow obstruction due to aortic "stenosis." Therefore an echocardiogram may be necessary to differentiate between sclerosis and stenosis and to quantify the degree of stenosis.

If the patient is asymptomatic and has normal left ventricular function, periodic repeat echocardiography and close clinical follow-up may be all that is required. The mortality rate from sudden death in this asymptomatic group with no intervention is less than the perioperative mortality rate with aortic valve replacement (Duncan and Vittone, 1996). However, when angina or CHF develops with aortic stenosis, the prognosis for survival falls dramatically. If there are symptoms such as chest pain or pressure, dyspnea, syncope, evidence of pulmonary vascular congestion on examination or chest x-ray, or evidence of ischemia on ECG with symptoms, it is time to plan for aortic valve replacement. Echocardiography with Doppler flow studies can give very good estimations of valve orifice area and even of the pressure gradient across the aortic valve, in addition to estimations of ejection fraction. However, with surgery planned, cardiac catheterization is usually required for exact data and to evaluate the coronary arteries as well. A valve orifice with an area of less than 0.75 cm^2 or a peak systolic pressure gradient over the valve of more than 50 mm Hg is an indicator for surgical valve replacement. Ideally, replacement is done before any significant left ventricular dysfunction develops.

For patients who do not undergo surgery but who have severe aortic stenosis and angina or CHF, prognosis for survival is approximately 2 years. Balloon valvuloplasty, a less invasive procedure, is available for correction of aortic stenosis. Balloon valvuloplasty has a high rate of restenosis, however, and should not be considered definitive therapy (Duncan and Vittone, 1996). It has been used for patients with severe aortic stenosis who are not candidates for aortic valve replacement surgery but require other surgical procedures and need to have their cardiovascular status improved before surgery. An example would be the elderly patient with a fractured hip who needs surgery but has a significant increase in risk for perioperative mortality because of tight aortic stenosis.

In patients with aortic stenosis, noncritical and asymptomatic, up to 10% develop atrial fibrillation. Some may also throw off calcific emboli, which are usually small and rarely cause any clinical sequelae. Subacute bacterial endocarditis (SBE) is not common, but it is common practice to use SBE prophylaxis with patients with aortic stenosis, although it is not necessary with aortic sclerosis (Duncan and Vittone, 1996).

Aortic Insufficiency

In the Helsinki Aging Study population of 75- to 86-year-olds, 29% had some degree of aortic insufficiency (Duncan and Vittone, 1996). In the elderly mild aortic insufficiency may be chronic, and a compensatory increase in ventricular systolic ejection fraction may occur, resulting in little or no hemodynamic compromise. Over time, left ventricular hypertrophy may result. At the point that significant left ventricular hypertrophy develops, the stiffened, thickened ventricular walls might lend to diastolic dysfunction (i.e., decreased filling), or left ventricular wall hypertrophy could result in outflow tract obstruction, compromising the ability of the heart to increase ejection fraction and compensate for the aortic insufficiency. If there is hypertension that is not optimally controlled, this increased peripheral resistance also negatively affects the ability of the heart to increase ejection fraction and compensate for the aortic insufficiency. In general, the aging heart is less able to increase ejection fraction with exercise.

Therefore therapy for aortic insufficiency is focused on preventing left ventricular hypertrophy or reducing it, optimizing hypertension treatment, and even further decreasing peripheral resistance, if tolerated. Calcium channel blockers are appropriate agents in chronic asymptomatic aortic insufficiency. They may actually decrease left ventricular hypertrophy and peripheral resistance. Vasodilator drugs also decrease peripheral resistance.

Mitral Regurgitation

Again, degenerative changes in the mitral valve can lead to mitral valve insufficiency with aging. This degeneration may be accompanied by calcification of the mitral valve annulus or calcium deposits in the submitral areas of the left ventricular wall. The latter actually cause more trouble than regurgitation, being implicated in the etiology of atrial fibrillation. In patients with mitral valve calcifications in the submitral area, there is a twelvefold increase in the incidence of atrial fibrillation (Duncan and Vittone, 1996). In the elderly, degeneration of valvular components can lead to mitral valve prolapse as a cause of mitral valve insufficiency. Ischemic heart disease can cause papillary muscle dysfunction and subsequent mitral valve insufficiency.

Surgical correction of mitral insufficiency can and should be done before there is irreversible left ventricular dilation and dysfunction, but it carries a higher risk than aortic valve replacement. Procedures to reconstruct rather than replace the valve carry less risk. For the elderly, reconstruction procedures with simultaneous CABG are associated with 13% mortality compared with 22% mortality for mitral valve replacement with simultaneous CABG. However, when the mitral insufficiency is due to calcification of the mitral valve annulus, the reconstruction procedure is technically more difficult and carries higher operative risk.

Pericarditis and Endocarditis

Although pericarditis and endocarditis are not frequently seen, they do occur, and the practitioner must be alert to the possibility. In the elderly, pericarditis and accompanying pericardial effusion are most commonly secondary to CHF or malignancy. If infectious, pericarditis is less likely viral and more likely TB in an elderly person. Other causes of pericarditis in the elderly include acute MI, acute pulmonary embolus, and uremia.

It is important to be aware of the incidence of bacterial endocarditis in the elderly. The source of the bacteria in the elderly is likely to be mouth organisms, including viridans streptococci, because of poor dentition, or bacteremia introduced via surgical procedures. Because of the higher incidence of aortic sclerosis and stenosis, the site is usually the aortic valve in the elderly patient. Surgical procedures that occur more frequently in the elderly and place the elderly patient at risk for bacteremia are multiple dental extractions and oral surgery for extraction of impacted, fractured, decayed teeth; cystoscopy in men; and repair of hip fractures in both men and women. Prophylaxis of endocarditis is usually penicillin V 2 g orally 1 hour before a dental procedure and 1 g 6 hours after the procedure. For penicillin-allergic patients, erythromycin is used, 1 g orally 1 hour before and 0.5 g orally after the procedure (Andreoli et al., 1990).

Congestive Heart Failure

Epidemiology

CHF is the end stage of heart disease. The heart is unable to pump enough blood to supply the vital organs and the body tissues with enough oxygen and nutrients to meet their metabolic demands. Most CHF is a result of CAD. The Framingham 32-year follow-up study showed that some 76.4% of the men and 79.1% of the women with long-standing hypertension developed CHF, whereas 45.8% of men and 27.4% of women with CAD developed CHF. Elderly patients with chronic CHF have a very poor prognosis and high mortality. There is a high incidence of ventricular arrhythmias leading to sudden death. The 5-year mortality with chronic CHF is greater than 50%, and there is a twofold increase in mortality in persons over age 60 (Kannel, 1989). The annual mortality is as high as 50% in those with end-stage (ejection fraction less than 20%) or functional class IV CHF. The prevalence of CHF more than doubles with each decade of age, starting in the 40s. The incidence of heart failure doubles every 10 years in men and doubles every 7 years in women. By age 80 or older, 10% of all people have CHF. Three million Americans have CHF, and 400,000 new cases are diagnosed yearly. It is the most common reason for hospitalization and repeat hospitalization in Medicare patients. At least 50% of those over age 65 who are hospitalized for CHF are hospitalized again within 6 months after their first discharge for CHF. The cost of treatment is from $10 to $30 billion per year (Tresch, 1997). The number of outpatient visits from CHF, more than 11 million per year, is second only to visits for hypertension (Senni and Redfield, 1997).

Etiology

No matter what the etiology of the CHF, age-related changes in the cardiovascular system contribute to the development of CHF (see Box 8-8).

In addition to these aging changes, cardiac conditions in the patient can lead to CHF acutely or gradually. Three-fourths of all CHF is associated with either hypertension or CAD. Causes of acute CHF are listed in Box 8-9.

Box 8-8

Age-Related Changes Contributing to Congestive Heart Failure

- Increased peripheral vascular resistance because of arterial noncompliance
- Decreased left ventricular compliance
- Decreased maximum cardiac output
- Decreased maximum oxygen consumption
- Decreased peak heart rate with exercise
- Decreased glomerular flow rate

Box 8-9

Causes of Acute Congestive Heart Failure

- Acute hypertensive episodes
- Ischemic episodes or acute MI
- Acute onset of arrhythmias
- Volume overload as in intravenous fluid therapy
- Pulmonary embolism
- Tamponade from pericardial effusion
- Acute decompensation (e.g., anemia or hyperthyroidism)
- Acute illnesses such as pneumonia or other infection
- Drugs (e.g., beta blockers and some calcium channel blockers)

More gradual development of CHF can occur in chronic hypertension, chronic ischemic heart disease, valvular disease such as aortic stenosis, hypertrophic cardiomyopathy, diabetic cardiomyopathy, restrictive cardiomyopathy such as infiltrative myocardial disease from amyloid, constrictive pericardial disease, and drugs such as nonsteroidal antiinflammatory drugs (NSAIDs) and corticosteroids, which may cause increased sodium and water retention (Levy and Larson, 1996; Tresch, 1997; Wei, 1992). Because of the improvement in the therapy of hypertension, CAD and ischemia are now the main causes of chronic CHF. Ischemia with or without actual myocardial infarct leads to ventricular remodeling with scar and fibrosis, which ultimately affect both systolic and diastolic function (Duncan and Vittone, 1996).

Pulmonary hypertension causes right heart failure. Some other conditions that cause or mimic right heart failure are pulmonic stenosis, right ventricular infarction, right atrial myxoma, and intracardiac shunts. Some conditions mimic left heart failure, such as left ventricular outflow obstruction, left atrial abnormality, and acute or chronic volume overload (Vasan and Benjamin, 1996). Any of these conditions over time could cause such increased strain on the heart as to contribute to the development of true left ventricular heart failure, or CHF. If the right heart is continuously contracting against increased pulmonary vascular bed pressures, there is decreased venous return and eventually decreased filling of the left ventricle. This decreased filling increases demand on the left ventricle, requiring increased rate or increased ejection fraction and stroke volume to deliver the same cardiac output. Over time, the left ventricle might be expected to hypertrophy; even without hypertrophy, there would be increased oxygen demand. In the presence of CAD, this could result in relative ischemia of the left ventricular myocardium and eventual failure of the pump function and CHF. Conditions that mimic left ventricular failure do so because there is obstruction to systolic outflow, resulting in the same kind of demand on the left ventricle to keep the cardiac output stable and eventually the same physiologic pattern.

Many comorbid states contribute to the development of CHF. Any condition that results in decreased coronary blood flow, decreased heart muscle function, decreased ventricular filling, and decreased ventricular contraction, along with increased heart rate and increased oxygen demand, contributes to the development of CHF. Therefore any acute infection or other acute physiologic stress such as surgery can contribute to the development of CHF. Box 8-10 lists the common cardiac etiologies of heart failure.

Systolic vs. Diastolic Congestive Heart Failure

CHF can be the failure of contraction, systolic failure, or the failure of filling, diastolic failure. Both increase with age. In CHF diagnosed before age 60, 94% are systolic dysfunction. Between the ages of 61 and 70, 79% of the CHF diagnosed are systolic dysfunction. After age 70, the percentage of patients with systolic dysfunction as the major component of their CHF is 59% (Tresch, 1997). After age 80, more patients have diastolic dysfunction than systolic dysfunction. In fact, of patients developing CHF after age 80, more than 50% have normal or near normal systolic function as defined by a left ventricular ejection function of greater than or equal to 50% (Senni and Redfield, 1997; Wei, 1992). It is important for therapeutic decisions to differentiate between diastolic dysfunction and systolic dysfunction as the type of CHF.

Systolic dysfunction is very familiar. The left ventricle loses its strength of contraction. The ventricle may be thinned and dilated, the musculature "floppy." Thus contractions are weak and ineffective in delivering the stroke volume. The ejection fraction falls to less than the normal 45% to 50%. When ejection fraction falls below

Box 8-10

Cardiac Etiologies of Heart Failure

Ventricular overload
- Pressure—aortic and pulmonary stenosis, systemic and pulmonary hypertension
- Volume—valvular incompetence shunt defects, hyperthyroidism

Coronary artery disease
- Myocardial infarction
- Myocardial ischemia

Cardiac muscle disease
- Infiltrative cardiomyopathy—amyloid, sarcoid
- Hypertrophic cardiomyopathy
- Restrictive cardiomyopathy
- Congestive cardiomyopathy

Mechanical diastolic restrictive disorder
- Mitral valvular stenosis
- Constrictive pericarditis

From Tresch D: The clinical diagnosis of heart failure in older patients, *J Am Geriatr Soc*, 45:1128-1133, 1997.

20%, it is considered end-stage CHF with very poor prognosis. There is impaired contraction at rest, which worsens with any increase in demand. The causal factor in chronic, irreversible systolic dysfunction is most often CAD with previous myocardial damage from infarction, clinical or subclinical, resulting in hypokinesis of segments of the ventricular wall. Some dilated cardiomyopathies, as opposed to hypertrophic cardiomyopathies, have other causes, such as alcoholic cardiomyopathy (which shows components of both dilation and hypertrophy on autopsy) or viral cardiomyopathies. However, in elderly patients the cause of dilated cardiomyopathy is overwhelmingly ischemic disease with prior MI.

Diastolic dysfunction results in poor filling of the ventricle, usually during the early rapid filling phase or diastole, but can affect filling throughout the entire diastolic period. Systemic hypertension leading to left ventricular hypertrophy and underlying ischemic heart disease are the most common causes of diastolic heart failure. In the first case the hypertrophied ventricle is stiff and thickened because of increased connective tissue matrix. With increased exercise this stiff ventricle cannot stretch to accommodate a larger filling volume, so there is no increased stroke volume and no increased cardiac output.

In the second case, both transient and sustained ischemia can lead to profound alteration in left ventricular diastolic function. As mentioned earlier, chronic ischemia causes remodeling of the left ventricle, with scarring and fibrosing. However, acute transient ischemia can cause sudden compromise of the hypertrophied, scarred ventricle. In acute stress the ventricle has impaired relaxation and decreased compliance, and extremely high pressures are necessary to fill the ventricle during diastole. Thus acute stresses such as demand ischemia, tachycardia, and tachyarrhythmias can result in decompensation and acute CHF, even with normal systolic function. In fact, acute reversible CHF associated with an acute stress is often diastolic dysfunction alone. Diastolic dysfunction can occur alone, whereas systolic dysfunction never occurs without concomitant diastolic dysfunction (Senni and Redfield, 1997).

The phenomenon known as flash pulmonary edema is usually due to acute ischemia in patients with severe CAD, hypertension, and left ventricular hypertrophy. It can happen with normal systolic function, meaning "flash pulmonary edema" may be diastolic dysfunction alone. In fact, abrupt-onset CHF, prominent jugular venous distention (JVD) and prominent crackles or rales in the lungs, with little or no edema, in a setting of an acute stress, are characteristic of diastolic CHF. In treating this acute CHF, presume that myocardial ischemia is part of the picture and treat for it.

In some elderly people with diastolic dysfunction, the hypertrophied left ventricle may resemble the hypertrophic cardiomyopathy patient. There may be asymmetric basal and septal hypertrophy. The left ventricle, if studied by echocardiography, appears small, hypertrophied, and hyperdynamic; there may even be left ventricular outflow tract obstruction during systole; and there may be left atrial enlargement. Yet these changes are the result of long-standing hypertension and not idiopathic changes such as the asymmetric hypertrophic cardiomyopathy of younger patients. In obese or diabetic patients, a type of cardiomyopathy that leads to diastolic dysfunction can develop even in the absence of hypertensive history (Vasan and Benjamin, 1996). Box 8-11 lists those cardiovascular changes that occur with aging that affect diastolic dysfunction. Box 8-12 is a summary of the disorders that are known to be associated with the development of diastolic dysfunction.

Box 8-11

Normal Aging Changes Affecting Diastolic Function

Increase in systolic blood pressure
Increase in ventricular wall thickness
Decrease in left ventricular cavity size
Decrease in rate of ventricular filling
Increase in myocardial interstitial fibrosis
Ventricular relaxation prolonged
Increase in left atrial size

From Tresch D: The clinical diagnosis of heart failure in older patients, *J Am Geriatr Soc* 45:1128-1133, 1997.

Box 8-12

Disorders Associated with Diastolic Dysfunction

Systemic hypertension
Coronary artery disease
Hypertrophic cardiomyopathy
Diabetes
Chronic renal disease
Infiltrative cardiomyopathy
Idiopathic restrictive cardiomyopathy
Aortic stenosis
Atrial fibrillation

From Tresch D: The clinical diagnosis of heart failure in older patients, *J Am Geriatr Soc* 45:1128-1133, 1997.

Assessment

Clinical findings to look for in CHF include JVD, rales or crackles in the lungs, an S_3 gallop on heart auscultation, displacement of the point of maximal impulse (PMI) compatible with cardiomegaly, possibly hepatojugular reflux, and peripheral edema. Other data helpful to diagnosis include chest x-ray examination, ECG, and echocardiography. Clues to etiology may be obtained from a CBC, thyroid function tests, and chemistries.

In the elderly looking for JVD may have less yield, as an uncoiled aorta may impair venous outflow from the neck and cause a false-positive JVD. Then, flattened neck veins obliterated by fibrosis can cause a false-negative JVD (Schneiderman, 1993). Likewise, in the elderly, the sign of leg edema is less useful because of the high incidence of venous insufficiency. Cardiac enlargement on chest x-ray film and left ventricular hypertrophy (LVH) by voltage on an ECG are both independently associated with increased risk for CHF. In hypertensive elderly patients LVH on echocardiography is also an independent risk factor for CHF (Vasan and Benjamin, 1996). The ECG may also show ST and T wave changes compatible with ischemia to lend weight to the likelihood that CHF is present. The chest x-ray film may also show increased pulmonary vasculature, pulmonary vascular congestion, and the presence or absence of other pulmonary disease.

An echocardiogram can confirm the diagnosis of systolic or diastolic left ventricular dysfunction and provide clues to the etiology. Chamber size and configuration and ejection fraction on echocardiography help to differentiate between systolic and diastolic dysfunction. Echocardiography can differentiate between a hypertrophied left ventricle and a dilated one. Dimensions of the ventricle can be obtained. Echocardiography can estimate the ejection fraction, which is a measure of systolic contractile function. A normal ejection fraction is 45% to 50%. With Doppler flow studies and echocardiography, diastolic filling can be evaluated. Impaired relaxation can be seen, which affects the early phase of diastolic filling, or impaired distensibility can be detected, which affects late-phase ventricular diastolic filling. A left ventricle that is normal in size and contractility or that is hypertrophied but not dilated, along with an ejection fraction that is normal but left ventricular relaxation and distensibility that are abnormal, indicates that the patient's symptoms of CHF are due to diastolic dysfunction. The typical patient with diastolic dysfunction has these echocardiography findings and, in addition, is likely to have a history of hypertension, CAD, or valvular disease; be of advanced age; be female; have diabetes; and have chest x-ray film findings compatible with CHF. With the availability of age-standardized reference values for Doppler indexes of left ventricular filling, the diagnosis of diastolic CHF in the elderly may soon become even more precise (Vasan and Benjamin, 1996).

A dilated left ventricle on echocardiography with a less than normal ejection fraction indicates systolic dysfunction. This patient probably has left atrial enlargement and regional wall motion abnormalities on echocardiography as well.

Additional information can be obtained from an echocardiogram about valvular disease and even ischemic disease. Valve orifice diameter and pressure gradients across the valves can be estimated with Doppler flow echocardiography. Also, the direction of flow can be determined, so valvular regurgitation can be seen. If valvular disease is shown on echocardiography, heart catheterization may be necessary later to further evaluate the degree of valvular disease. An echocardiogram can also give information about the presence or absence of prior ischemic muscle injury. Wall motion abnormalities suggest areas of prior infarct. Stress echocardiography with Doppler can give even more information about areas of wall motion abnormality, such as whether these abnormalities change with exercise. Such data might suggest still viable myocardium that is jeopardized during exercise. Similar data can be obtained from radionucleotide ventriculography, MUGA testing, and stress thallium testing, but these tests have the disadvantage of not providing the information about the heart valves that echocardiography can.

An echocardiogram can also diagnose hypertrophic cardiomyopathy and identify left ventricular outflow obstruction and subvalvular obstruction. There are other conditions that can mimic CHF, when there is neither systolic nor diastolic dysfunction. Any condition that causes increased left atrial pressures can result in pulmonary vascular congestion without left ventricular dysfunction. Valvular disease such as mitral stenosis and aortic stenosis can do this. Chronic renal failure, with accompanying volume overload and high-output states such as thyrotoxicosis and anemia can also do this. Pericardial disease and restrictive heart disease can mimic CHF as well. Fortunately, echocardiography with Doppler is able to detect these conditions and thus is an excellent tool for diagnosis.

In diagnosing CHF, noncardiogenic causes of pulmonary edema must be ruled out. Adult respiratory distress syndrome results in pulmonary edema because the abnormal permeability of pulmonary capillaries causes leakage of fluid from the blood vessels into the extravascular space. Direct pulmonary injury such as inhalation injury, chemical pneumonitis, aspiration, or trauma can cause pulmonary vascular congestion secondary to the inflammatory process. Sepsis, pancreatitis, high altitude, narcotic overdose, and disseminated intravascular coagulation are all associated with pulmonary edema. One factor that differentiates these conditions from CHF is that in these conditions, if the pulmonary capillary wedge pressure (PCWP) is measured, it is normal (Vasan and Benjamin, 1996). Actually, the definitive diagnosis of diastolic CHF requires findings of elevated PCWP, elevated left ventricular end diastolic pressures, normal systolic function, and normal ejection fraction. To take these measurements, cardiac catheterization is necessary. Short of that invasive test, diagnosis of CHF, diastolic and systolic, can be made with a high level of reliability by using history, physical examination, ECG, chest x-ray examination, and echocardiography with Doppler flow studies. *The Mayo Clinic Proceedings* published a handy algorithm for the diagnosis of diastolic heart failure in its review of CHF in the elderly (Figure 8-2).

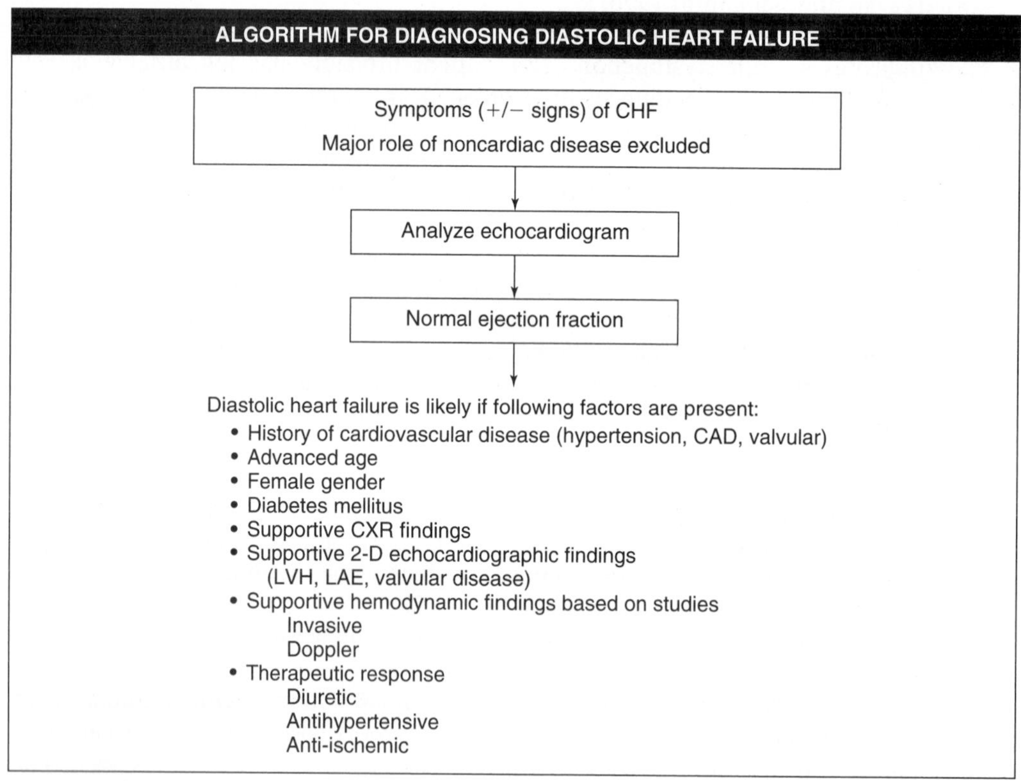

Figure 8-2 Algorithm for diagnosing diastolic heart failure. (From Senni M, Redfield M: Concise review of primary care physicians: congestive heart failure in elderly patients, *Mayo Clin Proc* 72:453-460, 1997.) *CHF,* Congestive heart failure; *CXR,* chest x-ray examination; *LVH,* left ventricular hypertrophy; *LAE,* left atrial enlargement.

Presentation of Congestive Heart Failure in the Elderly

Before an elderly person becomes symptomatic from CHF, there may be signs that are a manifestation of deteriorating myocardial function. There may be an enlarged heart detectable by a displaced PMI on physical examination. There may be an enlarged cardiac silhouette on chest x-ray film. The patient may have a rapid resting heart rate. Hematocrit may be elevated, reflecting erythrocytosis that is compensatory for decreased cardiac output. There may be decreased exercise tolerance. As the patient develops either increased pulmonary venous pressure or increased systemic venous pressure because of CHF, other signs and symptoms appear.

With increased pressure and congestion in the pulmonary vascular tree, there may be rales in the lungs, cough, wheezing, paroxysmal nocturnal dyspnea, an inability to recline in a flat position without dyspnea that leads patients to prop themselves up on pillows to sleep (orthopnea), insomnia, and dyspnea on exertion. Wheezing as a manifestation of pulmonary vascular congestion and the presence of fluid in the pulmonary alveoli are sometimes called "cardiac asthma." These are the usual manifestations of left-sided heart failure.

With increased systemic venous pressure come edema of the lower extremities, edema in the gut, JVD, and total body weight gain. Edema in the gut can cause nausea, indigestion, anorexia, and even vomiting. When pressure on the liver causes a visible increase in jugular venous distention, or hepatojugular reflux, it is a sign of edema in the liver due to increased systemic venous pressure. There may be abnormal liver function tests such as elevated transaminases, elevated alkaline phosphatase, and elevated total bilirubin, as well as abnormal coagulation functions associated with congestion of the liver due to CHF. These are the usual manifestations of right-sided heart failure.

Whether the CHF is primarily systolic or diastolic, pulmonary vascular congestion usually develops first; then, because of back pressure and back flow, eventually systemic venous congestion develops. In other words, the most common cause of right heart failure is left heart failure. The exception is the case of primary right heart failure. In right heart failure, as in primary and secondary lung diseases, there is increased resistance in the pulmonary vascular bed without any congestion. For instance, in primary pulmonary hypertension, acute pulmonary embolus, or COPD, increased pulmonary vascular pressure develops before and independent of any cardiac dysfunction. In such cases the right ventricle may fail. Failure of either pump or filling function of just the right ventricle presents first with the signs of systemic venous congestion. Lower extremity edema develops first, progressing to abdominal wall and visceral edema. Because the circulation is circular, with the heart in the middle as the pump, any right heart failure eventually leads to left heart failure, and the reverse is also true.

It is also true that with CHF, as with other disorders, the elderly may present atypically. With some elderly patients, the signs and symptoms of decreased cardiac output from CHF may be subtle. There may be only somnolence, fatigue, weakness, and motor retardation. Often there is confusion or increased confusion, and it may be the only major presenting symptom. Elderly patients are also likely to be diagnosed at a more advanced stage of their CHF. At earlier stages, when elderly people experience increased fatigue, increased dyspnea on exertion, and decreased physical stamina, they may simply decrease their activities and become more sedentary. As a result, their average cardiac demand falls, and their CHF continues to go unnoticed and undiagnosed. These vague complaints are the predominant presentation of CHF in the very elderly. Thus CHF must be on the differential diagnosis list for an elderly patient who becomes confused rather acutely, stops eating, or stops being active on account of being "too tired." Their worsening air exchange while recumbent may lead to nocturnal anxiety, and poor sleep and nightmares are common. Nocturia with daytime oliguria is a frequent early complaint in the elderly. It occurs because in the recumbent position, venous return is no longer in an against-gravity direction and therefore increases. Increased venous return, with decreased cardiac demand from lack of muscular activity, results in increased renal perfusion and output at night. These vague complaints may be the first clue, before any dyspnea, rales, cough, wheezes, edema, or similar signs and symptoms appear, or they may be the only clue. As dyspnea in the elderly is often the predominant symptom with CAD, dyspnea in a setting of new ECG changes or in the absence of any other signs and symptoms of CHF should be considered a possible anginal equivalent. Anorexia and a resultant weight loss can be such a striking sign in CHF in the elderly that the term "cardiac cachexia" has developed. This hepatic and gut congestion is a frequent cause of weight loss in the elderly (Cuffe and Rao, 1997). Cough and wheezing in the elderly person with CHF are often mistakenly attributed to COPD. However, when a patient has COPD and is experiencing frequent exacerbations or repeated pulmonary infections, the possibility of concomitant CHF should be strongly considered. Echocardiogram findings, and perhaps pulmonary function tests in addition, can help differentiate between the possible etiologies. In some cases stress testing, if necessary, with the several nonexercise nuclear stress tests that are available, can also be helpful.

Other comorbidities can confuse evaluation of the symptoms of CHF in the elderly. The patient with dyspnea on exertion may simply be deconditioned or have orthopedic limitations, obesity, or the pulmonary fibrosis with restriction that can be a physiologic aging change in the lungs. The patient with edema may have venous insufficiency, renal disease, or fluid retention in response to medications such as some of the calcium channel blockers, NSAIDs, or hormones. Patients may simply be obese and inactive. Again, echocardiography is a simple, accessible, usually fast, noninvasive way to evaluate heart function.

Diastolic CHF may not be distinguishable from systolic CHF clinically. There are no ECG distinguishing factors. The chest x-ray film might show an enlarged heart, but this can be a finding with systolic or diastolic CHF. It is usually not possible to distinguish between cardiomegaly due to hypertrophy vs. that due to dilation on chest x-ray film. A hugely enlarged heart on x-ray may be a dilated heart or may represent pericardial effusion. A history of hypertension or CAD in patients with CHF may be a useful clue but does not distinguish between diastolic and systolic CHF with any certainty. In fact, the history of hypertension, the history of CAD, a third heart sound, and a fourth heart sound are all findings that occur with equal frequency in diastolic and systolic CHF (Vasan and Benjamin, 1996). The pattern of presentation can be helpful. Diastolic CHF is likely to be the cause when CHF develops abruptly with acute stresses such as pneumonia, surgery, or acute arrhythmias, in the absence of acute MI. Again, the most useful tool for determining the difference is an echocardiogram. The echocardiogram with Doppler flow studies is necessary to assess diastolic function.

Treatment of Congestive Heart Failure

In general, treatment consists of inotropic support where needed, fluid mobilization accomplished by preload reduction, afterload reduction, and relief of ischemia. In terms of drug therapy, this translates into digoxin, diuretics, vasodilators such as hydralazine and nitrates, and ACE inhibitors. In the elderly the effective doses of each are usually lower. The first, digoxin, is given in systolic dysfunction to increase inotropism, or the strength of ventricular contraction. Because of the decrease in renal function that occurs with normal aging, the elderly are at greater risk for digoxin toxicity. Therefore it is prudent to use lower maintenance doses of digoxin in treating the geriatric patient. The goal of digoxin therapy is control of heart rate and symptoms. It is not necessary to achieve a therapeutic laboratory level of digoxin if these goals are achieved. However, it is still important to monitor the digoxin level at least every 6 months once the condition is stabilized to monitor for toxicity.

This same decreased renal function can make the elderly rather resistant to the effect of diuretics. Often it is necessary to use loop diuretics to achieve effective diuresis. Yet in using these loop diuretics, use the minimum dose necessary. If adequate diuresis is still not achieved, it often helps to add metolazone (Zaroxolyn), a thiazide diuretic, to the loop diuretic. Giving the metolazone 30 to 60 minutes before the loop diuretic results in a synergism that can be very effective. This regimen can result in severe hypokalemia, so adequate potassium supplementation must be supplied. Any diuretics in the elderly may quickly deplete the intravascular volume faster than fluid in the interstitial spaces of the tissues (edema) can be mobilized and resorbed, resulting in intravascular dehydration, decreased renal perfusion, prerenal azotemia, and hypotension. If there is hypotension, perfusion simply becomes worse. The balance between too "wet" and too dry can be a very delicate one in the elderly. To achieve this delicate balance, start with low doses of medications, and increase or decrease minimally while observing the effects on urinary output, BUN and creatinine levels, and BP.

The elderly, likewise, may be more sensitive to the effect of decreased volume from the decreased sodium and fluid retention ACE inhibitors cause. Renal function on ACE inhibitors must be monitored closely as well. They reduce the preload by reducing volume, and they also reduce afterload as they have a vasodilating effect. Generally they are a great asset, even a necessity in the successful treatment of CHF. Some current clinical pathways developed by various medical communities for the treatment of CHF now consider the use of ACE inhibitors for the treatment of CHF the standard of practice. If decreased renal function or development of cough or angioedema precludes the use of ACE inhibitors, hydralazine and nitrates can be used for their vasodilating effect. Angiotensin II receptor blockers are now available as an alternative in blocking sodium and fluid retention, although they, too, might cause the same side effects as ACE inhibitors. Although the worsening renal function with ACE inhibitors and angiotensin II receptor blockers might be dose related, cough seems to be an idiosyncratic reaction. Therefore it is entirely possible that a patient who gets a cough with ACE inhibitors might not do so with angiotensin II receptor blockers. Table 8-7 gives suggested dosage ranges for vasodilator therapy in the elderly.

Calcium channel blockers may be indicated in the treatment of CHF if coronary artery insufficiency coexists. The chief contraindication to their use in CHF has been the

TABLE 8-7 Suggested Dosages of Vasodilators in the Treatment of Systolic Congestive Heart Failure

Vasodilator	Dosages	
	Initial	Goal
Captopril	6.25 mg t.i.d.	50 mg t.i.d.
Enalapril	2.5 mg b.i.d.	10 mg b.i.d.
Lisinopril	5 mg/day	20 mg/day
Hydralazine/isosorbide dinitrate	10/5 mg t.i.d.	75/40 mg t.i.d.

From Senni M, Redfield M: Concise review of primary care physicians, congestive heart failure in elderly patients, *Mayo Clin Proc* 72:453-460, 1997.
b.i.d., Twice a day; *t.i.d.*, three times a day.

depressive effect on strength of contraction or inotropy that some have. Verapamil, diltiazem, and nifedipine all have some negative inotropic effect. There are newer alternatives, however. Amlodipine (Norvasc) has not been demonstrated to have any negative inotropic effect. When CAD coexists, beta blockers, which reduce mortality in CAD patients in part because they decrease myocardial oxygen demand, would be a desirable part of the treatment regimen. However, their known negative inotropic effect has caused them to be considered contraindicated in patients with CHF. Some recent studies, nevertheless, have shown that more than 95% of CHF patients are able to tolerate at least small doses of beta blockers. Several small studies even suggest that besides decreasing mortality from CAD, they improve symptoms, and in some they may even result in improved systolic function. Their potential for benefit is even more understandable in treatment of CHF from diastolic dysfunction.

Other measures important in the treatment of CHF include elevating edematous legs, wearing compression (or TED) stockings, avoiding complete bedrest, and, if hospitalized, using subcutaneous heparin to reduce risk of deep vein thrombosis. In patients with chronic CHF and dilated cardiomyopathy, long-term anticoagulation with warfarin may be indicated. Oxygen supplementation may be important to relieve symptoms as well.

Diastolic dysfunction requires adjustments in the therapeutic approach. In the patient with normal systolic function but CHF from diastolic dysfunction, small changes in intravascular volume can result in large changes in filling pressures. Therefore reducing the preload, which reduces the volume that reaches the left ventricle, can actually further reduce filling pressures and cardiac output. Thus diuretic therapy, although perhaps necessary initially to control symptoms, can actually worsen the failure. Just as in hypertrophic cardiomyopathy, the stiff, noncompliant ventricle that does not relax and accommodate adequate filling volumes may need more volume to overcome that stiffness, "stretch" the ventricle, and fill adequately. Just as in aortic stenosis, there is already decreased stroke volume, so further decreasing preload can further compromise stroke volume and cardiac output. Therefore diuretics must be used with extreme caution.

Digoxin should be avoided. The stiff, noncompliant ventricle has a problem relaxing and stretching to fill. Increasing the strength of contraction is not necessary and may be counterproductive. The need is to improve relaxation. Again, a parallel can be seen in hypertrophic cardiomyopathy, in which digoxin is contraindicated.

The mainstay of therapy for diastolic dysfunction should be ACE inhibitors. As they dilate both the venous and arterial tree, ACE inhibitors reduce preload, but they also reduce afterload, with a resultant increase in cardiac output. There is evidence that over time ACE inhibitors actually induce the regression of left ventricular hypertrophy (Senni and Redfield, 1997). They may accomplish this result by lessening the accumulation of myocardial collagen over time (Cuffe and Rao, 1997). Both the symptoms of CHF in the short term and survival in the long term may be increased by the use of ACE inhibitors in diastolic heart failure (Duncan and Vittone, 1996). The usual precautions in the elderly hold. Start with the smallest effective dose. Watch for renal insufficiency. The initial dose can cause marked drops in BP within the first 3 hours after it is given. This drop in BP is even more dramatic in patients who already are on diuretics. It may be wise to stop diuretic therapy while initiating ACE inhibitor therapy in the elderly, or at least to decrease the diuretic dose. For treatment of CHF with ACE inhibitors, the therapeutic goal is the maximum tolerated dose. Stop the ACE inhibitor only for symptomatic hypotension, rather than holding it for arbitrary BP limits (Senni and Redfield, 1997).

In diastolic heart failure calcium channel blockers and beta blockers may have an even greater role. The negative inotropic effect of a particular calcium channel blocker may make it more desirable therapy. Reduced contractility may result in greater relaxation and therefore greater filling. At least one calcium channel blocker contraindicated in systolic dysfunction because of its suppression of ventricular contraction may have benefit in diastolic dysfunction. Verapamil not only has significant negative inotropism but also causes the regression of left ventricular hypertrophy. However, this benefit may not be lasting with long-term use (Duncan and Vittone, 1996). Beta blockers would be useful for the same reason, negative inotropic effect. Yet it is useful to remember that one of the physiologic changes in normal aging is decreased responsiveness to beta-adrenergic stimuli, so beta blockers may not be as effective in the elderly.

As in systolic dysfunction, it is important to treat and control coexisting disorders. If a patient is in atrial fibrillation, restoring normal sinus rhythm and thereby restoring the elderly person's "atrial kick," the final and active phase of diastolic filling, may be the most effective therapy of all. Hypertension must be controlled. Angina needs to be treated.

For any patient with CHF of either modality, diet should be low in sodium, the exercise level should be maintained or increased if possible, and calorie supplementation may be necessary for "cardiac cachexia." If the patient's CHF is primarily systolic and the patient is severely compromised functionally or has an ejection fraction of less than 20%, fluid intake may need to be restricted as well.

The Sequelae of Congestive Heart Failure in the Elderly

The incidence of CHF increases with age. Therefore as the population of older adults increases, more and more patients will require treatment for CHF. There is a high mortality from CHF. For patients with CHF as a primary diagnosis, mortality is 58%

higher than average. For patients for whom CHF is a secondary diagnosis, mortality is 29% higher. The 1-year mortality rate for elderly with CHF in one study was 20% (Senni and Redfield, 1997). In elderly patients with CHF followed over 5 years, the mortality rate was 76% for men and 69% for women (Levy and Larson, 1996). There is increased hospitalization and, perhaps with more impact, increased functional decline because of CHF (Wolinsky, et al., 1997). Patients with primarily diastolic dysfunction did better in some studies, with a 1-year mortality as low as 10% and a 5-year mortality of 62%. Age, comorbid conditions, and the etiology do make a difference. With systolic dysfunction and coexisting CAD, short-term mortality may be as high as 85% (Cuffe and Rao, 1997). Women and diabetic patients with CHF and ischemia do worse than others. Those with CHF with LVH have an increased incidence of sudden death phenomena (Wei, 1992). Patients with ejection fractions less than or equal to 20%, even if they are already on maximum medical therapy with ACE inhibitors, diuretics, and vasodilators, have increased early mortality. The mortality rates in these patients increase even more in the presence of supraventricular tachyarrhythmias; ventricular arrhythmias; or a history of syncope, stroke, or previous cardiac arrest and cardiopulmonary resuscitation. The incidence of stroke in CHF increases fourfold. The incidence of ischemic events increases 2.5 to 5 times. Overall, the prognosis for CHF is little better than that for cancer (Kannel, 1989). The functional disability that results from heart failure may be the most important factor for older patients. They lose function in mobility and independence in activities of daily living. In addition, these losses are often associated with additional financial burdens. Currently, studies of cardiovascular physiology that seek to refine preventive therapy for CHF focus on measures to reduce cardiac muscle stress, lower cardiac oxygen demand, and suppress norepinephrine.

Summary

Cardiovascular disease is the most common cause of disease and disability in the older adult. The practitioner must understand cardiovascular physiology and pathophysiology. Presenting symptoms can be vague or misleading, and the possible causes can be numerous. The practitioner must be skillful in history taking and physical examination to differentiate the possibilities, initiate the appropriate diagnostic evaluation, and refer when appropriate. Treatments for various conditions are often influenced by comorbidities, and it may take much consideration to determine the appropriate intervention. Education for the patient, family, and caregiver is critical to ensure the best possible outcome.

Resources

American Heart Association
7320 Greenville Avenue
Dallas, TX 75231
(214) 373-6300
http://www.americanheart.org

National Heart, Lung, and Blood Information
P.O. Box 30105
Bethesda, MD 20824-0105
(301) 251-1222

References

Andreoli TE et al: *Cecil essentials of medicine*, Philadelphia, 1990, WB Saunders.

Applegate W: Review: hypertension in elderly patients, *Ann Intern Med* 110:901-914, 1989.

Cuffe M, Rao S: Heart failure and special therapeutic considerations in older patients, *Clinical Geriatrics* 5:56-71, 1997.

Duncan A, Vittone JM: Cardiovascular disease in elderly patients, *Mayo Clin Proc* 71:184-196, 1996.

Fauci A et al: Electrocardiography: acute MI. In Isselbacher, KJ, editor: *Harrison's principles of internal medicine*, ed 13, New York, 1994, McGraw-Hill.

Kannel W: Epidemiological aspects of heart failure, *Cardiol Clin* 7:1-9, 1989.

Kannel W, Dawber TR, McGee DL: Perspective in systolic hypertension: the Framingham study, *Circulation* 71:1179-1182, 1980.

Kannel W, Gordon T, Schwartz MJ: Systolic versus diastolic BP and risk of coronary heart disease: the Framingham Study, *Am J Cardiol* 27:335-346, 1971.

Levy D Larson M: The progression from hypertension to congestive heart failure, *JAMA* 275: 1557-1562, 1996.

Massie BM, Amidon TA: Heart. In Tierney LM, McPhee SJ, Papadakis MA, editors: *Current medical diagnosis and treatment*, ed 36, Stamford, Conn, 1997, Appleton & Lange.

National Institutes of Health: *The sixth report of the Joint National Committee on prevention, detection, evaluation, and treatment of high blood pressure*, Bethesda, Md, 1997, International Medical.

Reardon M, Camm J: Atrial fibrillation in the elderly, *Clin Cardiol* 19:765-775, 1996.

Ryan T et al: ACC/AHA guidelines for the management of patients with acute myocardial infraction: executive summary, *Circulation* 94:2341-2350, 1996.

Schneiderman H: Physical examination of the aged patient, *Conn Med* 57:317-324, 1993.

Senni M, Redfield M: Concise review of primary care physicians: congestive heart failure in elderly patients, *Mayo Clin Proc* 72:453-460, 1997.

Stemmer E, Aronow W: Surgical treatment of coronary artery disease in the elderly, *Clin Geriatrics* 5:19-38, 1997.

Stuart B et al: Medical guidelines for determining prognosis: heart disease. *Medical guidelines for determining prognosis in selected non-cancer diseases*, ed 2, Arlington, Va, 1996, National Hospice Organization.

Tresch D: The clinical diagnosis of heart failure in older patients, *J Am Geriatr Soc* 45:1128-1133, 1997.

Vasan R, Benjamin E: Congestive heart failure with normal left ventricular systolic function, *Arch Intern Med* 156:146-157, 1996.

Wei J: Age and the cardiovascular system, *N Engl J Med* 327:1735-1739, 1992.

Wolinsky F et al: The sequelae of hospitalization for congestive heart failure among older adults, *J Am Geriatr Soc* 45:543-666, 1997.

9

Gastrointestinal Conditions

As our population ages, more and more attention is being directed toward providing care to persons of advanced age. It is important not to relate different manifestations of gastrointestinal (GI) diseases in the elderly simply to the aging process (Brody and Schneider, 1986).

Age-related Changes

Age-related changes in the GI system include decreased saliva flow; in the stomach there is a decrease in production of acid and an increase in gastrin production. In the small intestine transit time is increased with an accompanying increase in motility, but the absorption of vitamin D and B_{12}, folate, calcium, and iron are decreased; for fat-soluble vitamins the absorption rate is increased. In the colon the mucosa, musculature, and transit time are all decreased with an increase in diverticular disease. The size of the liver decreases along with hepatic blood flow (Baime et al., 1994). The changes in the GI system along with the progressive age-related decrease in creatinine clearance increase the possibility of adverse drug reactions in the older adult.

Gastroesophageal Reflux Disease

More than 40% of the adult population of the United States complain of heartburn at least once a month (The Gallop Organization, 1988), about 7% of those complain of reflux at least once a day, and a total of 7% of adult Americans have erosive esophagitis. It is noted that the incidence of advanced esophageal involvement seems to increase substantially after age 40. Reflux disease is more common in white males (Spechler, 1992).

The lower esophageal sphincter is a physiologic barrier to the transfer of gastric acid secretions from the stomach to the esophagus. However, this high-pressure zone has episodes of transient relaxation, which is thought to be the main etiology behind gastroesophageal reflux disease (GERD) (Mittal and McCallum, 1987).

History

Heartburn is the most common manifestation of reflux esophagitis. Neither its severity nor its frequency predicts the degree of severity of the tissue damage seen on endoscopy. Solid food dysphagia indicates peptic stricture more commonly than carcinoma in a Barrett's esophagus. Reflux can also present with nonesophageal symptoms such as in noncardiac chest pain, chronic sinusitis, globus hystericus, hoarseness, wheezing, asthma, aspiration pneumonia, and poor dentition (Gaynor, 1991). Rarely, reflux esophagitis can present with upper GI bleeding or iron deficiency anemia as seen with ulcerative esophagitis.

Reflux esophagitis is found more frequently in the elderly patient and is more severe than in younger patients. Although the degree of symptom manifestation was similar between the elderly and nonelderly with high-grade esophagitis, elderly patients with mild reflux esophagitis were less symptomatic than younger patients (Maekawa et al., 1998). Older symptomatic patients had longer reflux episodes, manifested by 24-hour pH manometry with pH less than 4.0 (Ter, Johnston, and Castell, 1998).

Differential Diagnosis

Diagnosis of tissue injury is best made by upper endoscopy with biopsies. Biopsies would also rule out the presence of Barrett's or any malignant transformation. The 24-hour continuous intraesophageal pH monitoring provides the ability to correlate symptoms with episodes of acid reflux, especially in the presence of atypical symptoms (Demeester, Cimochowski, and O'Drobinak, 1982).

Treatment

Treatment should be conservative at first, starting with lifestyle modifications that include elevating the head of the bed at least 6 inches and avoiding late-night snacks, alcohol, smoking, caffeine derivatives, and any food that makes the patient symptomatic, including citrus juices or carbonated beverages. Weight reduction, along with reduction of dietary fat and meal size, appears to be beneficial.

When lifestyle modifications fail, drug therapy is recommended. It may be limited to oral antacids or H_2 blockers that help in cases with symptomatic reflux that cause no significant tissue damage. With an advanced degree of esophagitis, proton pump inhibitors are needed for healing and maintenance. These may be coupled with a prokinetic agent such as cisapride, which is shown to increase the lower esophageal sphincter pressure. When medical management fails or if the patient is young and lifelong medical treatment is not preferred, antireflux surgery is indicated. Antireflux surgery is also safe and effective in treating the elderly (Trus et al., 1998). When compared with different modalities of medical management, it was found to be superior in preventing symptom relapse (Spechler, 1992).

Peptic Ulcer Disease

Risk Factors

Of all the suspected risk factors, nonsteroidal antiinflammatory drug (NSAID) intake and the presence of *H. pylori* gastritis provide unequivocal causal association with peptic ulcer disease (Schubert et al., 1993). It has been suggested that cigarette smoking increases the incidence of peptic ulcer disease. The estimated lifetime prevalence of peptic ulcer disease in the United States is 10% (Monson and McMahan, 1969).

History

The most common presenting symptom is burning epigastric pain that is nocturnal or postprandial and nonradiating. Pain that awakens the patient from sleep is highly suggestive of duodenal ulcer but can also be seen in nonulcer dyspepsia and gastric ulcers. About 10% of patients with peptic ulcer disease present with complications (i.e., GI bleed and perforation) without any prior history of epigastric pain.

Differential Diagnosis

The differential diagnosis of epigastric pain is vast and should include pain of esophageal, biliary, pancreatic, cardiac, and intestinal origin.

Osteoarthritis is more common in elderly individuals, and the use of NSAIDs is particularly toxic in the elderly. If NSAIDs are required, propionic acid derivatives are better tolerated. Examples include naproxen, oxaprozin, and ibuprofen. A new generation of COX-2 (cyclooxygenase-2 inhibitors) such as Celebrex has become available.

Elderly patients have the highest risk of rebleeding, which is related to ulcers greater than 2 cm in size (Chow et al., 1998). Also, the 30-day mortality in bleeding peptic ulcer increases in the elderly (Hasselgren et al., 1998). Clinically suspected peptic ulcer disease may be confirmed by a barium study. However, upper endoscopy remains the gold standard because it has been shown by multiple studies to be more sensitive and specific. In addition, it provides the opportunity to obtain tissue for histologic diagnosis. The diagnosis of *H. pylori* can be made histologically by Giemsa stain and a Clotest or by the breath test and determining the *H. pylori* antibody titers in the serum.

Treatment

In treating peptic ulcer disease, one should eliminate the offending factors such as the NSAIDs and smoking and also eradicate *H. pylori* infection, which is found to be responsible for 90% of duodenal ulcers in patients who do not use NSAIDs. Such eradication helps decrease the relapse rate and prevent the possible transformation to mucosa-associated lymphoid tissue (MALT) lymphoma seen in the stomach. Several therapy regimens have been found to be highly effective in eradicating *H. pylori,* all of which should include an antisecretory agent with either one antibiotic plus bismuth or two antibiotics. One such plan consists of a 14-day regimen (taken before eating) of:

One Prevacid (lansoprazole) 30-mg capsule PO twice a day
Two amoxicillin 500-mg capsules PO twice a day
One Biaxin (clarithromycin) 500-mg tablets PO twice a day

Follow-up upper endoscopy may be indicated in cases in which healing needs to be documented.

Diverticular Disease

Risk Factors

Diverticulosis of the colon is a disease that affects mainly the elderly, presenting in up to 20% of this age group (Lux et al., 1998). In developed countries, it is present in more than 40% of people older than 50 (Parks, 1975). This increase in prevalence is thought to be due to the decrease in fiber intake seen in the industrialized world (Gear et al., 1979). More than 90% of all patients with diverticular disease have sigmoid colon involvement (Parks, 1969).

About 70% of patients with diverticulosis are either asymptomatic or have infrequent symptoms and rarely seek medical care. About 20% of symptomatic patients present with diverticulitis; 5% present with lower GI bleed; and the rest may complain of abdominal pain, constipation, or bloating (Thompson, 1986). In the symptomatic patient, colon cancer should be ruled out.

Differential Diagnosis

Diagnosis is best made by barium enema, which shows outpouching of the colonic wall. This also helps to rule out an obstructing lesion. Colonoscopy may miss mild diverticular disease because of the hypertrophy of the muscularis layer in the colonic wall or because of spasm. Therefore, lower endoscopy is helpful mainly in ruling out a coexisting lesion or in the setting of lower GI bleed.

When microperforation of the diverticulae occurs, it starts an inflammatory process in the peridiverticulum area and causes diverticulitis. This inflammation may extend further and cause abscess formation that may, in turn, encase the colonic lumen and cause obstruction. One should differentiate this from acute appendicitis, inflammatory bowel disease, Crohn's colitis, infectious colitis, ischemic colitis, or any other process causing pericolonic abscess.

When hemorrhage complicates diverticular disease, it presents with a painless, self-limited rectal bleeding in the majority of the cases, but in about 5% bleeding may be massive and require urgent intervention (Browder et al., 1986).

Treatment

The main treatment of uncomplicated diverticulosis is a high-fiber diet (Brodrib, 1977). Antispasmodic agents may be tried in patients with chronic, intermittent, nonspecific abdominal pain. When diverticulitis occurs, management should include fluid replacement and bowel rest. Seven to 10 days of broad-spectrum antibiotic coverage should be used intravenously to cover colonic pathogens. Nasogastric suction may be needed in the presence of mechanical or functional obstruction.

Surgical resection is necessary in about 20% of patients with diverticulitis (Parks, 1969). Indications are peritonitis, perforation, colonic obstruction, poor response to conservative management, or recurrent diverticulitis, which may occur in 30% of patients (Ertan, 1990).

The management of diverticular bleeding should be directed first toward volume replacement and resuscitation, to be followed by a colonoscopy. Angiography may be necessary if bleeding recurs or continues with the failure to identify the bleeding site by colonoscopy. Angiography should be the first step if the patient presents with a major persisting bleed. Localizing the bleeding site and colonic involvement with diverticular disease helps the surgeon direct the treatment plan to segmental colectomy vs. total abdominal colectomy. In cases in which the bleeding ceases spontaneously, as seen in the majority of the cases, surgery is not needed, and the prognosis is good.

Colorectal Cancer

Risk Factors

The estimated yearly incidence of colorectal cancer is more than 150,000 new cases per year. Colorectal cancer represents more than 12% of all cancer deaths in the United States (Boring, Squires, and Tong, 1993). The long exposure to environmental carcinogens resulting in the neoplastic clone increases the incidence exponentially (Schottenfeld, 1981). Factors such as alcohol use, particularly beer; tobacco smoking (Neugut, Jacobson, and DeVivo, 1993); and dietary habits such as a high-fat, low-fiber or a red meat–rich diet have been implicated in adenoma or adenocarcinoma of the colon. Other factors, including the P53 genes and the APC gene, have also been implicated in the adenoma to carcinoma sequence. Inflammatory bowel diseases, colonic adenomas, and prior exposure to radiation increase the risk for colorectal cancer.

A family history of colorectal polyps increases the risk of cancer by about the same amount as a family history of colorectal cancer. The increased risk seen with a positive family history of polyps does not appear to decrease with age (Kerber et al., 1998).

Occult GI bleeding is generally the only manifestation of early colon cancer. Bright red blood per rectum may be seen with more distal lesions. In advanced cases, colonic obstruction, abdominal pain, and symptoms of local and distant invasion may be found. Wasting syndrome has been described even with small early tumors (Theologids, 1979).

Screening

The American College of Gastroenterology has announced recent recommendations to screen the asymptomatic population starting at age 50 with annual occult fecal blood testing. If heme negative, then periodic flexible sigmoidoscopy is indicated at 5-year intervals. If the stool is positive for occult blood, a colonoscopy vs. a flexible sigmoidoscopy with air contrast barium enema is indicated.

The adenoma carcinoma sequence takes an average of 15 years to occur (Kozuka et al., 1975). Therefore, screening asymptomatic patients is a crucial first step in diagnosing adenocarcinoma in the colon. It is estimated that 50% of positive hemoccult tests are indicative of a neoplastic process that includes adenomatous polyps in 38% and adenocarcinoma in 12% (Winawer, Schottenfeld, and Flechinger, 1991). Annual fecal occult blood testing has reduced mortality from colorectal cancer by at least 33.4% (Ederer, Church, and Mandel, 1997). The most sensitive and specific test available, especially in patients with small polyps or early cancers, is colonoscopy, which also provides the opportunity to obtain tissue biopsies. Barium enema is helpful in more advanced cases.

Treatment

Adenomatous polyps are treated with polypectomy or polyp fulguration based on the polyp size. Some large polyps may require segmental resection. Surgery is the mainstay treatment for adenocarcinoma. Adjuvant chemotherapy with fluorouracil (5-FU) plus levamisole increases survival in patients with Duke's C colon cancer (Lauri et al., 1989). Self-expanding colonic metallic stent placement is a minimally invasive and cost-effective palliative approach (Binkert et al., 1998). Elderly patients with comorbidities who have colon perforation and obstruction due to colon cancer and require emergency surgical intervention may benefit from conservative surgery followed by staged resection. The same may be said for patients with intraoperatively established greater spread of tumor. This procedure permits delayed radical resection at the lowest rate of clinical mortality and is especially suitable for frail elderly patients in poor condition (Koperna, Kisser, and Schulz, 1997).

Acute Abdomen

Especially in the elderly, the GI and hepatobiliary systems are responsible for a wide range of pathologies resulting in an acute abdomen. These include appendicitis, diverticulitis, perforated peptic ulcer disease, intestinal ischemia, obstruction and perforation, acute pancreatitis, acute cholangitis, acute cholecystitis, hepatic abscess, and ruptured hepatic neoplasm.

Because early diagnosis is essential in directing treatment, one should start first with a thorough history and physical examination that should provide clues to the diagnosis in most cases. One should pay attention to the pain characteristics and the presence of peritoneal irritation signs, masses, or GI bleeding.

Acute Appendicitis

Acute appendicitis has increased in incidence in the last decades, in part because of the increased longevity in the general population (Moro et al., 1996). Appendicitis is prevalent in the elderly population, accounting for up to 14% of all cases of acute abdomen (Reiss and Deutch, 1985). Mortality is reported to be higher in the elderly because of the nonclassical presentation, delayed diagnosis, and higher rate of complication in a patient with multiple preexisting diseases.

History

Typically the pain starts in the periumbilical area and is associated with nausea and possibly vomiting. This is thought to be due to the obstruction of the appendiceal lumen by a fecalith, a foreign body, or lymphatic hyperplasia. If the obstruction continues, the inflammation becomes transmural, resulting in serosal inflammation and then to pain localization in the right lower quadrant.

Differential Diagnosis

The diagnosis of appendicitis is often made on clinical examination. It can be supported by leukocytosis, small bowel ileus, the presence of the appendicolith on the abdominal flat plate, the presence of pneumoperitoneum indicating a perforation, or the presence of a dilated appendix with a thickened wall on ultrasound. The accuracy of ultrasonography in nonperforated appendix is 93%, with a negative predicted value of 97% (Fa and Cronan, 1989). In the elderly, the diagnosis is often made very late, with 40% to 80% of cases already perforated. The reasons for delayed hospitalization include atypical course, reduction in sensitivity to pain in old age, and inadequate ability to communicate (Zachert and Meyer, 1998).

Treatment

The treatment for acute appendicitis is emergent appendectomy. Delayed diagnosis or presentation may lead to increased mortality due to appendiceal perforation. The overall mortality increases with age, reaching up to 16% in patients above the age of 70 (Louis et al., 1975). Postoperative complications occurred much more frequently in the elderly, resulting in an increased morbidity and prolonged hospital stay (Moro et al., 1996).

Mesenteric Ischemia

The diagnosis of mesenteric ischemia requires a high degree of suspicion in the patient with abdominal pain. It is associated with a high mortality rate. It can result from an occlusive or a nonocclusive process and can be arterial or venous in origin. Acute occlusive arterial ischemia is a result of an embolic phenomenon most commonly caused by a mural thrombus from an underlying cardiac disease or an aortic embolus.

Presentation and Differential Diagnosis

Patients present with acute sudden onset of severe midabdominal pain that may be associated with peritoneal irritation and occult GI bleeding. The diagnosis is made clinically, but the presence of leukocytosis, hemoconcentration, and metabolic acidosis with increase in serum lactate levels (Meyer et al., 1998), which usually indicates a late presentation, is helpful. Once the diagnosis is suspected, emergent angiography is indicated. Once the embolus is identified, intraarterial injection of urokinase and systemic intravenous heparin may spare the patient from an emergent surgery, which includes embolectomy and resection of necrotic bowels.

In cases of the low flow state, nonocclusive mesenteric ischemia is due to vasoconstriction as a result of decreased cardiac output, hypovolemia, or medications such as digoxin. Angiography shows mesenteric vasoconstriction with a pruned appearance. Treatment is directed toward fluid and volume resuscitation. Surgery is reserved for necrotic bowel resection.

Mesenteric Thrombosis

Mesenteric thrombosis can present with acute abdominal pain but more commonly presents as a chronic postprandial abdominal pain, resulting in decreased food intake and weight loss. Diagnosis is made angiographically, and treatment can be achieved by intraarterial stenting or surgical bypass. Patients older than 75 with mesenteric ischemia have a higher overall mortality after exploratory laparotomy (Bronner and Boissel, 1997).

Hepatobiliary Pancreatic Diseases

Isolated abnormalities of liver enzymes have been noted occasionally in the elderly. Isolated elevation of alkaline phosphatase is related to osteomalacia in 50% of patients and to liver disease in 25% and is idiopathic in 25%. An isolated elevation of serum bilirubin may reflect congestive hepatopathy seen with congestive heart failure (Lubin et al., 1982). Hepatocellular dysfunction and cholestatic damage are also seen in the elderly and may reflect conditions such as hepatitis, drug toxicity, and hepatocellular carcinoma.

Cholelithiasis and Choledocholithiasis

The prevalence of cholelithiasis increases with age to as much as 30% of the geriatric population. It commonly presents with acute cholecystitis or acute cholangitis secondary to choledocholithiasis and biliary obstruction (Mee et al., 1981).

Presentation

Biliary colic is characterized by an epigastric or right upper quadrant abdominal pain that gradually worsens before reaching a plateau of constant severe pain that may last for several hours. Spontaneous resolution of biliary colic reflects the dislodgment of the impacted stone from the cystic duct. The pain is most commonly postprandial, especially after a fatty meal, and is associated with nausea and vomiting.

Cholecystitis occurs as a result of the continued obstruction of the cystic duct leading to gallbladder wall inflammation. When the inflammation reaches the serosal surface of the gallbladder, peritoneal irritation signs occur, leading to localization of the pain in the right upper quadrant. Murphy's sign is described as the inhibition of deep inspiration secondary to pain produced by the movement of an inflamed gallbladder against the parietal peritoneum. Fever, leukocytosis, and elevation of liver enzymes, including bilirubin, alkaline phosphatase, and transaminases, may be seen. Ultrasonographic findings may include gallstones, biliary obstruction and dilation, thickened gallbladder wall, or pericholecystic fluid.

Differential Diagnosis

In the proper clinical setting and in the presence of gallstones, a positive sonographic Murphy's sign predicts acute cholecystitis in 90% of the cases (Ralls et al., 1985). When acalculus cholecystitis is suspected, cholescintigraphy can help in the diagnosis.

Treatment

Management includes fluid resuscitation, intravenous antibiotics, and cholecystectomy, which is the most effective management. When laparoscopic cholecystectomy was studied in patients over age 85, it was found to have an overall morbidity of 9.8% and no increased mortality when compared to the general population (Barrat et al., 1996). Therefore, laparoscopic cholecystectomy should be undertaken with caution in geriatric patients with acute cholecystitis in view of other comorbid diseases. In this setting when patients are poor surgical candidates, percutaneous cholecystostomy is a safe, effective treatment for acute cholecystitis. For acalculus cholecystitis, cholecystostomy can be followed by elective surgery (Sujiyama, Tokuhara, and Atomi, 1998). Biliary obstruction may be complicated by acute pancreatitis, termed *biliary pancreatitis*. If acute pancreatitis is severe, the abdominal pain may be periumbilical or midabdominal, radiating to the back; some relief may be obtained by adopting the fetal position. Acute pancreatitis is usually associated with amylase and lipase elevation.

When biliary pancreatitis and continued biliary obstruction are suspected, endoscopic retrograde choledochopancreatography (ERCP) with sphincterotomy and stone removal is indicated within the first 24 hours of admission. This results in substantial improvement in the outcome of acute biliary pancreatitis (Pezzilli et al., 1998).

Liver Disease

Viral Hepatitis

The widespread availability and recommended usage of hepatitis A and B vaccines have resulted in decreasing the incidence of these diseases and of hepatitis D, a coinfection with hepatitis B. Hepatitis E virus (associated with pregnancy) should not represent a major morbidity for elderly patients. The clinical significance of the newly discovered hepatitis G is yet to be defined.

Hepatitis B virus is usually transmitted by inoculation of infected blood or blood products. The incubation period of hepatitis B is 6 weeks to 6 months (average 12 to 14 weeks) but may be prolonged by the administration of hepatitis B immune globulin. See Table 9-1 for recommended postexposure prophylaxis for exposure to hepatitis B

TABLE 9-1 Recommended Postexposure Prophylaxis for Percutaneous or Permucosal Exposure to Hepatitis B Virus, United States

Vaccination and Antibody Response Status of Exposed Person	Treatment When Source Is: HBsAg* Positive	HBsAg Negative	Source Not Tested or Status Unknown
Unvaccinated	HBIG† × 1; initiate HB vaccine series‡	Initiate HB vaccine series	Initiate HB vaccine series
Previously vaccinated:			
Known responder§	No treatment	No treatment	No treatment
Known non-responder	HBIG × 2 or HBIG × 1 and initiate revaccination	No treatment	If known high-risk source, treat as if source were HBsAg positive
Antibody response unknown	Test exposed person for anti-HBs‖ 1. If adequate,§ no treatment 2. If inadequate,§ HBIG × 1 and vaccine booster	No treatment	Test exposed person for anti-HBs 1. If adequate,§ no treatment 2. If inadequate, initiate revaccination

From Centers for Disease Control and Prevention: Immunization of Health-Care Workers, *MMWR* 46: No. RR-18, pp 1-42, 1997.

*Hepatitis B surface antigen.

†Hepatitis B immune globulin; dose 0.06 ml/kg intramuscularly.

‡Hepatitis B vaccine.

§Responder is defined as a person with adequate levels of serum antibody to hepatitis B surface antigen (i.e., anti-HBs ≥10 mIU/ml); inadequate response to vaccination defined as serum anti-HBs <10 mIU/ml.

‖Antibody to hepatitis B surface antigen.

virus. Table 9-2 outlines the interpretation of the hepatitis B panel to determine the patient's immune or infection status.

Hepatitis C virus is a ribonucleic acid virus that was first identified in 1989 and currently affects about 2% of the American population and 4.1% of patients over age 60. In the subgroup of geriatric patients, risk factors for acquiring hepatitis C are blood transfusion, surgical intervention, and the use of nondisposable syringes (Monica et al., 1998). The most prevalent route of transmission is through parenteral transmission, in the elderly population most commonly from a blood transfusion before 1990. After exposure to hepatitis C, more than 80% of patients develop chronic hepatitis C, which has an insidious course and is usually discovered when abnormal liver enzymes are found and further investigated or when the patient with the chronic hepatitis C decompensates with cirrhosis.

Symptoms are usually very mild and are most commonly fatigue and malaise. Change of sleep pattern, easy bruisability, altered mental status due to hepatic encephalopathy, and GI bleeding are seen in the late stages when cirrhosis is present.

Diagnosis is made clinically and by laboratory values. Liver biopsy may be needed if treatment is planned or to assess the severity and stage of the liver involvement. Patients over age 60 were found to have mild histologic changes, which were thought to be related to the higher prevalence of genotype IIA found in the majority of these patients (Monica et al., 1998).

TABLE 9-2 Interpretation of the Hepatitis B Panel

Tests	Results	Interpretation
HBsAg anti-HBc anti-HBs	Negative Negative Negative	Susceptible
HBsAg anti-HBc anti-HBs	Negative Negative or positive Positive	Immune
HBsAg Anti-HBc IgM anti-HBc Anti-HBs	Positive Positive Positive Negative	Acutely infected
HBsAg Anti-HBc IgM anti-HBc Anti-HBs	Positive Positive Negative Negative	Chronically infected
HBsAg Anti-HBc Anti-HBs	Negative Positive Negative	Four interpretations possible*

From Hepatitis B Coalition website: http://www.immunize.org, 1998.

*1. May be recovering from acute HBV infection.
2. May be distantly immune and test not sensitive enough to detect very low level of anti-HBs in serum.
3. May be susceptible with a false-positive anti-HBc.
4. May be undetectable level of HBsAg present in the serum and the person is chronically infected with HBV.

It is generally accepted that 10% to 20% of patients with chronic hepatitis C will develop cirrhosis within 10 years of first infection (Dusheiko, 1998). The recommended treatment for naïve patients is interferon in subcutaneous injections for 12 to 18 months. Patients older than 65 years of age have been found to have a 30% virologic/complete response (Eyigun, Van Thiele, and De Maria, 1998). Some studies have recommended postponing treatment in asymptomatic patients if liver biopsy specimens show no more than grade I necroinflammatory activity or stage I fibrosis (Levine, 1998). Therefore, one would argue that in a geriatric patient who fits the preceding description, clinical monitoring is a reasonable course of action.

In patients with decompensated cirrhosis, the only treatment that would improve the 5-year survival rate is liver transplantation, which is less frequently done in the geriatric population because of the comorbid conditions that would make such a major intervention futile. Therefore, conservative management with diuretics for fluid retention in ascites and lactulose for portosystemic encephalopathy is indicated.

With the increased incidence of hepatocellular carcinoma in cirrhotics who do not tolerate surgical resection because of advanced cirrhosis, new modalities of treatment have recently been described that include thoracoscopic microwave coagulation therapy for tumor ablation (Asahara et al., 1998) and percutaneous ethanol injection (Bartolozzi et al., 1998), both of which have resulted in partial or complete resolution of liver lesions.

Summary

Several GI disorders are very common in the older population. It is important to be able to perform the appropriate evaluation to distinguish among them, especially the acute or malignant conditions. There are numerous special considerations for diagnosing and treating GI conditions such as the presence of *H. pylori* in ulcer disease or the risk of hepatitis. Several laboratory and diagnostic examinations are available. The ability to determine the appropriate one (and to know when to refer) can save much discomfort and expense. In addition, the practitioner must be able to prescribe the appropriate treatment or intervention and provide adequate teaching to the patient or caregiver.

Resources

American Institute for Cancer Research
http://www.aicr.org

National Cancer Institute
http://www.nci.nih.gov

GERD Information Resource Center
http://www.gerd.com

American College of Gastroenterology
http://www.acg.gi.org

Hepatitis B Immunization Action Coalition
1573 Selby Avenue
St. Paul, MN 55104
(651) 647-9009
http://www.immunize.org

References

Asahara T et al: Thoracoscopic microwave coagulation therapy for hepatocellular carcinoma, *Hiroshima J Med Sci* 47(3):125, 1998.

Baime M, Nelson J, Castelli D: Aging of the gastrointestinal system. In Hazzard W et al, editors: *Principles of geriatric medicine and gerontology*, ed 3, New York, 1994, McGraw-Hill.

Barrat C et al: Is there an age limit for cholecystectomy? Aprospos of 61 patients over 85 years of age, *J Chir (Paris)* 133(9-10):414, 1996.

Bartolozzi C et al: Hepatocellular carcinoma treatment with percutaneous ethanol injection: evaluation with contrast enhanced Doppler sound, *Radiology* 209(2):387, 1998.

Behrman SW et al: Laparoscopic cholecystectomy in geriatric population, *Am Surg* 62(5):386, 1996.

Binkert CA et al: Acute colonic obstruction: clinical aspects and cost effectiveness of preoperative and palliative treatment with self-expanding metallic stent: a preliminary report, *Radiology* 206(1):199, 1998.

Bird HA: When are NSAIDs appropriate in osteoarthritis? *Drugs Aging* 12(2):87, 1998.

Boring CC, Squires TS, Tong T: Cancer statistics, 1993, *CA Cancer J Clin* 43(1):7, 1993.

Brodrib AGM: Treatment of symptomatic diverticular disease with high-fiber diet, *Lancet* 1:664, 1977.

Brody JA, Schneider EL: Diseases and disorders of aging: an hypothesis, *J Chron Dis* 39:871, 1986.

Bronner JF, Boissel P: Acute ischemia in arterial mesenteric infarction in patients over age 75: apropos of comparative series of 38 cases, *J Chir (Paris)* 134(3):109, 1997.

Browder W et al: Impact of emergency and geography in massive lower GI bleeding, *Ann Surg* 204:530, 1986.

Chow LW et al: Risk factors for rebleeding and death from peptic ulcer in the very elderly, *Br J Surg* 85(1):121, 1998.

Demeester TR, Cimochowski GE, O'Drobinak J: Esophageal function in patients with angina type chest pain and normal coronary angiograms, *Ann Surg* 196:488, 1982.

Dusheiko GM: The natural course of chronic hepatitis C: implications for clinical practice, *J Viral Hepat* 5(suppl 1):9, 1998.

Ederer F, Church TR, Mandel JS: Fecal occult blood straining in the Minnesota study: role of chance detection of lesions, *J Natl Cancer Inst* 89(19):1423, 1997.

Ertan A: Colonic diverticulitis: recognizing and managing its presentation and complications, *Postgrad Med* 88:67, 1990.

Eyigun CB, Van Thiele DH, De Maria N: Use of interferon for the treatment of chronic hepatitis C in the elderly, *Hepatogastroenterology* 45(20):325, 1998.

Fa EM, Cronan JJ: Compression ultrasonography as an aid in the differential diagnosis of appendicitis, *Surg Gynecol Obstet* 169:290, 1989.

The Gallop Organization: A Gallop Organization national survey: heartburn across America, Princeton, NJ, 1988, The Gallop Organization.

Gaynor E: Otolaryngologic manifestations of gastroesophageal reflux, *Am J Gastroenterol* 86:801, 1991.

Gear JSS et al: Symptomless diverticular disease and intake of dietary fiber, *Lancet* 1:511, 1979.

Hasselgren G et al: Short and long-term course of elderly patients with peptic ulcer bleeding: analysis of factors influencing fatal outcome, *Eur J Surg* 164(9):685, 1998.

Kerber RA et al: Risk of colon cancer associated with a family history of cancer or colorectal polyps: the diet, activity, and the production in the colon cancer study, *Int J Cancer* 5:78(2):157, 1998.

Koperna T, Kisser M, Schulz F: Emergency surgery for colon cancer in the aged, *Arch Surg* 132(9):1032, 1997.

Kozuka S et al: Prevalence of the mucosal polyp in the large intestine. II. Estimation of the periods required for malignancy transformation of mucosal polyps, *Dis Colon Rectum* 18:494, 1975.

Lauri A et al: Surgical adjuvant therapy of large bowel carcinoma: an evaluation of levamisole and combination of levamisole and fluorouracil, *J Clin Oncol* 7:1447, 1989.

Levine RA: Treating histologically mild chronic hepatitis C: monotherapy, combination therapy or tincture of time, *Ann Intern Med* 15: 129(4):323, 1998.

Louis FR et al: Appendicitis: a critical view of diagnosis and treatment in 1,000 cases, *Arch Surg* 110:677, 1975.

Lubin JR et al: The value of profiling liver function in the elderly, *Postgrad Med J* 49:763, 1982.

Lux G et al: Diverticulosis and diverticulitis in the elderly, *Forschr Med* 30:116(9):26, 1998.

Maekawa T et al: Relationship between severity and symptoms of reflux esophagitis in elderly patients in Japan, *J Gastroenterol Hepatol* 13(9):927, 1998.

Mee AS et al: An operative removal of bile duct stones by duodenoscopic sphincterotomy in the elderly, *Br Med J* 283:P521, 1981.

Meyer T et al: How can the prognosis of acute mesenteric artery ischemia be improved: results of retrospective analysis, *Zentralb L Chirr* 123(3):230, 1998.

Mittal RK, McCallum RW: Characteristics of transient lower esophageal sphincter relaxation in humans, *Am J Physiol* 252:G636, 1987.

Monica F et al: Hepatitis C virus infection and related chronic liver disease in a resident elderly population: the Silea study, *J Viral Hepat* 5(5):345, 1998.

Monson RR, McMahan B: Peptic ulcer in Massachusetts physician, *N Engl J Med* 281:11, 1969.

Moro MJ et al: Appendicitis in the elderly: delay between the first symptoms and clinical procedure, *Am Med Int* 13(12):580, 1996.

Neugut AI, Jacobson JS, DeVivo I: Epidemiology of colorectal adenomatous polyps, *Cancer Epidemiol Biomarkers Prev* 2:159, 1993.

Parks TG: Natural history of diverticular disease: a review of 521 cases, *Br Med J* 4:639, 1969.

Parks TG: Natural history of diverticular disease of the colon, *Clin Gastroenterol* 4:53, 1975.

Pezzilli R et al: Effect of early ductal decompression in the human biliary acute pancreatitis, *Pancreas* 16(2):165, 1998.

Ralls PW et al: Sonography in suspected acute cholecystis: perspective evaluation of primary secondary signs, *Radiology* 155:767, 1985.

Reiss R, Deutch A: Emergency abdominal procedures in patients above 70, *J Gerontol* 40:154, 1985.

Schottenfeld D: Epidemiology of cancer: an overview, *Cancer* 47:1108, 1981.

Schubert TT et al: Ulcer risk factors: interactions between *Helicobacter pylori* infection, nonsteroidal use and age, *Am J Med* 94:413, 1993.

Spechler SJ: Comparison of medical and surgical therapy for complicated gastroesophageal reflux disease in veterans, *N Engl J Med* 326:786, 1992.

Spechler SJ: Epidemiology and natural history of gastroesophageal reflux disease, *Digestion* 51(suppl 1): 24, 1992.

Sujiyama M, Tokuhara M, Atomi Y: Is percutaneous cholecystostomy the optimal treatment for acute cholecystitis in the very elderly? *World J Surg* 22(5):459, 1998.

Ter RB, Johnston BP, Castell DO: Influence of age and gender on gastroesophageal reflux in symptomatic patients, *Dis Esophagus* 11(2):106, 1998.

Theologids A: Cancer cachexia, *Cancer* 43:2004, 1979.

Thompson WG: Do colonic diverticula cause symptoms (editorial A), *M J Gastroenterol* 81:613, 1986.

Trus TL et al: Laparoscopic anti-reflux surgery in the elderly, *Am J Gastroenterol* 93(3):351, 1998.

Winawer SJ, Schottenfeld D, Flechinger BJ: Colorectal screening, *J Natl Cancer Inst* 83:243, 1991.

Winne HA et al: The effect of age upon liver volume and apparent liver blood flow in healthy men, *Hepatology* 9:297, 1989.

Zackert HR, Meyer HJ: Acute appendicitis in advanced age, *Fortshr Med* 116(9):36, 1998.

10

Endocrine Conditions

This chapter discusses the care of older adults who have significant but common disturbances within their endocrine system. The focus of this chapter is on the assessment, diagnosis, and treatment of three conditions of the endocrine system. The condition that occurs most frequently is diabetes mellitus followed by thyroid conditions, which are frequent but at times undiagnosed and, third, conditions of the parathyroid gland, which are uncommon but often misdiagnosed.

Diabetes Mellitus

Diabetes mellitus is a heterogeneous group of metabolic disorders characterized by hyperglycemia secondary to defects in insulin secretion, insulin action, or both.

Sixteen million people, or approximately 5.9% of the population of the United States, have diabetes mellitus. Each year an additional 800,000 people are diagnosed with the disease—more than 2000 people per day or 90 people per hour (Peterson and Vinicor, 1998). The rate of diagnosed diabetes mellitus rises with age from less than 1% among people 45 years of age and younger to a plateau of 10% among people 65 years of age and older. Another 9.3% of the population 65 years of age and older met the criteria for diabetes but had not been diagnosed, and 22.7% of people 65 years of age and older had an impaired glucose tolerance (Harris, 1988). Diabetes is the seventh leading cause of death in the United States and a major contributor to disability and impaired quality of life (Peterson and Vinicor, 1998).

Clinical Features

Diabetes in the elderly is characterized by a variety of nonspecific clinical manifestations (see Box 10-1 for common symptoms of diabetes in older persons). The classical polyuria, polydipsia, and polyphagia are uncommon in the elderly population (Goldberg and Coon, 1994).

Box 10-1

Common Symptoms of Diabetes in the Older Person

General
- Unexplained weight loss
- Fatigue
- Slow wound healing
- Mental status changes
- Recurrent bacterial or fungal infections

Eyes
- Cataracts
- Retinal detachment, hemorrhages
- Microaneurysms
- Macular disease

Gastrointestinal
- Gastroparesis

Neuromuscular
- Paresthesias
- Cranial nerve palsies
- Pain
- Muscle weakness

Cardiovascular
- Angina
- Silent cardiac ischemia
- Myocardial infarction
- Transient cerebral ischemia
- Stroke
- Diabetic foot ulcers

Renal
- Proteinuria
- Glomerulopathy
- Uremia

Classifications of Diabetes

Type 1 Ketosis-prone Diabetes

With type 1 ketosis-prone diabetes, there is insulin deficiency secondary to islet cell loss. It is often associated with specific human leukocyte antigen (HLA) types, with predisposition to viral insulitis or autoimmune (islet cell antibody) phenomena. It occurs at any age, but most commonly in young people.

Type 2 Ketosis-resistant Diabetes

Ketosis-resistant diabetes can occur at any age, but more frequently in adults. Patients have insulin resistance and usually have relative (rather than absolute) insulin deficiency (American Diabetes Association, 1998). The average age of patients at the time of diagnosis with type 2 diabetes is 60 years. Approximately 50% to 60% are obese. Hypertension is present in approximately 50% to 65%, and 20% to 40% already have clinically significant cardiovascular disease (Nuttall and Chasuk, 1998). It may be seen in family aggregates as an autosomal-dominant genetic trait. It frequently goes undiagnosed for many years because the hyperglycemia develops gradually. These patients are at increased risk of developing microvascular and macrovascular complications even before they are diagnosed. Insulin may be required for control of either chronic or acute hyperglycemia during stress. Diabetes mellitus type 2 is the more prevalent form of diabetes mellitus in the elderly population.

Of persons with type 2 diabetes, 50% to 80% exhibit what has come to be called syndrome X, or the insulin resistance syndrome. This syndrome consists of the following components: central obesity, hyperinsulinemia, hypertension, a dyslipidemia characterized by an increase in fasting triglycerides and a decrease in high-density lipoprotein cholesterol, a normal or only modestly increased low-density lipoprotein (LDL) cholesterol, hyperuricemia, microalbuminuria, and an increased plasminogen activator inhibitor-1 and fibrinogen concentration (Nuttall and Chasuk, 1998).

Diagnosis

The recent criteria for diagnosis of diabetes mellitus are:

- Symptoms of diabetes plus casual plasma glucose concentration >200 mg/dl. Casual is defined as any time, without regard to time since last meal.
  or
- Fasting plasma glucose concentration >126 mg/dl. Fasting is defined as no caloric intake for at least 8 hours.
  or
- 2-hour plasma glucose concentration >200 mg/dl during an oral glucose tolerance test (OGTT). The test should be performed as described by the World Health Organization, using a glucose load containing the equivalent of 75 g of anhydrous glucose dissolved in water (World Health Organization, 1985).

In the absence of unequivocal hyperglycemia with acute metabolic decompensation, these criteria should be confirmed by repeating testing on a different day. OGTT is not recommended for routine clinical use (American Diabetes Association, 1998).

Chronic Complications

Microangiopathy

Microvascular complications of type 2 diabetes cause significant morbidity, including renal failure, blindness, and lower extremity amputations (O'Connor, Spann, and Woolf, 1998). Older persons with diabetes have a high incidence of renal disease, retinopathy, and neuropathy, usually as a result of a long duration of untreated disease before detection (Goldberg and Coon, 1994).

Diabetic Nephropathy

Diabetes is the most common single cause of end-stage renal disease (ESRD) in the United States, accounting for close to one third of all cases. Approximately 20% to 30% of patients with diabetes develop evidence of nephropathy; more than half who begin dialysis have type 2 disease (O'Connor, Spann, and Woolf, 1998). Persistent albuminuria of 30 to 300 mg/24 hours has been shown to be the earliest stage of diabetic nephropathy. (American Diabetes Association, 1998). Hypertension can hasten the progression of renal disease. Intensive diabetes control and maintaining blood pressure at <130/85 will decrease the rate of progression of diabetic nephropathy.

Angiotensin-converting enzyme (ACE) inhibitors are recommended for all type 1 patients with microalbuminuria with or without hypertension, and for hypertensive type 2 patients with microalbuminuria. Protein restriction to 0.8 g/kg/day should be instituted with onset of overt nephropathy.

Diabetic Retinopathy

Retinopathy is a common microvascular complication and is estimated to be the most frequent cause of new blindness among Americans 20 to 74 years of age. Prevalence and severity of diabetic retinopathy depend on the duration of diabetes and an individual's control of glycosylated hemoglobin (Hb A_{1c}) (O'Connor, Spann, and Woolf, 1998). More than 60% of persons with type 2 diabetes show some degree of retinopathy. Optimal screening intervals have not yet been determined; however, most consensus-based guidelines call for yearly, dilated, comprehensive examinations by ophthalmologists or optometrists, beginning 3 to 5 years after diagnosis with type 1 diabetes, and beginning immediately on diagnosis in patients with type 2 diabetes (O'Connor, Spann, and Woolf, 1998).

Diabetic Neuropathy

Diabetic neuropathy may affect almost any part of the nervous system except the brain. It presents as peripheral polyneuropathy, mononeuropathy, radiculopathy, autonomic neuropathy, and amyotrophy (Foster, 1994). Peripheral polyneuropathy is the most common form, with sensory involvement being more common than motor. Peripheral neuropathy, combined with peripheral vascular disease, increases the risk of diabetic foot ulcers and amputations. Approximately 50% of lower extremity amputations in the United States are related to diabetes—almost 55,000 amputations per year. Patients who undergo an amputation are at greater risk for a second amputation on either the same leg or the other leg. The risk for amputation is 15 times that of persons without diabetes. Yet it has been estimated that half of the amputations in patents with diabetes are preventable (O'Connor, Spann, and Woolf, 1998).

Macroangiopathy

Macroangiopathy presents as silent myocardial ischemia, angina, myocardial infarction, cerebrovascular accidents, and peripheral vascular disease with foot ulcers. Diabetes doubles the risk for cardiovascular disease in the older person and is more pronounced in women with diabetes than in men (Goldberg and Coon, 1994). Cardiovascular mortality is higher in elderly persons with diabetes compared to the elderly without diabetes. More than 70% of adults with type 2 diabetes die of heart attacks or strokes (O'Connor, Spann, and Woolf, 1998). Hypertension and hyperlipidemia increase the risk of the patient with diabetes for cardiovascular disease complications (Bierman, 1992). Hyperinsulinemia, insulin resistance, and hereditary factors all increase the risk of atherosclerosis.

Assessment

History

A comprehensive history is important and should include presenting symptoms, family history, other medical conditions, surgical history, medications, allergies, and tobacco and alcohol use. Information should be obtained regarding any previous treatments for diabetes and success of glycemic control, cardiovascular risk factors, and presence of diabetic complications. Functional abilities, including vision and fine motor skills, and ability to manage medications will determine the patient's ability to self-manage his or her diabetes control via blood glucose monitoring and insulin administration, if necessary. A social history will help to ascertain who might be available to help the patient manage his or her diabetes treatments. Information regarding insurance coverage is helpful in ensuring the patient's ability to afford medications, diagnostics, and services that might be needed.

Physical Examination

The physical examination should include blood pressure determination with orthostatic measurements, ophthalmoscopic examination, cardiac examination, abdominal examination, evaluation of pulses, and foot examination. Current consensus-based guidelines recommend that comprehensive foot evaluations, including vascular, neurologic, musculoskeletal, and skin and soft tissue assessments, be performed at least annually. These guidelines recommend that once a high-risk abnormality is identified, the patient should have a foot examination at each visit (i.e., several times a year).

The vascular examination should involve palpation of lower extremity pulses and inspection of the legs and feet for ischemic changes.

The neurologic examination should include a sensorimotor test to ascertain whether protective sensation has been lost. A 10-g Semmes-Weinstein monofilament is recommended. This inexpensive but valuable tool is simple to use. It can be obtained from Sensory Testing Systems and Curative Health Services (see Resources). Patients identified as having loss of sensation should participate in a comprehensive, ongoing program of patient education concerning self-care and podiatric care and always wear appropriate footwear (O'Connor, Spann, and Woolf, 1998).

Laboratory Testing

The initial laboratory evaluation should include fasting plasma glucose, glycosylated hemoglobin level (HG A1c), fasting lipid profile, serum creatinine, urinalysis, test for microalbuminuria, and electrocardiogram. Hemoglobin A1c levels should be drawn every 3 to 6 months for ongoing monitoring.

Current consensus-based clinical guidelines recommend screening for microalbuminuria on a yearly basis to detect early diabetic nephropathy. Screening is recommended to begin 5 years after diagnosis in type 1 patients and immediately on diagnosis in patients with type 2 disease (O'Connor, Spann, and Woolf, 1998).

Treatment

The optimal strategy for a particular patient depends not only on research evidence, but also on other concerns, including timing of the intervention and its appropriateness to the patient's circumstances, other existing patient problems, medications the patient is taking, patient preference, and the anticipated adherence of the patient to the contemplated course of action (O'Connor, Spann, and Woolf, 1998).

The American Diabetes Association has recommended the following goals for glycemic control for all patients with diabetes:

Preprandial glucose of 80 to 120 mg/dl
Bedtime glucose of 100 to 140 mg/dl
Hemoglobin A1c of less than 7% (Kappel and Dills, 1998)

However, treatment goals should take into consideration the patient's ability to understand and carry out the management regimen, risk factors for severe hypoglycemia, patient factors that may increase risk or decrease benefit of tight glycemic control (such as advanced age, ESRD, or advanced cardiac or cerebrovascular disease), or other conditions that may shorten life expectancy (Kappel and Dills, 1998). It may be preferable to allow slightly higher glucose levels to minimize the risk of hypoglycemia.

Diet

In 1994 the American Diabetes Association recognized that the concept of a specific diabetic diet should be abandoned and that the dietary recommendations for patients must be individualized (Nuttall and Chasuk, 1998). The American Diabetes Association recommends a diet that contains 55% carbohydrates, 20% proteins, and less than 30% fat. Studies have shown that dietary therapy leads to weight loss and glycemic control in the elderly with diabetes (Reaven, 1985). Weight loss should be a goal for patients with diabetes who are overweight. A nutritionist or dietitian is an important member of the interdisciplinary team.

Exercise

Physical activity improves insulin sensitivity and enhances cardiovascular fitness. Although elderly persons with diabetes may find certain forms of exercise (such as brisk walking or swimming) difficult because of other comorbid conditions, it is important to encourage some sort of aerobic activity lasting at least 20 minutes three times per week. This may be as simple as wading in a pool, performing chair exercises, or walking at the mall (Lebovitz, 1995).

Smoking Cessation

Smoking cessation should be strongly recommended to reduce the risk of cardiovascular events, peripheral vascular disease and foot ulcers, retinopathy, and nephropathy.

Oral Hypoglycemic Agents

Currently there are five classes of oral hypoglycemic agents with different modes of action. These are the sulfonylureas, metformin, acarbose, troglitazone, and repaglinide.

Sulfonylureas

Mechanism of action:
- Stimulate insulin secretion

Examples:
- First generation (rarely used anymore)
  - Acetohexamide
  - Chlorpropamide
  - Tolazamide
  - Tolbutamide
- Second generation
  - Glipizide
  - Glyburide
  - Glimepiride

For many years sulfonylureas were the only oral agents available. They are most likely to be effective in patients who were diagnosed after the age of 40, have had the disease for fewer than 5 years, and are not overweight and whose initial fasting plasma glucose is less than 270 mg/dl (Ruoff, 1993). Treatment with sulfonylureas generally yields a mean decrease in fasting glucose of 60 mg/dl (Kappel and Dills, 1998). The major risk of sulfonylureas is hypoglycemia, and older patients appear to be at greater risk than younger patients. Other side effects include gastrointestinal discomfort, weight gain, and hyperinsulinemia.

Metformin

Mechanisms of action (proposed):
- Suppression of hepatic glucose output
- Increased glucose use and uptake
- Decreased fatty acid oxidation

Metformin is approved for use in the United States. Starting dose is 500 mg twice a day, titrated up to 2550 mg/day in divided doses. However, it is likely that the maximum effective dose is 2000 mg/day (Kappel and Dills, 1998). Metformin can be used in combination with a sulfonylurea. Side effects of metformin most commonly involve the gastrointestinal tract.

Diarrhea, abdominal pain, anorexia, nausea, and a metallic taste in the mouth usually decrease if the dose is reduced. Vitamin B_{12} and folate absorption may be decreased. The most serious complication of metformin is lactic acidosis. Lactic acidosis occurs at a rate of 0.03/1000 patient-years with 50% fatality.

Absolute contraindications to the use of metformin are renal dysfunction (creatinine greater than or equal to 1.5 mg/dl in men or 1.4 mg/dl in women), cardiac or pulmonary dysfunction severe enough to cause central hypoxia or decreased peripheral perfusion; history of lactic acidosis, abnormal liver function test, alcohol abuse with abnormal liver function; pregnancy, type 1 diabetes mellitus, severe infection or other acute illness, congestive heart failure, and use of radiocontrast agents (Kappel and Dills, 1998). Metformin should be withheld on the morning of a parenteral contrast x-ray film, to be resumed only after renal function has returned to baseline.

Alpha-glucosidase Inhibitors (Acarbose)

Mechanism of action:

Inhibits intestinal alpha-glucosidases
Interferes with hydrolysis of ingested disaccharides and complex carbohydrates
Impairs postprandial glucose excursion and insulin response

Approval for use in the United States occurred in 1996. Acarbose should be taken with the first bite of each meal. Recommended starting dose is 25 mg three times a day, titrated upwards to 50 mg three times a day in patients weighing less than or equal to 60 kg and to 100 mg three times a day in patients greater than 60 kg (Kappel and Dills, 1998). Gastrointestinal symptoms are the most common reactions to acarbose. These include diarrhea (33%), flatulence (77%), and abdominal pain (21%). In long-term studies, elevated liver enzymes occurred in 15% of patients taking acarbose. These elevations were asymptomatic, dose dependent, and reversible once acarbose was discontinued.

Acarbose is contraindicated in patient with cirrhosis, diabetic ketoacidosis, hypersensitivity to acarbose, inflammatory bowel disease, colonic perforation, partial intestinal obstruction and situations causing a predisposition to intestinal obstruction, chronic intestinal diseases associated with significant disorders of digestion or absorption, or conditions that may deteriorate due to increased intestinal gas formation (Kappel and Dills, 1998).

Troglitazone

Mechanism of action:

A thiazolidinedione
Acts as an insulin sensitizer to decrease insulin resistance
Inhibits hepatic gluconeogenesis

Troglitazone was approved by the Food and Drug Administration (FDA) in January 1997. Dosage begins at 200 mg per day and is titrated after 2 to 4 weeks to 400 mg per day. The maximal dose is 600 mg per day (Kappel and Dills, 1998). There has been a 2.6% incidence of abnormal liver function tests in patients who are taking this agent, and there have been reports of deaths due to liver failure. It is recommended that liver enzymes be checked every month for 6 months, then every 2 months for 6 months, and then periodically. Because of the risk involved and the inconvenience of frequent blood draws, this agent may not be considered preferable for the older population.

Repaglinide

Mechanism of action:
A benzoic acid derivative
Stimulates release of insulin

Repaglinide was recently approved by the FDA as: (1) first-line therapy for patients with type 2 diabetes uncontrolled by diet and exercise alone; and (2) combination therapy with metformin when therapy with either metformin or repaglinide alone is inadequate to control glucose levels. For patients not previously treated with oral antiglycemic agents and patients with hemoglobin A1c levels less than 8%, the starting dose is 0.5 mg taken preprandially anytime from 30 minutes to immediately before the meal. For patients previously treated with oral agents and those with a hemoglobin A1c greater than 8%, the starting dose is 1 mg before each meal. Dosage adjustments may be made as frequently as once per week (Kappel and Dills, 1998). Side effects may include hypoglycemia, headache, rhinitis, nausea, and arthralgias.

Insulin

Insulin preparations consist of either animal or human insulin. The short-acting insulins are regular, lispro, and Semilente. When given intravenously, they exert their effects within 10 to 15 minutes. When given subcutaneously, the regular and Semilente insulins reach peak effect in 2 to 3 hours, whereas the lispro reaches peak effect in 0.5 to 1.5 hours. The intermediate-acting insulins are NPH and Lente. Their peak effect is reached in 6 to 9 hours. Therapy is initiated with a dose of 5 to 10 U/day, to be increased by 2 to 3 U every 4 days until the fasting plasma glucose goal is reached. Insulin is relatively inexpensive. The major risk of insulin therapy is hypoglycemia.

Insulin regimens can range from a single dose of long-acting insulin (with a goal of preventing symptomatic hyperglycemia) to multiple doses of short- and long-acting insulin (with a goal of achieving normal levels of glycemia) (Morrow and Halter, 1993).

Initial treatment may be started by instituting a sliding scale administration of regular insulin based on fingersticks before each meal and at bedtime. For example:

Blood Sugar	Insulin Dose
<200	0 U
201 to 249	2 U
250 to 299	4 U
300 to 349	6 U
350 to 399	8 U
≥400	Call medical provider

Total amount of insulin administered within 24 hours is then added, and an initial dose of long-acting insulin is thereby determined. Patients receiving a bedtime insulin dose must be instructed to eat a bedtime snack, such as a piece of fruit or a half sandwich.

Management of Subsequent Health Risks

Attention must also be given to other health issues such as hyperlipidemia, coronary artery disease, renal disease, and stroke risk. These problems may exist independently or as a result of the diabetes. Recommendations include:

- Hyperlipidemia
  - Lowering LDL cholesterol below 130 mg/dl if no coronary artery disease is present and below 100 mg/dl if coronary artery disease is present.
  - Lower high triglyceride levels (>1000 mg/dl) to <400 mg/dl.
- Blood pressure
  - Maintain blood pressure at <130/85 mm Hg.
- Renal disease
  - Nephrology consult is necessary when glomerular filtration rate drops below 60 ml/min, serum creatinine rises to 2 mg/dl, or when difficulties occur in management of hypertension or hyperkalemia.
- Coronary artery disease and stroke risk
  - Daily aspirin administration has been shown to reduce adverse clinical outcomes, especially subsequent major cerebrovascular events (O'Connor, Spann, and Woolf, 1998).

Management

The management plan should include short- and long-term goals, medications, nutritional recommendations, home blood glucose monitoring, annual comprehensive dilated eye examinations, Pneumovax and yearly influenza vaccine administration, and follow-up plans.

Patients starting oral antidiabetic agents need to be in contact with their provider weekly until reasonable glucose control is achieved. Patients starting insulin therapy or having a major change in their regimen need to be in contact with their provider daily until glucose control is achieved. Patients are seen at least every 3 months until their treatment goals are achieved and then every 6 months (American Diabetes Association, 1998).

During follow-up visits an interim history is obtained that includes questioning about hypoglycemic episodes, results of self-monitoring blood glucose, current medications, and other medical illnesses. The health provider should examine the feet and measure weight and blood pressure. Hemoglobin A1c should be measured every 3 months; lipid profile, urinalysis, and microalbuminuria should be checked every year.

Managing Diabetes During Glucocorticoid Therapy

Although glucocorticoid therapy carries a risk of promoting or exacerbating hyperglycemia, there are currently no established medical guidelines for detecting or managing diabetes in patients starting such therapy. However, the importance of having a strategy to detect, monitor, and, if necessary, aggressively treat diabetes during glucocorticoid therapy is underscored by the potential seriousness of diabetic metabolic emergencies

TABLE 10-1 Medications or Agents That Alter Glucose Control

Drugs That Increase Blood Glucose	Drugs That Decrease Blood Glucose
Corticosteroids	Insulin
Thiazides	Oral hypoglycemic agents (sulfonylureas; acetohexamide, chlorpropamide, glipizide, glyburide, tolazamide, and tolbutamide)
Thyroid preparations	Alcohol
Phenytoin	Salicylates (high doses)
Epinephrine	Reserpine
Sugary preparations (many over the counter cold medications)	Clonidine
Estrogens	Phenylbutazone
Glucagon	Probenecid
Acetazolamide	Allopurinol
Caffeine	Pentamidine
Cyclophosphamide	Chloroquine
Ethacrynic acid	Dicumarol
Nicotine	Beta-blockers
Calcium-channel blockers	Clofibrate
Nonsteroidal anti-inflammatory drugs	Monoamine oxidase inhibitors
Phenobarbitol	Anabolic steroids
Chloramphenicol	Potassium salts

Modified from Steil D: Prescription drugs and diabetes, *Diabetes Spectrum* 3(2):119-122, 1990.

(Braithwaite et al., 1998). Glucocorticoid therapy makes patients insulin resistant. Therefore patients who have used insulin before moderate or high-dose glucocorticoid therapy often must increase insulin doses 1.5 to two times the previously established doses. Other medications and agents that alter glucose control are listed in Table 10-1.

Management of Hypoglycemia

Patients, caregivers, and family members must be educated regarding signs and symptoms of hypoglycemia, as well as how to manage this problem. Table 10-2 describes levels of hypoglycemia and the treatment of each.

Education

Patients should be given as much verbal and written information as they can manage to encourage self-care and prevention of complications. Education should include issues discussed previously such as diet, exercise, medication management, and glucose monitoring. The patient or caregiver must be able to administer the correct medication or insulin dosage, monitor blood sugar at home, and recognize symptoms of hypoglycemia and their management. Referral to a local home nursing agency can provide the patient and caregivers with at-home initial instruction and observation of blood glucose monitoring, medication and/or insulin administration, and nutrition counseling and

Table 10-2 Levels of Hypoglycemia and Treatment

Hypoglycemia Level	Symptoms	Treatment
Mild	Hunger, diaphoresis, nervousness, shakiness, tachycardia, and pale skin	15 g of carbohydrate (4 oz. of juice, no sugar added)
Moderate	Headache, irritability, fatigue, blurred vision, and mood changes	15 g of carbohydrate; may repeat
Severe	Unresponsiveness, confusion, coma, or convulsions	Glucagon, intravenous glucose

monitoring of complications. Patients must first purchase their own glucose monitoring machine and test strips (available from most pharmacies). The monitor, supplies, and nursing services are usually covered by Medicare.

Another important issue is foot care and prevention of foot ulcers. Teaching should include proper foot wear, avoidance of walking barefoot, and soaking the feet. Daily assessment of skin integrity of the feet should be performed by the patient using a mirror and flashlight to see all surfaces of the foot if necessary. If the patient is unable to do this, a caregiver should be taught how to do it. Feet should be washed daily in water that is not too hot, and lubrication applied to avoid skin cracks that can lead to infection. Regular evaluations by a podiatrist may be beneficial.

Thyroid Conditions

Thyroid disease is the second most frequent endocrine problem for older people. Many of the signs and symptoms of both hypothyroidism and hyperthyroidism in older persons are blunted in their presentation, or the presentation is atypical, or the presentation may be dismissed as a normal reaction to aging. Although laboratory tests are remarkably improved in reliability, they still can pose difficulties in reaching a firm diagnosis. Patients with thyroid disease need to be initially diagnosed and managed by a team of health professionals with expertise in this area. If the health care team does not include specialists, consultation with an endocrinologist is essential in managing patients with hyperthyroidism and selected cases of hypothyroidism.

Hypothyroidism

Epidemiology

The prevalence of hypothyroidism varies depending on ethnicity, the iodine content of the diet, and the criteria used to define the diagnosis. In the United States prevalence of hypothyroidism, as determined by elevated thyroid-stimulating hormone (TSH), varies from 4.4% to 7.3% in healthy adults above 55 years of age (Bagchi, Brown, and Parish, 1990; Sawin et al., 1985). In one study high TSH was more prevalent in Caucasians than African-Americans (8.8% vs. 5.8%), in women than men (5.95% to 8.5% vs. 2.3% to 4.4%), and in subjects older than 75 years of age (Bagchi, Brown, and Parish, 1990; Sawin et al., 1985).

Causes

Hypothyroidism is usually due to primary thyroid gland disorders. The most common cause of primary hypothyroidism is Hashimoto's thyroiditis, an autoimmune disorder with chronic lymphocytic infiltration of the thyroid gland. Bagchi found that 53.8% of subjects with elevated TSH level were positive for antimicrosomal or antithyroglobulin antibodies or both (Bagchi, Brown, and Parish, 1990). Other causes include prior treatment of Graves' disease; prior radiotherapy of Hodgkin's disease; previous thyroidectomy; and medications, especially lithium, amiodarone, and iodine (Reuben, 1993; Wallace and Hoffman, 1998). About 8% of patients taking amiodarone develop clinically significant hypothyroidism because of its high concentration of iodine, and 2.5% of patients taking high-dose amiodarone develop symptomatic hyperthyroidism (Fitzgerald, 1997).

Features

The signs and symptoms of hypothyroidism often develop insidiously. As many as 70% of elderly hypothyroid patients show typical symptoms and signs of hypothyroidism (Mokshagundam and Brazil, 1993). Common symptoms include dry skin, hair loss, cold intolerance, paresthesias, confusion, unsteadiness, constipation, fatigue, lethargy, hoarseness, slowed speech, depression and muscle cramps (Mokshagundam and Brazil, 1993; Wallace and Hoffman, 1998). Physical findings of hypothyroidism include delayed deep tendon reflexes, bradycardia, diastolic hypertension, hypoventilation, hypothermia, ataxia, carpal tunnel syndrome, cool pale skin, and puffy face and hands. Symptoms of peripheral neuropathy such as mild to severe burning and knifelike pain in the extremities may be the only symptoms in an elderly patient (Rizzolo, 1997). Hypothyroidism is a cause of reversible dementia; and even subclinical hypothyroidism may be associated with cognitive dysfunction, mood disturbance, and diminished response to standard psychiatric treatments (Smith and Ganja, 1992; Haggerty, 1990). Anemia may be the only manifestation in some cases (Mokshagundam, 1993). Clinicians need to be aware that many older people and family members may mistake the signs of hypothyroidism and consider that these are *only signs of aging*.

Diagnosis

There is inadequate evidence to support either screening or not screening for thyroid function in asymptomatic older adults (Goldberg and Chain, 1997). The best test for diagnosis of primary hypothyroidism is the serum TSH concentration (Mokshagundam and Brazil, 1993). The circulating TSH concentration is regulated by the circulating free thyroxine (T_4) concentration in a negative-feedback manner and is elevated in primary hypothyroidism. When serum thyroid hormone concentrations decrease below an individual's threshold for thyroid hormone sufficiency, serum TSH concentration increases. (Surks and Ocampo, 1996). Serum TSH levels will be elevated in subclinical and overt hypothyroidism. Free T_4 should be measured when TSH level is high. If free T_4 level is normal, TSH levels should be repeated in 4 to 6 weeks, since they may be transiently elevated during the recovery phase of nonthyroid illness (Hanishin et al., 1986).

The American Thyroid Association recommends the measurement of both TSH and free T_4 as initial tests in patients with suspected hypothyroidism (Hay et al., 1991). The American College of Physicians recommends a total T_4, free thyroxine index (T_4I), or sensitive TSH as the best initial test in patients with suspected hypothyroidism (Helfand and Crapo, 1991). Isolated elevated TSH levels should be repeated in 4 to 6 weeks.

Many sick and even normal elderly people may have abnormal levels of TSH. Furthermore, nonspecific illnesses, drugs, and decreased food intake may depress triiodothyronine (T_3) both in young and old people. TSH may show minor elevation during recovery from an illness, and T_4 can be affected by multiple factors (Table 10-3).

TABLE 10-3 Factors That Influence Thyroid Status

Factors Increasing T_4	Factors Decreasing T_4
Laboratory error	Severe illness (eg, chronic renal failure, major surgery, caloric deprivation)
Autoimmunity	Acute psychiatric problems
Acute illness (eg, viral hepatitis, chronic active hepatitis; primary biliary cirrhosis; acute intermittent porphyria; AIDS)	Cirrhosis
High-estrogen states (may also increase T_3)	Nephrotic syndrome
Oral estrogen-containing contraceptives	Hereditary TBG deficiency
Pregnancy	Drugs
Estrogen replacement therapy	Phenobarbital
Neonatal period	Phenytoin (T_4 may be as low as 2 μg/dL)
Acute psychiatric problems	Carbamazepine
Hyperemesis gravidarum and morning sickness (may also increase T_3)	Triiodothyronine (T_3) therapy
Familial thyroid hormone binding abnormalities	Androgens
Generalized resistance to thyroid hormone	Fluorouracil
Drugs	Halofenate (lowers triglycerides and uric acid; not marketed in USA)
Amiodarone	Mitotane
Amphetamines	Phenylbutazone
Clofibrate	Fenclofenac (nonsteroidal anti-inflammatory agent; not marketed in USA)
Heparin (dialysis method)	Salicylates (large doses)
Heroin	Chloral hydrate
Levothyroxine (T_4) replacement therapy	Asparaginase
Methadone (may also increase T_3)	
Perphenazine	

From Fitzgerald P: Endocrinology. In Tierney LM et al: *Current medical diagnoses and treatment,* ed 36, Stamford, Conn, 1997, Appleton & Lange.

Many of the laboratory tests may be misleading, and a combination of tests should still be used to define thyroid status (Gregerman and Katz, 1994).

Treatment

Thyroid hormone replacement therapy is the treatment of overt hypothyroidism. The goal should be full physiologic replacement. The preferred agent is levothyroxine (Synthroid) because of its long half-life and its conversion to T_3. Brand-name products are preferred over generic ones because they vary less in bioavailability from batch to batch (Barzel, 1995; Wallace and Hoffman, 1998). Levothyroxine requirements decrease with age (Sawin et al., 1995).

Levothyroxine therapy for hypothyroid elderly patients with or without overt heart disease should start at 25 μg/day. The dose is increased in increments of 25 μg at 8-week intervals until the serum TSH level returns to normal.

Precautions

Two areas of concern during thyroid hormone replacement in the elderly are the effects on the cardiovascular system and bone mineral density. Two percent of elderly patients developed new-onset angina during levothyroxine therapy (Mandel, Brent, and Reed, 1993). Thyroxine treatment with patients who have known coronary artery disease (CAD) need to be treated initially with caution. Thyroxine increases cardiac muscle demand and can precipitate angina or a myocardial infarction in patients with CAD (Rizzolo, 1997). If cardiac symptoms develop or worsen, therapy should be stopped pending the evaluation of the cardiac disease.

In a study of postmenopausal women it was found that long-term levothyroxine therapy was associated with decreased bone density of the spine and hip. Of the 19 subjects, sixteen had normal serum thyroxine levels, and 13 of 19 had low TSH levels, suggesting supraphysiologic levothyroxine treatment (Adlin et al., 1991). To protect women from bone loss, the dosage of levothyroxine should not suppress the TSH below normal even if T_4 levels are normal (Fitzgerald, 1997).

Subclinical Hypothyroidism

Of people with subclinical hypothyroidism, 20% to 50% develop overt hypothyroidism within 4 to 8 years. Overt hypothyroidism develops within 4 years in 80% of those above the age of 65 with subclinical hypothyroidism and elevated antithyroid antibodies (Wallace and Hoffman, 1998). Treatment of subclinical hypothyroidism must be individualized and considered a strong possibility in the presence of antithyroid antibodies (Wallace and Hoffman, 1998). Patients with subclinical hypothyroidism may notice increased energy, decreased skin dryness, and constipation after treatment with thyroxine (Surks and Ocampo, 1993). Once a decision is made to treat the person with subclinical hypothyroidism, the same treatment plan as for overt hypothyroidism is followed.

Hyperthyroidism

Prevalence

Hyperthyroidism is a metabolic disorder that results when tissues are exposed to excess thyroid hormone. The prevalence of hyperthyroidism in older persons (55 years of age and older) has been reported to be 0.5 to 2.3%, depending on the population studied and the criteria used for diagnosis (Bagchi, Brown, and Parish, 1990). Approximately 15% of all patients with hyperthyroidism are above the age of 60 years (Berglund, Christensen, and Hallengren, 1990).

Causes

Graves' disease is the most common cause of hyperthyroidism in the elderly. In a study of 25 hyperthyroid patients, Tibladi and associates (1986) found that 21 had Grave's disease, three had multinodular goiter, and one had a toxic nodule. Other rare causes of hyperthyroidism in the elderly are thyroid carcinoma, excess TSH secretion, thyroiditis, and a large iodine load (Mokshagundam and Brazil, 1993).

Clinicians need to be aware that radiographic examinations that use iodine-containing contrast materials (gallbladder and others) may contribute to an increased risk of an elderly person developing iodine-induced thyrotoxicosis such as that caused by amiodarone (Gregerman and Katz, 1994).

Clinical Manifestations

Elderly patients with hyperthyroidism have fewer signs and symptoms than their younger counterparts (Nordyke, Gilbert, and Harada, 1988). Weight loss and nonspecific failure to thrive are the most common manifestations of hyperthyroidism in older persons. The common signs and symptoms of hyperthyroidism are weight loss (44%), palpitations (36%), weakness (32%), heat intolerance (4%), constipation or diarrhea, anorexia, depression and apathy, tachycardia (28%), atrial fibrillation (32%), lid lag (12%), fine skin (40%), and tremor (36%) (Mokshagundam and Brazil, 1993). Atrial fibrillation may be the only manifestation of hyperthyroidism in the elderly.

Diagnosis

TSH measurement, using one of the newer, sensitive TSH assays, is the preferred test for hyperthyroidism. The American Thyroid Association recommends free T_4 and a sensitive thyrotropin assay for hyperthyroidism measurement (Hay et al., 1991). The American College of Physicians recommends the free T_4 index as the best initial test (Helfand and Crapo, 1991). However, Drinka et al. (1991) found that free T_4 index is not a good test for hyperthyroidism in chronically ill, institutionalized elderly patients. Patients with hyperthyroidism will have TSH levels below the detection limit of the assay. If TSH levels

TABLE 10-4 Thyroid Testing

Purpose	Test	Comment
Screening	Serum TSH (sensitive assay)	Most sensitive test for primary hypothyroidism and hyperthyroidism
	Free T_4	Excellent test
	T_4 (RIA)	Varies directly with TBG
	T_3 resin uptake (T_3RU)	Varies inversely with TBG
	Free thyroxine index	Useful combination of T_4 and T_3U
For hypothyroidism	Serum TSH	High in primary and low in secondary hypothyroidism.
	Antithyroglobulin and antithyroperoxidase antibodies	Elevated in Hashimoto's thyroiditis
For hyperthyroidism	Serum TSH (sensitive assay)	Suppressed except in TSH-secreting pituitary tumor or hyperplasia (rare)
	T_3 (RIA)	Elevated
	^{123}I uptake and scan	Increased diffuse vs. "hot" areas
	Antithyroglobulin and antimicrosomal antibodies	Elevated in Graves' disease
	TSH receptor antibody (TSH-R Ab [stim])	Usually positive in Graves' disease
For nodules	FNA	Best diagnostic method for thyroid cancer
	^{123}I uptake and scan	Cancer is usually "cold"; less reliable than FNA
	^{99m}Tc scan	Vascular versus avascular
	Ultrasonography	Solid versus cystic; pure cysts are usually not malignant

From Fitzgerald P: Endocrinology. In Tierney LM et al: *Current medical diagnoses and treatment,* ed 36, Stamford, Conn, 1997, Appleton & Lange.
FNA, Fine-needle aspiration; *RIA,* radioimmunoassay; T_3, triiodothyronine; T_4, thyroxine; *TSH,* thyroid-stimulating hormone; *TBG,* thyroxine-binding globulin.

are low, free T_4 index should be measured and, if it is normal, T_3 should be measured. If free T_4 and T_3 levels are normal, the TSH measurement should be repeated in 4 to 6 weeks (Mokshagundam and Brazil, 1991). Radioactive iodine uptake will help in identifying the cause of hyperthyroidism (see Table 10-4 for screening using thyroid tests).

Treatment

Radioactive iodine therapy is the preferred treatment of hyperthyroidism in the elderly. It carries the risk of a transient worsening of the hyperthyroidism. Some recommend achieving a euthyroid state using anti-thyroid drugs before the iodine radiotherapy

(Mokshagundam and Brazil, 1993). After completing radioactive iodine treatment, 80% of the patients will be euthyroid, 10% will be hypothyroid, and 10% will remain hyperthyroid. Propylthiouracil and methimazole are the most widely used antithyroid drugs in the United States. Their major side effects include skin rash, fever, agranulocytosis, arthritis, and hepatitis. The major concern of treatment of elderly patients with hyperthyroidism is to eliminate the hyperthyroidism before any complications arise. Patients will be followed closely during therapy (Gregerman and Katz, 1994).

Primary Hyperparathyroidism

Hyperparathyroidism is a metabolic disorder of calcium, phosphorus, and bone metabolism caused by increased circulating levels of parathyroid hormone (PTH) (Lyles, 1994).

Epidemiology

Hyperparathyroidism occurs with increasing frequency in older people (Lyles, 1994). Its average annual incidence was 7.8/100,000 population in the sixties. During the early 1970s the introduction of the technology of multichannel autoanalyzers appeared to increase the incidence to an annual average of 51/100,000 population. The annual incidence rate remained the same for people below 39 years of age at <10/100,000, but increased sharply in people above 40 years of age to reach a rate of 188/100,000 in women over 60 years of age and 92/100,000 in men over 60 years of age (Heath, Hodgson, and Kennedy, 1980).

Causes

Hyperparathyroidism is considered primary when there is autonomous excessive secretion of PTH and consequent hypercalcemia. Single adenomas cause 80% to 85% of cases of primary hyperparathyroidism. Hypertrophy of all four parathyroid glands causes hyperparathyroidism in 15% of patients. A very small number of cases of hyperthyroidism result from parathyroid carcinomas and multiple adenomas (Allerheiligen, 1998). No etiologic agent is identified in the majority of cases. However, previous neck exposure to radiation and lithium intake has been associated with hyperparathyroidism. Multiple endocrine neoplasia syndromes (I and II) and familial hyperparathyroidism cause a few number of cases of hyperparathyroidism.

Clinical Features

The presenting signs and symptoms of patients with hyperparathyroidism vary from lack of symptoms to the rare hypercalcemic crisis. Currently hyperparathyroidism presents as an unexpected elevation in calcium found incidentally on a serum chemistry profile in an asymptomatic person. Most of the specific signs and symptoms involve the skeleton or the kidneys.

Hyperparathyroidism causes an increased bone remodeling that leads to the rare pathologic diagnosis of osteitis fibrosa cystica. It causes osteopenia or osteosclerosis, which has the "salt and pepper" appearance on a skull X-ray. However, there has been no increased incidence of vertebral fractures with primary hyperparathyroidism. (Lyles, 1994) The effects of hyperparathyroidism include nephrolithiasis, proximal renal tubular acidosis, nephrocalcinosis, and nephrogenic diabetes insipidus.

Most of the other signs and symptoms associated with hyperparathyroidism can be attributed to the resultant hypercalcemia. These include headaches, fatigue, nausea, vomiting, constipation, peptic ulcer disease, memory loss, cognitive dysfunction, lethargy, depression, paresthesias, proximal muscular weakness, pseudogout, and pain in the extremities. The varied symptoms of hyperparathyroidism place it in the differential diagnosis of most chief complaints.

Diagnosis

Hypercalcemia in the presence of elevated PTH measured by double immunoradiometric assay confirms the diagnosis of primary hyperparathyroidism (Allerheiligen, 1998). The scattergram plot of PTH vs. calcium provided by the laboratory helps to interpret the result. The differential diagnosis should include all causes of hypercalcemia. Common causes of hypercalcemia are primary hyperparathyroidism, humoral hypercalcemia of malignancy, renal failure, malignancy via direct bone destruction, and thiazide diuretics. Uncommon causes of hypercalcemia are immobilization, lithium use, hyperthyroidism, vitamin D toxicity, granulomatous diseases, and familial hypocalciuric hypercalcemia.

Treatment

Treatment of hyperparathyroidism depends on the presenting signs and symptoms. Since the majority of the cases are asymptomatic at presentation, no immediate treatment is needed.

Nonsurgical Management

Management of hypercalcemic crisis should take precedence over diagnostic workup. This involves intravenous hydration; diuresis with fluids and furosemide; and administration of pamidronate, calcitonin, glucocorticoids, and mithramycin.

At this time there is no effective medical therapy for primary hyperparathyroidism; the current and acceptable treatment is surgery. However, diagnosis of hyperparathyroidism in an asymptomatic patient does not in all cases mandate referral for surgery. Asymptomatic patients with calcium levels below 11 mg/dl and no evidence of disease can be followed safely with serum calcium, serum creatinine, creatinine clearance, urinary calcium, bone density, and kidney-ureter-bladder x-ray (NIH, 1991). Although there is still no agreement on how often these tests should be done, some have recommended doing them on an annual basis (Lyles, 1994; NIH, 1991). There is no evidence that surgery will improve symptoms or neuropsychiatric disturbances in patients with serum calcium below 11 mg/dl (Lyles, 1994). During medical management avoidance of dehydration and immobilization, maintenance of a modest dietary calcium intake, treatment of hypertension, cautious use of diuretics, and estrogen replacement in postmenopausal women are advised.

Surgical Management

Computed tomographic scan, magnetic resonance imaging, ultrasonography, and radionuclide scans have been used to locate adenomas before surgery. Some studies have found that preoperative localization decreased the time and lowered the incidence of complications (Lundgren et al., 1995). However, the NIH stand is that preoperative localization in patients without a previous neck operation is rarely indicated and has not proven to be cost-effective (NIH, 1991). A recent NIH consensus conference has identified 10 indications for surgical treatment of hyperparathyroidism: (1) typical parathyroid-related symptoms; (2) markedly elevated serum calcium level (1 to 1.6 mg/dl above accepted normal range); (3) history of an episode of life-threatening hypercalcemia; (4) reduced creatinine clearance (30% less than expected), markedly elevated urinary calcium excretion (greater than 400 mg/day); (5) substantially reduced bone mass; (6) significant neuromuscular or psychologic symptoms; (7) patient requests surgery; (8) consistent follow-up is unlikely; (9) coexistent illness complicates management; (10) patient is young (<50 years of age).

Parathyroid surgery has the following complications: (1) damage to the recurrent laryngeal nerve; (2) transient hypocalcemia in the immediate postoperative period; (3) recurrence of symptoms. Recurrence of hyperparathyroidism is less likely after a solitary adenoma than after multiglandular disease (Allerheiligen, 1998).

Summary

Endocrine disorders such as thyroid disease and diabetes are common in the older population. However, they may present in a somewhat vague fashion, making them more difficult to diagnose. It is important to be adept in obtaining history that will lead the practitioner to the appropriate diagnostic evaluation. Several medications have recently been added to the available options for managing diabetes. Although many of these are promising, most have special considerations for use in the older population. Hypothyroidism is often well managed in the primary care setting, whereas hyperthyroidism requires evaluation and treatment by a specialist. Referral to an endocrinologist or other specialist may be necessary to ensure the best outcome for the patient's health. Management, monitoring, and education of endocrine disorders require ongoing care; these disorders are often ideally managed by a multidisciplinary team.

Resources

Sensory Testing Systems
1815 Dallas Dr., Suite 11A
Baton Rouge, LA 70806-1454
1-888-289-9293

Curative Health Services
150 Motor Pkwy.
Hauppague, NY 11788
1-800-966-5656, ext. 7078

American Diabetes Association
National Office
1660 Duke Street
Alexandria, VA 22314
http://www.diabetes.org
1-800-DIABETES

Diabetes Related Sites on the Internet
http://www.diabetes.org/internetresources.asp

References

Adlin EV et al: Bone mineral density in post-menopausal women treated with L-thyroxine, *Am J Med* 90:360-366, 1991.

Allerheiligen DA et al: Hyperparathyroidism. *Am Fam Physician* 57(8):1795-1802, 1998.

American Diabetes Association: Clinical practice recommendations. *Diabetes Care* 21:S5-S31, 1998.

Bagchi N, Brown TR, Parish RF. Thyroid dysfunction in adults over age 55 years: a study in urban US community, *Arch Intern Med* 150:785-787, 1990.

Barzel US: Hypothyroidism: diagnosis and management, *Clin Geriatr Med* 2:239-249, 1995.

Berglund J, Christensen SB, Hallengren B: Total and age specific incidence of Grave's thyrotoxicosis, toxic nodular goiter, and solitary toxic adenoma in Malmo, 1970-1974, *J Intern Med* 227:137-141, 1990.

Bierman EL: George Layman Duff Memorial Lecture: Atherogenesis in diabetes, *Arterioscler Thromb* 6:647-656, 1992.

Braithwaite SS et al: Managing diabetes during glucocorticoid therapy, *Postgrad Med* 104(5):163-176, 1998.

Drinka PJ et al: Misleading elevations of free thyroxine index in nursing home residents, *Arch Pathol Lab Med* 115:1208-1211, 1991.

Fitzgerald P: Endocrinology. In Tierney LM et al: *Current medical diagnosis and treatment 1997*, ed 36, Stamford, 1997, Appleton & Lange.

Foster D: Diabetes mellitus. In Isselbacher KJ et al, editors: *Harrison's principles of internal medicine*, ed 13, New York, 1994, McGraw-Hill.

Gregerman R, Katz M: Thyroid disease. In Hazzard WR et al, editors: *Principles of geriatric medicine and gerontology*, ed 3, New York, 1994, McGraw-Hill.

Goldberg AP, Coon PJ: Diabetes mellitus and glucose metabolism in the elderly. In Hazzard WR et al, editors: *Principles of geriatric medicine and gerontology*, ed 3, New York, 1994, McGraw-Hill.

Goldberg TH, Chain SI: Preventive medicine and screening in older adults, *J Am Geriatr Soc* 45:344-354, 1997.

Haggerty JJ et al: Subclinical hypothyroidism: a review of neuropsychiatrics aspects, *J Psychiatry Med* 20:193-208, 1990.

Hanishin PS et al: Relationship between thyrotropin and thyroxin changes during recovery from severe hypothyroxinemia of systemic illness, *J Clin Endocrinol Metab* 62:717-722, 1986.

Hay ID et al: American Thyroid Association of current free thyroid hormone and thyrotropin measurements and guidelines for future clinical assays, *Clin Chem* 37(11):2002-2008, 1991.

Heath H III, Hodgson SF, Kennedy MA: Primary hyperparathyroidism incidence, morbidity, and potential economic impact in a community, *N Engl J Med* 302:189-193, 1980.

Helfand M, Crapo LM: Screening for thyroid disease. In Eddy DM, editor: *Common screening tests,* Philadelphia, 1991, American College of Physicians.

Kappel C, Dills DG: Type 2 diabetes: update on therapy, *Compr Ther* 24(6/7):319-326, 1998.

Lebovitz HE: Rationale in the management of noninsulin-dependent diabetes. In Leslie RD, Robbins DC, editors: *Diabetes: clinical science in practice,* New York, 1995, Cambridge University Press.

Lloyd WH, Goldberg IJL: Incidence of hypothyroidism in the elderly, *Br Med J* 2:1556-1559, 1961.

Lundgren E et al: The role of preoperative localization in primary hyperparathyroidism, *Am Surg* 61:393-396, 1995.

Lyles KW: Hyperparathyroidism. In Hazzard WR et al, editors: *Principles of geriatric medicine and gerontology,* ed 3, New York, 1994, McGraw-Hill.

Mandel SJ, Brent GA, Reed LP: Levothyroxine therapy in patients with thyroid disease, *Ann Intern Med* 119:492-502, 1993.

Mokshagundam S, Brazil US: Thyroid disease in the elderly, *J Am Geriatr Soc* 41:1361-1369, 1993.

Morrow L, Halter J: Diabetes mellitus. In Yoshikawa TT, Cobbs EL, Brummel-Smith K, editors: *Ambulatory geriatric care,* St Louis, 1993, Mosby.

NIH Conference: Diagnosis and management of asymptomatic primary hyperparathyroidism: consensus development conference statement, *Ann Intern Med* 114:593-597, 1991.

Nordyke RA, Gilbert FL, Harada ASM: Grave's disease: influence of age on clinical findings, *Arch Intern Med* 148:626-631, 1988.

Nuttall FQ, Chasuk RM: Nutrition and the management of type 2 diabetes, *J Fam Pract* 47(5)(suppl):S45-S53, 1998.

O'Connor PJ, Spann SJ, Woolf SH. Care of adults with type 2 diabetes mellitus: a review of the evidence, *J Fam Pract* 47(5)(suppl):S13-S22, 1998.

Peterson KA, Vinicor F. Strategies to improve diabetes care delivery, *J Fam Pract* 47(5)(suppl):S63-S64, 1998.

Reaven GM: Beneficial effect of moderate weight loss in older patients with noninsulin-dependent diabetes mellitus poorly controlled with insulin, *J Am Geriatr Soc* 33(2):93-95, 1985.

Rizzolo P: Thyroid disease. In Ham R, Sloane P, editors: *Primary care geriatrics,* ed 3, St Louis, 1997, Mosby.

Reuben DB: Thyroid disorders. In Yoshikawa TT, Cobbs EL, Brummel-Smith K, editors: *Ambulatory geriatric care,* St Louis, 1993, Mosby.

Ruoff G: The management of noninsulin dependent diabetes mellitus in the elderly, *J Fam Pract* 36(3):329-335, 1993.

Sawin CT et al: The aging thyroid: thyroid deficiency in the Framingham study, *Arch Intern Med* 145:1386-1388, 1985.

Sawin CT et al: Subclinical hypothyroidism in older persons. *Clin Geriatr Med* 11(2):231-238, 1995.

Smith CL, Ganja CV: Hypothyroidism producing reversible dementia: a challenge to medical rehabilitation, *Am J Phys Med Rehabil* 71:28-30, 1992.

Surks MI, Ocampo E: Subclinical thyroid disease, *Am J Med* 100:217-223, 1996.

Tibladi JM et al: Thyrotoxicosis in the very old, *Am J Med* 81:619-622, 1986.

Wallace K, Hoffman MT: Thyroid dysfunction: how to manage overt and subclinical disease in older patients, *Geriatrics* 53:32-41, 1998.

World Health Organization: Diabetes mellitus: report of a WHO study group (Technical Report Ser., no. 727), Geneva, 1985, World Health Organization.

11

Osteoporosis

Osteoporosis is the fourth most common and the eighth most expensive disease to treat in the United States. Annually, 1.3 million fractures related to osteoporosis occur, the most frequent being 300,000 hip and 700,000 vertebrae fractures (Siris, 1997). The cost of this untreated disease is approximately $14 billion annually, but rarely do primary care providers talk about this disease to their patients. Although many women report thinking about osteoporosis often, few ask questions about it.

Osteoporosis is a disease that increases in frequency with advancing age, especially in the female population. In women 13% to 18% (4 to 6 million) have osteoporosis, and 37% to 50% (13 to 17 million) have osteopenia. In men 3% to 6% (1 to 2 million) have osteoporosis, and 28% to 47% have osteopenia (Looker et al., 1997). Thirty-seven percent of visits for osteoporosis occur between the ages of 71 and 80, 28% between the ages of 61 and 70, 20% after age 80, and only 10% between the ages of 51 and 60. Fifty-nine percent of the visits for osteoporosis are to primary care physicians, but it is generally other specialists who prescribe therapy for osteoporosis.

Why has osteoporosis been traditionally underdiagnosed and undertreated? This fact can be explained by one of or a combination of factors:

- Osteoporosis has traditionally been thought to be a consequence of "normal" aging.
- Although it is a common disease, osteoporosis symptoms are seldom a complaint until complications such as hip and vertebral fractures develop and therefore are perceived by health care professionals as unimportant to treat.
- Until recently there has been a lack of practical and short-term treatment for asymptomatic disease.
- Health care providers experience too little satisfaction in treating osteoporosis because often they are not convinced they are helping the patient by preventing morbidity and mortality.
- Osteoporosis is asymptomatic until late in the disease.

- Health care professionals and the public lack education about osteoporosis.
- There is confusion among health care professionals related to the lack of clear guidelines for primary care providers regarding when and whom to treat.
- There is confusion as to the appropriate laboratory and radiologic tools to make the diagnosis.
- Osteoporosis is seemingly unimportant, as reflected in the lack of malpractice claims; therefore concern about early treatment and prevention diminishes.

Age-related Changes

The process of osteoporosis involves increased bone resorption over bone formation. Physiologically, bone is continuously turning over, with the bony skeleton acting as a reservoir for calcium. The increase in bone resorption that causes osteoporosis is primarily mediated by the osteoclast and normally initiates bone remodeling. Increased bone formation, which is mediated primarily by the osteoblast, follows 40 to 60 days afterward. The process of osteoporosis may be primary or secondary. Primary osteoporosis is usually senile or postmenopausal and is mediated by estrogen. Estrogen receptors have been found in osteoclastic-like cells. Estrogen decreases bone resorption by decreasing responsiveness of the osteoclast (Chestnut, 1994). Secondary osteoporosis may be mediated by one of several factors: vitamin D metabolites (osteomalacia), calcitonin (Paget's disease), parathyroid hormone (hyperparathyroidism or malignant tumors), thyroxine (hyperthyroidism), cortisol (Cushing's disease or exogenous cortisol excess), and other biomarkers.

Screening

Screening for primary osteoporosis in women should be initiated at least once after the natural or surgical menopause. The most practical and cost-effective method of screening the general population includes a thorough history and physical examination, with a particular focus on those women with a family history of osteoporosis, who are therefore at a greater risk of developing the disease. Caucasian women, women who are thin and tall, and those with low weight also have a high risk of developing the disease. Other women at risk include those who have experienced an early menopause, the advanced elderly, those who are sedentary, those who smoke, those who regularly drink alcohol, those with a history of diabetes, and those with a history of inadequate calcium intake, as represented by dairy products (cheese, milk). In elderly men risk factors include a history of diabetes and testosterone deficiency. Alternatively, African-Americans, those of short stature, the obese, regular exercisers, those who take calcium and vitamins regularly, and those who use estrogen regularly are protected.

Serum calcium and phosphorus levels are usually normal with primary osteoporosis, and 30% of bone loss must occur before routine radiologic evidence appears. Signs and symptoms of advanced osteoporosis include loss of height, chronic pain secondary to muscle spasm, kyphosis with abdominal protuberance and constipation (as a result of spine curvature), pulmonary insufficiency secondary to thoracic cage deformity, painful rubbing of the ribs on the iliac crest with severe disease, and pain secondary to vertebral or hip fracture. Nursing home residents are at high risk because of the lack of sunlight that converts the inactive form of vitamin D to the active form involved in calcium absorption from the gut.

Secondary osteoporosis should be a consideration in the patient, male or female, who presents with a pathologic fracture (one not associated with significant trauma or incidental findings of advanced osteoporosis noted when the patient is evaluated by radiology for other medical reasons). Other indications include chronic smokers, patients with diabetes, patients who use steroids chronically, patients with hyperparathyroidism or hyperthyroidism, those on oral thyroxine, patients with Paget's disease, multiple myeloma, hypercalcemic states, patients with malabsorption syndromes, and immobilized patients.

Focused Physical Examination

Evaluation should include a determination of osteoporosis risk according to history and physical examination findings. Serum calcium, vitamin D, phosphorus, and alkaline phosphate levels and routine radiology are usually normal with primary osteoporosis. Radiography usually shows evidence of reduced bone density after 30% of bone mass is lost.

Laboratory evaluation should be performed in male or female patients with radiologic evidence of osteoporosis as noted on routine radiology or in patients with the indications listed previously. It should include a serum calcium, cortisol level, parathyroid hormone level, thyroxine, hemogram, determination of Bence Jones protein in the urine, vitamin D levels, renal function studies (blood urea nitrogen and creatinine level), testosterone level, and serum alkaline phosphatase level (Chestnut, 1994).

In addition, confirmatory evidence for osteoporosis can be provided by comparing the actual amount of bone content with that expected at various bone sites throughout the body through bone densitometry. The bony skeleton is composed of two types of bone. Trabecular bone, found mostly in the spine and hip, is metabolically more active than cortical bone and is altered more in osteoporosis than cortical bone. Densitometry types vary by principal site measured and thus percent cortical to trabecular bone content determined, radiation exposure, and cost (Chestnut, 1994). Indications for its use include the following:

- Selected perimenopausal or postmenopausal patients with previous fracture if combined with history of risk factors
- When assessing the need for prophylactic (preventive) treatment
- When assessing response to treatment at regular intervals (e.g., every 2 years)
- When assessing for osteoporosis associated with various secondary states

Types of bone densitometry include the following:

- Single-energy photon absorptiometry (SPA) measurement of the radius and ulna, os calcis, or spine involving the first to fourth lumbar vertebrae

- Dual-energy photon absorptiometry (DPA-DEXA) measurement of the neck or trochanter of the femur, SPA measurement of the spine at the level of the twelfth thoracic to fourth lumbar vertebrae
- Computed tomography (CT) dual-energy evaluation of the spine at the level of the twelfth thoracic to the fourth lumbar vertebrae
- Ultrasound of the patella or os calcis

The SPA measurement is more specific for osteoporosis because it involves approximately 85% to 95% cortical vs. 20% to 25% trabecular bone determination. At the other end of the spectrum, ultrasound provides the least specific method, measuring 5% cortical vs. 95% trabecular bone determination. The percent radiation emitted for the SPA and DPA-DEXA methods is low as opposed to the CT or ultrasound methods, which emit very high levels of radiation. Usually, CT scanning is the most expensive method, ranging in cost from $350 to $500, and ultrasound is the cheapest at $25 to $50; SPA is about $75 to $200, and DPA-DEXA is $50 to $175, depending on the site.

Treatment

Initial treatment of osteoporosis should be modification of risk factors such as cessation of smoking and moderation of alcohol consumption, regular (weight resistance) exercise, and adequate dietary calcium and vitamin D intake (1500 mg daily for the postmenopausal and 1000 mg daily for the premenopausal female) and 400 IU of vitamin D. Secondary causes of osteoporosis should be treated by treating the underlying disease process (Chestnut, 1994) (Table 11-1).

Studies indicate the process of primary osteoporosis can be slowed and to some extent prevented through regular exercise, regular calcium and vitamin D intake, and weight bearing. Immobilization and lack of exercise can hasten its onset. Prevention of osteoporosis is obviously less expensive and associated with better quality of life than treatment of hip and vertebral fractures, with their associated morbidity and mortality (Reid, 1996).

Treatment of hip and vertebral fractures usually involves acute hospitalization and subsequent transfer to a rehabilitation hospital or free-standing or hospital-based skilled nursing unit, followed by a period of skilled home health therapy. However, primary and secondary interventions (medications) to prevent osteoporosis have not been the focus of routine office visits by health care providers until recently. In the past there has been controversy among experts as to whether primary osteoporosis is a "normal" consequence of aging or a "disease." Furthermore, the lack of studies related to the benefit of estrogen and the lack of alternative therapies other than estrogen, as well as some side effects and the cost of other pharmacologic agents shown to be of benefit, all add to the debate surrounding the treatment of osteoporosis.

Estrogen

Traditional estrogens are useful for 3 to 5 years after either natural or surgical menopause, with the maximum effect during a hypothetic window of opportunity of 15 to 20 years or more, even though specifics are unknown and studies are ongoing. Estrogen has been shown to significantly increase bone density at all bone sites and to

TABLE 11-1 Treatment Options for Osteoporosis

Modality	Benefits	Adverse Sequelae	Side Effects	Special Considerations
Risk factor modification	Retards bone loss			Smoking cessation, reduction in alcohol intake
Exercise	Increased bone density, reduced risk for falls and fractures			Frequency of 30-45 minutes per week recommended: walking, jogging, bicycling, weight resistance exercises
Calcium and vitamin D	Increased bone density		Constipation, excess vitamin D intake associated with toxicity	1000 mg per day recommended for premenopausal and 1,500 mg per day for postmenopausal women; 400-800 international units (IU) of vitamin D recommended
Estrogens	Increased bone density at all bone sites, reduced risk of vertebral and hip fracture; reduced cholesterol, increased HDL and reduced LDL cholesterol; possible link to reduced risk for dementia; increased quality of life; reduced risk of ASHD	Unopposed use associated with vaginal bleeding and uterine cancer; does not reduce risk of cardiac events in women with heart disease	Breast swelling and tenderness, edema, hypertension, abnormal glucose tolerance, headache, nausea, fluid retention, gall stones, increased triglyceride level, stimulation of uterine myoma, darkening of skin	Used sequentially or in combination with progesterone nullifies risk of uterine cancer but reduces slightly the benefits of estrogen's effect on lipid profile; relative contraindications: congestive heart failure, hypertension, migraine headache, previous myocardial infarction, angina, stroke, chronic renal failure; absolute contraindications: family history of (first-degree relatives) or history of breast cancer, history of pelvic cancer, suspected pregnancy, active thrombophlebitis or thromboembolic disorders; combination with calcium and vitamin D

ASHD, Arteriosclerotic heart disease; *HDL*, high-density lipoprotein; *LDL*, low-density lipoprotein.

Continued

TABLE 11-1 Treatment Options for Osteoporosis—cont'd

Modality	Benefits	Adverse Sequelae	Side Effects	Special Considerations
Calcitonin	Increase in bone density at hip and lumbar spine at 1 year	Allergy	Nasal irritation, epistaxis, sinusitis	Expensive; given by subcutaneous injection 3 times per week or nasal spray (daily to every other nostril); indicated for women intolerant to or in whom estrogen is contraindicated 5 years after the menopause; given with calcium and vitamin D
Sodium fluoride		Gastric upset, arthritis, fasciitis		Bone formed is more brittle and subject to fracture; experimental use only
Anabolic steroids		Reduced HDL; increased risk of ASHD in men	Masculinization; weight gain, fluid retention, HBP	Not recommended
Testosterone	Increased bone density and muscle mass; increased potency	Stimulates growth of prostate cancer and hypertrophy; suppresses clotting factors and increases prothrombin time	CHF, fluid retention, hair loss, weight gain, hepatitis and cholestatic jaundice	Indicated in the presence of impotency, testicular atrophy and reduced testosterone levels only
Etidronate	Increase in bone density; prevents recurrent vertebral fractures	GI irritation and bleeding, osteomalacia with continuous use	Heartburn	Must be used cyclically for 2 weeks with 13 weeks of calcium and vitamin D

Alendronate	Increase in bone density	GI bleeding in patients with history, increased incidence of GI bleeding in patients using NSAIDs	Abdominal pain, nausea, dyspepsia, constipation, diarrhea, reflux	Should not be given simultaneously with calcium (chelates); expensive; must be given with 8 oz water on empty stomach sitting up before food or other drink
Raloxifene	Increase in bone density of hip, lumbar spine, and total body; reduces cholesterol and LDL, no effect on HDL; no increase in triglyceride level; decrease in fibrinogen level	Hot flashes	Similar to estrogens	Bone density effect in 24 months; no vaginal bleeding or endometrial thickening noted in studies at 39 months follow-up; effect on cardiovascular profile unknown at this point, expensive

GI, Gastrointestinal; *NSAIDs,* nonsteroidal antiinflammatory drugs.

reduce spine and hip fracture risk in the long term (Chestnut, 1994). A minimum dose of 0.625 mg of conjugated estrogen is recommended. Estrogen has also been shown to retard the development of osteoarthritis of the hip in postmenopausal Caucasian women (Nevitt et al., 1996). Other nonskeletal benefits provided by regular estrogen use include a short-term (1 to 2 years) significant reduction in cardiovascular morbidity and mortality (heart attack and stroke), mediated by its effect on a reduction in total cholesterol and an increase in high-density (HDL) cholesterol (Stampfer et al., 1991; Goldman and Tosteson, 1991; Psaty et al., 1994; Finucane et al., 1993). Other beneficial effects include reduction in the frequency of urinary tract infection in women with atrophic vaginitis (Raz and Stamm, 1993) and increased quality of life through relief of symptoms of estrogen deficiency (Daly et al., 1993).

The use of estrogen does carry risks and may be relatively or absolutely contraindicated in some women. Bothersome side effects include breast tenderness and swelling, abnormal glucose tolerance, headache, nausea, fluid retention, edema, development of gallstones, elevated triglycerides, enlargement of benign tumors of the uterus, and darkening of the skin. Relative risks include use in patients with congestive heart failure, hypertension, migraine headache, previous myocardial infarction, angina, stroke, or chronic renal failure because of the fluid retention associated with its use. Absolute contraindications include suspected pregnancy, active thrombophlebitis or thromboembolic disorders, suspected breast carcinoma, undiagnosed vaginal bleeding, previous pelvic carcinoma, or a patient's first-degree relatives with breast carcinoma (*Physicians Desk Reference*, 1998). Unopposed estrogen use continuously in women with an intact uterus has been shown to significantly increase the risk of uterine adenocarcinoma with subsequent death (Voight et al., 1991). Studies have shown that the addition of progesterone on a cyclic or continuous basis to the estrogen regimen in older women with an intact uterus effectively nullifies the risk of uterine adenocarcinoma but also partially nullifies the positive effects of estrogen on the lipid profile (Chestnut, 1994). When estrogen is used either by itself or with progesterone, the fear of uterine adenocarcinoma prompted by vaginal bleeding makes estrogen use impractical in older women for the treatment of osteoporosis, especially considering its lack of short-term benefit in preventing osteoporosis. As a result, a significant percentage of women fail to get a prescription filled or quit taking estrogen.

Other Treatments

For the patient who has traditionally been intolerant to estrogen or in whom it is contraindicated, physicians advise treating osteoporosis with regular exercise, adequate calcium intake, and cessation of smoking and alcohol intake or with other alternatives mentioned previously. One study recently indicated that combined estrogen and progesterone use for up to 4.1 years does not decrease the risk of cardiovascular events in patients with cardiovascular disease, but it significantly increases the risk of gallbladder disease and thromboembolic disease (Hulley et al., 1998).

Other agents that have been used to treat osteoporosis include calcitonin, sodium fluoride, and anabolic steroids. Calcitonin is expensive and until recently had to be administered by subcutaneous injection. Bothersome side effects include local skin irritation, flushing, and occasional anaphylaxis. A new formulation uses the nasal mucosa for administration and once-daily dosing (alternating nostrils) with the side effects of nasal irritation and rare sinusitis, epistaxis, or rhinitis. Studies show it causes a significant increase in bone mineral density at 2 years when measured at the lumbar spine and at 1 year when measured at the hip, with a trend toward nonsignificance at 2 years. It is recommended for women 5 years after menopause and only in patients who are intolerant to estrogen or in whom estrogen is contraindicated. Calcitonin should be used in conjunction with calcium and vitamin D (*Physicians Desk Reference,* 1998).

Sodium fluoride is still considered experimental, with a significant side effect profile, including gastric upset, tendinitis, arthritis, and plantar fasciitis. The bone that is produced is brittler, and subsequently there is a greater risk of fracture. Chronic anabolic steroid administration can cause a significant reduction in high-density lipoprotein levels and increase the risk of premature atherosclerosis, liver toxicity, and masculinization (Chestnut, 1994).

Testosterone injection is beneficial in increasing bone mineral density in men with senile osteoporosis. It also significantly increases muscle mass, with side effects of weight gain, increased appetite, hypercalcemia, increased hematocrit leading to polycythemia, gynecomastia, fluid retention, congestive heart failure, and cholestatic hepatitis and jaundice. It is indicated in the presence of reduced testosterone levels associated with impotence and testicular atrophy. It may stimulate the prostate gland, increasing the risk for prostate hyperplasia and carcinoma. The drug also suppresses clotting factors and increases prothrombin time. It is contraindicated in patients with known or suspected prostate or breast cancer, hypercalcemia, nephrosis, or pregnancy (*Physicians Desk Reference,* 1998).

Recent events that have revolutionized the awareness and treatment of osteoporosis include published guidelines for the evaluation and management of osteoporosis, Medicare reimbursement of densitometry, and the advent of the biphosphonates and estrogen designer drugs. Of academic interest is the study showing that thiazides can reduce the risk of hip fracture in older women with hypertension treated with thiazide diuretics (Jones et al., 1995). The mechanism of action is postulated to be secondary to the effect of thiazide at the kidney in preventing calcium loss in the urine and thereby retarding osteoporosis.

Etidronate has been used for many years for the treatment of Paget's disease. Cyclic etidronate (400 mg per day for 2 weeks, followed by 11 weeks of calcium supplementation alone) was shown to prevent recurrent vertebral compression fractures in older women with osteoporosis. However, subsequent continuous use was associated with the development of osteomalacia (Reuben, Yoshikawa, and Besdine, 1996). Subsequently, alendronate was the first biphosphonate approved for prevention and treatment of primary osteoporosis several years ago. For primary osteoporosis, results can be seen as early as 3 months, with a significant increase in bone mineral density at the femoral neck, trochanter, and lumbar spine at 3 years' follow-up. It also has been shown to be effective in reducing the incidence of new vertebral fractures at 3 years' follow-up. The mechanism of action of the biphosphonates is inhibition of osteoclast function, but there is no inhibition of fracture healing, such as hip fractures. There is no evidence for the development of osteomalacia with continuous use after 3 years, but long-term evidence is lacking. The combined use of biphosphonates and nonsteroidal antiinflammatory drugs can increase the incidence of gastrointestinal bleeding and side effects (*Physicians Desk Reference,* 1998).

A dose of 10 mg daily of alendronate is initially recommended for treatment of postmenopausal osteoporosis, and 40 mg daily for 6 months is indicated for treatment of Paget's disease. Factors limiting its use are cost, the common side effect profile of gastrointestinal irritation in 6% of patients (abdominal pain, nausea, dyspepsia, constipation, diarrhea, reflux), and rarely peptic ulceration and bleeding. Another limitation for its use is compliance with medication administration. The drug should be taken 30 minutes before food with 8 oz of water in the morning while the patient is standing upright for 30 minutes to prevent reflux. Alendronate should not be administered simultaneously with calcium because chelation in the gastrointestinal tract may occur and cause lack of absorption. No dosage reduction is necessary with mild to moderate renal disease, but it is contraindicated with hypocalcemia (*Physicians Desk Reference*, 1998).

Another biphosphonate, risedronate, was released by the Food and Drug Administration (FDA) in the late 1990s for prevention and treatment of osteoporosis. It has the potential advantage of a better gastrointestinal side effect profile than alendronate. Biphosphonates should be given with supplemental calcium and vitamin D. Biphosphonates may be used in combination with estrogens for the treatment of osteoporosis and especially to reduce cardiovascular risk, but whether the two have an additive effect on the reduction in the incidence of osteoporosis is unknown at this point. However, there is little rationale to use these drugs in combination because biphosphonates, estrogens, and calcitonin all are antiresorptive drugs (Reuben, Yoshikawa, and Besdine, 1996).

The FDA approval in 1998 of raloxifene, the first in a series of estrogen designer drugs, offers clinical advantages over estrogen. Raloxifene significantly increased bone mineral density of the hip, spine, and total body at 24 months' follow-up in 601 postmenopausal women but to a lesser extent than estrogen when used in doses of 30, 60, and 150 mg per day when compared with placebo. There was no difference in the frequency of hot flashes, vaginal bleeding, or thickness of the endometrium in women taking raloxifene compared with placebo. The drug also had a positive effect on the lipid profile similar to that of estrogen (except with no increase in the HDL fractions) (Delmas et al., 1997). In a study involving 390 healthy postmenopausal women involved in a double-blind, randomized, parallel trial, raloxifene did not increase the triglyceride level and significantly decreased fibrinogen levels by 12% to 14% at 3 and 6 months' follow-up. Its overall effect on the cardiovascular profile is unknown at this point, and studies are ongoing (Walsh et al., 1998). There is no difference in the incidence of the side effects of hot flashes or vaginal bleeding compared with placebo at 24 months' follow-up. Raloxifene has a profile like estrogen regarding relative contraindications, including deep venous thrombosis or history of the disease, and previous pulmonary embolus.

Summary

Just as the cardiovascular era raised interest in cholesterol, the next several years and beyond will be a period of transition during which the public will be bombarded from the news media and public awareness campaigns about the benefits of prevention and the deleterious effects of untreated osteoporosis. Health care professionals will be bombarded by medical journals and the pharmaceutic industry regarding new therapies for osteoporosis promoting pharmacologic agents with better side effect profiles, more efficacy, lower cost, and better compliance. During and after this period, health care providers who fail to address osteoporosis may find themselves in precarious medicolegal situations as a result of the adverse consequences of the untreated disease.

Resources

National Institutes of Health
Osteoporosis and Related Bone Diseases
National Resource Center
http://www.osteo.org

Doctor's Guide to Osteoporosis: Information and Resources
http://www.pslgroup.com/osteoporosis.htm

References

Chestnut CH: Osteoporosis. In Hazzard WR et al: *Principles of geriatric medicine and gerontology*, ed 3, New York, 1994, McGraw-Hill.

Daly E et al: Measuring the impact of menopausal symptoms on quality of life, *Br Med J* 307:836-840, 1993.

Delmas PD et al: Effects of raloxifene on bone mineral density, serum cholesterol concentrations, and uterine endometrium in postmenopausal women, *N Engl J Med* 337:1641-1647, 1997.

Finucane FF et al: Decreased risk of stroke among postmenopausal hormone users: results from a national cohort, *Arch Intern Med* 153:73-79, 1993.

Goldman L, Tosteson ANA: Uncertainty about postmenopausal estrogen—time for action, not debate, *N Engl J Med* 325:800-802, 1991.

Hulley S et al: Randomized trial of estrogen plus progestin for secondary prevention of coronary heart disease in postmenopausal women, *JAMA* 280(7):605-613, 1998.

Jones G et al: Thiazide diuretics and fractures: can metaanalysis help? *J Bone Miner Res* 101(1):106-111, 1995.

Looker AC et al: Prevalence of low femoral bone density in older U.S. adults, *J Bone Miner Res* 12(11):1761-1768, 1997.

Nevitt MC et al: Association of estrogen replacement therapy with the risk of osteoarthritis of the hip in elderly white women, *Arch Intern Med* 156:2073-2080, 1996.

Physicians Desk Reference, ed 52, Montvale, NJ, 1998, Medical Economics.

Psaty BM et al: The risk of myocardial infarction associated with the combined use of estrogens and progestins in postmenopausal women, *Arch Intern Med* 154:1333-1339, 1994.

Raz E, Stamm WE: A controlled trial of intravaginal estriol in postmenopausal women with recurrent urinary tract infections, *N Engl J Med* 329:753-756, 1993.

Reid IR: Therapy of osteoporosis: calcium, vitamin D, and exercise, *Am J Med Sci* 312(6):268-286, 1996.

Reuben DB, Yoshikawa TT, Besdine RW: *Geriatric review syllabus: a core curriculum in geriatric medicine*, ed 3, New York, 1996, American Geriatrics Society.

Siris E: Arthritis and osteoporosis. Women's Health Seminar, March 6, 1997. http://www.nih.gov/niams/healthinfo/orwhseminar.htm

Stampfer MJ et al: Postmenopausal estrogen therapy and cardiovascular disease: ten year follow-up from the nurses' health study, *N Engl J Med* 325:1189-1195, 1991.

Voight LF et al: Progesterone supplementation of exogenous estrogens and risk of endometrial cancer, *Lancet* 338:274-277, 1991.

Walsh BW et al: Effects of raloxifene on serum lipids and coagulation factors in healthy postmenopausal women, *JAMA* 279(18):1445-1451, 1998.

12

Musculoskeletal: Common Injuries

Age-related Changes

Musculoskeletal problems are among elderly patients' most common complaints, affect quality rather than quantity of life, and often lead to disabilities that are costly to manage. From a skeletal standpoint, the major problem in the elderly is loss of bone mass (osteopenia); this leads to the clinical syndrome of osteoporosis, which affects 40% to 50% of women over the age of 50 with fractures of the vertebral bodies, hip, wrist, and shoulder (Wilson and Lin, 1997). Cartilage loss, which produces osteoarthritis, is extremely common in the weight-bearing joints of the elderly.

Muscular changes include a significant decrease in the strength and speed of contraction of the muscles in the extremities, although overall muscle endurance is minimally affected. Bone mass decreases significantly after the age of 30, with declines of 0.5% to 1% per year. There is a 2% loss per year in postmenopausal women. By age 80 gender differences in bone mass have almost disappeared (Wilson and Lin, 1997).

Organ systems lose approximately 1% of their function per year, beginning about the age of 30 (Wilson and Lin, 1997). Age-related changes in laboratory values may occur. For example, older patients may have normal serum creatinine despite a significant reduction in renal function because lean body mass and endogenous creatinine production decline with age. Interpretation of physical findings requires an awareness of age-related physical changes. It is of particular importance that elderly patients about to undergo orthopedic operative procedures be thoroughly assessed if significant problems exist in other organ systems. Although no studies have shown convincingly that age alone increases surgical morbidity and mortality, these outcomes are affected by systemic illnesses such as cardiac or renal failure, obstructive pulmonary disease, and anemia. Medications must be scrutinized to determine what modifications, if any, are necessary before and after surgery. Prophylaxis for infection and thromboembolic disease should be strongly considered, especially if there is a history of these disorders. Only with a full understanding of the patient's general health can the appropriateness and risk-benefit ratio of the proposed surgery be assessed accurately. Particular caution should be exercised when operating on patients who have sustained a myocardial infarction within the past 6 months or who have pulmonary edema, unstable angina, or aortic stenosis. In addition, renal function must be known for patients in whom the use of nephrotoxic or renally excreted drugs is anticipated (Wilson and Lin, 1997).

There is a common misconception that regional anesthesia is preferred for the elderly because of the increased risks from general anesthesia in this group. However, data do not support this contention, especially because many elderly patients require added intravenous sedation or analgesia. Because significant cardiovascular changes may take place during regional anesthesia, invasive monitoring may be required as well (Wilson and Lin, 1997).

Degenerative arthritis is a disorder of movable joints resulting from cartilage degeneration. It is associated with mild, inflammatory degeneration in the synovium and with faulty bone and cartilage regeneration. Between one third and half of the adult population have radiographic evidence of osteoarthritis, with a striking rise in prevalence that parallels advancing age. Men and women are affected with equal frequency, but the findings are more advanced and generalized in women.

Musculoskeletal disease is not an inevitable consequence of aging and thus should be regarded as a specific disease process and not just the result of normal aging.

Neck Pain

Neck pain is a common problem. Nearly 50% of individuals age 50 and over experience neck pain at some time. Because there are multiple sources of referred pain, as well as many structures in the neck that may cause pain when diseased, patients who complain of new or persistent neck pain should be systematically evaluated.

The cervical spine consists of seven vertebral bodies connected by an anterior and posterior longitudinal ligament. These ligaments provide stability when the neck is flexed and extended. The vertebral bodies are joined by intervertebral disks composed of a gel-like material (the nucleus pulposus) that absorbs increased pressure applied to the spine. The nucleus pulposus is contained within an annulus fibrosus, a fibrous structure ringing the outer margin of the disk. During the fourth decade of life, both the nucleus pulposus and the annulus fibrosus undergo progressive degeneration, which is seen microscopically as a loss of the fibrous pattern and the collagen alignment. As a result, the ability of the disk to absorb shocks is reduced.

There are facet joints between vertebral elements posteriorly, one on each side of the spine; they are apophyseal (projecting) joints with a synovium-lined capsule. Osteoarthritis (a breakdown of the articular cartilage within the joints) can occur within these small joints in the posterior spine. The intervertebral neural foramina, located laterally on either side of the vertebral bodies, are the canals through which the individual nerve roots emerge from the spinal canal. Eight pairs of nerve roots arise from the cervical spinal cord. Each nerve exits above the vertebra of the same number. Thus the sixth nerve root exits at the C5-6 disk space. Except for the first two pairs, each nerve leaves the spinal column by passing through an intervertebral foramen (Figures 12-1 and 12-2). The spinal canal and the foramina can be encroached on by a bulging intervertebral disk or an osseous proliferation (bony spur) originating in a vertebral body, by a facet joint, or from the bony

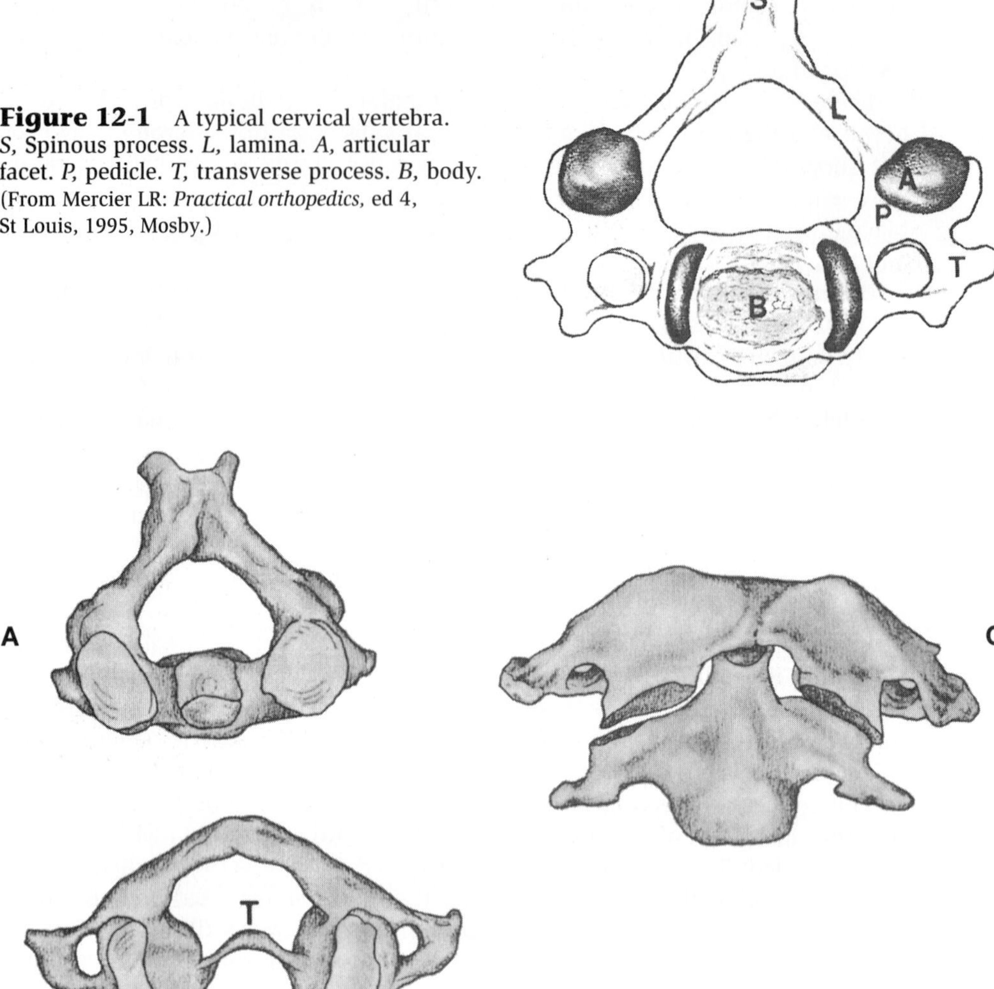

Figure 12-1 A typical cervical vertebra. *S,* Spinous process. *L,* lamina. *A,* articular facet. *P,* pedicle. *T,* transverse process. *B,* body. (From Mercier LR: *Practical orthopedics,* ed 4, St Louis, 1995, Mosby.)

Figure 12-2 **A,** The axis. **B,** The atlas and transverse ligament *(T).* **C,** The articulation of the atlas and the axis. (From Mercier LR: *Practical orthopedics,* ed 4, St Louis, 1995, Mosby.)

margin of a neural foramen. When the encroachment involves a nerve root, pain in the distribution of that root (radicular pain) may occur. The facet joint capsules and the intervertebral disk are innervated by fine nerves with simple nerve endings. When these nerve endings are stimulated by degenerative disease within the disk or joint capsules, the patient may experience pain that is referred to the posterior aspect of the neck at any level. The pain felt in the neck may not be at the cervical level from which the nerve is arising. In addition, stimulation of the nerves can cause pain to be referred to the interscapular area, superiorly and laterally over the shoulders. Spasm of any of the many muscles of the neck region is also a common source of pain (Barker, Burton, and Zieve, 1995).

Neck Ache or Neck Strain

Neck ache or neck strain involves nonradiating discomfort or pain around the neck area and is associated with loss of motion or stiffness. It may present as a headache, but most often the pain is located in the middle or lower portion of the back of the neck. The source of the pain is often the ligaments of the cervical spine or surrounding muscles. Patients involved in rear-end automobile accidents, in which a relaxed person in the stationary car is struck from behind and the torso moves forward as the neck is hyperextended, may suffer acute hyperextension injuries to the neck, commonly called *whiplash*. Recoil forward flexion occurs, and the chin strikes the chest. Individuals often feel little discomfort at the scene but develop neck stiffness 12 to 14 hours after the accident.

History

Area of maximal tenderness
Radiation of pain
Presence of numbness or weakness in the extremities
Precipitating events (e.g., car accident or prolonged hyperextension such as painting the ceiling)
Past history of similar problems
Headache or migraine
Dizziness with lateral rotation
Meningeal irritation signs (e.g., photophobia, fever)
Gradual or sudden onset
Constant or intermittent pain
Alleviating or exacerbating activities: rest, motion
Proper or improper neck positions at home or at work
Bruxism (grinding or clenching the teeth) at night or jaw complaints after sleep
Sensory impairment (vision, hearing) that causes unconscious head tilting
Previous trauma
Occupation
Hobbies
Changes in daily activity patterns

Symptoms

Headache
Dull, aching pain exacerbated by neck motion
Pain abated by rest or immobilization
Pain that may be referred to other structures: scapula, posterior shoulder, occiput, or anterior chest wall
Dysphagia (may result from an esophageal tear with hyperextension)
Hoarseness (may result from a laryngeal tear)
Pain in the temporomandibular joint
Neck ache
Neck stiffness

Focused Physical Examination

If a fracture is suspected, do not test range of motion (ROM).
Assess for localized tender area of neck lateral to the spine.
Assess for loss of cervical motion.
Pain on neck motion may be variable.
The presence of true spasm rare, except in severe cases where the head may be tilted to one side (torticollis).
Perform a neurologic examination (usually normal).
Horner's syndrome, nausea, and dizziness may result from longus colli muscle tears.
Assess strength of contraction of trapezius and sternocleidomastoid muscles.
Inspect for laceration, swelling, or bruising.
Palpate lymph nodes for enlargement and tenderness.

Differential Diagnoses

Muscle strain
Muscle spasm
Cervical spondylosis
Cervical root compression
Lymphadenopathy
Thyroiditis
Angina pectoris
Meningitis
Trigger points
Tumor
Infection

Diagnostic Tests

Plain x-ray films are usually not warranted at the first visit unless the patient presents with a history of trauma or neurologic findings. If pain continues for longer than 2 weeks or the patient develops other physical findings, x-ray films should be obtained to rule out other conditions such as neoplasia or instability.

It is essential to visualize the cervical spine radiologically down to C7-T1. If plain x-ray films are normal, flexion-extension x-ray films should be obtained. **Any patient with neurological findings in these circumstances should be immobilized in a collar and seen immediately by a neurosurgeon or othopedic surgeon before flexion extension x-ray films are taken.**

A complete blood count (CBC) with differential is useful when infection or inflammatory arthritis is suspected.

Treatment

Therapeutics

Immobilization in a cervical collar for no more than 2 to 4 weeks to prevent atrophy of nonworking muscles.

Box 12-1
Muscle Relaxants

Cyclobenzaprine (Flexeril) 10 mg q8h *or*
Methocarbamol (Robaxin) 750 mg to 1.5 g qid *or*
Metaxalone (Skelaxin) 400-800 mg tid-qid *or*
Carisoprodol (Soma) 350 mg qid *or*
Chlorzoxazone (Parafon Forte) 500 mg qid

From Georgetown University Medical Center Orthopaedic Spine Clinic, Washington, DC, 1998.

Analgesics such as acetaminophen or nonsteroidal antiinflammatory drugs (NSAIDs).
Heat, either moist or dry, may provide symptomatic relief but does not speed healing.
Restrict activity based on severity of symptoms. "Let pain be your guide."
Avoid narcotics; they may be administered for the first 2 weeks if necessary.
Muscle relaxants: Use with caution (Box 12-1).

Education. Encourage the patient to perform work and daily activities as much as possible. When the pain subsides and the patient has full ROM without muscle spasm, the cervical collar can be gradually discontinued. Initially decrease the length of time the collar is worn during the day; however, instruct the patient to continue using the collar at night, when the neck is unprotected and subjected to awkward movements. Once the patient is pain-free, use of the cervical collar may be discontinued.

Once patients are pain-free, they should begin a program of isometric strengthening exercises. Using the hand for resistance, the muscles controlling flexion, extension, rotation, and lateral bend should be strengthened.

If the patient has severe pain and muscle spasm at the initial injury, the clinical course will probably last 4 to 6 weeks.

If headaches persist, consider head computed tomography (CT) studies.

If arm or shoulder pain persists, consider a neck and thoracic CT to rule out conditions such as mass or brachial plexus injury.

If tests are negative for organic causes of pain, consider emotional overlay.

Although medications such as NSAIDs and muscle relaxants may be adjuncts to pain relief, they do *not* alter the natural history of the disorder.

The patient should avoid driving during the acute phase, when neck mobility is limited.

Teach the patient proper body mechanics for sitting, standing, lifting, and so on.

Follow-up. Because this condition is usually self-limited, follow-up or referral to a specialist is dictated by either worsening symptoms or the persistence of symptoms after 4 to 6 weeks (Figure 12-3).

Cervical Spondylosis

Degenerative disease of the disk and facet joints is included under this heading because it occurs simultaneously and may be difficult to distinguish clinically. This condition is very commonly encountered in people over age 45.

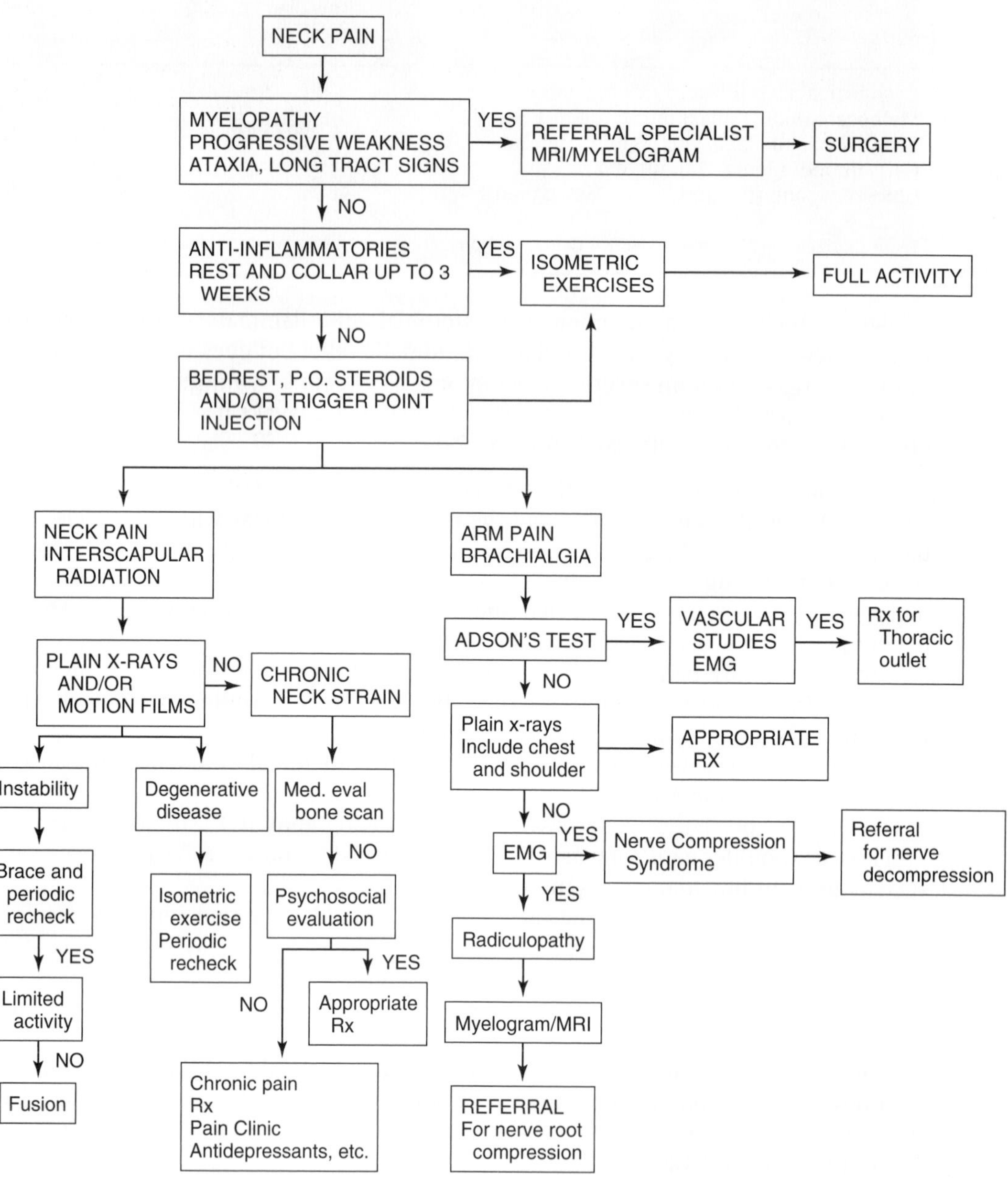

Figure 12-3 Cervical spine algorithm.

Cervical spondylosis is a chronic process defined as the development of osteophytes and other stigmata of degenerative arthritis as a consequence of age-related disk disease. This process may produce a wide range of symptoms. However, an individual may have significant spondylosis and be asymptomatic (Wiesel and Delahay, 1997).

Cervical spondylosis is thought to be the direct result of age-related changes in the intervertebral disk. These changes include desiccation of the nucleus pulposus, loss of annular elasticity, and narrowing of the disk space with or without disk protrusion or rupture. Secondary changes include overriding of facets, increased motion of the spinal segments, osteophyte formation, inflammation of synovial joints, and even microfractures. These macroscopic and microscopic changes can result in various clinical syndromes (Wiesel and Delahay, 1997).

History

Past history of neck pain
Onset of symptoms that is usually insidious but may be acute, with exacerbations and remissions
Acute exacerbations that may be brought on by excessive activity, such as reading (especially with bifocals) or painting a ceiling with the neck in extension
Pain that is aggravated by movements and may be worse after activities
Pain that is relieved by lying down and avoiding certain activities
Symptoms that improve when the patient is at rest or asleep
Proper or improper neck positions at home or at work
Bruxism (grinding or clenching the teeth) at night or jaw complaints after sleep
Sensory impairment (vision, hearing) that causes unconscious head tilting
Previous trauma
Motor vehicle accident
Occupation
Hobbies
Changes in daily activity patterns

Symptoms

Headache
Neck pain with referred pain patterns
Occipital headaches
Pain in the shoulder or arm with possible radiation to one side
Pain in the suboccipital region, intrascapular areas, and anterior chest wall
Vague symptoms suggestive of anatomic disturbances (e.g., blurring of vision, tinnitus)

Focused Physical Examination

Inspection: Patient avoids all movements of the neck and holds it still and straight.
Normal lordosis of the cervical spine is lost.
Paraspinal muscles may be tender and firm because of muscle spasms.
There are coexisting localized trigger points.
Compression test: **This test should not be performed if instability of the cervical spine is suspected.** While the patient is in a sitting position, downward pressure is exerted with the palms of the examiner's hands placed on the patient's head. This test may reproduce the pain if there is narrowing of the intervertebral foramen and pres-

sure on the nerve root. If there is no pain, the patient is asked to bend the neck to the affected side, and similar pressure is exerted.

A neurologic examination is performed.

Differential Diagnoses

Trigger points of the paraspinal muscles
Carpal tunnel syndrome
Peripheral neuropathy
Prolapsed intervertebral disk
Tumor
Infection

Diagnostic Tests

Anteroposterior (AP), lateral, and oblique radiographs of the cervical spine in cervical spondylosis show varying degrees of changes: disk space narrowing, osteophytosis, foraminal narrowing, degenerative changes of the facets, and instability. However, these findings do not necessarily correlate with symptoms. In large part, the radiographs serve to rule out more serious causes of neck and referred pain, such as tumors.

Further diagnostic testing is usually not warranted.

Treatment

Therapeutics

Rest
Immobilization in a cervical collar
Analgesics: aspirin, acetaminophen, or NSAIDs; must often be administered on a chronic basis or at least intermittently
Muscle relaxants: used with caution (see Box 12-1)
Trigger point injections with local anesthetics (lidocaine) and corticosteroids (triamcinolone)
Isometric exercises for neck strengthening: using the hand for resistance, strengthening of the muscles controlling flexion, extension, rotation, and lateral bend
Restricted activity based on severity of symptoms; "Let pain be your guide."
(Georgetown University, 1998)

Education. Educate the patient regarding proper sleep positions (e.g., side-lying vs. prone) and proper body mechanics for sitting, standing, lifting, and so on.

When the patient's pain subsides, the cervical collar may be gradually discontinued. Initially decrease the length of time the collar is worn during the day; however, instruct the patient to continue using the collar at night, when the neck is unprotected and subjected to awkward movements. Once the patient is pain-free, use of the collar may be discontinued.

Although medications such as NSAIDs or muscle relaxants may be adjuncts to pain relief, they do *not* alter the natural history of the disorder.

Follow-up. Follow-up or referral to a specialist is dictated by either worsening or persistence of symptoms.

Cervical Spondylosis with Radiculopathy

Aching or burning pain that follows a radicular distribution (dermatome) is cervical spondylosis with radiculopathy. Most often the C5-6 and C6-7 interspaces are involved, with compromise of the sixth and seventh cervical roots, respectively.

History

Aching or burning pain that follows a radicular or dermatomal distribution
Symptoms that are worse at rest or asleep than at other times
Proper or improper neck positions at home or at work
Bruxism (grinding or clenching the teeth) at night or jaw complaints after sleep
History of migraine
Sensory impairment (vision, hearing) cause unconscious head tilting
Previous trauma
Motor vehicle accident
Occupation
Hobbies
Changes in daily activity patterns

Symptoms

Pain in neck, shoulder, medial border of scapula, lateral arm, and dorsal forearm, with sensory changes in the thumb and index finger (compromise of C6 nerve root).
Pain plus sensory changes in the index and middle finger suggests a C7 lesion.

Focused Physical Examination

Neurologic examination: Motor and reflex changes involving the biceps indicate C6 compromise; vs. triceps changes indicate C7 compromise (Table 12-1).

Differential Diagnoses

Trigger points of the paraspinal muscles
Cervical spondylosis
Carpal tunnel syndrome
Peripheral neuropathy
Prolapsed intervertebral disk
Radiculopathy
Tumor
Infection

Diagnostic Tests

AP, lateral, and oblique radiographs of the cervical spine show varying degrees of changes with cervical spondylosis: disk space narrowing, osteophytosis, foraminal narrowing, degenerative changes of the facets, and instability. However, these findings

TABLE 12-1 Symptoms and Findings in Cervical Radiculopathy

Disk Level	Nerve Root	Symptoms and Findings
C2-3	C3	**Pain:** Back of neck, mastoid process, pinna of ear **Sensory change:** Back of neck, mastoid process, pinna of ear **Motor deficit:** None readily detectable except by EMG **Reflex change:** None
C3-4	C4	**Pain:** Back of neck, levator scapula, anterior chest **Sensory change:** Back of neck, levator scapula, anterior chest **Motor deficit:** None readily detectable except by EMG **Reflex change:** None
C4-5	C5	**Pain:** Neck, tip of shoulder, anterior arm **Sensory change:** Deltoid area **Motor deficit:** Deltoid, biceps **Reflex change:** Biceps
C5-6	C6	**Pain:** Neck, shoulder, medial border of scapula, lateral arm, dorsal forearm **Sensory change:** Thumb and index finger **Motor deficit:** Biceps **Reflex change:** Biceps
C6-7	C7	**Pain:** Neck, shoulder, medial border of scapula, lateral arm, dorsal forearm **Sensory change:** Index and middle finger **Motor deficit:** Triceps **Reflex change:** Triceps
C7-T1	C8	**Pain:** Neck, medial border of scapula, medial aspect of arm and forearm **Sensory change:** Ring and little finger **Motor deficit:** Intrinsic muscles of hand **Reflex change:** None

Adapted from Wiesel SW, Delahay JN: *Essentials of orthopaedic surgery,* ed 2, Philadelphia, 1997, WB Saunders.

do not necessarily correlate with symptoms. In large part, radiographs serve to rule out more serious causes of neck and referred pain, such as tumors.

Treatment

Therapeutics

Rest: Restricted activity based on severity of symptoms; "Let pain be your guide"
Immobilization in a cervical collar
Analgesics: acetaminophen or NSAIDs
Trigger point injections with local anesthetics (lidocaine) and corticosteroids (triamcinolone)
Isometric exercises for neck strengthening: using the hand for resistance, strengthening of the muscles controlling flexion, extension, rotation, and lateral bend
Possible use of cervical traction, in slight flexion, of 5 to 10 pounds
Heat, either moist or dry, which may provide symptomatic relief
Muscle relaxants: used with caution (see Box 12-1)

Education. Educate patient regarding proper sleep positions (e.g., side-lying vs. prone) and proper body mechanics for sitting, standing, lifting, and so on. Chiropractic manipulation is contraindicated.

In 75% to 80% of individuals with radiculopathy, nonsurgical interventions are successful in relieving pain.

When the patient's pain subsides, the cervical collar may be gradually discontinued. Initially decrease the length of time the collar is worn during the day; however, instruct the patient to continue using the collar at night, when the neck is unprotected and subjected to awkward movements.

Although medications such as NSAIDs or muscle relaxants may be adjuncts to pain relief, they do *not* alter the natural history of the disorder.

Follow-up. With failure of these therapeutic measures, consider referral to a neurosurgeon or orthopedist for intervention.

Cervical Myelopathy

When the secondary bony changes of cervical spondylosis encroach on the spinal cord, a pathologic process called *myelopathy* develops. If this process involves both the spinal cord and nerve roots, it is called *myeloradiculopathy*. Regardless of its etiology, radiculopathy causes shoulder or arm pain (Wiesel and Delahay, 1997).

Myelopathy is the most serious sequela of cervical spondylosis and is the most difficult to treat effectively. Fewer than 5% of patients with cervical spondylosis develop myelopathy, and they are usually between 40 and 60 years old. The changes of myelopathy are most often gradual and associated with posterior osteophyte formation (spondylitic bone or hard disk) and spinal canal narrowing (spinal stenosis). Acute myelopathy is most often the result of a central soft disk herniation that produces a high-grade block that may be visualized on myelogram.

History

Cervical spondylosis

Symptoms

Patients gradually notice a peculiar sensation in the hands that is associated with clumsiness and weakness.

Lower extremity symptoms may include difficulty in walking, peculiar sensations, leg weakness, and spasticity. These symptoms may antedate the upper extremity findings.

Neck pain is not a prominent feature of myelopathy.

Abnormal urination indicates more severe disease.

Focused Physical Examination

Stooped posture; gait that is wide stance

Possible hyperreflexia or clonus

Upper extremity weakness

Loss of vibration and position sense that is more common in feet than in hands and may be unilateral
Possible electric sensation down the spine when neck is flexed (Lhermitte's sign)
Signs of cord compression: increased reflexes in the upper and lower extremities with a positive Babinski's sign

Differential Diagnoses

Cervical spondylosis
Myelopathy
Herniated nucleus pulposus
Peripheral neuropathy
Multiple sclerosis
Localized compression of vascular structures
Peripheral nerve entrapment
Spinal stenosis
Tumor
Infection

Diagnostic Tests

X-ray films of the cervical spine often reveal advanced degenerative disease, including spinal canal narrowing by prominent posterior osteophytosis, variable foraminal narrowing, disk space narrowing, facet joint arthrosis, and instability.

Congenital stenosis of the cervical canal is often seen; this condition predisposes the patient to the development of myelopathy.

Consider a myelogram. Consider magnetic resonance imaging (MRI).

Treatment

Therapeutics. Conservative therapy that consists of immobilization and rest with a soft cervical collar and cervical pillow offers a viable option to the patient with myelopathy who is not a good operative risk. In general, myelopathy is a surgical disease but not an absolute indication for surgical decompression. Surgery is clearly indicated if the myelopathy is progressive despite a trial of conservative treatment (Wiesel and Delahay, 1997). Surgical decompression yields satisfactory results in 75% to 80% of cases (Wilson and Lin, 1997).

Local heat
Gentle range-of-motion exercises
Analgesics: acetaminophen or NSAIDs, which may help relieve pain
Injection of trigger points with local anesthetic agents (lidocaine), which provides immediate relief of pain
Physical therapy
(Georgetown University, 1998)

Education. Educate the patient regarding proper sleep positions (e.g., side-lying vs. prone) and proper body mechanics for sitting, standing, lifting, and so on.

Chiropractic manipulation is contraindicated.

Although medications such as NSAIDs may be adjuncts to pain relief, they do *not* alter the natural history of the disorder.

Follow-up. Refer to an orthopedist or neurosurgeon if symptoms persist despite conservative measures.

Cervical Herniated Nucleus Pulposus

Protrusion of the nucleus pulposus through the fibers of the annulus fibrosus produces cervical herniated nucleus pulposus. Most acute disk herniations occur posterolaterally and around the fourth decade of life, when the nucleus is still gelatinous. The most common areas of disk herniation are C5-6 and C6-7. Unlike the lumbar herniated disk, the cervical herniated disk may cause both myelopathy and radiculopathy because of the presence of the spinal cord in the cervical region (Wiesel and Delahay, 1997).

Disk herniation usually affects the root numbered lowest for the given disk level (e.g., the C5-6 disk affects the sixth cervical root, and the C6-7 disk affects the seventh cervical root).

Not every herniated disk is symptomatic. The presence of symptoms depends on the spinal reserve capacity, the presence of inflammation, the size of the herniation, and the presence of concomitant disease, such as osteophyte formation.

History

Symptoms that are worse when at rest or asleep than at other times
Proper or improper neck positions at home or at work
Bruxism (grinding or clenching the teeth) at night or jaw complaints after sleep
History of migraine
Sensory impairment (vision, hearing) that causes unconscious head tilting
Previous trauma
Motor vehicle accident
Occupation
Hobbies
Changes in daily activity patterns

Symptoms

The major complaint is arm pain, not neck pain. The pain is often perceived as starting in the neck area, but it radiates from this point down the shoulder, forearm, and usually into the hand, commonly in a dermatomal distribution.

The onset of radicular pain is often gradual, although there can be a sudden onset associated with a tearing or snapping sensation.

As time passes, the magnitude of the arm pain clearly exceeds that of the neck or shoulder pain. The arm pain may vary in intensity from severe enough to preclude any use of the arm without severe pain, to a dull cramping ache in the arm muscles with use of the arm. The pain is usually severe enough to wake the patient at night.

Focused Physical Examination

There is motion limitation in the neck. Occasionally, the patient may tilt head in a "cocked robin" toward the side of the herniated disk.

Extension of the spine often exacerbates the pain because it further narrows the intervertebral foramina. Axial compression, the Valsalva maneuver, and coughing may also re-create or exacerbate the pain pattern.

Palpate the posterior neck muscles for spasm and symmetry. See if shoulder ROM elicits pain within the shoulder itself.

The presence of a positive neurologic finding is the most helpful aspect of the diagnostic workup, although the neurologic examination may remain normal despite a chronic radicular pattern. To be significant, the neurologic examination must show objective signs of reflex diminution, motor weakness, or atrophy. An objective sensory deficit is one that conforms to a dermatomal distribution.

Differential Diagnoses

Herniated nucleus pulposus
Cervical myelopathy
Cervical radiculopathy
Shoulder impingement
Carpal tunnel syndrome
Infection
Tumor

Diagnostic Tests

Plain x-ray films are usually not diagnostic. However, disk space narrowing may be visualized in the AP view. The value of an x-ray examination is to exclude other causes of neck and arm pain. Tests such as an electromyogram (EMG) or MRI are confirmatory examinations and should not be used as screening tests because misinformation may ensue.

Treatment

Therapeutics
Immobilization in a soft cervical collar and rest
Decreased activity for at least 2 weeks
Muscle relaxants: used with caution (see Box 12-1)
Analgesics: acetaminophen or NSAIDs
Avoid narcotics; may be administered for the first 2 weeks if necessary
(Georgetown University, 1998)

Education. A well-informed patient who is willing to follow through on suggestions will have improved outcomes.

Educate the patient regarding proper body mechanics, such as sitting, standing, and lifting.

Educate the patient regarding proper use of the cervical collar: Wear it 24 hours/day for the first 2 weeks.

When the pain subsides and the patient has full ROM without muscle spasm or radicular pain, the cervical collar can be gradually discontinued. Initially decrease the length of time the collar is worn during the day; however, instruct the patient to continue using the collar at night, when the neck is unprotected and subjected to awkward movements. Once the patient is pain-free, use of the cervical collar can be discontinued.

Although medications such as NSAIDs or muscle relaxants may be adjuncts to pain relief, they do *not* alter the natural history of the disorder.

Follow-up. Most patients respond to a 4- to 6-week course of conservative treatment. Follow-up or referral to a specialist is dictated by either worsening or persistence of symptoms.

Shoulder Pain

Shoulder pain is one of the most commonly encountered complaints in adult primary care practice (Millstein, 1997). A proper diagnosis requires (1) a sound understanding of the anatomy of the shoulder region, (2) a realistic differential diagnosis, and (3) a focused history and physical examination.

Pain originating in the shoulder region, as opposed to referred pain, is typically exacerbated by activities requiring ROM. The shoulder is best described as a region (Figures 12-4 to 12-6) of three large bones (the scapula, clavicle, and humerus) and four joints (the glenohumeral, sternoclavicular, acromioclavicular [AC], and scapulothoracic). Most of the shoulder's stability depends on muscular and ligamentous attachments. The acromion projects from the scapula to form the roof of the shoulder. Together with the coracoid and attaching ligaments, it forms a socket called the glenoid fossa. The ball-like head of the humerus is cradled here, forming the glenohumeral joint, or shoulder joint. The shallow glenohumeral joint, the lax ligamentous capsule, and the interplay of the other regional joints allow maximum mobility.

However, this mobility comes at a price. The shoulder's dependence on soft tissue articulation makes it vulnerable to injury and accounts for the relatively high prevalence of problems in this region. The most significant shoulder stabilizers are the four scapulohumeral muscles collectively known as the rotator cuff. These supraspinatus, infraspinatus, subscapularis, and teres minor muscles function in countertraction to

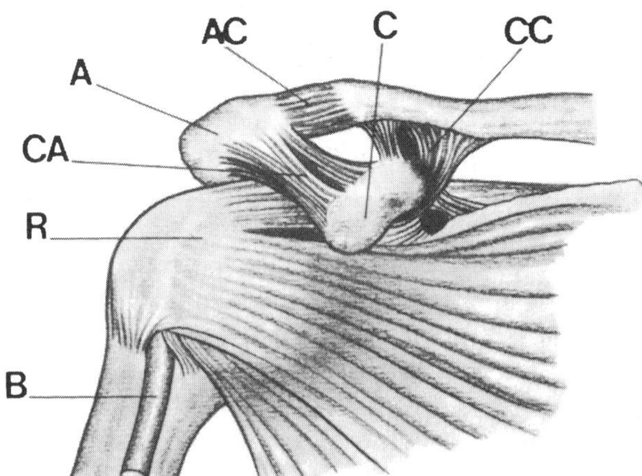

Figure 12-4 Bones and ligaments of the shoulder. *R,* rotator cuff. *B,* long head of the biceps. *AC,* acromioclavicular joint capsule. *CC,* coracoclavicular ligaments. *A,* acromion. *C,* coracoid process. *CA,* coracoacromial ligaments. (From Mercier LR: *Practical orthopedics,* ed 4, St Louis, 1995, Mosby.)

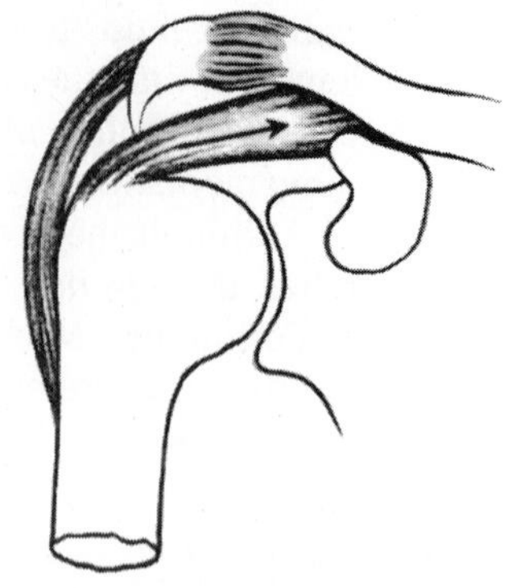

Figure 12-5 Abduction of the shoulder. By stabilizing the humeral head in the glenoid *(arrow)*, the superior portion of the rotator cuff prevents it from being forced into the acromion by the deltoid muscle. (From Mercier LR: *Practical orthopedics,* ed 4, St Louis, 1995, Mosby.)

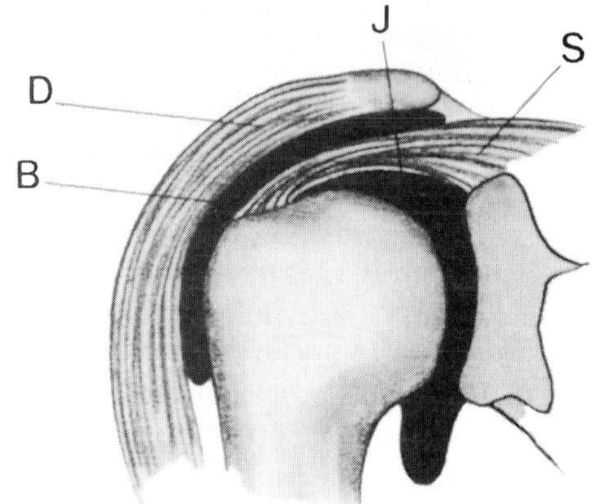

Figure 12-6 The subacromial bursa *(B)* is shown between the deltoid *(D)* and supraspinatus *(S)* muscles. Deep to the rotator cuff is the glenohumeral joint cavity *(J)*. (From Mercier LR: *Practical orthopedics,* ed 4, St Louis, 1995, Mosby.)

abduction by the deltoid muscle. The tendons of these muscles converge under the acromion and coracoid processes and attach to the capsular ligaments. The tendon of the long head of the biceps runs through the joint capsule and along the bicipital groove of the humerus. Between the acromion and the rotator cuff lies a bursa that cushions the tendon from the bone. This small sac is a common trouble spot. The shoulder anatomy is unique in that surrounding bursae communicate with the joint, thus providing a pathway for extraarticular infection to invade the joint (Sykes, 1997).

Dermatomes represented in the shoulder area are those originating from C4, C5, and T1-4. In addition, the sensory branch of the axillary nerve (C5) supplies the area over the deltoid.

A rotator cuff tear should be considered in all patients over age 40, even though they may not complain of severe pain or limitations in activity. For individuals under age 70, the prevalence is 30%. For individuals age 71 to 80 the prevalence is nearly 60%, and for those over 80, nearly 70%. Older patients who have mild chronic impingement symptoms but sustain an episode of trauma may experience tears of the rotator cuff. The most common differential diagnosis in individuals who experience shoulder pain with exertion of the joint is rotator cuff tear. Another key point to keep in mind during the evaluation of shoulder pain is that disorders can coexist (Millstein, 1997).

With the anatomy of the shoulder region in mind, the practitioner can arrive at a differential diagnosis by examining the pathophysiology and clinical epidemiology of shoulder pain in the adult patient population. Despite advances in sophisticated imaging studies, the history and physical examination remain the benchmark of diagnostic success (Wiesel and Delahay, 1997).

History

The most common complaints are pain, stiffness, instability, and weakness. In reviewing the history, consider the following points:

Whether the pain has a sudden or insidious onset
Whether it is a burning pain or a dull ache over the shoulder
Cervical spine symptoms: neck pain, neck stiffness, paresthesias (Figure 12-7)
Pain that occurs during a specific activity or with a particular position
Nocturnal awakening
Pain at rest
Stiffness
Weakness (the least common complaint)
Activities the patient is unable to perform: lift arm over head, wash under opposite axilla
History of trauma: whether or not the patient experienced a snapping, popping, or tearing sensation
Gastrointestinal, pulmonary, or cardiovascular symptoms
Arm dominance
Current medications
Allergies
Occupation
Hobbies
Alleviating factors

Focused Physical Examination

There are five components to the physical examination: inspection, palpation, ROM, strength, and neurovascular examination.

Inspection. Check for shoulder symmetry, masses, swelling, erythema, ecchymosis, and muscular atrophy.

With an AC joint separation, there is a step-off at the AC joint.

With an anterior shoulder dislocation, there is anterior fullness and lateral flatness.

With a posterior shoulder dislocation, there is flattening of the anterior aspect of the shoulder, which is best seen from above as the patient sits on a stool.

With a tear of the long head of the biceps, there is a globular appearance to the biceps muscle.

Note the position of the scapula in relation to the thorax and spine (Figure 12-8).

Observe spinal curvature.

Palpation. Palpate for tenderness, masses, warmth, and crepitus. Begin at the sternoclavicular joint and follow along the clavicle to the acromioclavicular joint, the coracoid, the acromion, and the scapular spine. Also palpate the trapezius and deltoid muscles. Note any focal tenderness over the sternoclavicular or acromioclavicular joint, which indicates joint strain. Palpate for trigger points along the superior border of the trapezius, paraspinal, supraspinatus, and infraspinatus muscles. Palpate axillae for enlarged or tender lymph nodes.

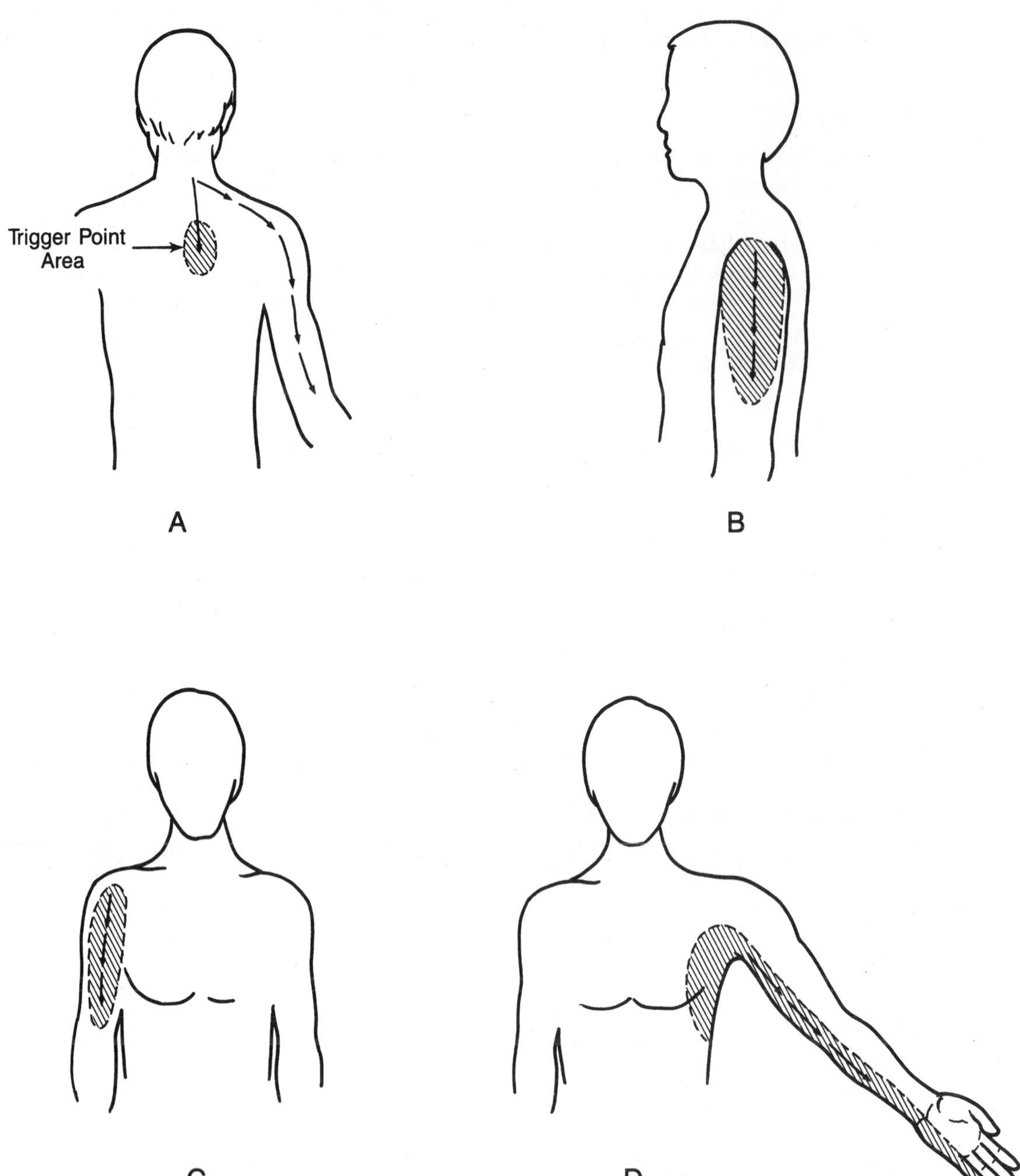

Figure 12-7 General pain distribution of common neck and arm disorders. **A,** Cervical disk syndrome. **B,** Rotator cuff syndrome. **C,** Bicipital tendinitis. **D,** Disorders involving the lower portion of the brachial plexus (Pancoast tumor, thoracic outlet syndrome). When the shoulder pain has a visceral origin, the patient sometimes recognizes it as "deep" and perhaps not arising in the exact region where it is felt. (From Mercier LR: *Practical orthopedics,* ed 4, St Louis, 1995, Mosby.)

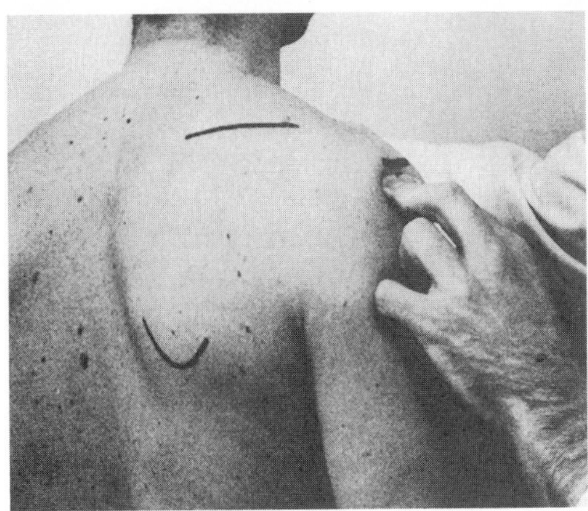

Figure 12-8 Superficial landmarks of the shoulder. The spine of the scapula lies at the level of the third dorsal vertebra. The inferior angle lies at the level of the seventh rib and eighth dorsal vertebra. The rotator cuff is palpated just distal to the acromion process. (From Mercier LR: *Practical orthopedics,* ed 4, St Louis, 1995, Mosby.)

Range of Motion. *Do not perform ROM in a traumatized, obviously fractured, or dislocated shoulder until x-ray films have been obtained.*

ROM of the shoulder is measured from the neutral position with the arm by the side of the body. Evaluate forward elevation by asking the patient to lift the arm overhead. Evaluate external rotation by having the patient stand with elbows at the side and rotate the arms out as far as possible. Evaluate internal rotation by asking the patient to put hand behind body and touch that hand as high as possible with the thumb on the spinal column. Note the level of the spinal column reached. (The tip of the scapula is T7.) If a discrepancy is noted in comparing either side, have the patient lie supine and perform passive ROM, which disallows spine or trunk compensation. Mild restriction is common following immobilization, trauma, arthritis, or rotator cuff pathology.

Strength. Ask the patient to perform a wall pushup and to shrug shoulders to assess strength of the scapular rotators.

Two tests are used to assess the rotator cuff muscles. To evaluate the supraspinatus, have the patient elevate both arms to 90 degrees, point thumbs down, and hold arms at 90 degrees against resistance. If the patient exhibits weakness or an arm drops, it is considered cuff pathology. To evaluate the infraspinatus and teres minor, ask the patient to put elbows at the side, with forearms parallel to the floor, and externally rotate against resistance.

Neurovascular Examination. Perform thorough reflex and sensory testing. The biceps tendon correlates with the C5 nerve, the brachioradialis correlates with C6, and the triceps correlates with C7.

Sensory: Evaluate light touch over the thumb web space (radial nerve), the radial aspect of the index finger (median nerve), and the ulnar aspect of the little finger (ulnar nerve).

Differential Diagnoses

Rotator cuff tendinitis or tear
Subdeltoid or subacromial bursitis
Adhesive capsulitis (also known as frozen shoulder)
Acromioclavicular arthritis or strain
Biceps tendinitis

Cardiac sources (referred pain)
Carpal tunnel syndrome (referred pain)
Cerebral vascular accident with hemiparesis (referred pain)
Cervical and neck disorders (referred pain)
Neoplasm (local or referred pain)
Fracture
Dislocation
Arthritis
Infection
Polymyalgia rheumatica
Reflex sympathetic dystrophy
Nerve entrapment
Visceral sources (referred pain)

Most commonly, shoulder pathology falls in one of three areas: trauma (dislocations, fractures, sprains, strains), inflammation (acute rotator cuff tear or tendinitis, bursitis, adhesive capsulitis), and infection.

Trauma

Dislocation

Dislocation most commonly occurs following an outstretched hand with forceful abduction, extension, and external rotation of the shoulder. Anterior dislocation accounts for 95% of shoulder dislocations; posterior dislocations account for 5%, are less obvious, and are more likely to be overlooked on examination and on x-ray films. Posterior dislocations result from direct or indirect trauma that forces the humeral head posteriorly out of the glenoid fossa and may follow an electrical shock or convulsion.

Focused Physical Examination

Anterior Dislocation. The finding of a sulcus or hollow in the skin beneath the acromion, together with fixed external rotation of the arm, should be easily diagnostic. In addition, there is displacement of the humeral head, which is seen and felt inferior to the clavicle.

The patient may have a positive apprehension test. With this test, the arm is abducted and externally rotated. Just before the joint is about to dislocate, an expression of anxiety appears on the patient's face, because the patient knows the joint is about to dislocate.

Posterior Dislocation. The arm is adducted and fixed in internal rotation. Anteriorly, there is flattening of the shoulder contour and prominence of the coracoid process. Posteriorly, there is more prominence and rounding of the shoulder than normal. There is markedly limited external rotation and elevation of the arm.

Differential Diagnosis

Shoulder dislocation

Diagnostic Tests

The findings on standard AP x-ray films are subtle. An additional axillary lateral view should also be ordered to assist in revealing posterior displacement of the humeral head.

If the diagnosis is still in question after an axillary view, a CT scan should be ordered.

Dislocations may be accompanied by rotator cuff injury, neurovascular compromise (commonly the axillary nerve in anterior dislocation), or fracture; therefore posttreatment x-ray films should be obtained to evaluate these complications and ensure the adequacy of the reduction (Barker, Burton, and Zieve, 1995).

Treatment

Therapeutics. Treatment of dislocations requires prompt reduction and referral to an orthopedist or emergency department.

Education. Postreduction immobilization in a sling allows capsular structures to tighten. This is followed by physical therapy to build strength. Passive exercises are started early to prevent stiffness. The range and intensity are increased as tolerated by the patient.

Follow-up. Reevaluate the patient at completion of the course of physical therapy. In the event of recurrent dislocation, consider a referral for possible surgical intervention.

Fractures

The constriction around the articular surface of the proximal end of the humerus is the anatomic neck of the humerus. The surgical neck is the region where the expanded proximal end meets the shaft of the humerus. Fractures commonly occur at the surgical neck (Figure 12-9). In the elderly, fractures usually occur after a fall, although they may accompany traumatic dislocation.

Symptoms

Pain occurs in the shoulder region after a fall or dislocation. The severity of pain depends on the severity of trauma; in the elderly, osteoporotic patient with an impacted fracture, there may not be much pain.

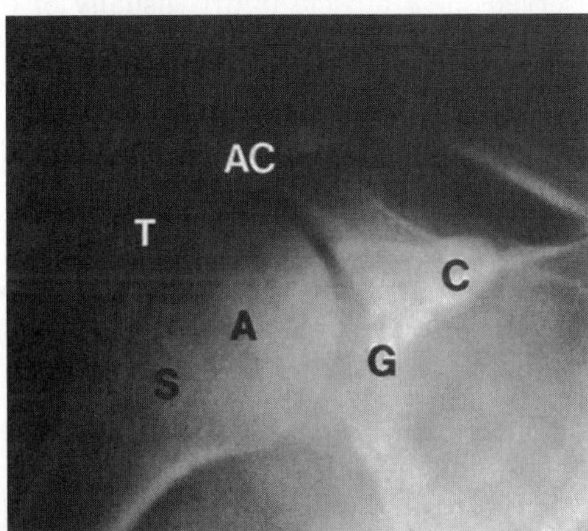

Figure 12-9 Roentgenographic anatomy of the shoulder. *S*, surgical neck of the humerus. *A*, anatomic neck of the humerus. *T*, greater tuberosity. *C*, coracoid process. *AC*, acromion process. *G*, glenoid fossa. (From Mercier LR: *Practical orthopedics*, ed 4, St Louis, 1995, Mosby.)

Focused Physical Examination

The injured arm is supported by the other hand, and swelling is visible in the upper arm. Later, ecchymosis appears, which may track down to the elbow or forearm (within 1 to 2 days after fracture). There is localized tenderness at the fracture site. All active and passive movements are painful.

Evaluate neurologic examination and radial and ulnar artery pulsations to rule out axillary artery injury.

Differential Diagnosis

Humoral fracture

Diagnostic Tests

Plain x-ray film establishes the diagnosis.

Treatment

Therapeutics

Referral to an orthopedist for definitive treatment
Analgesics to control pain
Support in a sling until evaluation by an orthopedist

Education. Gentle passive ROM exercises are started as soon as pain permits. Later, pendulum exercises and active exercises against gravity are started. Pendulum exercises may be performed with a weight (an iron works well). Patients are instructed to bend over and stabilize themselves by holding onto an object, such as a chair. They then move the arm back and forth, sideways, and in clockwise and counterclockwise circles.

Follow-up. Reevaluate the patient at completion of the course of physical therapy.

Strains and Sprains

The diagnosis of shoulder strain is reserved for a muscle injury, usually of the large deltoid muscle, and is a diagnosis of exclusion. When all other conditions have been ruled out and the shoulder is sore from an acute injury, look to the muscles as the cause, and look to rest, ice, and compression as the treatment (Sykes, 1997).

Inflammation

Rotator Cuff Tendinitis

Tendinitis is the most common cause of shoulder pain. The tendonous fibers of the rotator cuff muscles undergo degenerative changes with advancing age. The tendons, particularly the supraspinatus (which are the most superior), are thought to be worn down by repetitive excursion between the greater tuberosity of the humerus and the acromion and the acromioclavicular ligament. Pain is caused by edema, hemorrhage, and inflammation associated with the repeated trauma. *Impingement syndrome* and *pericapsulitis* are less specific terms applied to these degenerative and inflammatory disorders of the tendons and bursae. Risk factors for tendinitis include repetitive overhead work or activities and increasing age (Barker, Burton, and Zieve, 1995).

Symptoms

Acute severe pain occurs in the shoulder.
Radiation of pain depends on the severity of the lesion.
Initially, all movements may be painful.
Pain radiates laterally to the deltoid insertion.

Focused Physical Examination

Pain on resisted abduction

Painful Arc Sign. Have patient perform abduction from the rested position. At 45 degrees of abduction, pain is felt as inflamed tissue is forced under the acromion. Pain persists until the 120-degree portion of the arc is reached. The tissue has now moved from under the acromion. There is no pain from 120 to 180 degrees. Passive ROM is normal or exceeds active ROM, which may or may not be limited by pain.

Drop Sign. The arm is passively abducted to 180 degrees, and the patient is asked to let it come down slowly to the neutral position. At about 90 degrees of abduction, the arm falls abruptly because of weakness. The smooth lowering of the arm is replaced by sudden drop.

Differential Diagnoses

Rotator cuff tendinitis
Rotator cuff tear
Subacromial bursitis
Bicipital tendinitis

Diagnostic Tests

Plain x-ray films are usually normal. Degenerative changes, such as sclerosis and cysts, appear on the undersurface of the acromion and over the greater tuberosity of the humerus. Consider MRI to evaluate rotator cuff tear.

Treatment

Therapeutics
NSAIDs help reduce pain and inflammation.
Local injection of steroids may be used to reduce inflammation and pain.
Local ice or heat may be applied.

Physical therapy: Start with passive exercises to increase ROM (Wiesel and Delahay, 1997).

Education. Continue with exercises. As pain decreases and ROM increases, integrate active assisted exercises to strengthen various muscle groups. If pain worsens with exercise, withhold until pain decreases and then restart. "Let pain be your guide."

Follow-up. Failure to resolve symptoms with conservative therapy warrants referral to an orthopedist.

Subacromial Bursitis

The subacromial bursa and rotator cuff are squeezed between the head of the humerus and the coricoacromial arch when the arm is abducted beyond 45 to 60 degrees. Normally, full abduction is achieved by external rotation of the humerus, which helps to ease the subacromial bursa under the coricoacromial arch. Abduction of the arm becomes painful if there is swelling or inflammation in the subacromial region because of increased pressure on the inflamed structures. Clinically, subacromial bursitis, rotator cuff tendinitis, painful arc syndrome, and other impingement syndromes may present with similar symptoms, and these conditions may be difficult to distinguish from one another. However, management of all these conditions is conservative and similar (Mehta, 1997).

Symptoms

A dull ache is felt in the shoulder region and may extend down to the middle of the arm or even the wrist, depending on the severity of the condition.

Pain is worse at night and may interfere with sleep. Movements of the shoulder, especially abduction, aggravate the pain. Sometimes the pain may be severe enough to compel the patient to go to an emergency room in the middle of the night.

The patient may describe an inability to comb hair or hook bra.

Focused Physical Examination

Inspection: There may be wasting of the deltoid and supraspinatus muscles due to disuse.

There may be tenderness in the subacromial region over the lateral aspect of the shoulder.

There may be pain with active abduction beyond 50 to 60 degrees.

Active abduction of the arm against resistance produces pain.

A painful arc is demonstrated.

Differential Diagnoses

Subacromial bursitis

Calcific tendinitis

Fracture of greater tuberosity

Bicipital tendinitis

Degenerative joint disease of AC joint
Cervical radiculopathy

Diagnostic Tests

Plain x-ray films are usually normal. Degenerative changes, such as sclerosis and cysts, appear on the undersurface of the acromion and over the greater tuberosity of the humerus.

Consider MRI to evaluate rotator cuff tear.

Treatment

Therapeutics

NSAIDs to help reduce pain and inflammation
Local injection of steroids to reduce inflammation and pain
Local ice or heat
Physical therapy, with passive exercises to increase ROM

Education. Continue with exercises. As pain decreases and ROM increases, integrate active assisted exercises to strengthen various muscle groups. If pain worsens with exercise, withhold until pain decreases and then restart. "Let pain be your guide."

Follow-up. Failure to resolve symptoms with conservative therapy warrants referral to an orthopedist.

Bicipital Tendinitis

With aging the biceps tendon, like the rotator cuff tendons, is subject to inflammation, erosion, and rupture. Because the biceps tendon runs through the joint space and next to the rotator cuff and subacromial bursa, bicipital tendinitis may coexist with inflammation of these structures.

Symptoms

Pain

Focused Physical Examination

Palpation elicits tenderness over the biceps tendon in the bicipital groove. The elbow is flexed to 90 degrees with the shoulder in a neutral rotation, and the palpating finger moves over the anterior aspect of the shoulder. The forearm is moved gently to rotate the humerus into a position of external and internal rotation. The long head of the biceps will slip under the palpating fingers and give rise to pain if there is bicipital tendinitis.

Tenderness over the lateral aspect of the shoulder may also be felt if there is coexisting rotator cuff pathology or subacromial bursitis. Have the patient flex the elbow to 90 degrees and supinate the forearm against resistance. Have the patient flex the shoulder forward against resistance to elicit reproducible pain over the anterior shoulder.

Differential Diagnoses

Bicipital tendinitis
Rotator cuff pathology
Degenerative arthritis of the AC joint

Diagnostic Tests

None: Diagnosis is mainly clinical.

Treatment

Therapeutics. NSAIDs or local injection of long-acting steroid.

Education

Rest. Discontinuation of activities that precipitate tendinitis; "Let pain be your guide."
Heat
Gentle, passive ROM exercises; active exercises as tolerated by the patient

Follow-up. Persistence or worsening of symptoms warrants further evaluation or referral.

Adhesive Capsulitis

Adhesive capsulitis, or frozen shoulder, is of uncertain etiology but may be a sequela of shoulder pain of diverse causes, such as diabetic neuropathy, reflex sympathetic dystrophy, or previous shoulder trauma. Progressive restriction of motion occurs with this condition, usually after prolonged immobility. The glenohumeral capsule thickens, and adhesions to the humeral head form. The elderly are at especially high risk to develop adhesive capsulitis.

This disorder is somewhat more common in women than in men and generally occurs in the fifth decade or later (Sykes, 1997).

Symptoms

There is insidious onset of diffuse pain and limitation of motion in the shoulder. The patient notes difficulty with reaching arm overhead, reaching the hip pocket, or hooking the bra. Pain subsides in very late stages, but stiffness persists.

Focused Physical Examination

The normal swing of the arm during walking may be limited on the affected side. Later, when the shoulder has lost all movements, there may be wasting of the deltoid and other muscles because of disuse atrophy. The arm is kept adducted and close to the body in a neutral or internally rotated position.

There is tenderness in the shoulder area with palpation. However, tenderness and pain subside when inflammation is controlled.

Initially, active ROM is affected more than passive ROM. External rotation and abduction are restricted to a greater extent than other movements.

During the stage of inflammation, movements are restricted and painful. When inflammation subsides and fibrosis sets in, all movements are restricted and there may be little pain.

Differential Diagnosis

Subacromial bursitis
Adhesive capsulitis

Diagnostic Tests

Plain x-ray films are not very helpful because there are no abnormal findings.

Treatment

Therapeutics. NSAIDs: Injection of an anesthetic agent into the glenohumeral joint may result in improved pain control but does not result in improved ROM. Intraarticular and periarticular corticosteroid injections, weekly for several weeks, may assist in pain control and patient progress in mobility.

Physical therapy: During the acute painful stage, very gentle exercises are prescribed. Exercises are stepped up as the patient is able to tolerate increased activity.

Education. In mostly uncontrolled trials, a combination of corticosteroid injections and progressive exercise has been associated with recovery periods of 4 to 8 weeks. In contrast, treatment with analgesics yields a recovery rate only within 2 to 3 years. Therefore the value of passive and active exercise, either with or without the guidance of a physical therapist, must be stressed as an important tool in recovery.

Follow-up. In the past, referral to an orthopedist to free capsular adhesions by manipulation of the shoulder under anesthesia was commonly recommended for patients who did not improve with conservative management. However, the efficacy of this treatment has not been studied in a controlled fashion; it is generally not recommended and should be considered only in recalcitrant cases (Barker, Burton, and Zieve, 1995).

Infection

Infection is uncommon, but any patient with immune system depression should be considered at risk. This category includes all patients with rheumatoid disease, diabetes, vascular disease, and human immunodeficiency virus. The shoulder anatomy is unique in that surrounding bursae communicate with the joint, thus providing a pathway for extraarticular infection to invade the joint. The devastating effects of irreversible cartilage damage in a septic joint make early diagnosis and treatment mandatory (Sykes, 1997).

Symptoms

Pain
Loss of motion
Effusion

Increased temperature in the joint
Arm that is usually adducted
Sudden onset of systemic symptoms

Focused Physical Examination

X-ray films that show a widened glenohumeral joint space
Erythematous, warm, swollen shoulder joint
Intense pain on palpation or any attempt at ROM
Constitutional symptoms such as fever and chills

Differential Diagnoses

Septic joint
Gout
Rotator cuff tear
Shoulder dislocation

Diagnostic Tests

CBC with differential is used to rule out systemic infection.
Blood cultures are obtained.
Joint fluid aspiration, with smear, culture, and sensitivity, is used.
Indium scan is probably the best indicator of sepsis. If the scan is negative, infection is unlikely.
Consider a CT scan, which is helpful in identifying small lytic lesions often missed by plain films.

Treatment

Therapeutics. Consult with specialist regarding course and treatment plan. The initial antibiotic of choice is a broad-spectrum cephalosporin followed by the appropriate antibiotic as determined by sensitivity studies. The antibiotic regimen should be altered if the condition does not respond.

Rest the affected joint until the acute episode subsides. To avoid the development of adhesive capsulitis, introduce gentle, passive ROM exercises until the patient can tolerate more active ROM without pain.

For an analgesic, consider narcotics.

Education

Instruct in the appropriate use of antibiotics.
Instruct in ROM exercises to prevent loss of motion.
Stress the importance of follow-up.

Follow-up

Daily phone follow-up
Office visit in 3 days
Follow-up with referring practitioner as necessary

Low Back Pain

Low back pain is second only to the common cold as a cause for primary care office visits. More than 75% of people over age 75 have one or more episodes of low back pain secondary to disorders of the intervertebral disk; these episodes vary in intensity and frequency. Low back pain can be medically and economically devastating. It is the number one cause of disability in patients younger than age 45 and the number three cause of disability in patients older than age 45.

Acute low back problems are defined as activity intolerance due to lower back or back-related leg symptoms of less than 3 months' duration. Back pain may be due to a variety of disorders, including gynecologic, genitourinary, and gastrointestinal diseases, but the most common causes are disorders of the lumbar disk (Mercier, 1995). Many nonspinal conditions may masquerade as low back pain or create symptoms analogous to those commonly originating from the lumbar spine:

1. Sacroiliac joint pain: Pain is referred into the gluteal area, similar to facet joint pain.
2. Piriformis syndrome: Pain is referred in the distribution of the sciatic nerve, particularly an S1 distribution.
3. Myofascial pain: Pain referral can be radicular in quality and mimic a lumbar radiculopathy.
4. Peroneal nerve root entrapment at the fibular head: Pain referral in the peroneal nerve distribution may mimic an L5 radiculopathy (Cole and Herring, 1997).

An additional life-threatening cause of low back pain may be an abdominal aortic aneurysm, and careful evaluation of individuals is important to exclude this diagnosis.

The structure of the lumbosacral spine is complex. The lumbar spine is composed of five vertebrae with interposed intervertebral disks that consist of a gelatinous nucleus pulposus and a surrounding annulus fibrosus (Figure 12-10). The vertebrae and disks are supported by strong ligamentous structures and paraspinous muscles. The posterior aspects of the vertebrae surround the spinal canal, form the neural foramina, and

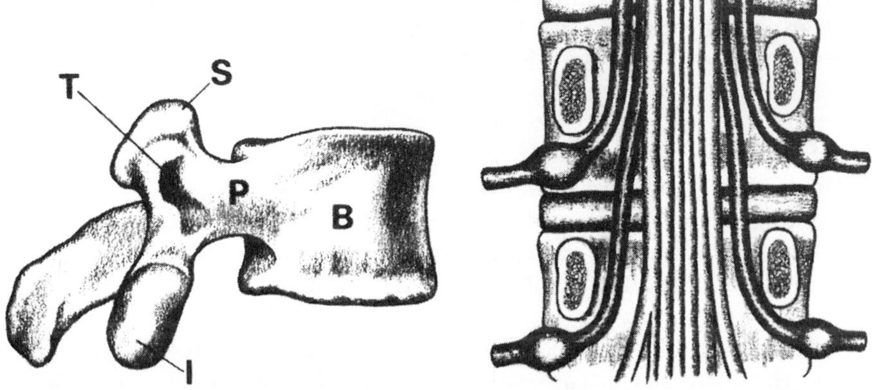

Figure 12-10 **Left,** A typical lumbar vertebra: *S,* superior articular facet; *I,* inferior articular facet; *P,* pedicle; *T,* transverse process; *B,* body. **Right,** Relationship of nerve roots to disks in the lumbar spine. (From Mercier LR: *Practical orthopedics,* ed 4, St Louis, 1995, Mosby.)

interlock to form apophyseal (facet) joints, whose main purpose is motion. The sacrum is the part of the spine that interdigitates with the iliac bones to form part of the pelvis.

An understanding of the nerve supply to the lumbosacral spine is essential in recognizing the patterns of pain associated with disease processes that affect individual anatomic components of the back. The sinuvertebral nerve is the major sensory nerve supplying structures in the lumbar spine.

Several organs are situated in the retroperitoneum, anterior to the lumbar spine. The kidneys, ureters, aorta, inferior vena cava, pancreas, and periaortic lymph nodes are retroperitoneal organs. Diseases that affect these organs may result in referred pain that is localized to the lumbar spine.

The lumbar vertebrae are exposed to tremendous forces, principally because of the magnification of stresses that result from the lever effect of the arm in lifting and the vertical forces associated with the human upright position. Because each intervertebral disk is a fluid system, hydraulic pressure is created whenever a load is placed on the axial skeleton. This hydraulic pressure magnifies three to five times the force that occurs on the annulus fibrosus. This force is akin to the hoop stress that occurs in a barrel when pressure is applied to its liquid content. The ability of the annulus fibrosus to withstand stress decreases significantly with age; by age 60, many individuals have only 50% of the strength in these fibers that they had at age 30 (Barker, Burton, and Zieve, 1995).

However, the lumbar spine is not just an isolated structure. Much support is obtained from the muscles and ligaments of the spine and by the muscles of the thoracic and abdominal cavities.

The natural history of low back pain is reported to be self-limited and to have a favorable prognosis. Approximately 90% of patients with acute low back problems spontaneously recover activity tolerance within 1 month. In primary care, the task is to accurately distinguish between the 90% of low back complaints that are the result of simple strain or overuse and the 10% that may be caused by serious pathology (McIntosh, 1997).

As a general guideline, the patient's age can yield the first clue to diagnosis. Diseases of middle age that can cause back pain include osteomyelitis, Paget's disease, and hemangioma. The elderly person with back pain is most likely to have underlying neuropathy, degenerative disease, metabolic disorder, or malignancy. However, disorders can be seen in any age group (O'Mara and Wiesel, 1997). A general medical review, especially in the older patient, is imperative. Metabolic, infectious, and malignant disorders may initially present as low back pain (Figure 12-11, Box 12-2).

History

The history is the most powerful diagnostic tool. A thorough history allows an accurate working diagnosis to be made in 90% of patients with low back pain. The history helps to determine the patient's current emotional state and the effect of pain on the patient's life. In reviewing the history, consider the following:

Past medical history: diabetes, hypertension, cardiac disease, cancer, infections, rheumatologic disease, gastrointestinal disorders (tolerance for NSAIDs)
Smoking
Past surgical history
Present medications
Allergies

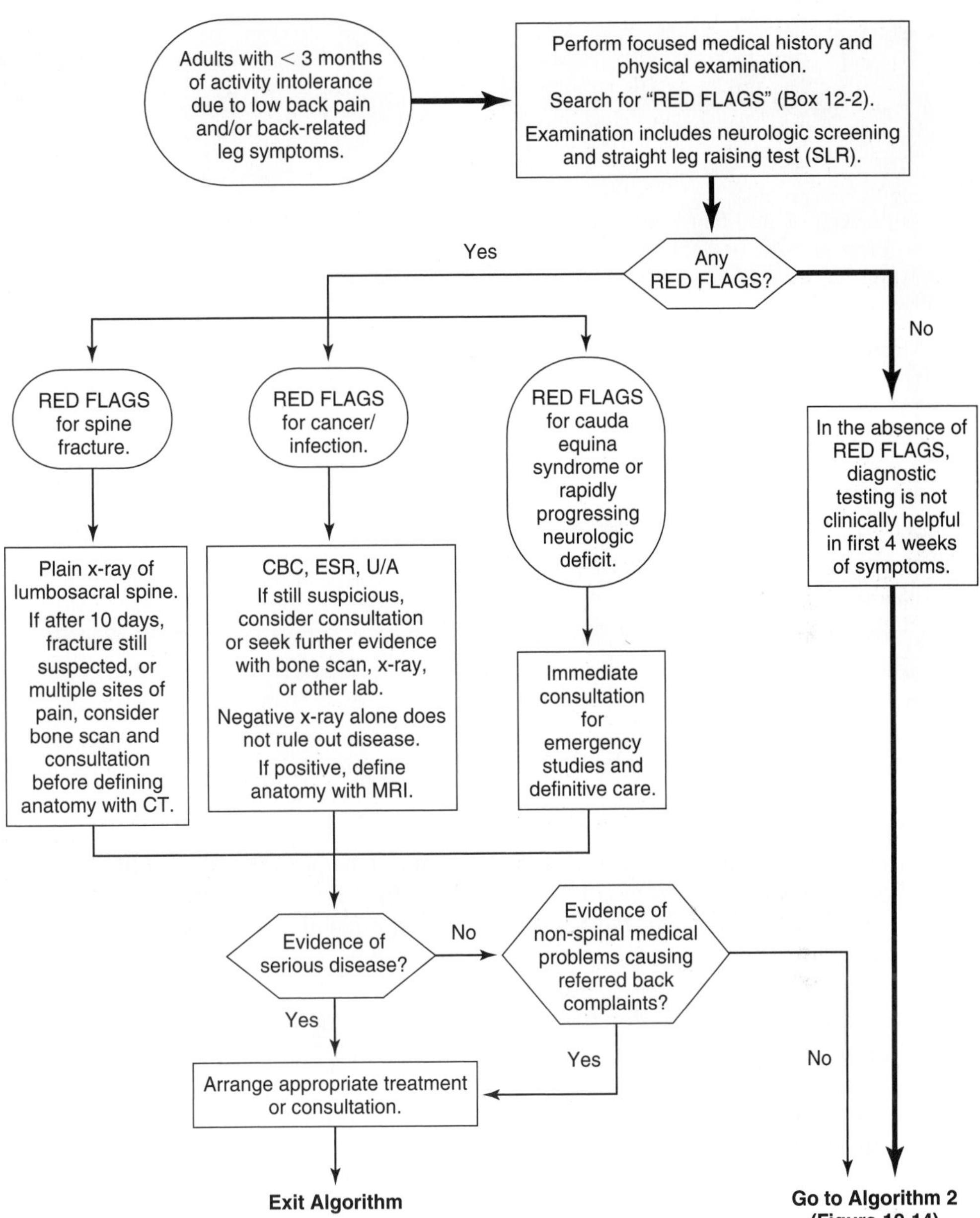

Figure 12-11 Algorithm 1. Initial evaluation of acute low back problem. (Modified from Bigos S et al: *Acute low back problems in adults: clinical practice guideline, quick reference guide,* AHCPR Pub. No. 95-0643, Rockville, Md, 1994, US Department of Health and Human Services.)

Operations, injuries, and previous hospitalizations
Onset of pain: when it began
How pain began: spontaneously with sudden or gradual onset, or traumatically via a motor vehicle accident or other mechanism (e.g., flexion, extension, twist, lift, fall, sneeze, cough, strain)

Box 12-2

Red Flags in Initial Evaluation of Acute Low Back Problem

Spinal Fractures

Significant trauma
Motor vehicle accident
Fall from height
Minor fall
Heavy lifting

Cancer/Infection

Unexplained weight loss
Immunosuppression
Intravenous drug use
Pain increased by rest
Presence of fever

Cauda Equina Syndrome

Bladder dysfunction
Saddle anesthesia
Major limb motor weakness

Modified from Bigos S et al: *Acute low back problems in adults: clinical practice guidelines, quick reference guide,* AHCPR No. 95-0642, Rockville, Md, 1994, US Department of Health and Human Services.

Work-related injury: details of specific injury, pending litigation, compensation for time off work

Sports-related injury

Intensity of pain: Have patient assign a numeric or percent value to pain.

Location: A pain diagram is helpful. If the patient describes primarily back pain, think of annular tear, facet syndrome, local muscular pathology, bony lesion. If the patient describes primarily distal lower extremity pain, think of extruded or lateral herniated nucleus pulposus (HNP), stenosis, nerve lesion.

Whether or not the location has changed over time and in response to specific treatments

Relationship of pain to daily routine: positions that increase pain. If the answer is "prone," think of facet pain, lateral HNP, systemic process. If the answer is "sitting," think of annular tear, paramedian HNP. If the answer is "standing," think of central stenosis, facet syndrome, lateral HNP.

Whether or not there is pain on arising from a seat, which is typical of discogenic pain

Relationship of walking and pain: Consider distance walked, posture with walking, and whether walking up or down hills aggravates or alleviates the pain. If pain is less while walking uphill, think of stenosis because the lumbar spine is flexed, which increases the foraminal and central canal space. If pain is less walking downhill, think of discogenic symptoms because the lumbar spine is extended and disks are unloaded. If pain is less with spinal flexion, think of stenosis.

Time of day: If pain awakens patient from sleep, think of systemic process; if there is morning stiffness of a duration of 20 to 30 minutes, think of discogenic source; if it lasts 2 hours, think of rheumatic process. Does pain increase or decrease as the day progresses?

Whether or not pain is intensified by coughing, sneezing, laughing, or Valsalva maneuver; think of discogenic source
Reproduction of distal pain strongly supports a discogenic source
Activities patient is unable to perform
Positions or maneuvers that relieve the pain
Associated neurologic symptoms: location of anesthesia, hypoesthesia, hyperesthesia, and paresthesias; regional, dermatomal, sclerotomal, or nonphysiologic
Weakness: Differentiate inability to perform a task because of pain vs. weakness.
Bladder, bowel, or sexual dysfunction: Think of cauda equina syndrome.
Review of systems: Include questions to investigate a differential diagnosis of organic problems such as aortic aneurysm, duodenal ulcer, abdominal tumor, fibroids, pelvic inflammatory disease, and prostate tumor.
Emotional issues: Recently published studies suggest that a history of emotional trauma contributes to an increased incidence of low back pain. Psychologic risk factors include physical abuse, sexual abuse, chemical dependency by primary caregiver, abandonment, and emotional neglect (McIntosh, 1997).

Focused Physical Examination

General Observation. Note how the patient walks into the office, the gait, how the patient sits, any expressions made and, if possible, how the patient undresses. Observe the patient's back to note alignment of the spine. Observe from the sides, noting normal cervical and lumbar lordosis and dorsal kyphosis. From the front, observe the head and neck, level of shoulders, anterior-superior iliac spines, and the relation of the trunk to the lower extremities.

Palpation. Palpate the spinous processes, supraspinous ligaments, paraspinous muscles, sacroiliac joints, coccyx, and greater trochanters. Note generalized or point tenderness, muscle spasm, and spinous process alignment. An infection, tumor, or fracture can cause localized soft tissue tenderness.

Evaluation of Range of Motion. The quality and the symmetry of movement are more important than the actual range (O'Mara and Wiesel, 1997). Evaluate flexion, extension, lateral bending, and rotation. Focus especially on the L5-S1 and L4-5 levels, where most movement occurs.

Testing for Muscle Strength with Neurologic Evaluation

Ability to toe walk: calf muscles, mostly S1 nerve root
Ability to heel walk: ankle and toe dorsiflexion muscles, L5 and some L4 nerve roots
Single squat and rise: quadriceps muscles and mostly L4 nerve root
Dorsiflexor muscles of the ankle and great toe: L5 and some L4 nerve root
Hamstring and ankle evertors: L5-S1
Toe flexors: S1

Reflexes. The reliability of reflex testing can be diminished in the presence of joint or muscle problems:

Ankle jerk: S1 nerve root
Knee jerk: L4 nerve root

Up-going toes in response to stroking the plantar footpad (Babinski's sign) may indicate upper motor neuron abnormalities (such as myelopathy or demyelinating disease) rather than a common low back problem (Cole and Herring, 1997).

Evaluate sensory examination via light touch and pressure: medial foot (L4), dorsal foot (L5), and lateral foot (S1) (Figure 12-12).

The straight leg-raising test (also known as a tension sign) is a maneuver that tightens the sciatic nerve and further compresses an inflamed nerve root against a herniated lumbar disk. It may be performed with the patient supine or seated at the edge of an examination table. The leg is then raised, in an extended position, by the heel. The test is positive if leg pain below the knee, not in the back and buttocks, is reproduced or intensified. Reliability is age dependent. Older patients who have desiccated disks have less disk volume to herniate and are therefore less likely to have a positive sign (Figure 12-13).

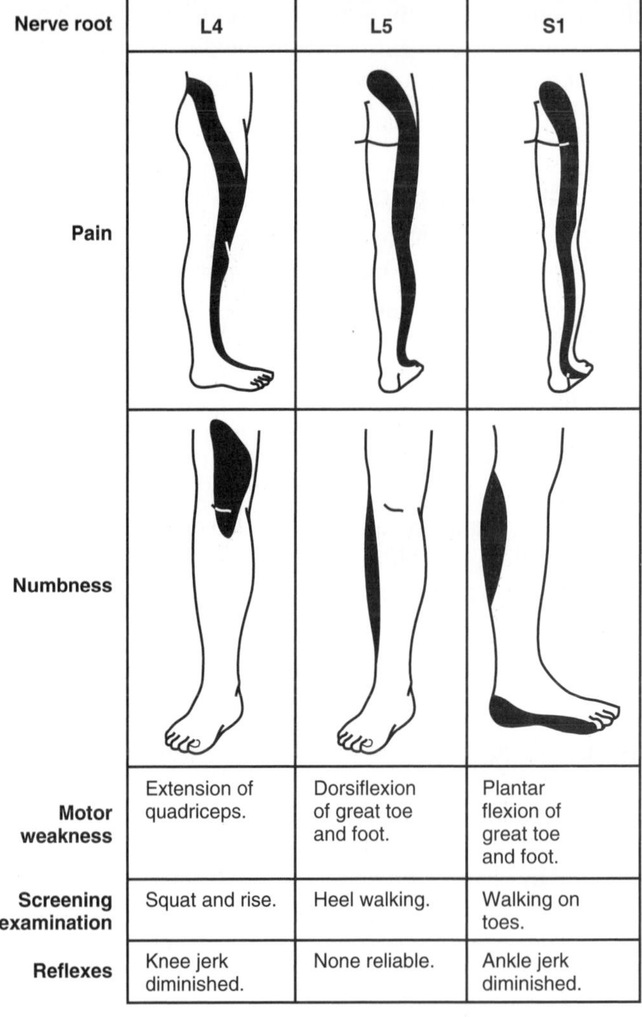

Nerve root	L4	L5	S1
Pain			
Numbness			
Motor weakness	Extension of quadriceps.	Dorsiflexion of great toe and foot.	Plantar flexion of great toe and foot.
Screening examination	Squat and rise.	Heel walking.	Walking on toes.
Reflexes	Knee jerk diminished.	None reliable.	Ankle jerk diminished.

Figure 12-12 Sensory examination. (Adapted from Bigos S et al: *Acute low back problems in adults: clinical practice guideline, quick reference guide,* AHCPR Pub. No. 95-0643, Rockville, Md, 1994, US Department of Health and Human Services.)

Patrick's or Faber's test to differentiate between hip problems and sacroiliac joint pain as the cause of low back pain involves maneuvers of flexion, abduction, and external rotation. Direct the supine patient to place heel on knee, and then place gentle downward pressure on the knee toward the table. The test is positive for hip pain if the patient complains of same-side hip pain. If the patient complains of pain in the ipsilateral pelvis, the sacroiliac joint may be the source of pain.

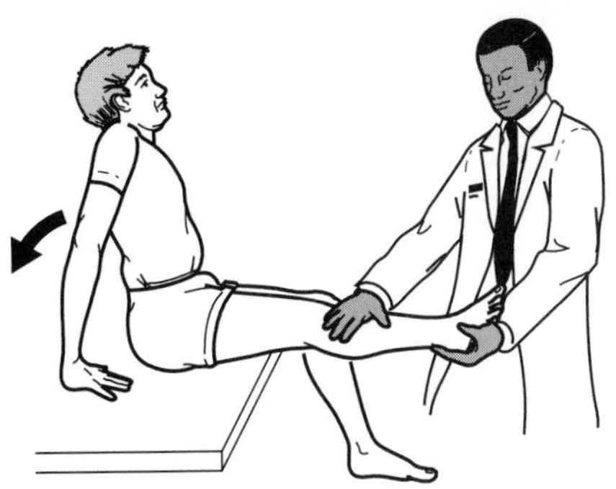

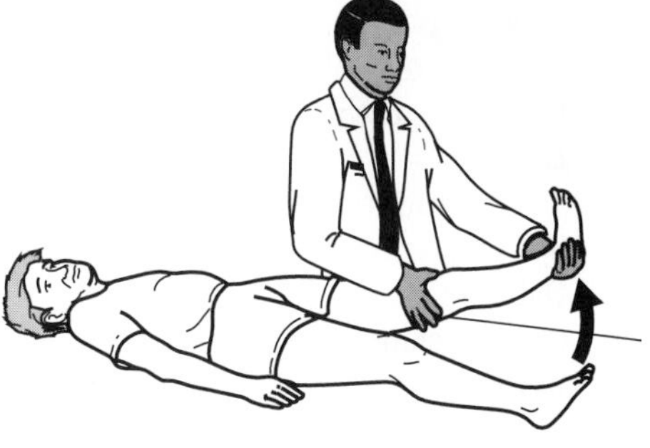

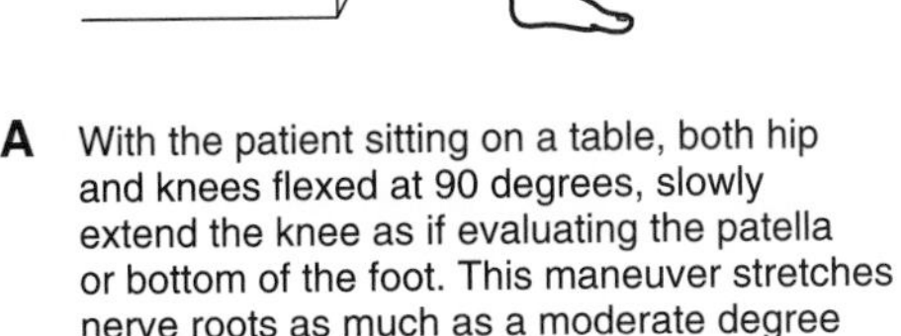

A With the patient sitting on a table, both hip and knees flexed at 90 degrees, slowly extend the knee as if evaluating the patella or bottom of the foot. This maneuver stretches nerve roots as much as a moderate degree of supine SLR.

B Ask the patient to lie as straight as possible on the table in the supine position. With one hand placed above the knee of the leg being examined, exert enough firm pressure to keep the knee fully extended. Ask the patient to relax.

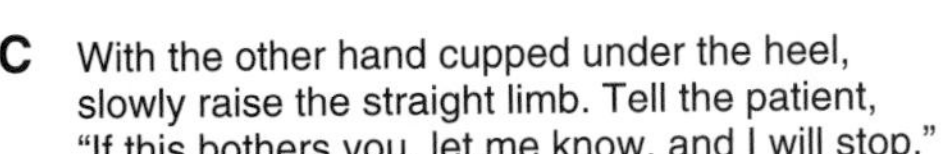

C With the other hand cupped under the heel, slowly raise the straight limb. Tell the patient, "If this bothers you, let me know, and I will stop."

D Monitor for any movement of the pelvis before complaints are elicited. True sciatic tension should elicit complaints before the hamstrings are stretched enough to move the pelvis.

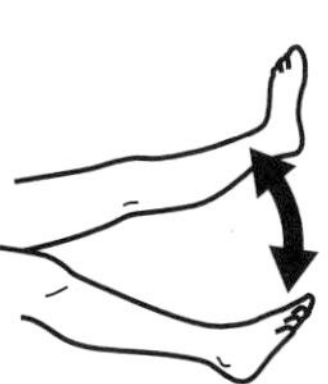

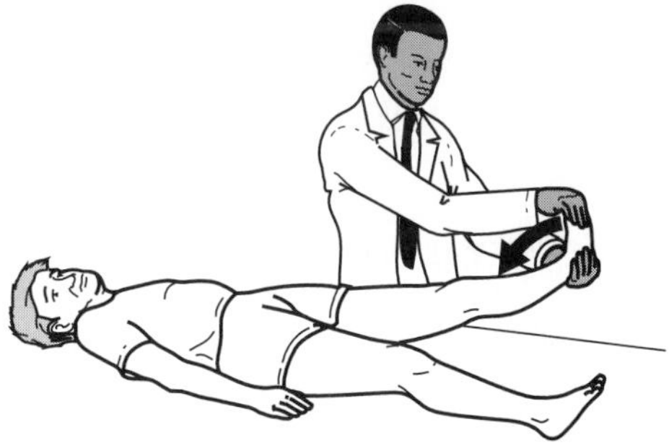

E Estimate the degree of leg elevation that elicits complaint from the patient. Then determine the most distal area of discomfort: back, hip, thigh, knee, or below the knee.

F While holding the leg at the limit of straight leg raising, dorsiflex the ankle. Note whether this aggravates the pain. Internal rotation of the limb can also increase the tension on the sciatic nerve roots.

Figure 12-13 Instructions for sitting knee extension test. (Adapted from Bigos S et al: *Acute low back problems in adults: clinical practice guideline, quick reference guide,* AHCPR Pub. No. 95-0643, Rockville, Md, 1994, US Department of Health and Human Services.)

Measure bilateral limb length.

Rectal examination for an enlarged prostate gland or a rectal carcinoma may suggest a cause for back pain. Abdominal examination is also appropriate.

Differential Diagnoses

Trauma: acute soft tissue strain, chronic strain
Overuse syndromes
Trigger points
Generalized inflammatory joint disease such as ankylosing spondylitis
Degenerative disk disease
HNP
Degenerative facet joint disease
Spinal stenosis
Osteoporosis
Compression fracture
Infection
Metastases, tumor
Spondylolisthesis
Viscerogenic source, such as abdominal aortic aneurysm, degenerative disease of the hip
Sacroiliitis
Cauda equina syndrome
Herpes zoster radiculopathy
Diabetic radiculopathy
Arachnoiditis
Sciatica
Psychogenic or nonorganic source
Vascular claudication

A number of conditions can present as low back pain in any given person. The following seven conditions are the most important of those typically evaluated in the primary care setting.

Back Strain

Back strain is ligamentous or muscular strain secondary to postural inadequacy, either continuously or with a single event. Pain may be limited to one spot or cover a larger area. Pain may radiate to the buttock or posterior thigh. However, pain referral does not necessarily indicate any mechanical compression of the neural element. The etiology is not always clear but may be related to muscular, ligamentous, or fascial strain. Attacks vary in intensity. Findings may include muscle spasm.

Symptoms

Pain that may be severe in the back, buttock, or one or both thighs
Recent increase in physical activity for the patient

Pain that begins 12 to 36 hours after an event
Muscular stiffness
Pain accentuated by standing and bending
Pain alleviated by rest and lying down

Focused Physical Examination

Tenderness over involved area
Muscle spasm
No evidence of nerve root impingement
Posture may be tilted forward or to side, with difficulty in ambulating

Differential Diagnosis

Lumbosacral strain syndrome

Diagnostic Tests

Routine lumbosacral spine films are generally not indicated at the first visit. However, if a patient fails to respond after 2 weeks of conservative therapy, consider lumbosacral x-ray films. Plain x-ray films do show the changes of degenerative disk and facet joint disease, but these conditions are so common after the fifth decade that x-ray films are not very useful in confirming the structure that is causing pain in a patient.

Treatment

Therapeutics
Limited physical activity, particularly bending, stooping, heavy lifting, twisting
Heat or ice
Analgesics: acetaminophen, or NSAIDs on a regular rather than on an as-needed basis
Muscle relaxants: used with caution (see Box 12-1)

Education. Patients with uncomplicated low back pain can be managed conservatively and directed toward exercise programs that provide acute treatment and long-term prevention of future injury. Patients should return to normal activity as soon as possible. Advise against activities such as vacuuming, which increase the force applied to the lower spine (Figure 12-14, Box 12-3).

Follow-up. Should the patient fail to respond or should pain recur, the patient ought to be reexamined 3 to 4 weeks later to investigate the possibility of a medical (systemic) cause of back pain.

Degenerative Disk Disease

The disk begins to degenerate early in life. According to autopsy studies, most patients over age 30 have pathologic evidence of disk degeneration (Cole and Herring, 1997). The intervertebral disk allows spinal mobility while retaining axial stability. Proteoglycan content decreases with age, leading to lower imbibition pressure, reduced water content,

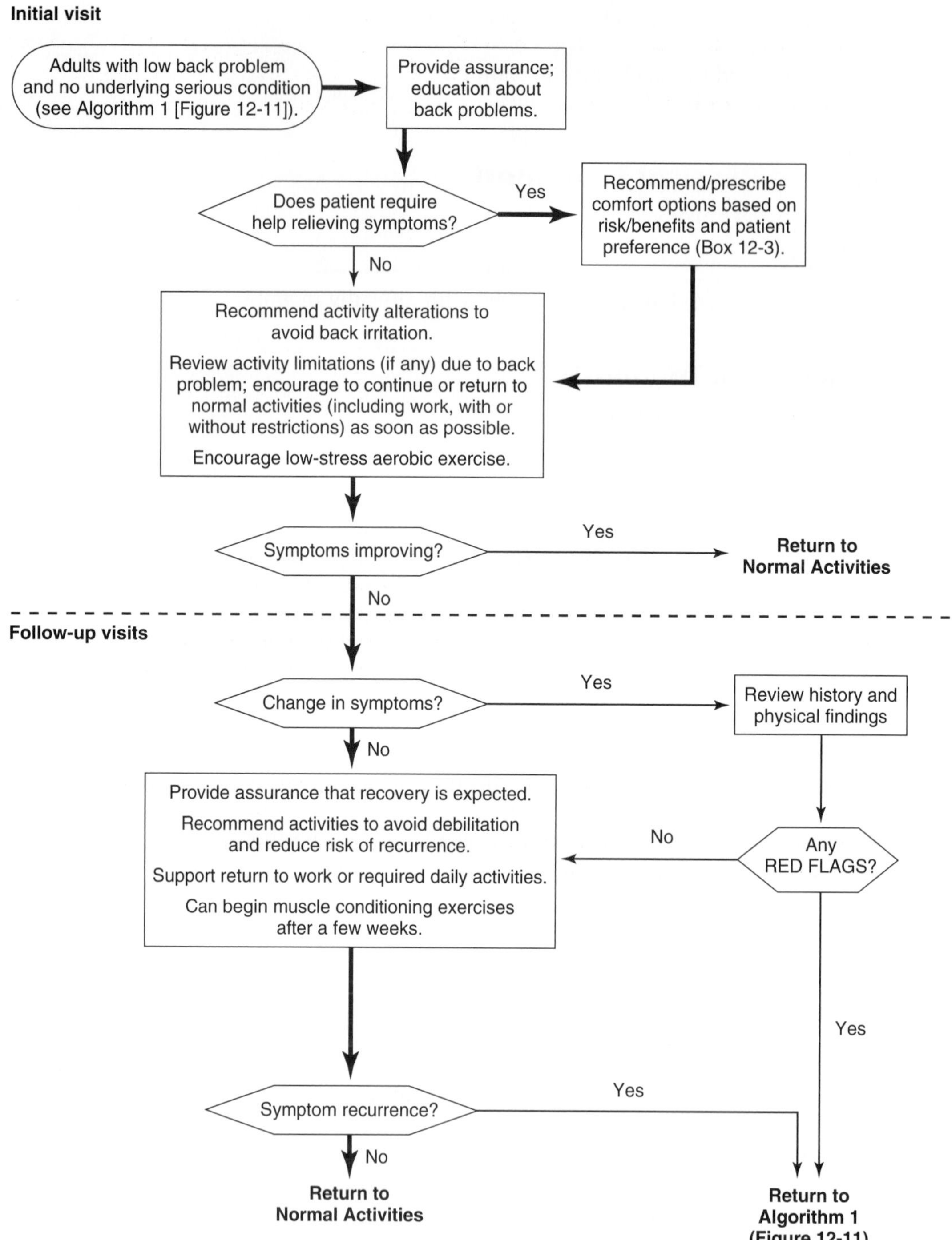

Figure 12-14 Algorithm 2. Treatment of acute low back problem on initial and follow-up visits. (Adapted from Bigos S et al: *Acute low back problems in adults: clinical practice guideline, quick reference guide,* AHCPR Pub. No. 95-0643, Rockville, Md, 1994, US Department of Health and Human Services.)

Box 12-3

Comfort Options for Patients with Acute Low Back Problem

Oral medications
  Acetaminophen
Gradual return to normal activity
  Bedrest not recommended
Exercise
  Low-stress aerobics
  Gradual increase to walking, biking, or swimming
Shoe insoles or shoe lifts
Ice or heat if patient finds comfort

Modified from Bigos S et al: *Acute low back problems in adults: clinical practice guidelines, quick reference guide,* AHCPR No. 95-0642, Rockville, Md, 1994, US Department of Health and Human Services.

and associated fibrous replacement of the nucleus pulposus. There are changes in the blood supply to the disk such that repair cannot keep pace with degeneration.

Degenerated disks have the following characteristics: decreased disk height, increased lateral bulging, reduced imbibition pressure, and increased mobility. Degenerative disk disease is a syndrome initiated by degenerative changes in the disk that secondarily involve other spinal elements that contribute to the symptom complex. Degenerative disk disease and prolapsed intervertebral disks are common causes of low back pain. Lumbar disk disease is most common at the L4-5 and L5-S1 levels and is less common between other vertebral bodies. Not all low back pains are due to prolapsed disk, and not all prolapsed disks need to be removed by surgery. At least 30% of asymptomatic individuals have abnormal imaging studies. Therefore treat the patient, not the imaging study. Most patients with back pain due to prolapsed disks can be treated successfully by conservative means.

History

Pain is usually located in the low back or gluteal region on one or both sides. Radiation of pain into the buttock or thigh is likely to be radiated from adjacent spinal joints or muscles rather than from the nerve root. Radiation of pain into the lower leg or foot may be caused by disk pressure on the nerve root.

Symptoms

Symptoms are of variable duration.
A traumatic event may precede pain. Coughing, sneezing, straining, lifting weight out in front of body, twisting, or bending at the waist may exacerbate the pain.
Bedrest may provide some relief from the pain.
There is muscle stiffness.

Focused Physical Examination

Pain with back flexion
Limited ROM
Muscle spasms
Possible neurologic signs with nerve root compression

Differential Diagnosis

Degenerative disk disease

Diagnostic Tests

Lumbosacral spine films: Disk space is narrowed, with horizontally directed osteophytes and reactive sclerosis of vertebral end plates. Vacuum phenomenon (description for a dark line seen in the intervertebral space) is considered a definite sign of disk degeneration. There are degenerative changes of the facet joints with osteophyte encroachment on the intervertebral foramen.

Consider MRI.

Treatment

Therapeutics
Rest: Limit activities that contribute to pain.
Analgesics: Consider NSAIDs.
Use local heat.
Consider local trigger point injections.
Muscle relaxants: Use with caution (see Box 12-1).

Education. Exercises to increase mobility and strengthen muscles begin after the acute pain episode or spasm is over. Continue for maintenance of benefits.

Avoid prone-lying activities, which accentuate lumbar lordosis. Consider lumbosacral support.

Follow-up. Should the patient fail to respond or should pain recur, the patient should be reexamined 3 to 4 weeks later to investigate the possibility of a medical (systemic) cause of back pain.

Herniated Nucleus Pulposus (HNP)

Most disk ruptures occur during the third, fourth, and fifth decades of life. More than 80% of all lumbar disk herniations occur at L4-5 and L5-S1.

Tears in the annulus fibrosus allow the contents of the nucleus pulposus to herniate beyond their normal confines. Tears in the annulus may be associated with transient episodes of low back pain. Herniation of the nucleus may result in sudden, severe pain if neural elements are compressed and inflamed by the nuclear contents. Sudden pressure placed on the lumbar spine that may occur with flexion (e.g., bending over to lift a heavy object or lifting with the arms extended) can precipitate the rupture. However, many patients who have a herniated disk do not give a history of injury or a sudden increase in pressure (Barker, Burton, and Zieve, 1995).

History

The major complaint is pain. Classic discogenic history factors that worsen the pain are sitting, standing, lying, arising from seated position, the first 20 to 30 minutes of the day, coughing, sneezing, straining, lifting weight out in front of body, twisting, and bending at the waist.

Features common to symptomatic presentations include prolonged sitting, twisting and rotation, occupations involving vibration such as truck drivers or operators of heavy machines, and chronic cough.

The patient may have a prior history of low back pain.

Symptoms

Onset is usually spontaneous. A sharp, lancinating pain may be insidious or sudden and is associated with a snapping or tearing sensation. Pain radiates from the back down the leg in the anatomic distribution of the affected nerve root. The patient may complain of thigh pain or calf pain, with accompanying numbness and paresthesias. Leg pain is usually more pronounced than back pain when herniation has occurred.

Focused Physical Examination

There is decreased ROM in flexion.

Pain may be so severe that the patient resists examination and splints the back in lateral lumbar flexion and hip flexion.

Patients tend to drift away from the involved side as they bend.

Antalgic gait: The patient holds the involved leg flexed to put as little weight as possible on the extremity.

The neurologic examination may be undependable because the nerve may still function or the patient may have a deficit from a previous injury (Table 12-2).

Reflex changes, weakness, atrophy, or sensory loss must conform to the rest of the clinical picture. The clinical picture varies depending on the level involved and the degree of herniation.

The straight leg-raising test is positive (see Figure 12-13).

Differential Diagnosis

Herniated lumbar nucleolus pulposus

Diagnostic Tests

The initial diagnosis of a herniated disk is ordinarily made on the basis of the history and physical examination. Plain x-ray films of the lumbosacral spine rarely help the diagnosis but should be obtained to rule out other sources of pain, such as infection or tumor.

TABLE 12-2 Symptoms and Findings in Lumbar Disk Syndromes

Disk Level	Nerve Root	Symptoms and Findings
L3-4	L4	**Pain:** Low back, posterolateral aspect of the thigh, across patella, anteromedial aspect of leg **Sensory change:** Anterior aspect of knee, anteromedial aspect of leg **Motor deficit:** Quadriceps (knee extension) **Reflex change:** Knee jerk
L4-5	L5	**Pain:** Lateral, posterolateral aspect of thigh, leg **Sensory change:** Lateral aspect of leg, dorsum of foot, first webspace, great toe **Motor deficit:** Great toe extension, ankle dorsiflexion, heel walking difficult (footdrop may occur) **Reflex change:** Minor (posterior tibial jerk depressed)
L5-S1	S1	**Pain:** Posterolateral aspect of thigh, leg, heel **Sensory change:** Posterior aspect of calf, heel, lateral aspect of foot (3 toes) **Motor deficit:** Calf, plantarflexion of foot, great toe; toe walking weak **Reflex change:** Ankle jerk
Cauda equina syndrome	Massive midline protrusion	**Pain:** Low back, thigh, legs; often bilateral **Sensory change:** Thighs, legs, feet, perineum, often bilateral **Motor deficit:** Variable; may be bowel, bladder incontinence **Reflex change:** Ankle jerk (may be bilateral)

Adapted from Bigos S et al: *Acute low back problems in adults,* 1994, AHCPR Publication No. 95-0642. Rockville, Md, US Department of Health and Human Services.

Other tests such as the EMG, CT scan, or MRI are confirmatory by nature and can be misinformative when they are used as screening devices.

Consider CBC, sedimentation rate, and chemistries to evaluate systemic illness in patients who have failed conservative therapy.

Treatment

Therapeutics

Controlled physical activity, sometimes bedrest; acute herniation usually requires 2 weeks of significant rest before pain substantially eases

Analgesics: NSAIDs

Muscle relaxants: used with caution (see Box 12-1)

Local heat

Education

Increase activity as pain improves.

Instruct patient in exercises for strengthening low back and abdominal musculature.

Instruct patient not to bend, twist, stoop, stretch, lift, sit for prolonged periods, or carry anything heavier than the Sunday newspaper.

The long-term prognosis for patients with disk herniation is quite good. Between 85% and 90% of patients respond to conservative measures. Patience is a virtue. It may take up to 6 weeks before there is any appreciable decrease in pain.

Lumbar Spinal Stenosis

Spinal stenosis is a narrowing of the spinal canal that leads to mechanical pressure on structures within the canal. Activities involved in extension, which narrows the foramina and spinal canal, are associated with increased symptoms. The narrowing is usually slowly progressive and gradually advances over several years unless other conditions intervene. Back and radicular symptoms increase with walking variable distances and are relieved by lumbar flexion or sitting. Stenosis may occur as early as the fourth decade but is uncommon before age 55. A history of significant prior disk or facet joint degenerative disease is common. The intermittent nature of symptoms may be due to increased venous congestion within the confined space of the spinal canal. Many patients with spinal stenosis have symptoms mimicking those of peripheral vascular insufficiency or claudication. These patients develop lower extremity pain while standing, walking, or hyperextending the spine in the absence of any evidence of peripheral vascular disease. Painful paresthesias are present in the feet or legs and may radiate to the hip girdle or lower trunk. Patients may experience lower extremity numbness and weakness. These symptoms are relieved by rest or flexion of the spine (the patient may report relief by bending forward as if to tie shoelaces) (Barker, Burton, and Zieve, 1995). With central canal stenosis, symptoms are generally noted bilaterally, fairly symmetrically, but in a nonspecific distribution. With lateral foraminal stenosis, symptoms are generally noted unilaterally in a fairly specific dermatomal distribution.

History

The history is the absolute key to diagnosis:

Obtain a medical history. Onset of pain: Gradual progression of pain is usual; sudden changes in symptoms require an explanation other than stenosis, such as HNP or tumor.

Symptoms: walking> standing> lying.

Sitting is often asymptomatic and relieves symptoms.

May complain of weakness, pain, tingling, or numbness of one or both legs after walking.

Legs feel "heavy" or rubbery.

Valsalva maneuver should not affect symptoms in pure stenosis.

While the patient is walking, relief is obtained with positions that increase lumbar flexion, such as squatting, stooping, going uphill, or leaning on a walker or cart.

Late in the course of the disease, patients walk with a kyphotic posture and spend most of their time sitting. Patients report sitting in a flexed position while sleeping. Sitting is comfortable until late in the course of the disease.

Bicycling and long car rides are well tolerated.

Symptoms

Back pain
Buttock pain
Radiating lower extremity pain or dysesthesias, which are worse with standing and walking
Main symptoms are sensory: vague dysesthesias, coldness, vague sense of weakness or "giving way," bizarre symptoms such as water trickling down leg

Focused Physical Examination

Muscle atrophy and asymmetric reflex changes may appear late in the course of the disease. Neurologic changes occur only after the patient is stressed. The following stress test can be used in an outpatient clinic: After a neurologic examination, the patient is asked to walk up and down the corridor until the symptoms occur or the patient has walked 300 feet. A repeat examination is then performed; in many cases the second examination is positive for a focal neurologic deficit when the first was negative.

ROM: Forward flexion is usually normal. At times, the patient is more supple and is able to touch the floor easily. Extension of the spine may be limited.

Straight leg-raising test is negative in most patients.

Differential Diagnosis

Lumbar spinal stenosis

Diagnostic Tests

Plain x-ray films of the lumbosacral spine, with AP, lateral, and oblique views, are usually sufficient for diagnosis. CT or MRI may be ordered to support clinical findings or if surgery is considered.

Treatment

Therapeutics

No treatment is necessary for asymptomatic patients.
Analgesics or NSAIDs are given as needed when patients are symptomatic.
A lumbosacral corset is used.
Relative rest (supine with slight lumbar flexion) is used. "Let pain be your guide."
Consider epidural steroid injections.
Use an exercise program to increase flexibility and strengthen abdominal and back muscles. Stationary bicycles and walking either on level surfaces or uphill are generally well tolerated (Georgetown, 1998).

Education

"Poor posture is acceptable."
Symptoms may be intermittent, and patients need encouragement to get through the episodes.

Have patients use chairs that place them in a flexed position.
Discuss potential surgery when conservative treatment fails to relieve symptoms and pain interferes with daily activities.

Follow-up. The patient should return to see the health care provider if symptoms persist or worsen. Refer for possible surgical intervention if symptoms persist despite aggressive conservative care.

Spondylolisthesis

Spondylolisthesis is a spinal condition in which all or part of a vertebra has slipped forward on another. There are several different types of spondylolisthesis, but in the most common the lesion is in the isthmus or pars interarticularis. In this type, symptoms appear in late childhood and adolescence. Most commonly, L5-S1 is involved, and the location of the pain is in the L5-S1 dermatome. The minority of patients have radicular symptoms. Consider this diagnosis in patients who have a history of involvement in sports with significant lumbar extension and rotation and that stress the pars interarticularis (e.g., gymnastics, dance, martial arts).

The next type of spondylolsthesis is degenerative and is the result of long-standing segmental instability with remodeling of articular processes. This type of spondylolisthesis presents in the fifth or sixth decade. Most commonly, L4-5 is involved, and pain is typically unilateral radicular, probably because of resultant foraminal stenosis. Bilateral calf pseudoclaudication is less common. The incidence increases with age; on rare occasions the onset can be as early as age 40. The female-to-male ratio is 6:1 (Cole and Herring, 1997). A slip of up to 10% (isthmic subtype) does not appear to increase the likelihood of back problems, but slippage beyond 25% increases the likelihood of low back symptoms, as does wedging of L5. In degenerative spondylolisthesis, slip rarely progresses past 33%. Footdrop may occur, but dural signs are rare. Most cases can be treated effectively with conservative measures (Figure 12-15).

History

Half of patients relate an acute episode of back and leg pain after a sudden twisting or lifting motion. Low back pain predominates initially, but over time leg pain develops and becomes the most annoying part of the problem. Pain is aggravated by activity and relieved by rest. The patient is seldom aware of any sensory or motor deficits. Occasionally, muscle spasm and local tenderness may be elicited.

Symptoms

Low back pain
Leg pain
Hamstring tightness
Acute back and leg pain after a sudden twisting or lifting motion

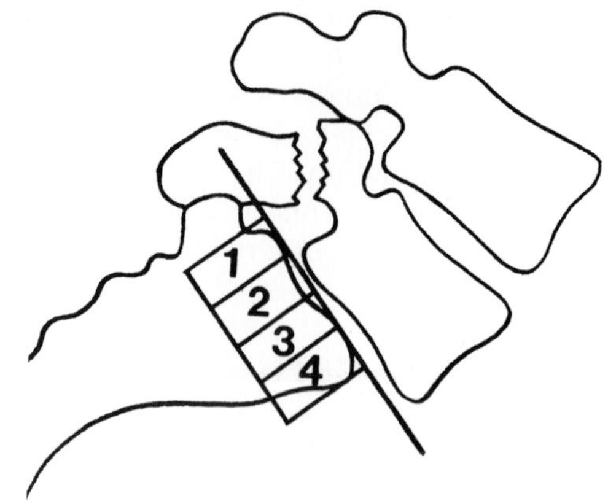

Figure 12-15 Meyerding's classification of spondylolisthesis. The amount of slippage is graded 1 to 4. Grade 1 represents 25% forward displacement; grade 2, 25% to 50%; grade 3, 50% to 75%; and grade 4, greater than 75%. (From Mercier LR: *Practical orthopedics,* ed 4, St Louis, 1995, Mosby.)

Focused Physical Examination

Exaggeration of the lumbar lordosis with a palpable step-off and a dimple at the site of the abnormality
Hamstring tightness
Normal ROM
Pain with back hyperextension
No postural scoliosis in the absence of any radicular pain
Morning stiffness
Mild muscle spasm

Differential Diagnosis

Spondylolisthesis, isthmic vs. degenerative

Diagnostic Tests

X-ray films, particularly the lateral views, confirm the diagnosis. Even the slightest amount of forward slipping of the body of the involved vertebra is readily discernible, and the oblique views disclose the actual defect in the pars.

Treatment

Therapeutics
Relative rest should be provided during times of flares.
Antiinflammatories or analgesics can be beneficial if leg pain is a significant problem.
Consider muscle relaxants.
Exercises, usually a flexion exercise program, should be started when the patient is asymptomatic.
Advise patients to own a lumbosacral corset or support for occasional use during strenuous activities (Georgetown University, 1998).

Education

Educate patient regarding proper body mechanics.

Reinforce the need to continue exercise program to prevent further injury or exacerbation of symptoms.

Follow-up. Patient should return to provider if symptoms persist or worsen. Refer for surgical intervention if symptoms persist despite aggressive conservative care.

Cauda Equina Syndrome

Cauda equina syndrome results from a mechanical compression of the neural elements, usually a result of an acute disk rupture at the L4-5 disk space. Only a small percentage of patients with low back pain have cauda equina, and it typically affects those in their third decade. The incidence is less than 1% of patients with lumbosacral pain. Because a missed diagnosis can have disastrous consequences, patients with suspected cauda equina syndrome require immediate referral to a specialist. This is the only entity affecting the lumbosacral spine that requires emergent operative intervention.

History

Pain as major complaint
Saddle anesthesia
Urinary retention
Bowel incontinence
Possible episode of trauma
Classic discogenic factors that worsen the pain: sitting > standing> lying; arising from seated position; coughing, sneezing, straining; lifting weight out in front of body; twisting; or bending at the waist
Possible prior history of low back pain

Symptoms

Severe low back pain
Bilateral lower extremity weakness
Bilateral sciatic pain
Saddle anesthesia
Bowel or bladder incontinence, with urinary retention the most common complaint
Frank paraplegia

Focused Physical Examination

Confirmation of the previous signs plus major progressive motor weakness
Neurologic abnormalities that are consistent with location of disk herniation

Differential Diagnosis

Cauda equina compression syndrome

Diagnostic Tests/Therapeutics/Education/Follow-up

Emergent advanced imaging (e.g., CT or MRI) and referral to a specialist for emergency decompression

Fractures of the Vertebrae

Vertebral fractures are common in the lower thoracic and upper lumbar regions. Most vertebral body fractures occur after some mechanical stress such as slipping on a stair, lifting, or jumping. Upper and middle thoracic regions are more stable and less prone to fractures because of the ribs, the shape of the articular processes, and the direction of the facets. Unique anatomic features of the thoracolumbar spine, T12-L1, predispose it to a high incidence of fracture. It is the junction between the relatively immobile thoracic spine (stabilized by the thoracic ribs) and the mobile lumbar spine (surrounded by soft tissue). It is also the junction between the kyphotic (forward curve) thoracic spine and the lordotic (reverse curve) lumbar spine. Change in facet orientation from the coronal plane (thoracic spine) to the sagittal plane (lumbar spine) predisposes the thoracolumbar junction to rotation and flexion strain (Cole and Herring, 1997).

Stable compression fractures of the vertebral bodies with intact spinal ligaments occur after a trauma such as a fall from a height and landing on the feet or buttocks. In addition, a downward blow to the shoulders may cause a fracture of the vertebral body. This force compresses the anterior part of the vertebra and leads to a compression fracture. Usually the force needed to compress the vertebral body in healthy bone is considerable. Sometimes the anterior and posterior surfaces of a vertebra are compressed to the same extent, especially in metastatic disease. In another type of injury, the spine remains straight instead of flexing and pushes the disk into the body of the vertebra above or below; the vertebral body explodes into small fragments that get displaced in all directions. This is a burst fracture (Mehta, 1997).

Vertebral compression fractures are common, especially among the elderly, and usually are the result of a flexion injury when the spine is abruptly flexed (Barker, Burton, and Zieve, 1995). Compression fractures may occur after only a minimum of trauma in diseased bone, as in osteoporosis, multiple myeloma, metastatic cancer, or hyperparathyroidism. Also, they may occur with minimal stress, such as with sneezing, bending, or lifting a light object. Back pain begins acutely and is sometimes associated with pain that radiates laterally and anteriorly. With multiple vertebral fractures, usually with anterior wedging, patients lose height and develop the characteristic dorsal kyphosis and cervical lordosis sometimes known as the "dowager's hump." At least one third of all vertebral compression fractures are asymptomatic. The overwhelming majority occur in people with osteoporosis. About 45% of patients with osteoporotic compression fracture experience another fracture in the next 12 months (Cole and Herring, 1997).

History

Mechanism of injury
History of osteoporosis, multiple myeloma, metastatic cancer, hyperparathyroidism
History of corticosteroid use
Positions such as sitting or walking that exacerbate pain

Cigarette smoking
Family history
Early or surgically induced menopause

Symptoms

In acute fracture, severe pain is localized over the affected vertebral body. Occasionally the pain radiates into the flanks, upper portion of the posterior thighs, or abdomen. Back motion, especially spinal flexion, aggravates the discomfort, as does prolonged sitting, standing, and the Valsalva maneuver.

The most common locations of painful vertebrae are T10, T11, T12, and L1 with resultant lumbar pain. Lumbar fractures may result in lower extremity pain and, occasionally, neurologic symptoms. Neurologic or radicular symptoms distant from an area of fracture are unusual; if they are present, other pathologic conditions must be considered.

Some patients are left with persistent nagging, dull spinal pain after a vertebral body fracture secondary to osteoporosis, and this pain may persist even in the absence of new fractures on x-ray films. The source of this pain may be microfractures too small to be detected by x-ray films or biomechanical effects of the deformity on the lumbar spine below.

Spasm of the paraspinous muscles contributes to the back pain.

Focused Physical Examination

Inspection. Abrasions and bruises indicate the direction and severity of forces involved. Visible deformity suggests a displaced, unstable fracture.

Palpation. Tenderness over the spinous processes helps localize the fracture. The interspinous ligament normally feels firm on palpation. When this ligament is torn, the interspinous space feels softer. In addition, palpation of the paraspinous muscles reveals spasm.

Range of Motion. These tests are *not* performed when a fracture is suspected to avoid damaging the spinal cord or cauda equina.

Special Tests. A detailed neurologic examination is carried out and is often normal. On abdominal examination, patients with severe pain secondary to an acute fracture may demonstrate a loss of bowel sounds, ileus, or bladder distention secondary to acute urinary retention (Borenstein, Wiesel, and Boden, 1995).

Differential Diagnoses

Vertebral compression fracture
Back strain
Tumor
Multiple myeloma

Diagnostic Tests

AP and lateral x-ray films: The AP view may appear nearly normal, whereas the lateral view shows wedging or compression of the normally square vertebra. A T12 fracture may be hidden by the liver and an underexposed lateral x-ray film. Compression of more than 20% should arouse suspicion that the fracture is an unstable burst fracture, and a CT scan should be obtained to check for fracture of the middle and posterior columns. The review of the CT scan is helpful in deciding on surgical intervention to relieve pressure on neurologic structures.

A bone scan is useful in demonstrating whether there are single or multiple fractures. A healing compression fracture may continue to be abnormal on bone scan for up to 2 years. The bone has healed before the bone scan becomes normal because of continued remodeling. More rapid resolution of an abnormal bone scan is usually seen in younger patients (Cole and Herring, 1997).

Treatment

Therapeutics. With lumbar or thoracic vertebral compression fractures, management includes rest, adequate analgesia, and gradual ambulation when the patient is free from severe pain. A lumbosacral support or, for the patient with thoracic vertebral fracture, a chairback or hyperextension brace may be helpful in alleviating pain. Bending and lifting activities should be restricted for 6 to 12 weeks (Barker, Burton, and Zieve, 1995).

Education. Instruct in appropriate use of the support or brace. Inform the patient that pain from a vertebral fracture may persist for several months, although the incapacitating component is usually only 2 to 3 weeks in duration (Barker, Burton, and Zieve, 1995). Instruct the patient to contact the health care provider immediately if neurologic symptoms develop.

Instruct the patient in proper body mechanics, including prevention of falls, if appropriate. Review the patient's home environment for safety issues.

Follow-up. Telephone follow-up in 2 to 3 weeks. Further evaluation or referral if symptoms persist or worsen.

Summary

Older persons are at high risk for musculoskeletal injury, which can lead to significant loss of function, pain, further morbidity, and even mortality. Age-related changes are significant, especially in bone mass and muscle strength. A history and physical examination are critical in localizing the area of injury and in determining whether the injury is muscular or skeletal in origin. The list of differential diagnoses can be significant. Diagnostic tests such as radiology studies, EMG, or MRI may be necessary to locate the source of pain and to determine appropriate therapy. Treatment often requires a multifaceted approach of medication, therapy, education, and surgery. The decision to pursue surgical intervention in a frail, older adult requires consideration of a number of issues, including comorbidities.

Resources

Healthwise Handbook
Neck and Back Pain
http://www.betterhealth.com

References

Barker LR, Burton JR, Zieve PD: *Ambulatory medicine,* ed 4, Baltimore, 1995, Williams & Wilkins.

Borenstein DG, Wiesel SW, Boden SD: *Low back pain: medical diagnosis and comprehensive management*, ed 2, Philadelphia, 1995, WB Saunders.

Cole AC, Herring SA: *The low back pain handbook: a practical guide for the primary care clinician*, St Louis, 1997, Mosby.

Georgetown University Medical Center Orthopaedic Spine Clinic (1998).

McIntosh E: Low back pain in adults: guidelines for the history and physical exam, *Adv Nurse Pract* 5(8):17-25, 1997.

Mehta AJ: *Common musculoskeletal problems,* Philadelphia, 1997, Hanley & Belfus.

Mercier LR: *Practical orthopedics,* ed 4, St Louis, 1995, Mosby.

Millstein JH: Three steps to diagnosing shoulder pain, *Intern Med* 18(11):14-30, 1997.

O'Mara JW, Wiesel SW: Initial diagnosis of low back pain, *J Musculoskel Med,* October, 10-33, 1997.

Sykes TF: A systematic approach to acute shoulder pain, *Patient Care* 11:34-51, 1997.

Wiesel SW, Delahay JN: *Essentials of orthopaedic surgery,* ed 2, Philadelphia, 1997, WB Saunders.

Wilson FC, Lin PP: *General orthopaedics,* New York, 1997, McGraw-Hill.

13

Musculoskeletal: Common Disorders

Physiologic Age-related Changes

With aging, there is a gradual loss of bone mass and an incremental process of bone resorption without successful formation of new bone mass. Bone mineral density has been shown to decrease in women with increasing age. Several factors appear to be predictive of bone mass: family and reproductive history, nutritional factors, medication use, and exercise. This loss of bone mass is combined with the diminished muscle strength that results from the age-related decrease in muscle fiber. However, studies have shown that regular exercise, especially resistance training, demonstrates a reduced rate of decline in muscle strength (Buchner et al., 1992). Function, rather than the negative results of age-related change or pathology, is the major defining characteristic of musculoskeletal health in older adults.

This chapter discusses the following conditions: osteoarthritis, rheumatoid arthritis, polymyalgia rheumatica, giant cell arteritis, and fibromyalgia.

Osteoarthritis

Epidemiology

Osteoarthritis (OA) is the most common form of joint disease. An estimated 15% of the population, 40 million U.S. adults, are afflicted with this condition. The projected prevalence for the year 2020 is that more than 18% of the population, 59.4 million people, will be affected (Lawrence et al., 1998). More than 80% of adults over age 55 have radiographic features of OA, and 90% of 40-year-olds have radiographic features of OA in weight-bearing joints (Hellmann, 1997; Brandt, 1996). However, there is no relationship between radiographic features of OA and symptoms; only 10% to 30% of the older group report symptomatic pain and disability. Primary idiopathic OA is one of the leading causes of disability in both men and women by age 65 (Ling and Bathon, 1998). The significant prevalence of OA brings a high cost to society through loss of productivity and loss of self-care abilities, with a resulting drain on health care costs (Levy et al., 1993).

Definition

Osteoarthritis is a chronic disease that involves the entire joint. It is characterized by dynamic biochemical and biomechanical changes that cause the central loss of articular cartilage and active remodeling, especially on subchondral bone, which affects the joint structures. Inflammation is usually minimal. The radiographic features of OA are joint space narrowing, osteophytes, subchondral sclerosis, and subchondral cysts. It affects weight-bearing joints (hip, knee, spine, hand, and feet) and is thought to result in part from mechanical wear and tear: however, the precise cause is unknown (Lozada and Altman, 1997; Brandt, 1996).

Pathology

With OA, the articular cartilage becomes thinner, tears, and disrupts the joint capsule, resulting in bone remodeling and deformity. As the cartilage wears away, less protection and reduced cushioning cause ulceration (eburnation), spurs (osteophytes), synovitis, hypertrophy of the capsule, and periarticular muscle wasting. There is general disruption of collagen and the other elements necessary for joint integrity. Joint inflammation is rare in OA, but soft tissue damage can result from osteophytes and bone remodeling.

Risk Factors

Although significant risk factors such as age and family history are not modifiable risks, obesity is also a significant risk for the development of OA in weight-bearing joints, especially in women. Primary care providers need to concentrate on the prevention of OA by addressing the association of obesity and OA with their obese patients. The protection of joints from joint trauma reduces the risk for OA, and this factor can be discussed with younger patients.

History

The frequent, classic, and clinical presentation of OA usually includes joint pain, swelling, decreased range of motion, and crepitus with movement. Pain and stiffness are the major complaints described by patients with OA. The practitioner gathers information concerning the dimensions of the pain and the description of affected joints and associated muscle spasms. An asymmetric joint pattern is typical of OA. Duration of morning stiffness is an important aspect; most OA patients report less than 30 minutes of morning stiffness (McCarty, 1997). Pain is usually relieved by rest, and pain at rest is often an indication of disease severity (Hellmann, 1997).

The practitioner needs to probe symptoms of fatigue, a vague general malaise, recent febrile illness, and general emotional state, with an awareness that some older patients may underreport by discounting symptoms. Osteoarthritis does not usually present with any systemic manifestations. During history taking, the differential diagnosis becomes paramount (Table 13-1).

Focused Physical Examination

Palpation for joint tenderness is an essential part of the examination. A grimace by the patient when shaking hands certainly is an indication of tenderness. The practitioner must exert sufficient pressure to elicit a painful response from a tender joint. Pressing gently is of no value and can lead to considerable confusion. Certainly good sense would dictate that a red, swollen joint is painful, and therefore there is no need to confirm this observation. In a systematic method, each joint is assessed for tenderness, swelling, skin temperature, the presence of crepitus, and muscle strength. Both passive and active range of motion of all joints are essential aspects of the focused physical examination. The characteristic distribution of involved joints is distal interphalangeal (Heberden's nodes), proximal interphalangeal (Bouchard's nodes), the thumb, carpal and metacarpal joints, the hallux metatarsophalangeal, and the hip, knee, and spine (Levy and Sethi, 1998) (Figure 13-1).

It is important to measure height accurately for baseline data. Observation of gait allows the practitioner to assess for limping or uneven gait, which is indicative of hip or knee involvement. Certain laboratory tests for osteoarthritis can be performed on a routine basis (Table 13-2).

For diagnostic tests for differential diagnosis, see Table 13-3.

Treatment

Pharmacologic Interventions

Nonsteroidal antiinflammatory drugs (NSAIDs) have been the most commonly prescribed pharmacologic agents for pain management of arthritis, but they should be avoided when treating older patients. The problem is that NSAIDs produce serious adverse side effects in the elderly population (precipitation of confusion, gastric bleeding, and renal insufficiency) and are known to have adverse interactions with multiple other drugs (Table 13-4 and Box 13-1).

In a recent study at McGill University, investigators commented that NSAID use "increases the risk for hospitalization and death from gastrointestinal bleeding and perforation" (McLeod et al., 1997). Unnecessary prescriptions for NSAIDs were written during 42% of visits, and suboptimal management of NSAID-related side effects was sufficiently common to raise questions about the use of NSAIDs in general (Tamblyn et al., 1997). The primary reason for using NSAIDs is to treat the inflammation associated with inflammatory arthritis, but they are also widely used as effective analgesic and antipyretic agents (Carson and Strom, 1994). The hazards of this category of drug are well described in the pharmacologic chapter in this book. (See Chapter 5.)

TABLE 13-1 Differential Diagnosis of Arthritis

	Degenerative	Inflammatory	Psychogenic
Symptoms			
Stiffness (duration)	Few minutes; "gelling" after prolonged rest	Hours (often); most pronounced after rest	Little or no variation in intensity with rest or activity
Pain	Follows activity; relieved by rest	Even at rest; nocturnal pain may interfere with sleep	Little or no variation in intensity with rest or activity
Weakness	Present, usually localized and not severe	Often pronounced	Often a complaint; "neurasthenia"
Fatigue	Not usual	Often severe with onset in early afternoon	Often in A.M. on arising
Emotional depression and lability	Not usual	Common; coincides with fatigue; often disappears if disease remits	Often present
Signs			
Tenderness localized over afflicted joint	Usually present	Almost always; the most sensitive indication of inflammation	Tender "all over"; "touch-me-not attitude"; tendency to push away or to grasp the examining hand
Swelling	Effusion common; little synovial reaction	Effusion common; often synovial proliferation and thickening	None
Heat and erythema (skin)	Unusual but may occur	More common	None
Crepitus	Coarse to medium	Medium to fine	None, except with coexistent arthritis
Bony spurs	Common	Sometimes found, usually with antecedent osteoarthritis	None, except with coexistent osteoarthritis

From McCarty D: Differential diagnosis of arthritis: analysis of signs and symptoms. In Koopman WJ, editor: *Arthritis and allied conditions,* ed 13, Baltimore, 1997, Williams & Wilkins.

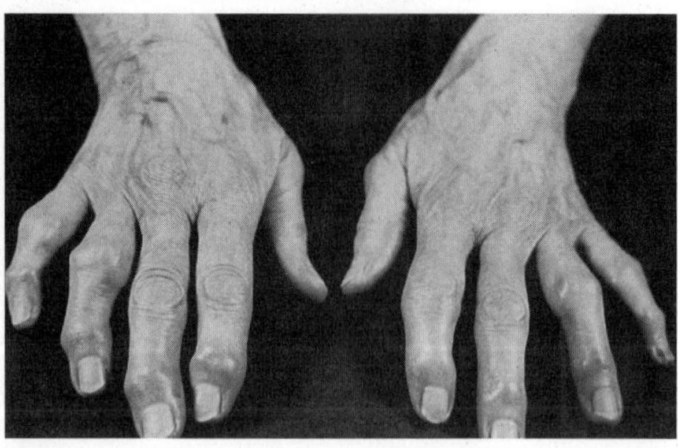

Figure 13-1 Degenerative joint disease; Heberden's nodes at the distal interphalangeal joints and Bouchard nodes at the proximal interphalangeal joints. (From the Clinical Slide Collection of the Rheumatic Diseases, copyright 1991. Used by permission of the American College of Rheumatology.)

TABLE 13-2 Laboratory Investigations

Test	Results
Erythrocyte sedimentation rate	Normal in osteoarthritis
	Elevated in polymyalgia rheumatica
	Elevated in rheumatoid arthritis
Rheumatoid factor	Negative in osteoarthritis
	Positive in rheumatoid arthritis
Antinuclear antibody	Negative in osteoarthritis
	20% of rheumatoid arthritis patients test positive
Uric acid	Elevated in gout
C-reactive protein	Elevated in rheumatoid arthritis

TABLE 13-3 Laboratory Findings in Arthritis

Class of Test	Category	Example of Abnormality
Hematology	Hemoglobin	Anemia in rheumatoid arthritis
	White cell count	Leukocytosis in septic arthritis
	Platelet count	Elevated in polymyalgia rheumatica
	ESR	
Biochemistry	Creatinine	High with involvement in systemic vasculitis
	Uric acid	Elevated in gout
	Creatine phosphokinase	
Immunology	Rheumatoid factor	Positive in rheumatoid arthritis
	Antinuclear antibody	Elevated in rheumatoid arthritis
	C-reactive protein	Elevated in Sjögren's syndrome
	Immunoglobulins	
	Complement C_3 and C_4	
Synovial fluid microscopy	Crystals	Present in gout and pyrophosphate crystal deposition disease
Culture	Bacteria in septic arthritis	

Adapted from Koopman WJ, editor: *Arthritis and allied conditions,* ed 13, Baltimore, 1997, Williams & Wilkins.

TABLE 13-4 Adverse Effects of NSAIDs

	GI Bleed	Peptic Ulcers	Abdominal Pain Heartburn, Dyspepsia	Rash	Dizziness, Headache	Tinnitus	Renal Failure	Blood Dyscrasias	Other
Placebo			++		+				
Aspirin	+	++	++++	+++	+++	++++	+		2, 4
Diclofenac	+	+	+++	+	++	+++		+	2, 4
Diflunisal	+	+	+++	+++	++	++			1
Etodolac	+	+	+++	++	+++	++	+		2
Fenoprofen	+	+	+++	++	+	++	+	+	1, 2
Flurbiprofen	+	+	++++	+++	+++	+++	+	+	2
Ibuprofen	+	+	+++	++	+	++		+	1
Indomethacin	+	+	++++	+	++++	++	+	+	1, 2
Ketoprofen	+	+	++++	+++	+++	++			1, 2, 3
Ketorolac	+	+	++++	+++	++++	+	+	+	1, 5
Meclofenamate	+	++	++++	+++	+++	++	+	+	1
Nabumetone	+	+	+++	+++	+++	++			1, 3
Naproxen	+	+	+++	+++	+++	+++	+	+	4
Oxaprozin	++	+	+++	+++		++	+	+	1, 2, 3
Phenylbutazone	+	+	+++	++	+	+	+	+	2, 5
Piroxicam	+	+	+++	++	++	++	+	+	2, 3
Salicylates (nonacetylated)	+	+	+++			++++			
Sulindac	+	+	+++	+++	+++	++	+	+	1, 3, 5
Tenoxicam		+	++++		+++				
Tiaprofenic Acid			+++	+	+++				3
Tolmetin	+	++	+++	+	+++	++	+	+	2

From Nishihara K, Furst D: Aspirin and other nonsteroidal antiinflammatory drugs. In Koopman WM, editor: *Arthritis and allied conditions,* ed 13, Baltimore, 1997, Williams & Wilkins.

+ = <1% incidence; ++ = 1%-4% incidence; +++ = >4%-9% incidence; ++++ = >9% incidence.

Blank spaces = insufficient data.

Other: 1 = diarrhea, 2 = hepatic toxicity, 3 = photosensitivity, 4 = colitis, 5 = pancreatitis.

Box 13-1
NSAID Drug Interactions

Cimetidine
Aluminum hydroxide
Gentamicin
Warfarin
Phenobarbital
Phenytoin
Estrogens
Furosemide
Hydrochlorothiazide
Acetaminophen
Digoxin
Lithium
Methotrexate
Prednisone
Probenecid

Adapted from Nishihara K, Furst D: Aspirin and other nonsteroid anti-inflammatory drugs. In Koopman WJ: *Arthritis and allied conditions,* ed 13, Baltimore, 1997, Williams & Wilkins.

Considerable evidence suggests that NSAIDs are no more effective than analgesics such as acetaminophen-propoxyphene (Brandt, 1996). In a randomized clinical trial comparing acetaminophen (4000 mg daily), low-dose ibuprofen (1200 mg daily), and high-dose ibuprofen (2400 mg daily) in patients with osteoarthritis of the knee, results after 4 weeks demonstrated 40% improvement in all three groups. However, the amount of improvement in overall pain, rest pain, and walking pain was generally small (Bradley et al., 1991; Bradley, 1992). The significance is that the side effects of acetaminophen are fewer, as are its adverse interactions with other drugs. Still, with acetaminophen there is an increased risk for hepatotoxicity in overdoses exceeding 10 g (2.5 times the normal dose). People with chronic high alcohol intake have been reported to be at risk for liver toxicity, and regular alcohol use increases the risk for induced liver damage. It seems best to discourage the use of alcohol by any patient who is prescribed either acetaminophen or NSAIDs. Because of the growing concern about the harmful effects of NSAIDs, the American College of Rheumatology guidelines for management of hip and knee OA recommend a daily dose of 4000 mg of acetaminophen as the initial drug therapy for the symptomatic patient (Hochberg et al., 1995a, 1995b).

Topical agents can be used in conjunction with other medications. Capsaicin is a nonprescription drug available in two strengths. It can be used two to four times a day, but to remain effective it should not be used continuously (McCarty and McCarty, 1992).

Intraarticular injection of depocorticosteroids is considered useful if there is evidence of inflammation. Synovial effusions should be removed prior to injection. There is no conclusive evidence that intraarticular injections of depocorticosteroids are of any benefit in OA. They should be limited to a maximum of four per year to an individual joint. A proper aseptic technique should be rigidly followed to prevent complications such as septic arthritis. If an infection is to occur, it usually develops 24 to 72 hours after the injection (Schnitzer, 1993).

Surgical intervention, usually joint replacement, is an elective orthopedic procedure

Box 13-2
Physical Interventions for Osteoarthritis

1. Exercise
   - Passive range of motion
   - Rest periods
   - Active range of motion
   - Isometric, isotonic, isokinetic
2. Support devices
   - Canes
   - Crutches
   - Collars
   - Shoe insoles
   - Knee braces
3. Modification of activities and environment
   - Proper positioning: sitting or driving
   - Adjustment of household furnishings
     - Use of chair with arms
     - Height of chairs
     - Raising toilet seat
     - Grab bars in shower and tub
     - Handrails: both sides of staircase
4. Thermal modalities
   - Hot packs
   - Deep heat (ultrasound)
   - Cold packs
5. Other
   - Transcutaneous electric nerve stimulation (TENS)
   - Acupuncture
   - Chiropractic
   - Massage
   - Yoga

Modified from Lozada C, Altman K: Management of osteoarthritis. In Koopman WJ, editor: *Arthritis and allied conditions,* ed 13, Baltimore, 1997, Williams & Wilkins.

performed for either intractable pain or restoration of compromised function. For most patients, the results are good to excellent and have long-term benefits. Arthroscopic intervention is usually limited to additional diagnosis, repair, lavage, and debridement.

Nonpharmacologic Interventions

Physical measures should always be the major aspect of a therapeutic management plan because they can relieve pain, reduce stiffness, and limit muscle spasm. Another major contribution of physical measures is to strengthen paraarticular structures and improve joint support through exercise, which adds to the patient's stability and reduces symptoms (Lozada and Altman, 1997). The physical interventions for OA are exercise, supportive devices, alterations in activities of daily living, and thermal modalities (Box 13-2).

An important aspect of a treatment program is the prevention of further injury. A joint protection program that reduces sudden impact loads and optimizes the patient's muscular capacity can be considered both as a treatment and as a preventive measure (Box 13-3).

Box 13-3
Joint Protection

1. Wear properly fitted shoes with well-cushioned soles.
2. Sit rather than stand for activities longer than 10 minutes.
3. Avoid low chairs, low beds, low toilet seats, bathtubs.
4. Do not kneel, squat, or sit cross-legged on the floor.
5. Do consider exercise by swimming or walking.

If the patient is obese, the primary care provider has an obligation to impress on the patient the health risks inherent in obesity as well as the relationship of obesity to the development and, most likely, the progression of OA (Felson et al., 1992). There is a need for compassionate consideration in such a warning. It is not appropriate to blame the victim for the disease; instead, the provider must recognize the importance of building a relationship with the patient to increase compliance and self-care abilities.

Exercise. The goals of an exercise program for patients with OA are to increase function and reduce joint pain. After pain relief has been achieved, a graded exercise program can begin. Depending on the severity of the functional limitations attributed to the disease, some patients need formal physical therapy to develop their program; others need only minimal instruction. The primary care provider needs to dispel the old myth that any exercise will exacerbate the already painful joints and should also stress that a graded exercise program does not cause pain and does not advance quickly. When pain occurs, the patient should be advised to stop. Swimming is an effective exercise method to alleviate pain and exercise multiple muscle groups. An expert should evaluate bicycle riding as exercise therapy for patients with knee involvement. Without a doubt, a regular exercise program that includes isometric exercises followed by resistance training will improve muscle tone and increase muscle strength, thereby reducing muscle spasm, preventing contractures, and improving the patient's quality of life (Brandt, 1996). Figure 13-2 shows strengthening exercises.

Rheumatoid Arthritis

Epidemiology

The prevalence rate of rheumatoid arthritis (RA) among adults in the United States is 10 per 1000, or approximately 2.1 million people—600,000 men and 1.5 million women. There is a declining incidence of RA in the United States, and these figures may not reflect this recent development (Lawrence et al., 1998). In the past, RA has been shown to increase with age: there is a 0.3% prevalence rate in individuals under age 35 and a 10% prevalence rate for individuals over age 65 (Mitchell, 1985). RA is known to be more prevalent in certain populations, such as the Chippewa and Pima Native American tribes, whose rate of RA exceeds 5% (Del Puente et al., 1989).

In a study of the resource utilization of 365 RA patients in one health maintenance organization, care was characterized by intensive treatment, frequent medications, and hospitalizations that accounted for 46% of total expenditures; the average individual cost

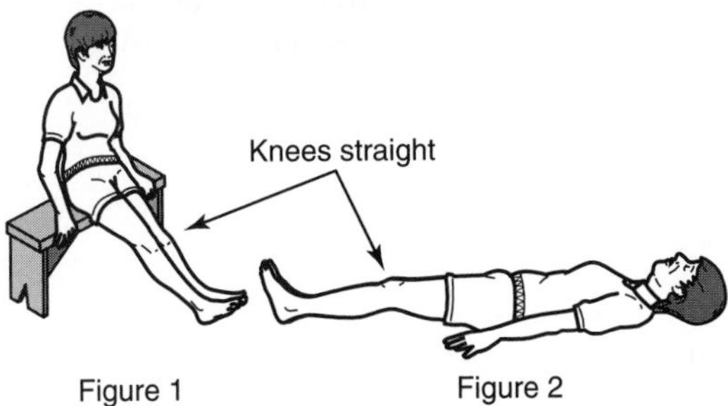

A

1. Sit on a firm surface (Figure 1) or lie flat in bed (Figure 2).
2. Perform this exercise in either of the following positions:
   a. Sit in a chair (Figure 1) with your legs straight, heels on the floor or on a footstool. Squeeze your thigh muscles, pushing your knees downward toward the floor.
   b. Lie in bed (Figure 2) with your legs straight and squeeze your thigh muscles, pushing the back of your knees into the bed.
3. Hold this position for a full 5 seconds. Use a clock or watch with a second hand, or count: one-one thousand, two-one thousand, three-one thousand, four-one thousand, five-one thousand.
4. Relax the muscles.

Instructions

If your arthritis is causing knee pain, apply heat to your knees for 15 to 20 minutes prior to performing your exercises.

Begin your strengthening program with 10 repetitions, holding each contraction for a full 5 seconds. Perform this exercise 7 times daily and increase the number of repetitions you perform with each set by three to five daily during the first week.

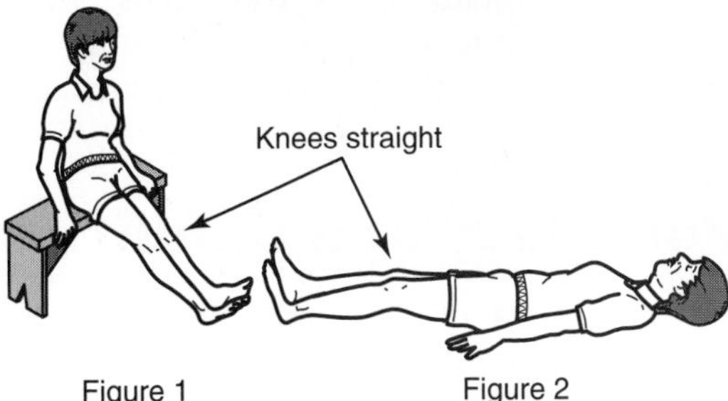

B

1. Sit on a firm surface (Figure 1) or lie flat in bed (Figure 2).
2. Cross your ankles with right leg above and left leg below. Legs should be stretched out straight.
3. With your heels on the floor or on the bed, push down with right leg, push up with left leg, squeezing your ankles together. (Pretend that you're crushing a walnut between your ankles.) There should be little actual movement except for the muscle tightening.
4. Hold this position for a full 5 seconds. Use a clock or a watch with a second hand, or count: one-one thousand, two-one thousand, three-one thousand, four-one thousand, five-one thousand.
5. Relax the muscles.
6. Reverse the position of the legs so that the leg that was on top is now on the bottom.
7. Repeat steps one, two and three.

Caution: In most patients, these knee exercises will not cause joint pain or increase the pain from your arthritis. If, however, you have significant pain lasting more than 20 minutes after you perform these exercises, decrease the number of repetitions by five per set. Maintain this number of repetitions until your knee discomfort subsides. Then, each day thereafter, increase the number of repetitions by three per set until you reach a maximum of 15 per set.

Figure 13-2 A, Quadriceps strengthening exercise. B, Quadriceps strengthening exercise concentrating on the vastus medialis oblique muscle. (Modified from Brandt KD: *Diagnosis and nonsurgical management,* Indianapolis, 1996, Professional Communications.)

rate was $2162 per year (Lane et al., 1997). A Canadian study performed over a 12-year period with a larger sample (1063) reported direct average individual costs to be $2165 (Canadian) in the late 1980s and $1597 in the early 1990s. Institutional stays and medications account for 80% of the total, with an increase in these costs for older and more disabled patients (Clarke et al., 1997).

Pathology and Definition

RA is a systemic autoimmune disorder of unknown origin (Weinblatt, 1997). Another definition of RA is a disorder of unknown cause characterized by a sterile inflammatory polyarthritis (Lawrence, 1998). Genetics may play a small role in that first-degree relatives are at increased risk; siblings of those with severe RA have the highest risk. Theories concerning the etiology of RA include a multifactorial system with autoimmune, inflammatory, and genetic elements. One major pathophysiologic difference between OA and RA is the presence of extensive synovial-based inflammation.

In 1987 the American Rheumatism Association established new criteria for RA (Table 13-5). RA can be considered a clinical syndrome with varying features between individual patients and also variations from time to time in the same patient.

TABLE 13-5 Revised Criteria for the Classification of Rheumatoid Arthritis

Criterion	Definition
Morning stiffness	Morning stiffness in and around the joints, lasting at least 1 hour before maximum improvement
Arthritis of 3 or more joint areas	At least 3 joint areas simultaneously with soft tissue swelling or joint fluid observed by a physician. The 14 possible areas are (right or left): PIP, MCP, wrist, elbow, knee, ankle, and MTP joints
Arthritis of hand joints	At least 1 area swollen in a wrist, MCP, or PIP joint
Symmetric arthritis	Simultaneous involvement of the same joint areas on both sides of the body (bilateral involvement of PIP, MCP, or MTP acceptable without perfect symmetry)
Rheumatoid nodules	Subcutaneous nodules over bony prominences or extensor surfaces, or in juxtaarticular regions, observed by a physician
Serum rheumatoid factor	Abnormal amount of serum rheumatoid factor by any method for which the result has been positive in <5% of control subjects
Radiographic changes	Erosions or unequivocal bony decalcification localized in or most marked adjacent to the involved joints (osteoarthritis changes excluded), typical of rheumatoid arthritis on posteroanterior hand and wrist radiographs

From Arnett FC et al: The American Rheumatism Association 1987 revised criteria for the classification of rheumatoid arthritis, *Arthritis Rheum* 31:315-324, 1988.

For classification purposes, a patient is said to have rheumatoid arthritis if 4 of 7 criteria are satisfied. Criteria 1-4 must have been present for at least 6 weeks. Patients with 2 clinical diagnoses are not excluded.

History

In three fourths of older people, the initial presentation of RA is an insidious process; in others, the onset is acute over a few days (Calkins, Reinhard, and Vladutiu, 1994). If the patient presents with polyarticular inflammatory arthritis, especially of the hands or feet, the primary care provider begins to consider a diagnosis of RA. Patients with early disease usually report a general malaise with fatigue, severe morning stiffness that lasts more than an hour, and joint swelling and tenderness. The initial presentation of RA may lack the aspect of symmetric involvement, but the symmetry becomes evident as the disease progresses. A definitive diagnosis of RA requires a period of 6 weeks with symptoms. The frequency of remission in the new-onset older patient is probably below 50%.

A baseline for functional status should be completed on the first visit. A four-point scale that rates limitations in self-care and vocational and avocational activities has been developed by the American College of Rheumatology for classification of functional status in rheumatoid patients (Table 13-6).

Focused Physical Examination

Examination of the affected joints for the signs of inflammation is important for early diagnosis because there are reversible aspects of inflammatory synovitis. RA criteria are to be considered only as guidelines for diagnosing RA. Essential for diagnosis is identification of inflammatory synovitis, which can be one of the following: synovial fluid leukocytosis (white blood cells >2000/mm^3), histologic demonstration of chronic synovitis, or radiologic evidence of characteristic erosions (Weinblatt, 1997). The presence of deformity in non–weight-bearing joints is highly indicative of RA unless there is a history of trauma.

TABLE 13-6 American College of Rheumatology Revised Criteria for Classification of Functional Status in Rheumatoid Arthritis

Class	Functional Status
Class I	Completely able to perform usual activities of daily living (self-care, vocational, and avocational)
Class II	Able to perform usual self-care and vocational activities but limited in avocational activities
Class III	Able to perform usual self-care activities but limited in vocational and avocational activities
Class IV	Limited in ability to perform usual self-care, vocational, and avocational activities

From Hochberg MC et al: The American College of Rheumatology 1991 revised criteria for the classification of global functional status in rheumatoid arthritis, *Arthritis Rheum* 25:498-502, 1992.

Usual self-care activities include dressing, feeding, bathing, grooming, and toileting. Avocational (recreational and/or leisure) and vocational (work, school, homemaking) activities are patient-desired and age- and sex-specific.

Laboratory Tests

Aspiration of a joint with a palpable effusion is a first consideration. Rheumatoid factor (RF) is found in the serum of approximately 85% of people with RA, but it is of little prognostic value and may present in other inflammatory processes. Titers of RF above 1:256 are more likely to be diagnostic of RA (Calkins, Reinhard, and Vladutiu, 1994). Some patients with early disease may be negative for RF but become positive as the disease progresses.

The erythrocyte sedimentation rate (ESR) varies from patient to patient and according to the degree of inflammation, but the rate is usually in the range of 20 to 60 mm/hr (Calkins, Reinhard, and Vladutiu, 1994).

Differential Diagnosis

Osteoarthritis
Polymyalgia rheumatica (Table 13-7)

Treatment

The goals of treatment are as follows:

To provide pain relief
To decrease joint inflammation
To maintain or restore joint function
To prevent bone and cartilage destruction

If at all feasible, patients should be followed either by a specialist or in a specialty clinic. An interdisciplinary team needs to be responsible for care given by primary care providers, who may at times be in charge of follow-up after the diagnosis is confirmed.

There is debate in the field of rheumatology over whether treatment should begin with second-step drugs and bypass the first step. For information purposes, the two steps are presented here, but the primary care practitioner will be following the recommendations of the specialist for the follow-up care of the patient with RA, or the patient will be under the direct care of the specialist.

After the diagnosis is confirmed, patients should be taught about all aspects of the disease, particularly the need for rest and exercise. Older patients with new-onset RA are often overwhelmed by the magnitude of the disease and need extra support from primary care providers. Motivation to continue the daily exercise prescription is essential to maintaining function and requires responsibility and sustained commitment by patients and their social support systems. Extensive bedrest, a usual component of early disease treatment, may be contraindicated in older people because periods of sustained inactivity may be hazardous to their ability to regain function. Limited rest with hot soaks and other physical measures and low-dose NSAIDs can be considered the first step in treatment (Calkins, Reinhard, and Vladutiu, 1994).

Referrals for physical therapy, occupational therapy, or both may be appropriate, depending on the severity of the disease. Orthopedic surgery is an option if warranted by

TABLE 13-7 Differential Diagnosis

	Pain Pattern	Common Systemic Symptoms	Onset and Course	Anatomy Affected	Laboratory Findings, X-Ray	Age at Onset
Rheumatoid arthritis	On arising, after prolonged inactivity	Fever, fatigue, weight loss, malaise, and organ-specific extraarticular symptoms such as shortness of breath	Acute or subacute onset, with chronic and variable course	Wrists, MCP joints, any synovial joints; symmetric; extra-articular (e.g., heart, lung, eye, integument)	Elevated ESR, +RA, +ANA; normochromic anemia; x-ray: joint changes and deformities; osteoporosis	Childhood to old age
Osteoarthritis	End of day or after heavy use of joints	Not prominent	Chronic, may emerge after injury	Weight-bearing joints, axial skeleton, distal hand joints; oligoarticular and asymmetric	Characteristic degenerative changes of joints on x-ray	>40 (unless posttraumatic)
PMR	On arising, after prolonged inactivity	Low-grade fevers, fatigue, general malaise, weight loss, depression, headache	Acute or subacute onset and chronic steady course	Proximal muscles, periarticular tissues of limb girdles	Elevated ESR, normochromic anemia	>55
Fibromyalgia	On arising and with active use	Insomnia, malaise, weakness, irritable bowel syndrome	Chronic but evanescent	Periarticular muscle insertion sites: "trigger points"	None	Middle age
Depression	Highly variable and changeable	Weakness, anxiety, malaise, insomnia, weight and appetite changes	Subacute to slow onset, with variable chronic course	Diffuse aches difficult to characterize; trigger points not prominent	No specific abnormalities	Childhood to old age
Chronic infection	Diffuse aching not clearly related to use	Spiking fevers, sweats, chills, malaise, anorexia, nausea, headache, weakness	Acute or subacute with variable course	Nonarticular diffuse aches and stiffness; varies with type of infection	Elevated ESR, elevated WBC; normochromic anemia; + skin test or serology; + cultures	Childhood to old age

Modified from Ham R, Sloane P: *Primary care geriatrics,* St Louis, 1997, Mosby.
ESR, Erythrocyte sedimentation rate; *MCP,* metacarpophalangeal joints; *RA,* rheumatoid factor; *ANA,* antinuclear antigen; *EMG,* electromyography.

Box 13-4
Drug Therapy in Rheumatoid Arthritis

First Line
- Aspirin
- NSAIDs

Second Line
- Antimalarials (chloroquine)
- Methotrexate
- Gold salts
- D-penicillamine
- Azathioprine
- Combination therapies
- Corticosteroids
  - Systemic steroids
    - Low dose oral
    - Parenteral pulse steroids
  - Intraarticular

Modified from Weinblatt M: Rheumatoid arthritis: the clinical picture. In Koopman WJ, editor: *Arthritis and allied conditions*, ed 13, Baltimore, 1997, Williams & Wilkins.

the severity of the disease. Reconstructive surgery and joint replacement have improved functional capacity for many patients. Patients' support systems may require assistance and counseling services.

The second step of a treatment regimen is an array of pharmacotherapeutics. (See Box 13-4 for a list of drugs and Table 13-8 for drug costs.) Because of the high toxicity of certain drugs used in this type of therapy, a specialist or at least an interdisciplinary team should oversee the care of RA patients. All providers need to stay informed about the latest clinical trials and reports regarding adverse reactions to RA drugs. The medication regimens of older adults are, indeed, different than those for younger RA patients because of the higher risk of adverse drug reactions (Weinblatt, 1997).

If the treatment plan includes low-dose prednisone, clinicians caring for older patients need to consider the risks and benefits of this treatment. The highest recommended daily dose that minimizes risk and optimizes benefits for elderly patients is considered to be 7 mg for women and 8 mg for men (Calkins, Reinhard, and Vladutiu, 1994). An important caveat to this therapy is that elderly patients, especially women, have a great risk of diminished bone mass without experiencing any overt symptoms. Needless to say, corticosteroids increase the risk of osteopenia, and patients should be closely followed.

If the treatment plan includes methotrexate, the practitioner needs to instruct the patient that it is given in a dose of 7.5 mg per week, either as three 2.5-mg tablets taken all at once or in three doses separated by 12-hour intervals. The effect is seen in most patients 3 to 5 weeks after starting the medication. Before starting this therapy, the provider should obtain a complete blood count, liver function tests, serum creatinine levels, urinalysis, and a chest x-ray film. Cell count needs to be followed monthly, and renal and liver studies should be performed at 3-month intervals. The provider should be aware that a small number of patients may develop hepatic fibrosis or pulmonary inflammation (Box 13-5). Chest x-ray examinations should probably be performed every

TABLE 13-8 Drug Costs

Drug Cost	Dose	Monthly ($)
First-line Therapy		
Ibuprofen	2400 mg/day	9
Indomethacin	150 mg/day	11
Naproxen	1500 mg/day	16
Choline magnesium trisalicylate	3000 mg/day	16
Piroxicam	20 mg/day	42
Diclofenac	150 mg/day	67
Nabumetone	1500 mg/day	91
Second-line Therapy		
Hydroxychloroquine	400 mg/day	73
Sulfasalazine	2000 mg/day	17
Methotrexate	15 mg/week	
	Oral	54
	Parenteral	15
Gold Salts		
Auranofin	6 mg/day	74
D-penicillamine	750 mg/day	126

Adapted from Weinblatt M: Rheumatoid arthritis: the clinical picture. In Koopman WJ, editor: *Arthritis and allied conditions,* ed 13, Baltimore, 1997, Williams & Wilkins.

2 years, and patients should be watched for the development of any pulmonary symptoms (Calkins, Reinhard, and Vladutiu, 1994; Nishihara and Furst, 1997). As with all drugs, the patient should be informed and understand all the risks and benefits of the therapy.

Alternative Therapies

Because RA and OA do not have a predictable disease course but rather an unpredictable pattern of flare-ups and remissions, patients may attribute remission to a variety of causes. Because health professionals are at a loss to explain the actual cause of either the positive or negative happenings, this chapter discusses a few of the alternative therapies that patients find and use in the informal health care system.

Copper bracelets were used by the ancient Greeks to relieve aches and pains, and many Americans wear copper bracelets for the same reason. Copper in the bracelets may be absorbed through the skin, but the effects of subjective well-being are considered a placebo effect. Copper salts have been used in the past, but there were severe adverse effects (Sorenson, 1981; Sorenson and Hangarter, 1977). Zinc has been tested and has shown no effect on the signs and symptoms of either RA or OA (Rasker et al., 1982).

Diet has been thought to play a role in a protective function and treatment of RA; the effects of fish and fish oil are not yet clear. A number of controlled small studies have shown improvement for some patients, with reduced morning stiffness and a reduction in the number of tender joints (Shapiro et al., 1996; Lau et al., 1993; Geusens et al., 1993).

Box 13-5

Recommendations for Monitoring for Hepatic Safety in Rheumatoid Arthritis Patients Receiving Methotrexate

A. Baseline
   1. Tests for all patients
      a. Liver blood tests (aspartate aminotransferase [AST], alanine amino-transferase [ALT], alkaline phosphatase, albumin, bilirubin), hepatitis B and C serologic studies
      b. Other standard tests, including complete blood cell count and serum creatinine
   2. Pretreatment liver biopsy (Menghini suction-type needle) only for patients with:
      a. Prior excessive alcohol consumption
      b. Persistently abnormal baseline AST values
      c. Chronic hepatitis B or C infection
B. Monitor AST, ALT, albumin at 4-8 week intervals
C. Perform liver biopsy if:
   1. Five of 9 determinations of AST within a given 12-month interval (6 of 12 if tests are performed monthly) are abnormal (defined as an elevation above the upper limit of normal)
   2. There is a decrease in serum albumin below the normal range (in the setting of well-controlled rheumatoid arthritis)
D. If results of liver biopsy are:
   1. Roenigk grade I, II, or IIIA, resume MTX and monitor as in B, C1, and C2 above
   2. Roenigk grade IIIB or IV, discontinue MTX
E. Discontinue MTX in patient with persistent liver test abnormalities, as defined in C1 and C2 above, who refuses liver biopsy

From Kremer JM et al: Methotrexate for rheumatoid arthritis: suggested guidelines for monitoring liver toxicity, *Arthritis Rheum* 37:316, 1994.

Some patients have maintained that food allergies contribute to the symptoms connected with RA. This hypothesis may have some validity in that food can evoke an immune response, but it seems relevant for only a very small number of patients (Panush, 1993).

The placebo effect is very strong in the course of treatment for arthritis patients—up to 50% of a sample in one clinical trial (Tilley et al., 1995). Again, practitioners must note the unpredictable pattern of the disease and understand the difficulty that patients have in bringing a sense of order and causality to their experience. The important aspect for the primary care provider is to stay informed about the latest trends in alternative therapies, read the research, and talk to the patient about the risks and benefits of unregulated drugs and untested therapies. If the therapy is safe and works for the patient, the practitioner should document it and ask about its use and any effects at the next visit.

Polymyalgia Rheumatica and Giant Cell Arteritis

Epidemiology

Polymyalgia rheumatica (PMR) and giant cell (temporal) arteritis (GCA) are closely related syndromes that occur in people over age 50. Polymyalgia rheumatica is 10 times more common in people after age 80. Prevalence estimates are higher in women, and it is much more common in Caucasians than in other racial groups. The PMR prevalence rate in the United States is estimated to be 700 per 100,000, and the GCA rate is estimated to be 200 per 100,000 (Lawrence et al., 1998; Levy and Sethi, 1998).

Definition

PMR is a syndrome of unknown origin that includes joint and muscle pain, muscle stiffness, and systemic illness; it precedes or follows GCA in up to 20% of cases but also exists independently. Genetic factors appear to be important, and PMR has also been linked with RA (Bahlas, Ramos-Remus, and Davis, 1998).

Clinical Features of Polymyalgia Rheumatica

Muscle pain in neck, shoulder girdle, or pelvic girdle (usually bilateral) for at least 4 weeks
Stiffness after rest
Elevated (>50 mm/hour) erythrocyte sedimentation rate (ESR)
Frequent general malaise, fever, weight loss
Clinical response to corticosteroid treatment (Labbe and Hardouin, 1998; Weyand and Goronzy, 1997)

Criteria for Classification of Giant Cell Arteritis

Age at disease onset >50 years of age
Headache of new onset or new type
Tenderness or decreased pulsation of temporal artery
Elevated (>50 mm/hour) ESR
Histologic changes of arteritis (Weyland and Goronzy, 1997)

Treatment

Patients with PMR and GCA need to be followed by a specialist or seen in a specialty clinic. An interdisciplinary team needs to be responsible for any care by primary care providers, who may at times be in charge of follow-up after the diagnosis is confirmed.

Treatment of Polymyalgia Rheumatica

If diagnosed and treated promptly, PMR has an excellent prognosis. Corticosteroids are the treatment of choice. The goal is to control the pain, stiffness, and general constitutional symptoms with low doses. However, the schedule for the initial dose, the duration of treatment, and the optimal tapering are much debated (Labbe and Hardouin, 1998). One current recommendation is to initiate treatment with 15 to 20 mg of prednisone per day, with the expectation that relief is obtained within either hours or days. Tapering of the daily dose needs to be supervised by the interdisciplinary team, but the recommended trial is a 2.5-mg reduction of the daily dose every 2 weeks until a dose of 10 mg daily is reached. After that level is reached, a 1-mg incremental reduction every 4 weeks can begin. Some patients cannot tolerate this reduction system, and the problem is that to regain control of the disease the dose of prednisone must be increased (Weyland and Goronzy, 1997). In a controlled 96-week study of 55 patients, side effects from oral prednisolone for the treatment of polymyalgia were weight gain, eight fractures, moon face, hypertension, cataracts, back pain, and depression; however, the numbers were small (Dasgupta et al., 1998).

Patients need to be followed for 6 to 12 months after treatment with corticosteroids has been discontinued. Every patient with PMR needs to be considered at increased risk for the development of GCA. Nonsteroid drugs are considered unsuitable for long-term treatment of PMR. Although long-term treatment with corticosteroids can lead to steroid side effects, they remain the mainstay of treatment (Labbe and Hardouin, 1998).

Treatment of Giant Cell Arteritis

High-dose corticosteroids in a range of 40 to 60 mg daily are the recommended treatment for GCA and need to be continued until reversible symptoms are in remission and laboratory values are normal. Tapering doses too rapidly may be harmful and has been associated with relapses. Treatment usually continues for 2 years, with clinical monitoring for an additional 6 to 12 years. Up to 50% of patients are unable to discontinue therapy in 2 years (Weyland and Goronzy, 1997). Again, the importance of a specialty or team approach to this type of patient must be noted.

Fibromyalgia

Fibromyalgia is a syndrome of unknown etiology, although it has been recognized for decades and has been described as nonarticular arthritis, psychogenic arteritis, and fibrositis. In 1990 the American College of Rheumatology established criteria that include pain over a wide area that persists for at least 3 months and specific point tenderness over at least 11 of 18 anatomic sites (Wolfe et al., 1990).

Epidemiology

Prevalence rates are difficult to approximate because many uninsured people do not seek care for this non–life-threatening condition and because it is a difficult condition to diagnose. However, available data suggest that prevalence rates are lower in men (0.5%) than in women (3.4%). The prevalence of fibromyalgia increases with age, with an estimate at age 80 of 59 per 100,000, compared with a rate of 34 per 100,000 at age 40 (Lawrence et al., 1998).

Clinical Characteristics

Widespread pain (Figure 13-3)
Decreased pain threshold

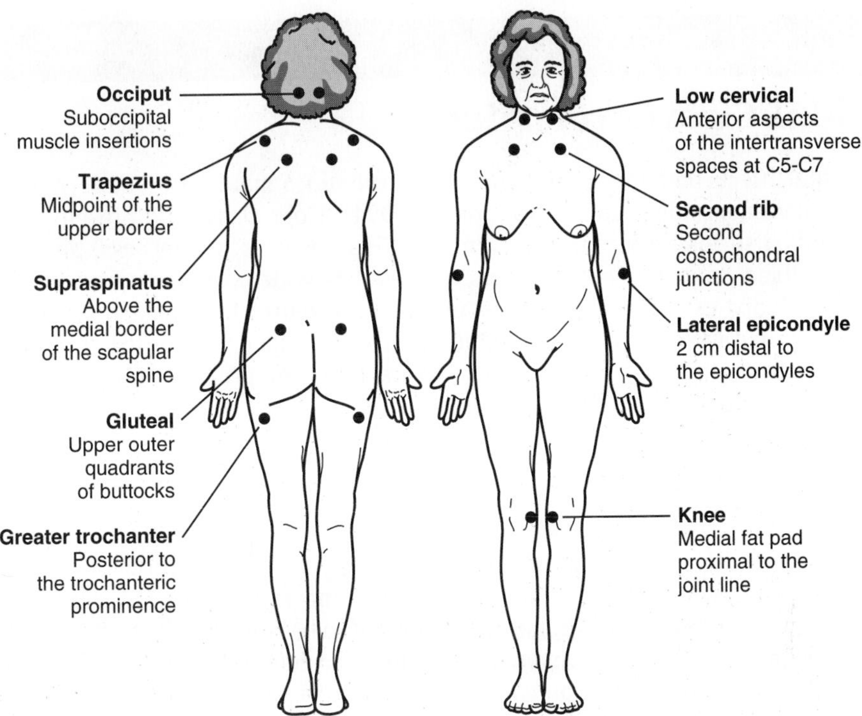

Figure 13-3 Location of tender points for diagnostic classification of fibromyalgia. (Redrawn from McCance KL, Huether SE: *Pathophysiology: the biologic basis for disease in adults and children,* ed 3, St Louis, 1998, Mosby.)

Sleep disturbance
Fatigue
Psychologic distress

Treatment

One aspect of treatment has been to increase deep sleep (stage IV) by prescribing amitriptyline or cyclobenzaprine. Outcome studies have demonstrated results, but the positive effects seem to diminish over time. Cardiovascular fitness training and flexibility exercises, physical therapy, and cognitive-behavioral therapy have shown improvements that were maintained over time. Most of the reported studies have methodologic problems of small sample size and few control groups (Bradley and Alarcón, 1997).

In general, there is no accepted pathway for the treatment of patients with fibromyalgia. Education of the patient and reassurance that the disorder is not life-threatening or associated with any type of joint deformity must be the first element of treatment. Training in pain management and coping skills may be helpful to many patients. Treatment is complex and should involve an interdisciplinary team, if available. If not, the primary care provider may need to enlist consultants to assist with the therapeutic plan.

Gout

Clinical Characteristics

Gout affects both men and women in a ratio of 1.5 males to 1 female, and it is seldom seen in patients under age 50 (Seegmiller, 1994). Gout classically presents as an acute distal monoarthritis with extreme pain, swelling, redness, tenderness, and warmth over the involved joint. The course of the disease has wide variations even if left untreated; the attack abates after 1 to 2 weeks and may not return for weeks or years. However, if left untreated in some patients, the progression includes joint destruction, progressive renal impairment, and hypertension. Factors that can precipitate an attack are uricosuric agents, alcohol, diuretics, and stress.

Diagnosis

The definitive diagnosis of gout is made by the observation of urate crystals in the aspirated synovial fluid from an involved joint. Hyperuricemia, defined as a serum uric acid value above 7 mg/dl, has been thought to be responsible for the development of gout (Seegmiller, 1994). However, an elevated uric acid level is not sufficient for a diagnosis. A 24-hour urine collection can be performed for uric acid levels.

Treatment

For the acute phase, treatment should include joint rest, cold compresses, and NSAIDs.

Long-term treatment after the acute phase is resolved most commonly involves allopurinol. It is to be used with some caution, because it can bring on a new attack of acute gout when used alone. For prevention, colchicine is usually prescribed along with the allopurinol. In some cases, uricosuric agents can be used in combination with allopurinol and colchicine (Sibbitt, 1996). The intent is to lower the uric acid level below 6 mg/dl. The toxicity of allopurinol is important because it can precipitate severe life-threatening reactions. Therefore the patient taking this drug needs to be monitored (Studenski and Laird, 1998).

Summary

A majority of older adults are affected by OA. In addition, RA, PMR, GCA, fibromyalgia, and gout cause severe pain, expense, and loss of function in a significant number of people in this population. Proper diagnosis requires knowledge of the risk factors and diagnostic criteria for each, a thorough history and physical examination, and use of the appropriate diagnostic tests. Treatment can involve both pharmacologic and nonpharmacologic interventions, including diet and alternative therapies. Proper use of assistive devices, exercise, and safety considerations can ease pain, prevent injury, and enhance function and independence.

Resources

Arthritis Foundation
1330 West Peachtree Street
Atlanta, GA 30309
(404) 872-7100
http://www.arthritis.org

Arthritis Net
http://www.arthritisnet.com

Polymyalgia rheumatica
http://www.plgrm.com/health/P/polymyalgia_rheumatica.HTM

References

Bahlas S, Ramos-Remus C, Davis P: Clinical outcome of 149 patients with polymyalgia and giant cell arteritis, *J Rheumatol* 25(1):99-104, 1998.

Bradley J: Treatment of knee osteoarthritis: relationship of clinical features of joint inflammation to the response to a nonsteroidal anti-inflammatory drug or pure analgesic, *J Rheumatol* 19:1950-1954, 1992.

Bradley J et al: Comparison of anti-inflammatory dose of ibuprofen, an analgesic dose of ibuprofen, and acetaminophen in the treatment of patients with osteoarthritis of the knee, *N Engl J Med* 325:87-91, 1991.

Bradley LA, Alarcón G: Fibromyalgia. In Koopman WJ, editor: *Arthritis and allied conditions*, ed 13, Baltimore, 1997, Williams & Wilkins.

Brandt KD: *Diagnosis and nonsurgical management*, Indianapolis, 1996, Professional Communications.

Buchner DM et al: Effects of physical activity on health status in older adults: two intervention studies, *Annu Rev Public Health* 13:469, 1992.

Calkins E, Reinhard J, Vladutiu A: Osteoarthritis. In Hazzard WR et al, editors: *Principles of geriatric medicine and gerontology*, ed 3, New York, 1994, McGraw-Hill.

Carson J, Strom B: Nonsteroidal anti-inflammatory drugs. In Hazzard WR et al, editors: *Principles of geriatric medicine and gerontology*, ed 3, New York, 1994, McGraw-Hill.

Clarke AE et al: Direct and indirect medical costs incurred by Canadian patients with rheumatoid arthritis: a twelve-year study, *J Rheumatol* 24(6):1051-1060, 1997.

Dasgupta B et al: An initially double-blind controlled 96 week trial of depot methylprednisolone against oral prednisolone in the treatment of polymyalgia rheumatica, *Br J Rheumatol* 37(2):189-195, 1998.

Del Puente A et al: High incidence and prevalence of rheumatoid arthritis in Pima Indians, *Am J Epidemiol* 129:1170-1187, 1989.

Felson DT et al: Weight loss reduces the risk for symptomatic knee osteoarthritis in women, *Arch Intern Med* 116:535-539, 1992.

Geusens P et al: Long-term effect of omega-3 fatty acid supplementation in active rheumatoid arthritis, *Arthritis Rheum* 37:824-829, 1993.

Hellmann D: Arthritis and musculoskeletal disorders. In Tierney LM, McPhee SJ, Papadakis MA, editors: *Current medical diagnosis and treatment*, ed 36, Stamford, Conn, 1997, Appleton & Lange.

Hochberg M et al: Guidelines for the medical management of osteoarthritis: part I, osteoarthritis of the hip, *Arthritis Rheum* 38:1535-1540, 1995a.

Hochberg M et al: Guidelines for the medical management of osteoarthritis: part II, osteoarthritis of the knee, *Arthritis Rheum* 38:1541-1546, 1995b.

Labbe P, Hardouin P: Epidemiology and optimal management of polymyalgia rheumatica, *Drugs Aging* 13(2):109-118, 1998.

Lane SF et al: Resource utilization and cost of care for rheumatoid arthritis and osteoarthritis in a managed care setting: the importance of drug and surgery costs, *Arthritis Rheum* 40(8):1475-1481, 1997.

Lau C et al: Effects of fish oil supplementation on non-steroidal anti-inflammatory drug requirement in patients with mild rheumatoid arthritis: a double-blind placebo controlled study, *Br J Rheumatol* 32:982-989, 1993.

Lawrence RC et al: Estimates of the prevalence of arthritis and selected musculoskeletal disorders in the United States, *Arthritis Rheum* 41(5):778-799, 1998.

Levy J, Sethi P: Joint pain in the elderly patient, *Journal of the American Academy of Orthopaedic Surgeons* 2(1):66-73, 1998.

Levy J et al: Socioeconomic costs of osteoarthritis in France, *Rev Rheum Engl Ed* 60:63S-67S, 1993.

Ling SM, Bathon JM: Osteoarthritis in older adults, *J Am Geriatr Soc* 46(2):216-225, 1998.

Lozada C, Altman R: Management of osteoarthritis. In Koopman WJ, editor: *Arthritis and allied conditions*, ed 13, Baltimore, 1997, Williams & Wilkins.

McCarty D: Differential diagnosis of arthritis: analysis of signs and symptoms. In Koopman WJ, editor: *Arthritis and allied conditions*, ed 13, Baltimore, 1997, Williams & Wilkins.

McCarty GM, McCarty DJ: Effects of topical capsaicin in the therapy of painful osteoarthritis of the hand, *J Rheumatol* 19:604-607, 1992.

McLeod PJ et al: Defining inappropriate practice in prescribing for elderly people: a national consensus panel, *CMAJ* 156(3):385-391, 1997.

Mitchell D: Epidemiology. In Utsinger PD et al, editors: *Rheumatoid arthritis: diagnosis and treatment*, Philadelphia, 1985, JB Lippincott.

Nishihara K, Furst D: Aspirin and other nonsteroid anti-inflammatory drugs. In Koopman WJ, editor: *Arthritis and allied conditions*, ed 13, Baltimore, 1997, Williams & Wilkins.

Panush R: Is there a role for diet and other questionable therapies in managing rheumatic disease? *Bull Rheum Dis* 42:1-4, 1993.

Rasker JJ et al: Lack of beneficial effect of zinc sulfate in rheumatoid arthritis, *Scand J Rheumatol* 11(3):168-170, 1982.

Schnitzer TJ: Osteoarthritis treatment update, *Postgrad Med* 93:89-93, 1993.

Seegmiller J: Gout. In Hazzard WR et al, editors: *Principles of geriatric medicine and gerontology*, ed 3, New York, 1994, McGraw-Hill.

Shapiro JA et al: Diet and rheumatoid arthritis in women: a possible protective effect of fish consumption, *Epidemiology* 7(3):256-263, 1996.

Sibbitt W: Approach to a patient with arthritis. In Rubin R et al, editors: *Medicine: a primary care approach*, Philadelphia, 1996, WB Saunders.

Sorenson J: Development of copper complexes for potential therapeutic use, *Agents Actions Suppl* 8:305-325, 1981.

Sorenson J, Hangarter W: Treatment of rheumatoid and degenerative diseases with copper complexes, *Inflammation* 2:217-238, 1977.

Studenski S, Laird R: Joint problems. In Yoshikawa TT, Brummel-Smith K, Cobbs EL, editors: *Practical ambulatory geriatrics*, St Louis, 1998, Mosby.

Tamblyn R et al: Unnecessary prescribing of NSAIDs and the management of NSAIDs-related gastropathy in medical practice, *Ann Intern Med* 127(6):429-438, 1997.

Tilley BC et al: Minocycline in rheumatoid arthritis: a 48-week, double-blind, placebo-controlled study, *Ann Intern Med* 122:81-89, 1995.

Weinblatt M: Rheumatoid arthritis: the clinical picture. In Koopman WJ, editor: *Arthritis and allied conditions*, ed 13, Baltimore, 1997, Williams & Wilkins.

Weyland C, Goronzy J: Polymyalgia rheumatica and giant cell arteritis. In Koopman WJ, editor: *Arthritis and allied conditions*, ed 13, Baltimore, 1997, Williams & Wilkins.

Wolfe F et al: The American College of Rheumatology 1990 criteria for the classification of fibromyalgia: report of the multi-center criteria committee, *Arthritis Rheum* 33:160-172, 1990.

14

Reproductive: Benign Prostatic Hyperplasia

Background

Benign prostatic hyperplasia (BPH) is a nearly ubiquitous development in men who have testes and live long enough. The condition is characterized by regional, nodular growth in the transition zone of the prostate gland that may impinge on the function of the urinary tract and lead to symptoms of obstruction and irritation (Grayhack, 1992). The condition is not a premalignant state, nor is it related to the development of cancer in any way. It is defined in a variety of ways: by postmortem weight of the prostate, by digital palpation, by suggestive urinary symptoms, and by objective measures based on urinary flow rate or transrectal ultrasonography. Despite the criteria used to define the condition, the overall prevalence of BPH invariably increases with age (Guthrie, 1997).

The prostate gland undergoes two periods of growth as a man ages. The first is a period of normal growth and maturation during puberty, which continues until around age 20. At the end of this growth episode, the average gland weighs around 20 g. During the second phase of growth, which begins around age 40, BPH develops. It is caused by the presence of testosterone and the normal processes of aging. Unlike the first episode, this pattern of growth is pathologic rather than normal (Reilly, 1997). The enlargement associated with BPH takes place in the transition zone of the prostate gland and results in the formation of nodules. After the nodules form, they begin to enlarge, leading to compression of the surrounding tissue and urethra, which passes through the transition zone. Simultaneously, growth of the fibromuscular stroma causes the transition zone to enlarge. The combination of these two processes varies in extent from patient to patient, but together they lead to compression of the urethral lumen and obstructive urinary symptoms (Reilly, 1997). This pattern of growth continues and eventually results in overall hypertrophy of the gland that is palpable on digital rectal examination. Surprisingly, the size of the prostate is not directly related to the presence or degree of obstruction and cannot be used to predict the presence or absence of symptoms in an individual. Not all men with BPH develop symptoms, and some, with minimal enlargement, experience severe disturbances in function. Therefore the size and growth of the prostate are considered irrelevant as independent predictors of urinary flow rates (Lepor, Oesterling, and Wasson, 1996).

Only two risk factors have been identified for the development of BPH: increasing age and male sex. Predisposition cannot be predicted, and its development is not related to sexual activity, vasectomy, improper diet, substance abuse, socioeconomic status, or unhealthy lifestyle (Lepor, Oesterling, and Wasson, 1996). The hormone dihydrotestosterone is known to play a role in the development of the prostate, and its presence is required in the process leading to BPH. Men without an indigenous source of testosterone and those who receive drugs that result in androgen deprivation do not develop BPH and in the latter instance can actually experience a decrease in the size of the prostate (Reilly, 1997) (Figure 14-1).

At least half of men older than 50 have BPH, and the percentage increases with age (Hicks and Cook, 1995). Autopsy data indicate that BPH is seen in approximately 8% of men in their 30s, 40% at ages 50 to 60, more than 70% at ages 61 to 70, and more than 80% in men older than 80. The prevalence of BPH increases in every decade from the fourth to the ninth (Grayhack, 1992). In one study focusing on men age 50 and older, 75% had some sign or symptom of enlargement, and 50% were at least moderately symptomatic. In 25% the symptoms had become so severe that surgery had been required to relieve them (Bruskewitz, 1992). The mortality rate for BPH is improving, dropping from 7.5 per 100,000 in the 1950s to 0.3 per 100,000 in the 1980s (Lepor, Oesterling, and Wasson, 1996). Many factors have contributed to improved morbidity and mortality associated with BPH, including more effective medical management and less destructive surgical procedures.

The cost for treatment of BPH is influenced by the two major factors: the patient and the health care system. Medical intervention for 2 years costs $2,000 in comparison with surgical intervention such as a transurethral resection (TURP) for $9,000 or an open prostatectomy for $13,000. The other salient factors influencing cost are the age, medical condition, and socioeconomic status of the patient (Clinical Practice Guidelines, 1998).

History

The majority of men who seek treatment for BPH do so because symptoms interfere with their activities or their quality of life. For some this interference means the inability to complete a game of golf or to engage in any other long-term activity without devising a strategy for voiding at intervals throughout the afternoon or evening. For others, multiple trips to the bathroom during the night lead to sleep disturbances. The characteristic complex of symptoms associated with BPH is known as *prostatism*, and these symptoms have been characterized as irritative or obstructive. Symptoms that develop initially in the course of BPH are usually caused by obstruction of the flow of urine from the bladder. The growth of the prostate gland exerts pressure on the urethra, which passes through it, and symptoms include a decreased force of stream, urinary hesitancy, dribbling at the end of urination (terminal dribbling), double voiding, and straining to urinate. These symptoms generally occur earlier in the course of the condition than irritative urinary symptoms, which include nocturia, urinary frequency, urinary urgency, dysuria, and urge incontinence (Hicks and Cook, 1995). As the urethra and bladder neck

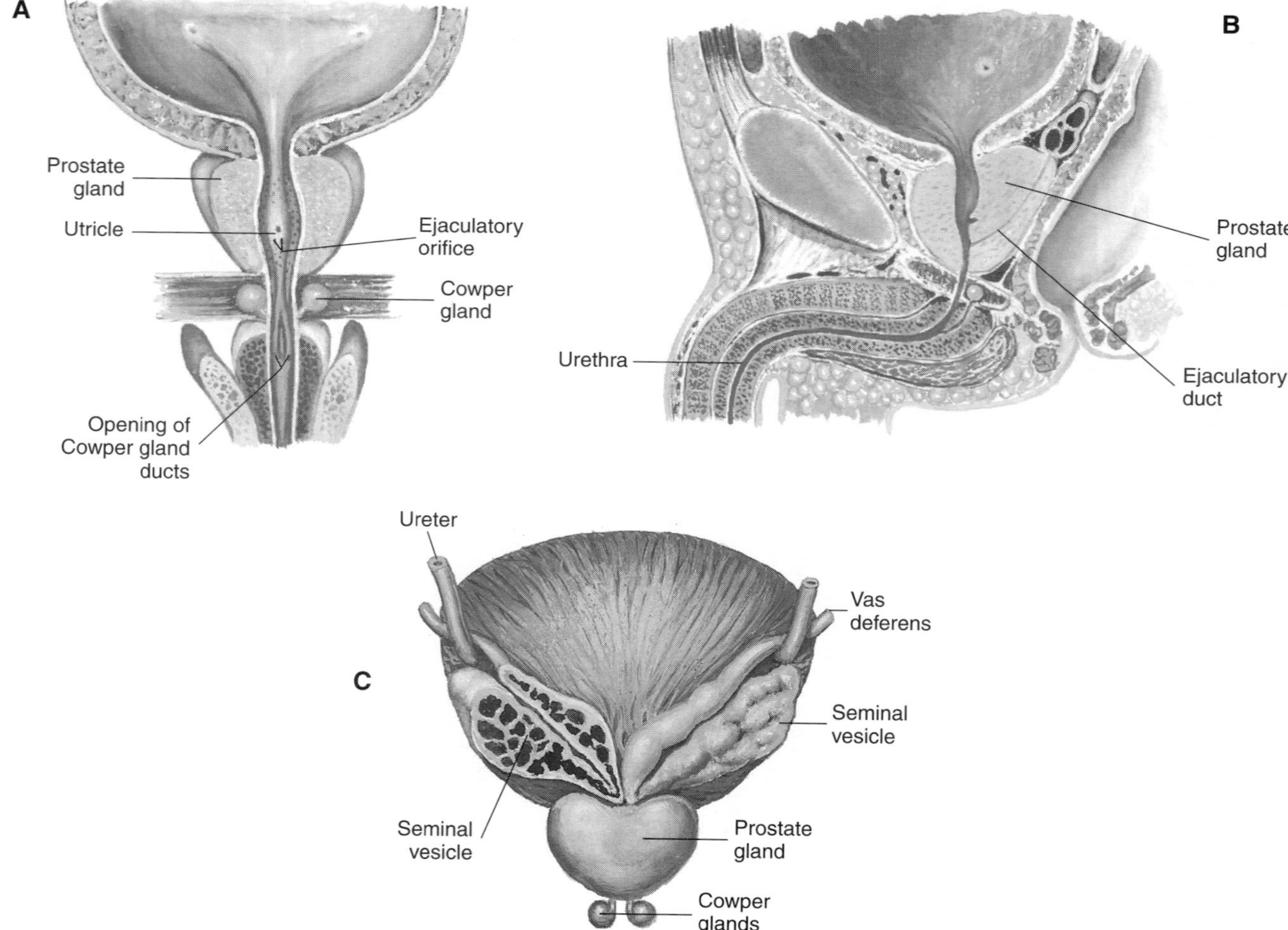

Figure 14-1 Anatomy of the prostate gland and seminal vesicles. **A,** Cross section. **B,** Lateral view. **C,** Posterior view. (From Seidel HM et al: *Mosby's guide to physical examination,* ed 4, St Louis, 1999, Mosby.)

occlusion continues, the bladder must overcome increasing resistance to empty; it may begin to hypertrophy and gradually fail to function. Should this occur, one of two clinical scenarios often develops: the bladder may fail to empty, leading to increased postvoid residual volumes, or it develops a condition known as *detrusor hyperreflexia*, in which it begins to contract involuntarily at a set volume, leading to urge incontinence. Needless to say, not all men with BPH report all symptoms or develop them equally from each category, and men frequently report a waxing and waning of symptom severity. In fact, studies of BPH have shown that disease progression is not inevitable without treatment; urinary flow rates and symptoms may improve over time in some individuals (Reilly, 1997).

Questioning men with BPH may elicit information about strategies used to compensate for certain symptoms. For example, sitting on the toilet, which appears to promote an increased volume voided, may reduce urinary frequency. Many individuals reduce their intake of liquids on days when they have to be out of the house, and some men resort to wearing dark-colored pants to disguise slight incontinence following urination (Hicks and Cook, 1995). Finally, men avoid ingesting certain substances, such as caffeine or over-the-counter (OTC) cold medications, that frequently exacerbate symptoms.

A short questionnaire devised by the American Urological Association (AUA) assesses severity of the reported symptoms. The AUA Symptom Index is the preferred instrument to gauge an individual's level of adjustment to symptoms and guide decision making about interventions. The self-administered tool has seven questions about the symptoms of prostatism, and the scoring system classifies symptoms as mild, moderate, or severe (Benign Prostatic Hyperplasia Guideline Panel, 1994). It helps the practitioner decide on the level of intervention to be used in each individual case: from watchful waiting to surgical intervention (Table 14-1).

Physical Examination

The physical examination focuses on the abdomen and genitalia and includes evaluation of the kidneys, bladder, penis, and scrotal contents. The bladder is palpated to assess the presence of distention and the need for further upper urinary tract evaluation. Individuals with BPH commonly suffer from incomplete emptying of the bladder, but residual urine volume does not necessarily correlate with the reported severity of symptoms, and percussion is generally not revealing.

A digital rectal examination (DRE) is mandatory to assess the size of the prostate and to identify any induration or nodules that might indicate the presence of cancer (Calciano et al., 1993). During the examination, the rectum is examined for polyps or internal hemorrhoids; the posterior and lateral lobes and borders of the prostate are examined for size, consistency, symmetry, and mobility, and the presence of nodules or masses is noted. The normal gland feels smooth and rubbery and does not extend into the rectum more than 1 cm (Lazzaro and Thompson, 1997). A gland with BPH often feels enlarged, smooth, and firm but somewhat elastic, and it protrudes further into the rectum. This is not always the case, however, because the growth of the prostate may be such that the urinary flow is obstructed before hyperplasia is detectable on DRE.

TABLE 14-1 American Urological Association Symptom Index for Evaluating Benign Prostatic Hyperplasia

Questions	Not at All	Less Than 1 Time in 5	Less Than Half the Time	About Half the Time	More Than Half the Time	Almost Always	Score
Over the past month, how often have you had a sensation of not emptying your bladder completely after you finished urinating?	0	1	2	3	4	5	____
Over the past month, how often have you had to urinate again less than 2 hours after you had finished urinating?	0	1	2	3	4	5	____
Over the past month, how often have you found you stopped and started again several times when you urinated?	0	1	2	3	4	5	____
Over the past month, how often have you found it difficult to postpone urination?	0	1	2	3	4	5	____
Over the past month, how often have you had a weak urinary stream?	0	1	2	3	4	5	____
Over the past month, how often have you had to push or strain to begin urination?	0	1	2	3	4	5	____
Over the past month, how many times did you most typically get up to urinate from the time you went to bed at night until you got up in the morning?	None 0	1 Time 1	2 Times 2	3 Times 3	4 Times 4	5 or more times 5	____
						TOTAL SCORE	____

From Barry MJ et al: The American Urological Association Symptom index for benign prostatic hyperplasia, *J Urol* 148:1549-1557, 1992.
Scoring Key:
Mild symptoms: 0 to 7 total points; moderate symptoms: 8 to 19 total points; severe symptoms: 20 to 35 total points.

Diagnostics

Baseline diagnostics include urinalysis to rule out infection and hematuria and blood urea nitrogen and creatinine levels to assess renal function. An increased serum creatinine level is an indication for imaging of the upper renal structures (Guthrie, 1997). This recommendation is not universally accepted.

Prostate-specific antigen (PSA) is believed to leak from the prostatic ductal system into the prostatic stroma and then the bloodstream via capillaries and lymphatics after the prostate gland is damaged by trauma or disease (Oesterling, 1996). The role of PSA in the routine workup of BPH is controversial. According to the guidelines developed by the Agency for Health Care Policy and Research (AHCPR), a PSA study should be optional, although the agency concedes that, when used with DRE, PSA tests improve the detection of cancer (Alexander, 1994). Routine PSA is not recommended by AHCPR because serum levels overlap in BPH and organ-confined prostate cancer, leading to a large number of false positives and false negatives. Because similar PSA levels are possible in patients with BPH and early prostate cancer, screening can result in unnecessary prostate biopsies and other tests. However it is generally accepted that a level above 10 mg/ml is suggestive of cancer (Reilly, 1997). Periodic PSA levels that are trending upward should also be suspect. Because of the recent discovery that several molecular forms of PSA exist in serum, the ability to differentiate between BPH and cancer may be improved. It has been demonstrated that the ratio of two of these molecular forms, free and unbound (f-PSA) and total (t-PSA), increased the diagnostic specificity of the PSA test. In fact, prostate cancer detection by a f-PSA:t-PSA ratio of <18% increased the diagnostic specificity by 20% as compared with the diagnostic efficacy of the total serum PSA concentration alone (Oesterling, 1996) (Figure 14-2).

The position of the AHCPR is in contrast to that of the AUA and the American Medical Association, which advocate annual PSA tests for all men over the age of 50 and for individuals in high-risk populations (African-American men and those with a family history) after age 40 (Alexander, 1994). In practice, PSA testing is usually limited to individuals with a life expectancy of more than 10 years and those in whom a diagnosis of prostate cancer would change the treatment plan (Guthrie, 1997). It is not uncommon at autopsy, in fact, that some degree of prostate cancer is detected that was previously unsuspected and totally unrelated to the cause of death.

Further tests and procedures are reserved for men whose initial evaluation evokes suspicion of complications beyond simple BPH. Urethrocystoscopy is not recommended in the initial evaluation to determine the need for treatment of BPH. Imaging of the upper urinary tract by ultrasound or intravenous urography is not recommended unless the patient has one or more of the following conditions: hematuria, urinary tract infection, renal insufficiency, a history of urolithiasis, or a history of urinary tract surgery (Clinical Practice Guidelines, 1998).

Differential Diagnosis

The differential diagnosis for BPH includes a number of conditions. Disorders such as poorly controlled diabetes, peripheral edema, and diuretic use present with urinary frequency but are not typically associated with obstructive symptoms. Urinary tract

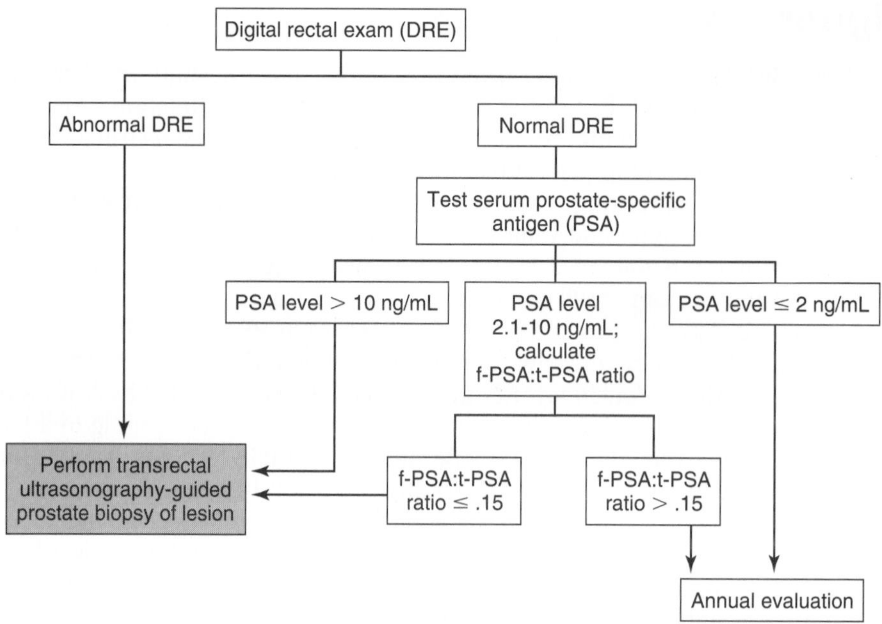

Figure 14-2 Prostate cancer detection algorithm. (From Oesterling JE: Molecular PSA: the next frontier in PCA screening, *Intern Med* 1[5 suppl]:52-68, 1996.)

infections have irritative symptoms, and urethral stricture causes both irritative and obstructive symptoms. Although BPH commonly causes hematuria, it is also associated with bladder cancer. Neurogenic bladder causes urinary frequency, urgency, and retention but not obstructive symptoms; it is associated with diabetes, cerebral infarction, Parkinson's disease, and spinal abnormalities. Finally, certain drugs and substances exacerbate prostatism, including alcohol, caffeine, first-generation antihistamines, and tricyclic antidepressants (Hicks and Cook, 1995).

Treatment

The treatment goals of clinical BPH are to improve symptomatology, relieve obstruction, improve bladder emptying, prevent urinary tract infection, and avoid renal deterioration (Beduschi, Beduschi, and Oesterling, 1998). The range of treatment options for men with BPH include watchful waiting, medication, surgery, and nonsurgical treatment. The presence of multiple disease processes in an individual is often a limiting factor in the development of a treatment plan, and involvement of the patient in the decision-making process is essential for the success of the intervention. A recently concluded 5-year AHCPR study of prostate disease treatment concluded that men with BPH should take a more active role in choosing treatment strategies and that facilitating their participation could result in a lower number of surgeries without sacrificing outcomes, ultimately reducing Medicare costs. The study challenged the conventional wisdom that mild symptoms of BPH always get worse. The study recommended that watchful waiting be made the standard strategy for men with mild symptoms of BPH and that management of

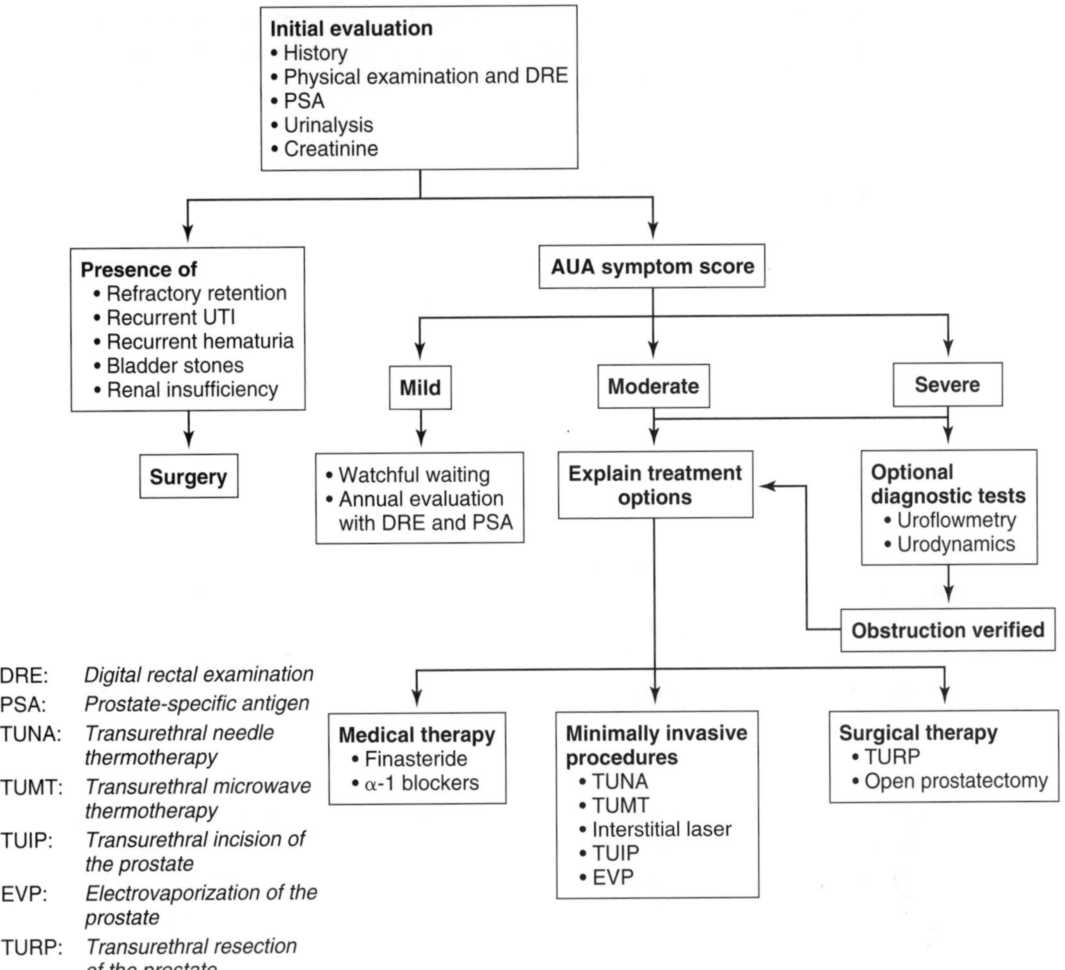

Figure 14-3 Management of BPH. (From Beduschi R, Beduschi M, Oesterling J: Benign prostatic hyperplasia: use of drug therapy in primary care, *Geriatrics* 53[3]:24-40, 1998.)

the condition be guided by the degree to which the individual is bothered by his symptoms (U.S. Public Health Service, 1995). Many urologists agree that watchful waiting is an appropriate strategy for men with very mild symptoms (AUA symptom score of less than 7) (Calciano et al., 1993; Clinical Practice Guidelines, 1998). (See Figure 14-3 for the management of BPH.)

Because BPH is characterized by a waxing and waning pattern of symptom severity, lifestyle changes can often reduce the bothersome factors. Suggested modifications include eating dinner early in the evening; avoiding fluids after 7 PM; taking time to void properly; avoiding excessive salt and diuretics (when possible); reducing caffeine, alcohol, and spices that tend to exacerbate symptoms; and avoiding OTC cold medications that contain adrenergic decongestants (Lepor, Oesterling, and Wasson, 1996). Although many "natural" remedies are touted for relief of urinary symptoms, only saw palmetto, by acting as a 5-alpha reductase inhibitor, is believed by some to provide any benefit in BPH. The benefits and risks of this substance are not well documented, however, and it does not approach the efficacy of the prescription drugs that are currently available (Reilly, 1997; Beduschi, Beduschi, and Oesterling, 1998).

Prescription Medications

Two types of medication are currently approved for treatment of symptomatic BPH. The 5-alpha reductase inhibitors are represented by a single drug, finasteride (Proscar), and act by inhibiting the conversion of testosterone to the prostatic androgen, dihydrotestosterone, leading to a suppression in androgenic stimulation to the prostate gland, a reduction in size, and decreased resistance to urinary flow. Because of its action on testosterone, its side effects potentially include reduced libido, impotence, and ejaculatory disorders (Hicks and Cook, 1995). Finasteride exerts its action slowly, with only mild improvement in symptoms after 6 months of treatment, but continuing efficacy over time. Indeed, in a recent Scandinavian study, additional improvement in symptom relief and urinary flow rates was noted during the second year of treatment with finasteride. A 4-year placebo-controlled study is currently under way to determine whether there is additional benefit associated with continuing treatment for more than 2 years (Eri and Kjell, 1997).

The second class of drugs used to treat BPH is the alpha-adrenergic antagonist group. These drugs decrease the smooth muscle tone of the bladder neck and prostate, resulting in increased relaxation and decreased resistance to urine flow through the urethra and a reduction in the symptoms of outflow obstruction. Symptom relief is achieved quickly, often within hours of the first dose, but a trial of 4 to 6 weeks is recommended to assess response. Terazosin (Hytrin) is widely used for BPH, but doxazosin (Cardura) and prazosin (Minipress) are also used, especially in individuals with coexisting hypertension. The most commonly encountered side effects of these drugs include initial dizziness and postural hypotension. Patients should be cautioned to take them at bedtime as they are preparing to turn out the light (bedside dosing) to reduce the risk of falls. Although approximately 10% of patients find it necessary to stop taking these medications because of side effects, initiating therapy with low dosages and careful titrating can reduce their severity (Lepor, Oesterling, and Wasson, 1996). It has also been noted that longer-acting agents have a more gradual onset of action, thus decreasing the risk of postural hypotension (Guthrie, 1997).

In 1995 the American Foundation for Urologic Disease reported findings of a study comparing the efficacy of finasteride and terazosin. By the AUA Symptom Index, symptoms were significantly reduced in patients given terazosin, but those taking finasteride failed to show any significant improvement over a placebo. The study concluded that terazosin was an effective therapy but finasteride was not, whether used alone or in combination with an alpha blocker. However, prostate size was not a consideration in this study, and participants tended to have smaller prostates. A metaanalysis of six previous studies of finasteride concluded that the effect of this drug is largely restricted to patients with prostates of at least 40 ml, thus explaining in part the poor showing of finasteride in the Veterans Administration Cooperative Study (Eri and Kjell, 1997). Comparative studies focusing on prostate size and duration of therapy are now underway, and their results should be helpful in clarifying the confusion over appropriate drug therapy (Table 14-2).

TABLE 14-2 Medications for the Treatment of Benign Prostatic Hyperplasia

Class/Drug	Dosage	Mechanism of Action	Comments
5-α Reductase Inhibitor			
Finasteride (Proscar)	5 mg/d	Impairs prostate growth by inhibiting the conversion of testosterone to DHT	Well-tolerated; does not affect sexual function in most patients May require up to 6 months to be effective Useful for men with large prostates (>40 g) who do not require acute intervention Affects serum PSA values
Long-acting Selective α-1 Blocker			
Doxazosin mesylate (Cardura)	1 to 8 mg/d	Relaxes prostate smooth muscle, decreasing bladder outlet resistance to urinary flow	Titration advised and once-daily administration at bedtime to minimize risk of side effects May lower blood pressure in men with hypertension Rapid onset of action Useful for men with smaller prostates (<40 g) and acute, mainly irritative symptoms Tamsulosin has no cardiovascular side effects and does not require titration
Terazosin (Hytrin)	1 to 10 mg/d		
Tamsulosin (Flomax)	0.1 to 0.8 mg/d		

DHT; Dihydrotestosterone; PSA; prostate-specific antigen.
From Beduschi R, Beduschi M, Oesterling J: Benign prostate hyperplasia: use of drug therapy in primary care, *Geriatrics* 53(3):24-40, 1998.

Patients who fail to improve significantly following 6 months on finasteride or 2 to 3 months on an alpha blocker should be referred to a urologist for further evaluation. Other indications for referral include an abnormal DRE, hematuria, or a finding of 300 ml or more on postvoid residual (PVR) evaluation.

Nonsurgical Treatments

Nonsurgical treatment options include balloon dilation, urethral stents, microwave thermotherapy and laser ablation. These options have the advantage of less risk than surgical intervention, require only outpatient treatment, and involve less blood loss.

Disadvantages include unknown long-term effects and the use of unproven devices. Balloon dilation involves the intraurethral placement and expansion of a balloon that was designed to split the anterior commissure of the prostate. Although symptomatic improvement has been shown to range from 50% to 70%, peak urinary flow rates tend to return to baseline levels by 1 year after treatment (Hicks and Cook, 1995). Intraurethral stents are used on a temporary basis in obstructed patients who are at high risk for developing complications from surgery. Although many patients report symptomatic relief, reports of urinary frequency and incontinence are not uncommon following the procedure. Microwave thermotherapy is an experimental therapy that has been associated with a 65% improvement in symptoms, but the urine peak flow rates improve only minimally. Transient postoperative obstruction occurs, and there is concern about the formation of fibrosis and scars associated with the procedure (Hicks and Cook, 1995). Other experimental procedures include laser prostatectomy, electrovaporization of the prostate, and transurethral needle ablation.

Surgery

Surgical intervention is recommended for patients with refractory urinary tract infections who have at least one failed attempt at catheter removal; recurrent urinary tract infections, recurrent gross hematuria; bladder stones; or renal insufficiency attributable to BPH (Clinical Practice Guidelines, 1998). The gold standard of BPH treatment remains the TURP because of its high success rate in relieving symptoms—success rates almost as high as those associated with an open prostatectomy, yet with much lower morbidity and mortality rates (Guthrie, 1997). In the United States 400,000 resections are performed each year, with a success rate of 80% to 90%. Despite this, complications such as bleeding, infection, stricture, retrograde ejaculation, impotence, and incontinence are associated with the surgery, making the decision to undergo it a serious one. Indications for this surgery include symptoms that are severe (a high "bother factor") and the presence of clinical conditions such as progressive azotemia, episodes of acute urine retention or bladder stones, PVR of 300 ml or more, or recurrent urinary tract infections secondary to bladder outlet obstruction. A newer surgical option is the transurethral incision of the prostate, which is simpler than a TURP and requires only an incision along the urethra from the bladder neck downward through the prostate. There is no tissue removal in this procedure, and it can be used only in patients with glands weighing 30 g or less. Because it uses telescopically guided technology, recovery is more rapid in most cases (Lepor, Oesterling, and Wasson, 1996). Although there is less risk associated with this procedure, the success rate is lower than that of TURP, and the improvements tend to be temporary.

Follow-up

Because BPH does not progress in a predictable manner, careful follow-up is required to assess the ongoing efficacy of the chosen treatment regimen. Patient monitoring is guided by the AUA Symptom Index, which should be administered every 6 months, or with reports by the patient of changes in symptomatology. Changes in an individual's score indicate the need to consider a revision in the treatment plan and also signal the appropriate time to involve a specialist in treatment planning. The digital rectal examination is mandatory on an annual basis, and the prudent provider will order a PSA at the same visit, despite the current conflict about its usefulness. Complications associated with BPH include urinary tract infection, bladder stones, and renal failure, and the patient should be assessed for these conditions during routine visits.

Education

Patient education is a critical component of the treatment process, especially with the current emphasis on patient involvement in decision making. The patient and family should be assured that the presence of BPH is in no way associated with the development of cancer. Further, they should be assured that BPH is a normal part of aging, much as menopause is for a woman, and that many treatment options are available to relieve the symptoms of prostatism. The patient and family should be aware of the possible complications of BPH and what symptoms require immediate attention. Relevant patient education information may be discussed at routine clinic visits, but a number of written resources are available and should be provided for the patient's later reference.

Summary

The significant prevalence of BPH makes it inevitable that practitioners caring for adult men will evaluate and treat this condition. It is important to know how to proceed with evaluation and to be able to distinguish BPH from cancer of the prostate. Treatment options have grown in recent years, and patients will need and expect information and assistance in choosing an intervention that is appropriate for them to maintain function and quality of life. Ongoing monitoring is also important to evaluate the efficacy of the treatment.

Resources

Health Topics
http://www.uro.com/prostate.htm

References

Alexander W: Practical briefings: new guidelines—and many options—for BPH, *Patient Care* 15:18, 23, 27, 1994.

Barry MJ et al: The American Urological Association symptom index for benign prostatic hyperplasia, *J Urol* 148:1549-1557, 1992.

Beduschi R, Beduschi M, Oesterling J: Benign prostatic hyperplasia: use of drug therapy in primary care, *Geriatrics* 53(3):24-40, 1998.

Benign Prostatic Hyperplasia Guideline Panel: Benign prostatic hyperplasia: diagnosis and treatment, *Clin Pract Guidel Quick Ref Guide Clin,* vol 8, 1994.

Bruskewitz RC: Benign prostatic hyperplasia: intervene or wait? *Hosp Pract (Off Ed)* 15:57-73, 1992.

Calciano RF et al: Finasteride and other options for BPH, *Patient Care* 15:14-40, 1993.

Clinical practice guidelines. Benign prostatic hyperplasia: diagnosis and treatment, *J Am Geriatr Soc* 46:1163-1165, 1998.

Cook WH, Roberts RG: Prostate disease, *Am Fam Physician Monograph* Winter:1-24, 1994.

Eri LM, Kjell JT: Treatment of benign prostatic hyperplasia: a pharmacoeconomic perspective, *Drugs Aging* 10(2):107-118, 1997.

Grayhack JR: Benign prostatic hyperplasia: the scope of the problem, *Cancer* 70(suppl):275-279, 1992.

Guthrie R: Benign prostatic hyperplasia in elderly men: what are the special issues in treatment? *Postgrad Med* 101(5):141-162, 1997.

Hicks RJ, Cook JB: Managing patients with benign prostatic hyperplasia, *Am Fam Physician* 52:135-142, 1995.

Lazzaro M, Thompson M: Update on prostate cancer screening, *Lippincott's Primary Care Practice* 1(4):408-418, 1997.

Lepor H, Oesterling JE, Wasson JH: BPH management: minimal to maximal, *Patient Care* 29:18-35, 1996.

Oesterling JE: Molecular PSA: the next frontier in PCA screening, *Intern Med* 1(suppl 5):52-68, 1996.

Peters S: For men only: an overview of three top health concerns, *Adv for Nurse Pract* 5(4):53-58, 1997.

Reilly NJ: Benign prostatic hyperplasia in older men, *Lippincott's Primary Care Practice* 1(4):421-430, 1997.

Simpson R: Benign prostatic hyperplasia, *Br J Gen Pract* 47:235-240, 1997.

US Public Health Service: Clinical information: prostate cancer patient involvement key to better prostate care, *New Mexico Nurse* 40(4):19, 1995.

15

Reproductive: Menopause

Epidemiology

Worldwide there are 719 million women over the age of 45 (Kronberg, 1990). At present more than 10 million postmenopausal women worldwide are taking some form of estrogen, accounting for sales figures of $2 billion. Conjugated estrogen, as the world's best-selling drug, has an enormous potential market (Calif i Alsina, 1997; Ettinger, 1998). Even though estrogen is widely prescribed, only 10% of postmenopausal women in Europe and 20% in the United States take estrogen replacement therapy (ERT), leaving room for a large increase in future users of ERT (Rees, 1997). Because it is widely agreed that menopause is not a disease and therefore does not need to be cured, ERT should be used for control of symptoms or for disease protection. Symptoms may be extremely bothersome to some. Because of the magnitude of the potential market, claims about the protective function of ERT must withstand the scrutiny of rigorous scientific examination. Clinicians need to approach the use of ERT with up-to-date evidence from clinical trials that investigate the benefits and risks associated with ERT.

Definition

Menopause is a normal physiologic transition that happens in women at an average age of 50 and typically between 45 and 55. Menopause occurs when the ovulation and menstrual cycles end, circulating estrogen and progesterone fall, and serum follicle-stimulating hormone and luteinizing hormone levels rise. This transition (perimenopause) develops over a period of time, with a progressive loss of ovarian function, although there are variations in estrogen production in postmenopausal women. The intervals between menses lengthen, and the postmenopausal period begins after there has been a cessation of menses for at least 6 consecutive months.

Age-related Changes

The physical changes that result from the decrease in estrogen include thinning of the vaginal mucosa, a decrease in vaginal secretions, and, often, urogenital atrophy. Vasomotor instability or hot flashes occur in 75% of postmenopausal women. The use of estrogen alleviates these symptoms. Physiologic and sociocultural influences, as well as personality traits, affect how an individual woman responds to these symptomatic changes (Marks and Shinberg, 1998).

Postmenopausal women who are 50 and older are at risk for osteoporosis and cardiovascular disease. There is significant evidence of an increase in loss of bone mass during the first 5 years after menopause. The incidence of death from cardiac disease for postmenopausal women equals that of men of the same age. The time of menopause marks a significant change in the ratio between men and women in terms of cardiac deaths, which has led to the premise that estrogen provides a protective function from cardiac disease in women. One rationale for the use of ERT has been the protective function in terms of development of either cardiovascular disease or osteoporosis.

Psychologic symptoms that may occur during menopause have reinforced a negative view of a normal physiologic transition period in the lives of older women. Within the youth-oriented culture of the United States, there are multiple negative images of older women (Gannon and Stevens, 1998). There is no consensus on the subject of menopausal causes of mood changes. Clinicians have differing views. Some consider the physical changes associated with menopause such as hot flashes as responsible for mood changes; others fault coincident life events. Providers must be aware of influences on their abilities to provide appropriate evidence-based care for older women (Marks and Shinberg, 1998; Wilbur and Miller, 1998).

History of Estrogen Replacement Therapy Use in the United States

In the 1960s unopposed estrogen was in wide use at a rate of one of every five prescriptions sold to American women; estimates were that a third of women over 50 were prescribed the drug. In 1975 it was found (confirmed in the 1990s by the Postmenopausal Estrogen/Progestin Interventions [PEPI] trials) that estrogen was a causal link to cancer of the uterus, and sales decreased by 40% (Voda, 1992). The 1980s found estrogen in use again, with the addition of progestin as a protective function against the effects of estrogen on uterine cancer. This new combined therapy was widely reported to protect women from heart disease and osteoporosis. Recently there have been claims that estrogen therapy has a protective function against cognitive decline. The risks of estrogen have also been reported: an increased risk for breast cancer, deep vein thrombosis, pulmonary embolism, and gallbladder disease. Estrogen is contraindicated in patients with liver disease.

Protective Benefits of Estrogen Replacement Therapy

Osteoporosis

Older postmenopausal women have an increased risk of sustaining hip fractures and compression fractures of the vertebrae because of the accelerated loss of bone mass during the early years of menopause. Bone loss in women is twice as great as that in men (Rosenthal, 1998).

The questions for clinicians to consider: Does the benefit of ERT's protective function outweigh the risks, and are there other protective functions and drugs? In the 3-year PEPI clinical trial, women assigned to the treatment arms of the protocol had significantly greater increases in hip and spinal bone density (3.5% to 5%) than those assigned to the placebo group, who lost bone density (spinal loss of 1.8% and hip loss of 1.7%) (Writing Group, 1996). Bone density treatment by ERT does provide a protective function and a decreased risk of hip fracture. Recent use of ERT provides protection, and the longer the duration of the therapy, the greater the decrease in risk. Five years after therapy is discontinued, however, the risk of fractures rises to the same level as would have occurred without therapy (Michaelsson et al., 1998). For maximum bone protection, therapy has been recommended to continue for at least 10 years, with the caveat that potential harms include breast cancer and endometrial cancer related to dosage and duration of therapy (Scientific Advisory Board of the Osteoporosis Society of Canada, 1996). Long-term use of ERT is associated with a rise in the occurrence of breast cancer, and compliance has been a major issue.

Lifestyle factors and risk factors not amenable to change, such as race, contribute to a woman's risk of osteoporosis. These issues and new therapies for osteoporosis are addressed in Chapter 11.

Heart Disease

Heart disease is the leading cause of death in older women. The lifetime probability of a woman developing coronary artery disease (CAD) is 46% (LaCharity, 1997). The primary and secondary protective effects of estrogen on heart disease have been a major reason that ERT is prescribed. In analyses of the PEPI trial data, the documented cardioprotective effects of ERT are on the lipid profile (Espeland et al., 1998; Barrett-Connor et al., 1997). Changes in the lipid profiles were associated with increased high-density lipoprotein (HDL) cholesterol, decreased low-density lipoprotein (LDL) cholesterol, and decreased total cholesterol in all treatment arms. The only trend to gain statistical significance was a larger increase in HDL cholesterol in the treatment arm of estrogen 0.625 mg daily only with no added drug (Barrett-Connor et al., 1997). This therapy has a high risk for endometrial cancer in women with an intact uterus.

In the Nurses Health 14-year study of 80,082 women that included 658 cases of nonfatal myocardial infarctions and 281 fatal cases, investigators reported interesting findings, including the following:

The risk of CAD increased by 17% with each increase of 5% of energy from saturated fat than from carbohydrates.

High intake of folate and vitamin B_6 halved the risk of disease and death.
One multivitamin a day had the same effect as long-term ERT.

These dietary primary prevention therapies are considerably less expensive and incur less risk than ERT (Rimm et al., 1998; Verhoef et al., 1998; Hu, 1997).

The 1998 clinical trial of "estrogen plus progestin for secondary prevention of CHD in postmenopausal women" reported by Hulley et al. (1998) does not support the claim of secondary protection from heart disease:

> In a 4.1-year treatment with oral conjugated equine estrogen plus medroxyprogesterone acetate did not reduce the overall rate of CHD events in postmenopausal women with established coronary disease. The treatment did increase the rate of thromboembolic events and gallbladder disease. (p. 605)

The 2,763 women, younger than 80 with a mean age of 66.7, with already established CHD and an intact uterus, were randomized into two treatments: placebo vs. equine estrogen 0.625 mg and 2.5 mg of medroxyprogesterone acetate daily. The study results demonstrated overall no significant differences between groups in the primary outcomes. One hundred seventy-two women in the hormone group and 176 women in the placebo group had a myocardial infarction or CHD death, despite a net 11% lower LDL and a 10% higher HDL in the hormone group than in the placebo group. There were more CHD first-year events in the hormone group, and more women in the hormone group than in the placebo group experienced venous thromboembolic events and gallbladder disease. On the basis of these results, the recommendation was not to start ERT for the purpose of secondary prevention of CHD (Hulley et al., 1998). A prudent practitioner takes into account all claims of protective functions of any drug and then pays close attention to clinical trials that investigate these claims with large and controlled populations.

Psychologic Symptoms

No support or relevant studies show that the use of ERT alleviates psychologic symptoms that may occur at the time of menopause. Furthermore, there is no scientific evidence of a causal link between the physiologic changes associated with menopause and psychologic symptomatology; rather, a reaction to negative life events or a depressive episode is probably being treated with ERT (Holte, 1998).

Cognitive Decline

A metaanalysis of studies dealing with cognitive function, dementia, and ERT counted five observational studies and eight trials that addressed cognitive function in healthy postmenopausal women, and there is no clear finding of benefit. Ten observational studies measured the risk of developing dementia. Analysis suggests a 29% decrease in risk among estrogen users, but the findings are not uniform. The conclusion of the metaanalysis was that all studies had substantial methodologic problems and have produced conflicting results. The recommendations were not to prescribe ERT because of the known risks and the need for adequate trials to investigate the relationship of ERT and cognition (Yaffe and Grady, 1998). Yaffee (1998) then reported on a prospective cohort study of 532 women with an average follow-up of 5 years who were enrolled in the ongoing Study of Osteoporetic Fractures. Three cognitive tests were administered at year 1 and then repeated in 5 years. The conclusions reached were the following:

> Endogenous estrogens are not consistently associated with cognitive performance or risk of cognitive decline . . . . Worse performance . . . among women with higher estrone levels . . . warrants further investigation.

Clinical Examination

History

Many perimenopausal and postmenopausal women seek medical care for symptom relief of the vasomotor experiences referred to as *hot flashes*. The usual description is a sudden feeling of warmth that increases in intensity in the area of the upper chest, neck, and face, followed, for many women, by profuse sweating or a visible erythema. It is quite frequent at night and may cause insomnia or disturbed sleep, which leads to daytime fatigue. Some women develop vaginal itching, stress incontinence, dysuria, and dyspareunia. Also, perimenopausal women may seek care and evaluation for what they consider irregular menstrual periods (Table 15-1).

The nature of the hot flashes, their duration, and associated factors need to be carefully assessed. Effects on the patient's function, especially regarding disruption in sleep pattern, need to be discussed. Other symptoms such as stress incontinence, vaginal dryness or irritation, and dyspareunia should be reviewed.

A complete menstrual and reproductive history, along with a complete medical history, should also note the following:

- Breast cancer
- Gynecologic cancer
- Cardiovascular disease
- Osteoporosis
- Gallstones
- Liver disease
- Migraine headache
- Lipid abnormalities

TABLE 15-1 Symptoms Experienced by the Menopausal Patient

Symptom	Rule Out
Irregular bleeding	Endometrial neoplasia Intrauterine tumor Unexpected pregnancy
Hot flashes	Tuberculosis Human immunodeficiency virus Hodgkin's disease

The family history ought to review breast cancers, gynecologic cancers, osteoporosis, and cardiovascular disease. Necessary lifestyle information includes smoking history, alcohol intake, dietary habits, level of exercise, and sexual activity. Current sexual activity is an important consideration for the practitioner to ascertain because postmenopausal women are at increased risk for contracting sexually transmitted human immunodeficiency virus; vaginal mucosa that is atrophic is easily torn (Janis, 1996). These items of inquiry assist the practitioner and the patient in reaching a decision about the risks ands benefits of taking ERT.

Focused Physical Examination

Baseline height should be recorded for future tracking of loss of height due to osteoporetic vertebral fractures. Breast and cardiovascular status need to be examined. The pelvic examination evaluates for enlargement of the uterus and ovaries, presence of cystocele or rectocele, and the condition of the vaginal mucosa.

Management

The decision to start or not to start hormonal therapy may depend on the severity of the symptoms that a woman may be experiencing. Alternatives to consider for alleviating hot flashes include daily exercise, relaxation practices, cotton clothing, layered clothing, and avoidance of caffeine and alcohol (MacKay, 1997; Miller, 1992). Vaginal atrophy can be alleviated somewhat by continued sexual activity or use of lubricants, such as estrogen cream (Premarin) or a water-based lubricant such as KY lubricant. Topical drugs have the same risks and contraindications as do all other forms of drug preparations.

Estrogen replacement therapy for symptom relief includes the following:

- Informed decision making to include understanding of the side effect of periodic bleeding and bloating, that localized skin irritation is common with the transdermal patch, and that side effects usually subside in a few months (Janis, 1996)
- Understanding and review of the risks and benefits of ERT
- Explanation to the patient that hot flashes may return on termination of ERT
- Common dosing regimens for ERT (Box 15-1)
- Explain that duration of treatment for symptoms is usually 2 years and will need to be tapered

Treatment by ERT for protective function needs to include an individual assessment of the woman's risk for osteoporosis or CHD, her risk factors for breast and uterine cancer, and her actual health practices in the realm of diet, exercise, smoking, and alcohol use. Persistent breakthrough bleeding on ERT needs to be evaluated to rule out endometrial cancer. The incidence of comorbid conditions also has to be considered. Follow-up of patients who are on ERT is an important aspect of primary care. Annual mammograms are a necessity, because long duration of ERT is associated with an increase in breast cancers (Giuliano, 1997).

Box 15-1
Common Dosing Regimens for Estrogen Replacement Therapy

Patient without a uterus
  Continuous estrogen:
    Conjugated estrogens (Premarin), 0.625 mg PO qd; or
    Estradiol (Estrace), 2 mg PO qd; or
    0.05 mg transdermal patch twice weekly
Patient with a uterus
  Cyclic therapy
    Conjugated estrogens, 0.625 mg PO qd, plus 5 to 10 mg medroxyprogesterone (Prempro) on days 1 to 10 of each month
  Continuous therapy
    Conjugated estrogens, 0.625 mg PO qd, plus 2.5 mg of medroxyprogesterone PO qd

Modified from Janis L: Menopause and postmenopausal symptoms. In Rubin R et al, editors: *Medicine: a primary care approach*, Philadelphia, 1996, WB Saunders; and Rousseau ME: Hormone replacement therapy, *Nurse Practitioner Forum* 9(3):147-153, 1998.

Summary

Because of the conflicting reports from retrospective studies and small observational studies, there has been an effort to fund prospective large studies to ascertain the evidence needed to protect the public and to help clinicians and patients make informed decisions. The astute practitioner will look for results from these studies: Women's Health Initiative, The Postmenopausal Estrogen/Progestin Intervention (PEPI) Trial, the Heart and Estrogen-Progestin Replacement Study (HERS), and the Women's International Study of Long Duration Oestrogen after Menopause (Wren, 1998).

Resources

The North American Menopause Society
P.O. Box 94527
Cleveland, OH 44101
(216) 844-8748
http://www.menopause.org

OBGYN Net
http://www.obgyn.net

References

Barrett-Connor E et al: The postmenopausal estrogen/progestin intervention study: primary outcomes in adherent women, *Maturitas* 27(3):261-274, 1997.

Calif i Alsina J: Benefits of hormone replacement therapy: overview and update, *Int J Fertil Womens Med* 42(Suppl 2)329-346, 1997.

Espeland M et al: Effect of postmenopausal hormone therapy on lipoprotein (a) concentration: PEPI investigators, postmenopausal estrogen/progestin interventions, *Circulation* 97(10):979-986, 1998.

Ettinger B: Overview of estrogen replacement therapy: a historical perspective, *Proc Soc Exp Biol Med* 217:2-5, 1998.

Gannon L, Stevens J: Portraits of menopause in the mass media, *Women's Health* 27(3):1-15, 1998.

Giuliano A: Breast. In Tierney LM, McPhee SJ, Papadakis MA: *Current medical diagnosis and treatment 1997*, ed 36, Stamford, Conn, 1997, Appleton & Lange.

Holte A: Menopause, mood, and hormone replacement therapy: methodological issues, *Maturitas* 29(1):5-18, 1998.

Hu FB: Dietary fat intake and the risk of coronary heart disease in women, *N Engl J Med* 337:1491-1499, 1997.

Hulley S et al: Randomized trial of estrogen plus progestin for secondary prevention of coronary heart disease in postmenopausal women and estrogen/progestin replacement study (HERS) research group, *JAMA* 280(7):650-652, 1998.

Janis L: Menopause and postmenopausal symptoms. In Rubin R et al, editors: *Medicine: a primary care approach*, Philadelphia, 1996, WB Saunders.

Kronberg F: Hot flashes: Epidemiology and physiology, *Ann N Y Acad Sci* 592:52, 1990.

LaCharity L: The experience of postmenopausal women with coronary artery disease, *West J Nurs Res* 19(5):583-602, 1997.

MacKay H: Gynecology. In Tierney LM, McPhee SJ, Papadakis MA, editors: *Current medical diagnosis and treatment 1997*, ed 36, Stamford, Conn, 1997, Appleton & Lange.

Marks NF, Shinberg DS: Socioeconomic status differences in hormone therapy, *Am J Epidemiol* 148(6):581-593, 1998.

Michaelsson K et al: Hormone replacement therapy and the risk of hip fracture; population based case-control study: The Swedish Hip Fracture Study Group, *Br Med J* 316(7148):1858-1863, 1998.

Miller F: Alternatives to estrogen for menopausal symptoms, *Clin Obstet Gynecol* 35:4, 1992.

Rees M: The need to improve compliance to HRT in Europe, *Br J Obstet Gynecol* 104:1-3, 1997.

Rimm EB et al: Folate and vitamin B6 from diet and supplements in relation to risk of coronary heart disease among women, *JAMA* 279:359-364, 1998.

Rosenthal R: Osteoporosis, *Arch Am Acad Orthop Surg* 1:52, 1998.

Scientific Advisory Board of the Osteoporosis Society of Canada: Prevention and management of osteoporosis: consensus statement, *Can Med Assoc J* 156(11):1530-1532, 1996.

Verhoef P et al: Folate and coronary heart disease, *Curr Opin Lipidol* 9(1):17-22, 1998.

Voda A: Menopause: a normal view, *Clin Obstet Gynecol* 35(4):923-933, 1992.

Wilbur J, Miller AM: Sociodemographic characteristics, biological factors and symptom reporting in midlife women, *Menopause* 5(1):43-51, 1998.

Wren B: Megatrials of hormonal replacement, *Drugs Aging* 12(5):343-348, 1998.

The Writing Group for the PEPI: Effects of hormone therapy on bone mineral density: results from the postmenopausal estrogen/progestin interventions (PEPI) trial, *JAMA* 276(17):1389-1396, 1996.

Yaffe K: Estrogen therapy in postmenopausal women: effects on cognitive function and dementia, *JAMA* 279(9):688-695, 1998.

Yaffe K, Grady D: Serum estrogen levels, cognitive performance, and risk of cognitive decline in older community women, *J Am Geriatr Soc* 46(7):816-821, 1998.

16

Neurologic: Parkinson's Disease

Parkinson's disease (PD), a neurodegenerative disorder, afflicts approximately 600,000 persons in the United States; 40,000 new cases are diagnosed each year (McDonald, 1994). Onset of symptoms usually occurs between the ages of 60 and 69, although in 5% of patients the first signs are seen before age 40. About 1% of those age 65 and older and 2.5% of those older than 80 have PD (Uitti, 1998). Incidence is greater in men by a ratio of 3:2 men to women (Tapper, 1997), and the highest prevalence of the disease is among nursing home residents, with rates reported as high as 10% of the population (Feinberg, 1998).

Parkinson's disease is very costly in terms of medications and caregiving. Antiparkinsonian medications alone cost $5,000 per year (Feinberg, 1998). This cost increases dramatically for patients who experience motor complications with progressive disease. In addition, there are very high indirect costs of care in loss of productivity for both the patient and the caregiver.

Pathophysiology

Although the exact cause of PD is unknown, research has concentrated on genetics, environmental toxins, endogenous toxins, and viral infection. The etiology of this progressive disease is thought to occur when the dopamine cells of the substantia nigra degenerate (Stern, 1997). There is an 80% to 90% loss of dopamine-producing cells by the time the patient becomes symptomatic. The result is an excessive inhibitory output from the basal ganglia to the thalamus. This change leads to decreased stimulation from the thalamus to the motor cortex, resulting in the characteristic bradykinesia of the disease (Feinberg, 1998). Imbalance between the levels of dopamine and acetylcholine, together with the loss of the dopamine receptor sites, affects the refinement of voluntary movement and causes the primary symptoms of PD: bradykinesia, resting tremor, and postural instability. The seven cardinal features of PD are tremor at rest, rigidity,

TABLE 16-1 Drugs That May Cause Parkinsonian Symptoms

Drug Category	Specific Drug
Antipsychotics	Haloperidol (Haldol), thioridazine (Mellaril), risperidone (Risperdal), chlorpromazine (Thorazine), lithium (Lithobid)
Antiemetics	Prochlorperazine (Compazine), metoclopramide (Reglan)
Antihypertensives	Methyldopa (Aldomet), verapamil (Calan), captopril (Capoten), reserpine
Antianginals	Diltiazem (Cardizem)
Antineoplastics	Cytarabine (Cytosar), vincristine (Oncovin)
Antiepileptics	Valproate (Depakote), phenytoin (Dilantin)

Modified from Kollar W, Montgomery E: Issues in the early diagnosis of Parkinson's disease, *Neurology* 49(suppl 1):10-25, 1997; and Moreau D: *Nursing 96 drug handbook,* Springhouse, PA, 1996, Springhouse.

bradykinesia, hypokinesia, flexed posture, loss of postural reflexes, and the freezing phenomenon.

Secondary PD may be caused by several medications, such as antipsychotic medications, antiemetic medications, antihypertensives, antianginals, antineoplastics, and antiepileptics (Table 16-1). Drugs and toxins such as 1-methyl-4-phenyl-1,2,3,6 tetrahydropyridine (MPTP), carbon monoxide, manganese, and alcohol withdrawal can also cause parkinsonian symptoms (Kollar, 1993). In the 1970s several young heroin addicts, using MPTP, a synthetic heroin, developed parkinsonian features. Their misfortune provided a major breakthrough for PD research, because animal models could now be made to further study this disorder (Stern, 1997). Another cause of parkinsonian symptoms is multiinfarcts to the substantia nigra. In this case symptoms are usually unresponsive to Parkinson's medication. Other possible causes of secondary parkinsonism to consider are parathyroid abnormalities, hypothyroidism, hepatocerebral degeneration, brain tumors, and normal-pressure hydrocephalus. Depression often accompanies PD and can mimic or enhance its symptoms. Parkinson plus syndromes are similar to PD but have additional neurologic abnormalities. Examples are progressive supranuclear palsy, Shy-Drager syndrome, and olivopontocerebellar palsy. Discussion of these diseases is beyond the scope of this chapter, but Table 16-2 summarizes symptoms associated with each condition.

Clinical Examination

History

For many, the onset of the disease is insidious, and this delays treatment. In early stages of the disease, the most common complaint is tremor. The Parkinson's tremor is most commonly a pill-rolling motion of the forefinger and thumb at rest, but tremor can also be seen in the head and feet. The patient may also complain of changes in handwriting, trouble with speech volume, stiffness, unusual fatigue, slowness of movement, difficulty in walking, falling, and difficulty in rising to a standing position or turning in bed. Symptoms progress over time as the disease progresses. Those with severe disease may become bedridden and require complete assistance with activities of daily living.

TABLE 16-2 Distinguishing Features

Neurologic Disorder	Distinguishing Features
Essential tremor	Kinetic tremor plus instability Frequent family history
Drug-induced parkinsonism	Antidopaminergic exposure Bilateral onset Reversibility
Progressive supranuclear palsy	Voluntary vertical gaze palsy Axial rigidity No tremor
Multiple system atrophy	Prominent dysautonomia (Shy-Drager syndrome) Cerebellar dysfunction (usually hereditable cerebellar atrophy) or peripheral neuropathy with brainstem/cerebellar atrophy
Striatal nigral degeneration	Akinetic-rigid No tremor Minimal or no benefit from levodopa
Alzheimer's disease with parkinsonism	Dementia more prominent than parkinsonism Dementia and parkinsonism probably related to the same pathologic process
Cortical basal ganglionic degeneration	Alien limb Dystonia Myoclonus Supranuclear gaze palsy Parietal sensory loss Asymmetric
Huntington's disease	Younger patient Positive family history No tremor Positively distinguished by DNA triplet code (CAG) repeat length
Toxin-induced parkinsonism	Exposure to carbon monoxide, manganese, cyanide, carbon disulfide, 1-methyl-4-phenyl-1,2,3,6 tetrahydropyridine (MPTP), n-hexane, methanol, or lacquer thinner

From Vitti RJ: Tremor: how to determine if the patient has Parkinson's disease, *Geriatrics* 53(5):34, 1998.

Physical Examination

On neurologic examination, look for evidence of the primary symptoms of PD: bradykinesia, resting tremor, and postural instability. In early disease patients exhibit bradykinesia (slowness of movement). They have masked facies, decreased blink rate, a monotonous tone, and low-volume speech. Frequent postural adjustments are not made; they seem to sit absolutely still. Muscular rigidity or cogwheeling can be found in all extremities and the neck. Testing for muscle tone can be followed by testing for cogwheeling: one hand is placed on the elbow or knee and the limb is moved; a cogwheeling or ratcheting of the limb is felt.

Tremor. Resting tremor may be noted in the hands, feet, or head. During movement the tremor diminishes. For example, during finger-to-nose testing, the tremor in the hand diminishes. This tremor is distinguished from an essential tremor because it diminishes with movement of the affected limb. Tremor can also be temporarily aggravated during stress (such as an argument) or with fatigue. Micrographia is present; handwriting is small and cramped. It may also be affected by tremor. Samples of handwriting in the chart are useful to monitor the progress of the disease or the effectiveness of medication.

Differentiation of tremors is an important aspect of securing a differential diagnosis, because one of the common errors in clinical practice is to diagnose PD on the basis of tremor alone. Frequently an essential tremor with a family history is mistaken for a resting tremor of PD (Whitehouse, 1997) (Table 16-3).

Tremor is defined as a rhythmic oscillation of a body part. The two most frequently encountered tremors in primary care are essential tremor and the tremor associated with PD. The characteristic tremor of PD is tremor at rest with pill rolling. A tremor maximally activated during maintenance of a posture is characteristic of essential tremor, and a tremor maximally activated during movement, a kinetic or intention tremor, is generally synonymous with cerebellar disease (i.e., secondary to trauma, tumor, multiple sclerosis, or stroke) (Reich, 1998).

TABLE 16-3 Parkinson's Disease vs. Essential Tremor

	Parkinson's Disease	Essential Tremor
History		
Age of onset	60, with limited variability	Variable, more common after 50
Duration of symptoms from prior presentation	Months-year	Years-decades
Family history	Generally negative	Generally positive (autosomal dominant)
Response to alcohol (small amount)	None	Improvement
Physical Examination		
Position of maximal activation	Rest	Maintenance of a posture
Frequency	3-6 Hz	6-12 Hz
Morphology	Pill rolling	Flexion and extension at shoulder, wrist
Anatomic	Unilateral	Bilateral, may be onset asymmetric
Body part affected	Upper limb> lower limb> chin=lips	Upper limbs>head> voice>chin=lips> lower limbs
Associated parkinsonian signs	Yes	No
Handwriting	Small, nontremulous	Normal size, tremulous
Natural history	Progressive	Insidiously progressive

Adapted from Reich SG: "Doctor, I shake." Presentation at Current Topics in Geriatrics, American Geriatric Society, Baltimore, 1998.

Postural Instability. Postural instability is easily examined by first watching the patient move from the waiting room. Patients have difficulty rising from a chair without pushing themselves up. Gait is difficult to initiate, slow and shuffling, with decreased arm swing. Posture is flexed, with a stooped trunk and arms semiflexed (Figure 16-1).

Turning is accomplished en bloc with small steppage in a circle (marche à petits pas). Propulsion (an inability to stop forward movement) or retropulsion (inability to stop backward movement) is present. Freezing of movement occurs as the disease advances. When negotiating a curb or a doorjamb or turning in a tight circle, patients are unable to lift their feet to walk. Freezing can be interrupted by initiating movement other than walking, such as touching another's arm, or taking a very large step or marching step. One patient studied had severe freezing, walked with the aid of a walker, and was able to walk by only kicking a small cigar box while walking. If the box was taken away, the patient was unable to walk.

Diagnostic Testing

For diagnostic testing, consider elimination of other causes of the patient's symptoms. Computed tomography (CT) or magnetic resonance imaging of the brain can rule out vascular disease, tumor, hydrocephalus, and other structural abnormalities. Repeat scanning during the course of the disease is indicated only when there has been a marked change in the person's condition and other causes should be considered. For instance, a person with PD who frequently falls may need to have a CT scan to rule out subdural hematoma. Complete blood count, chemistries, liver function testing, thyroid testing, and a drug screen should be obtained as necessary. Refer to Table 16-1 for drugs that may cause parkinsonian symptoms.

After the diagnosis of PD is made, no further diagnostic testing is necessary unless

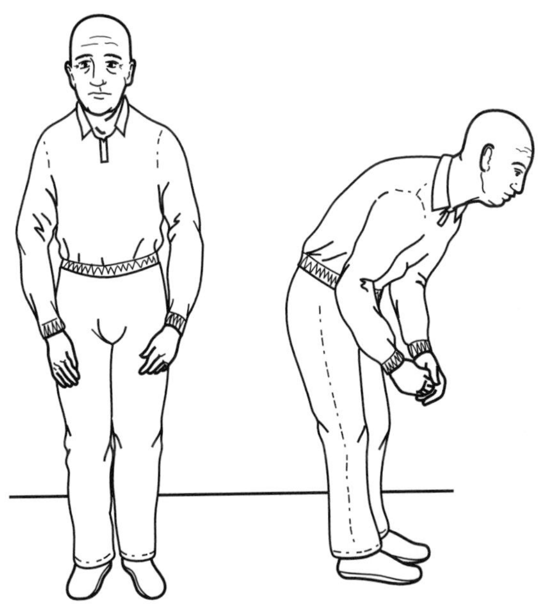

Figure 16-1 Parkinson patient body posture. (Modified with permission from Rowland LP: *Merritt's textbook of neurology,* ed 8, Baltimore, 1995, Williams & Wilkins, p. 715; In Tapper VJ: Pathophysiology, assessment, and treatment of Parkinson's disease, *Nurse Pract* 22[7]:85, 1997.)

there is a major change in the person's status. For instance, an increase in falling may be caused by orthostatic hypotension, development of hydrocephalous, or subdural hematoma. Appropriate diagnostic testing after examination should be ordered. The patient should continue to have annual physical examinations to monitor other age-related conditions or concurrent illness.

Consultation

A person suspected of having PD should always have a neurologic consultation to determine or confirm the diagnosis. If distance or availability impedes the care of a neurologist, the primary care provider can follow recommendations for treatment. When treatment is ineffective, new problems arise, or there is a marked change in the person's condition, the neurologist should be consulted or reevaluate the patient. Again, the diagnosis is based on history, neurologic examination indicating the clustering of the primary symptoms of PD (rigidity, tremor, bradykinesia, loss of postural reflexes), and elimination of other causes.

Treatment

PD is a chronic, progressive neurologic disease. Goals of therapy are to slow the progress of the disease, to maximize function to enable the patient to enjoy, as long as possible, a normal active life, and to minimize any disability that may result from the progression of the disease.

Therapeutic

There are many medications available to treat PD and several pending Food and Drug Administration (FDA) approval. When deciding among them, one must first consider the impact of the disease and symptoms on the person to determine which medication to use. Another important aspect of Parkinson's medication is compliance. Patients get the most benefit from their medications if they are taken on a regular schedule. Frequently symptoms improve when patients are asked to take their medications consistently at the same time, thus avoiding additional medication. See Table 16-4 for major drug classes used to treat PD.

Anticholinergics. Anticholinergics are used primarily for the treatment of tremor and early in the course of the disease. They block the action of the neurotransmitter acetylcholine, promoting a balance between acetylcholine and dopamine. The most commonly used anticholinergics are trihexyphenidyl (Artane), benztropine (Cogentin), and procyclidine (Kemadrin). The most common side effects of these medications are dry mouth, blurred vision, constipation, orthostatic hypotension, confusion, and hallucinations.

Amantadine. Early in Parkinson's disease, amantadine is also useful, but its usefulness tends to last only several months. It has anticholinergic and mild dopaminergic activity. Side effects are mild and include confusion and mottling of the skin. When discontinuing amantadine therapy, the patient must be weaned to avoid a sudden increase in PD symptoms.

TABLE 16-4 Parkinson Medications

Medications	Action	Dosage	Side Effects
Anticholinergics			
Trihexyphenidyl (Artane)	Blocks acetylcholine, thus promoting balance between acetylcholine and dopamine	2-20 mg/d	Dry mouth, blurred vision, constipation, orthostatic hypotension, confusion and hallucinations
Benztropine (Cogentin)		0.5-7 mg/d	
Symmetrel (amantadine)	Increases endogenous dopamine, prevents neuronal uptake of natural dopamine	100 mg bid	Mottling of skin, confusion
Levodopa			
Carbidopa (Lodosyn)	Levodopa crosses the blood-brain barrier and converts to dopamine inside the brain; carbidopa blocks conversion of levodopa outside the brain.	25-75 mg/d	Nausea and vomiting, orthostatic hypotension, and confusion and/or hallucinations. Long-term complications: dyskinesia, dystonias, motor fluctuations
Levodopa (L-dopa)		400-1000 mg/d	
Carbidopa-levodopa (Sinemet, Sinemet CR)		100-150/1000-1500 mg/d	
Dopamine Agonists			
Bromocriptine (Parlodel)	Dopamine synaptic agonists, decrease dopamine turnover.	2.5-100 mg/d	Dyskinesias, orthostatic hypotension, confusion and hallucinations
Pergolide (Permax)		0.05-5 mg/d	
Pramipexole (Mirapex)		0.1-5 mg/d	
Ropinirol (Requip)		3-24 mg/d	
MAO Inhibitor			
Selegiline (Eldepryl)	Inhibits MAO-B, thereby inhibiting dopamine metabolism	5-10 mg/d	
COMT Inhibitors			
Tolcapone (Tasmar)	Prolongs the effect of levodopa	100-200 mg/d	Mild headache, nausea, loose stools, changes in urine color, transient increase in dyskinesias

MAO, Monoamine oxidase, *COMT,* catechol-O-methyltransferase.

Levodopa or Carbidopa-Levodopa. Levodopa is the precursor to dopamine, the lacking neurotransmitter in PD. Levodopa crosses the blood-brain barrier and then is converted to dopamine inside the brain. Carbidopa blocks conversion of the levodopa outside the brain, decreasing the side effect of nausea and allowing more levodopa to enter the brain. Patients usually respond very quickly to carbidopa-levodopa (Sinemet) and can feel the onset within 60 minutes. Regular carbidopa-levodopa should be taken on an empty stomach, if tolerated, for the best absorption. Patients who cannot tolerate this should begin taking the drug with food and then change to taking it on an empty stomach later. Time-release carbidopa-levodopa (Sinemet CR) was developed to reduce motor fluctuations. To switch from Sinemet to Sinemet CR, increase the amount of levodopa by 10%. Changes in Sinemet CR may take 7 to 10 days to take effect; it is important to remind patients of this wait factor, because they will be used to receiving an immediate response to regular carbidopa-levodopa. Also, patients do not feel this form "kick in" after 30 minutes, and they may think it is ineffective. The time-release form should be taken on a full stomach and should not be crushed. Common side effects are nausea and vomiting, orthostatic hypotension, confusion, and hallucinations.

Long-term complications of this therapy are dyskinesias, dystonias, and motor fluctuations (the wearing-off phenomenon and the on-off phenomenon). Dyskinesias are the most common side effect; they are caused by too much dopamine in the brain and create symptoms opposite to the slow- and poor-moving patient with PD. Dyskinesias are choreoathetoid movements usually of the head, trunk, or extremities. They may be expressed as mild turning or tapping of the foot or hand or a twitching of the mouth, or they may be as dramatic as flinging of the extremities and trunk. When given a choice, most patients prefer to be mildly dyskinetic instead of bradykinetic. Dystonias are painful sustained muscle contractions that may occur with dyskinesias. They are difficult to treat but may respond to a decrease in levodopa-carbidopa or to an addition of the time-release form at bedtime to avoid early morning dystonias.

Motor fluctuations may present in two different ways: the wearing-off phenomenon or the on-off phenomenon. The wearing-off phenomenon occurs after several years of levodopa-carbidopa treatment (Kollar and Montgomery, 1997). The drug's effectiveness begins to wear off before the next dose is due. As the frequency of doses is increased, the on-off phenomenon begins to occur. The patient has periods of immobility lasting minutes to hours ("off"), followed by periods of mobility ("on"). These changes are not associated with medication doses. This phenomenon can be very dramatic; the patient may enter the office in a wheelchair, unable to move. Then, during the appointment, the patient gradually begins to move more freely and eventually walks out of the office unassisted.

Dopamine Agonists. Dopamine agonists act directly on the dopamine synapses and are useful adjunctive therapies to levodopa-carbidopa. They are effective to help control motor fluctuations and can reduce the total amount of levodopa-carbidopa dosage. The most common side effects are orthostatic hypotension, confusion, and hallucinations.

Monoamine Oxidase Inhibitor. The type B monoamine oxidase (MAO) inhibitor selegiline (Eldepryl) has been shown to delay the need for levodopa-carbidopa in the treatment of early disease and helpful in treating motor fluctuations. It stops the metabolism of dopamine. Patients do not need to follow the tyramine-free diet (or "cheese diet") recommended with the MAO inhibitor antidepressants because of its selectivity of MAO inhibition. It is given in a twice-daily dosage, one tablet in the morning and one at noon, because more MAO is available in the morning. This dosage also helps with the common side effect of insomnia. Other side effects are nausea, dizziness, dry mouth, abdominal pain, confusion, and hallucinations.

Catechol-O-Methyl Transferase Inhibitors. The Catechol-O-Methyl transferase (COMT) inhibitors (recently approved by the FDA) are the newest anti-PD medications. COMT is involved in the metabolism of levodopa and dopamine. Inhibition of this enzyme causes a decreased concentration of levodopa metabolite, 3-O-methyldopa, which may cause levodopa motor fluctuations. Also, levodopa blood levels are maintained for a longer time, resulting in a smoother effect from levodopa (Stern, 1993). Side effects are headache, dizziness, nausea, loose stools, change in urine color, and a transient increase in dyskinesias.

The drug therapies aim to control the symptoms and the progression of the disease. The next section deals with interventions that assist the patient in maintaining maximum function and preventing or alleviating disability (Boxes 16-1 and 16-2).

Box 16-1

Parkinsonism Teaching Plan

1. Assess the patient's and family's knowledge of, misconceptions about, and experiences with Parkinson's disease (PD).
2. Identify areas of concern to the patient and family regarding the disease, its treatment, and its impact on their lives.
3. Describe the incidence, etiology, pathophysiology, and primary and secondary symptoms of PD.
4. Describe the medical management of PD, including the various drug therapies.
5. Describe the common side effects of the drug therapies, their manifestations and measures that which minimize the side effects.
6. Discuss common self-care deficits of PD patients, and identify those the patient now has.
7. Teach methods to minimize or overcome the identified self-care deficits, and provide written information as needed.
8. Discuss common safety hazards faced by PD patients, and identify those presently existing for the patient.
9. Discuss measures to minimize or eliminate the identified safety hazards of the PD patient.
10. Instruct and provide information on a protein-restriction diet, as appropriate, to manage parkinsonism symptoms.
11. Provide written information regarding available PD community and national resources and organizations.
12. Assess the need for further education of the patient and family, and develop learning objectives if necessary.

Box 16-2

Guidelines for Managing Common Problems

1. If a patient is having a poor response to the medications, make sure the patient is taking the medications at regular intervals. Many times poor compliance with the prescribed regimen is the reason for inadequate medication response.
2. Educating the patient about the benefits of following the prescribed regimen (e.g., avoiding increased dosages or an increase in the number of drugs) is an early goal.
3. If the patient is experiencing confusion, hallucinations, or increasing memory problems, first review the patient's medication list to determine if these symptoms are a side effect.
4. Exercise is as important as medication in treating Parkinson's disease.
5. Stressful situations, such as anxiety or an argument, can increase symptoms temporarily.

Interventions for Managing Common Problems

Inability to Perform Activities of Daily Living

Encourage regular exercise within limitations.

Encourage realistic independence with activities of daily living.

Encourage use of affected hand unless tremor is extreme.

Provide nutritional counseling (e.g., protein redistribution diet), if indicated.

The patient who is not taking a decarboxylase inhibitor should omit any multivitamin containing B_6 and should limit intake of foods high in B_6 (e.g., milk, eggs, meat).

Avoid phenothiazines for nausea because they block dopamine action.

Evaluate effectiveness of drugs for rigidity, tremor, and bradykinesia.

Evaluate the need for devices to assist the patient or for physical and occupational therapy consultation, as needed.

Poor Speech

Encourage diaphragmatic speech.

Poor Handwriting

Encourage face and tongue exercises and massage.

Explore alternate methods of written communication.

Evaluate choreiform and athetoid movements (e.g., head dropping, facial grimacing, tongue protrusion, opening and closing mouth) in relation to medication.

Constipation

Provide nutritional counseling (e.g., high-residue diet, increased fluid intake).

Encourage exercise.

Establish defecation pattern.

Use stool softeners, laxatives, suppositories, and enemas, as needed.

Use warm liquids to stimulate peristalsis.

Evaluate constipation in relation to medication.

Monitor for signs of impaction or bowel obstruction.

Impaired Gait (Freezing, Propulsion, Retropulsion)

Evaluate symptoms (shuffling, tremor, freezing) in relation to medication.

Teach methods to facilitate rising from bed or chair (rocking back and forth before standing up).

Teach methods to assist with freezing (e.g., stepping over imaginary line, rocking).

Assess potential safety hazards in home.

Encourage regular exercise.

Physical therapy consultation for gait training and muscle-strengthening exercises, as needed.

Poor Sleep

Teach methods to promote a regular sleep pattern (e.g., daytime stimulus, exercise, quiet environment).

Sleep medication, as needed.

Evaluate sleep disturbance in relation to medication.

Dysphagia

Provide nutritional counseling (e.g., semisoft diet).

Teach measures that minimize problems associated with dysphagia (e.g., avoid thin liquids, cut food into small pieces, sit upright for meals).

Evaluate medication in relation to dysphagia.

Overweight or Underweight
Provide nutritional counseling, referral to nutritionist, as needed.
Increase activity as appropriate.
Establish short- and long-term goals for weight change.
Urinary Hesitancy, Urgency, and Incontinence
Establish bladder-emptying schedule.
Stimulation techniques to initiate voiding (Credé's reflex, Valsalva maneuver).
Use incontinence devices, as needed.
Evaluate urinary problems in relation to medication and to mobility.
Risk of Injury
Assess potential safety hazards in home.
Teach measures to minimize or eliminate safety hazards.
Evaluate need for supervision of patient.
Provide physical or occupational therapy consultation, as needed.
Poor Memory, Confusion, Hallucinations, Dementia
Evaluate symptoms in relation to medication.
Evaluate memory deficit, dementia symptoms, and disease progression through mental status tests, as needed.
Teach cognitive remediation techniques for memory problems.
Teach family and caregivers help strategies for specific dementia symptoms (such as confusion and hallucinations).
Evaluate need for family counseling, caregiver support, and community resources.
Depression
Assess the presence and degree of depressive symptoms.
Evaluate depressive symptoms in relation to medication.
Provide psychiatric consultation, as needed.
Educate about the disease and medications.
Provide written information regarding the disease and current regimens.
Provide information on community and national resources and organizations.

Summary

PD is a costly, disabling disorder that can be difficult to diagnose, especially early in its onset. The history and a skillful neurologic examination can provide the clues to detect this problem. Appropriate diagnostic testing and referral to a neurologist are important in establishing the diagnosis and treatment plan. Not only is pharmacologic intervention important but also focused education and therapies for managing problems common to PD can enhance successful management of the patient's overall functioning and well-being.

Resources

American Parkinson Disease Association
60 Bay Street
Staten Island, NY 10301
(718) 981-8001
(800) 223-APDA
http://www.APDAParkinson.com

National Parkinson Foundation, Inc.
1501 N.W. 9th Avenue (Bob Hope Road)
Miami, FL 33136-1494
(305) 547-6666
(800) 327-4545
(800) 433-7022 (in Florida)
http://www.parkinson.org

Parkinson's Support Groups of America
11376 Cherry Hill Road, Apt 204
Beltsville, MD 20705
(301) 937-1545

The Parkinson's Institute
1170 Morse Avenue
Sunnyvale, CA 34089-1605
(408) 734-2800

Parkinson's Educational Program (PEP) USA
3900 Birch Street
Newport Beach, CA 92660
(714) 250-2975
(800) 344-7872

United Parkinson Foundation
833 West Washington Boulevard
Chicago, IL 60607
(312) 733-1893

References

Bunting L, Fitzsimmons B: Degenerative disorders. In Barker E, editor: *Neuroscience nursing*, St Louis, 1994, Mosby.

Feinberg M: The role of COMT inhibitors in improving levodopa therapy in elderly patients with Parkinson's disease, *Annals of Long Term Care* 6(suppl F), 1998.

Hauser R, Zesiewicz T: Medications for the treatment of Parkinson's disease. In Hauser R, Zesiewicz T, editors: *Parkinson's disease questions and answers*, Hampshire, England, 1997, Merit.

Kollar W: Epidemiology of Parkinson's disease, *Am Parkinson's Disease Assoc Newsletter*, Fall: 1, 1993.

Kollar W, Montgomery E: Issues in the early diagnosis of Parkinson's disease, *Neurology*, 49(suppl 1):10-25, 1997.

Moreau D, editor: *Nursing 96 drug handbook*, Springhouse, PA, 1996, Springhouse.

Reich SG. "Doctor, I Shake" presentation at Current Topics in Geriatrics, Johns Hopkins Geriatrics Center and the American Geriatrics Society, Baltimore, October 1998.

Rowland LP: *Merritt's textbook of neurology*, ed 8, Baltimore, 1995, Williams & Wilkins.

Stern M: Contemporary approaches to the pharmacotherapeutic management of Parkinson's disease: an overview, *Neurology* 49(suppl 1):2-9, 1997.

Tapper VJ: Pathophysiology, assessment, and treatment of Parkinson's disease, *Nurse Pract* 22(7):76-80, 1997.

Uitti RJ: Tremor: how to determine if the patient has Parkinson's disease, *Geriatrics* 53:30-36, 1998.

Whitehouse PJ: Geriatric neurology. In Burton et al, editors: *Geriatrics and Gerontology 1997 Yearbook*, St Louis, 1997, Mosby.

17

Dementia

Dementia is an organic disorder with the loss of intellectual abilities of sufficient severity to interfere with social or occupational functioning. The deficit is multifaceted and involves memory, judgment, and abstract thought. Behavioral and personality changes also occur in an alert person.

Types of dementia are Alzheimer's type—50% to 60% cases, vascular dementia—15% to 20%, mixed dementia (a combination of the above)—20%, and Parkinson-associated dementia—10% to 15%.

The main etiologic factor in the development of primary dementia is advanced age. At the present time there is no known definite cause of most dementia-type illnesses, although infections, medications, metabolic disorders, toxic chemicals, neurologic disorders, nutritional disorders, vascular disorders, and space-occupying lesions can cause and/or contribute to the development of dementia (Box 17-1).

Age-related Changes

Cognitive ability is influenced by a person's state of health, genetic code, past experiences, educational background, cultural influences and beliefs, and current living conditions. Physical changes in the brain caused as a result of the normal process of aging and selected pathologic conditions may also affect the cognitive abilities of some elderly individuals. When cognitive abilities fall to a level that precludes a person's ability to care for himself or herself, health problems occur (Stockton and Burke, 1997).

Scientists disagree about what universal changes occur in the human brain and how these changes relate to cognitive function. There is agreement that the following changes do occur in association with aging: loss in brain volume and brain weight, enlargement of the ventricles, decrease in enzymes, loss of protein, loss of lipids, and alterations in the amount of and receptors for some neurotransmitters.

The extent of the contribution of these age-related changes to each aging person's cognitive abilities is unknown. The most significant functional loss related to neurologic change is the *slowed response time to tasks and the increase in time needed to recover from physical exertion*. Nonetheless, the ability of the human body to adjust to age-related

Box 17-1

Diseases and Disorders That Can Cause Dementia

Central Nervous System Disorders

Alzheimer's disease (primary degenerative dementia)
Huntington's disease
Pick's disease (primary degenerative dementia)
Parkinson's disease

Systemic Disorders

- Cardiovascular disease
  - Cerebral hypoxia or anoxia
  - Vascular dementia (including multi-infarct dementia)
  - Cardiac arrhythmias
  - Inflammatory diseases of blood vessels
- Deficiency states
  - Cyanocobalamin deficiency
  - Folic acid deficiency
- Effects of drugs
- Effects of toxins
- Endocrine and metabolic disorders
  - Thyroid disease
  - Parathyroid disease
  - Pituitary-adrenal disorders
- Infectious processes
  - Acquired immunodeficiency syndrome
  - Creutzfeldt-Jakob disease
  - Cryptococcal meningitis
  - Neurosyphilis
- Liver disease
  - Chronic progressive hepatic encephalopathy
- Neoplastic conditions
  - Intracranial tumors
- Pulmonary disease
  - Respiratory encephalopathy
- Urinary tract disease
  - Chronic uremic encephalopathy
  - Progressive uremic encephalopathy (dialysis dementia)

Miscellaneous Disorders

Hepatolenticular degeneration
Hydrocephalic dementia
Sarcoidosis

From Buckwalter K, Buchwalter J: Chronic cognitive dysfunction (dementia), *Arch Am Acad Orthop Surg* 2(1)20-32, 1998.

alterations and the ability of the human spirit to be resilient in the face of physical loss must not be overlooked or devalued.

Cognitive Changes

Cognitive changes or declines do not develop uniformly, either across all areas of cognitive functioning or at the same rate in all individuals. The diversity in older people is evident in this realm as loss begins from each person's level of acquired cognitive abilities.

Memory is the first area of cognition to be affected as the capacity of the brain to process, store, and retrieve information begins to function less efficiently. Because of this change, *word finding* becomes a slower and more difficult process for the individual person.

Psychologic Changes

For many older people advanced age is a period of adjustment that usually includes retirement, loss of status roles, financial change, risk of loss of health, loss of spouse, and cumulative losses.

How individuals adjust to these changes again varies considerably in relation to their personal and social resources. The role of the primary care provider is to recognize and augment the resources when appropriate.

Risk Factors

There is debate in the field of just what constitutes lifetime risk for the development of a dementia-type illness. The risk depends on life expectancy, gender, and disease incidence, since there is ample probability of mortality from other competing illness or injury (Jorm, 1997). Data from the Framingham longitudinal study projected the lifetime risk for a dementia-type illness for 65- to 80-year-old men at 10.9% and for women at 12%. The risk increased when the age was raised to include from 65 to 100, with men at 25.5% and women at 32.8%. The data project less of a risk than is hypothesized by other population models and supports advanced age and being female as risk factors (Seshadri et al., 1997).

Atrial fibrillation is an independent risk factor for vascular dementia by association with the risk of silent cerebral infarction. Antithrombotic therapy may protect patients at risk (O'Connell et al., 1998). Disorders that worsen cerebral blood flow such as head injury or coronary artery are considered risk factors by those who suggest that the pathogenesis of Alzheimer's disease (AD) is related to impaired vascular delivery of nutrients to the brain (de la Torre, 1997).

Apolipoprotein E has been studied and is universally accepted as an important risk factor for late-onset AD (Lopez et al., 1998; Wu et al., 1998).

Predictors of shorter survival time (i.e., at 3 and 7 years of a dementia-type disease) were older age, male, low education, comorbidity, and functional disability (Aguero-Torres et al., 1998).

Drugs now undergoing clinical trials to assess the possibility of delaying or eliminating the disease are estrogen replacement, nonsteroidal antiinflammatory drugs, and vitamin E (Hendrie, 1998).

Epidemiology and Economics

In a recent analysis of several epidemiologic studies, U.S. mortality rates, and U.S. Bureau projections, the prevalence of dementia in people over 65 years of age living in the United States was found to be 2.32 million, with 68% being female. With no new interventions, it is projected that the prevalence rates will nearly quadruple in the next 50 years, with 1 out of every 45 Americans being afflicted with the disease (Brookmeyer, Gray, and Kawas, 1998). This has occurred for two reasons:

1. Mortality rates in the elderly population have declined consistently over the past 30 years, leading to a major increase in the number of individuals ages 75 years and over, particularly those age 85 and older.
2. Those who develop the disease are likely to be diagnosed and live longer because care is available to treat infections and other life-threatening conditions.

Mortality attributed to dementia-type disease has significantly increased during the last 20 years. In an examination of 1979 to 1996 death rates in England and Wales, it was reported that death rates from AD for men had increased from 1 to 19 per 100,000 and for women to 21 per 100,000 (Kirby, Lehmann, and Majeed, 1998). In the United States dementia is an extremely frequent cause of morbidity and mortality. Rates vary widely, and death certificates grossly underestimate and underreport dementia as a cause of death (Lanska,1998).

The cost of dementia care in the United States is difficult to approximate because much of the care is done by the private and informal caregiving system of relatives and friends. The estimates of care from the formal system are derived from Medicare claims and self reports, both of which are problematic. The Medicare cost reports are used to document reimbursement and do not accurately reflect service use, by nature of the disease, and patient reports are usually from second sources rather than the care recipient (Fox, 1997). Data from Canada provide estimated costs of care based on use of nursing home care, medications, and community support services by caregivers, as well as unpaid caregiver time. The annual cost per patient expressed in 1996 Canadian dollars was as follows: for patients with mild disease, $9,451; mild to moderate disease, $16,054; moderate disease, $25,724; and severe disease, $36,794. Cost of institutional care for persons with severe disease accounted for 84% of their care (Hux et al, 1998).

In spite of differences between the U.S. and Canadian health care systems, it is clear that costs increase dramatically as the severity of the disease progresses. The ability to delay the onset of the disease or to delay the progression could have a major impact on the cost of care (Brookmeyer, Gray, and Kawas, 1998). Effectiveness of interventions can be measured not only by costs but also by changes in the patient's cognitive functioning, years of life gained, and quality of life in those years (Livingston, Manela, and Katona, 1997).

Diagnostic Criteria

Progression of the disease and the dimensions of any one symptom vary from person to person.

A. Development of multiple cognitive deficits is manifested by the following*:
   1. Memory impairment (short and long-term memory impairment)
   2. One or more of the following cognitive disturbances:
      a. *Aphasia*: Difficulty with the use of language, which may involve forgetting simple words or substituting one for another with a similar sound
      b. *Apraxia*: Difficulty in performing motor activities in spite of intact physical functioning
      c. *Agnosia:* Failure to recognize or identify objects in spite of intact sensory function
      d. *Disturbance in executive functioning*: Problem solving; the ability to plan, organize, or think in abstract terms—e.g., difficulty in defining words or detecting similarities, as in comparing a dog and a lion and clock drawing.

B. The cognitive deficits in A each cause significant impairment in social or occupational functioning and represent a significant decline from a previous level of functioning.

C. The course is characterized by gradual onset and continuing cognitive decline.

D. The cognitive deficits in A are not caused by any of the following:
   1. Other central nervous system conditions that cause progressive deficits in memory and cognition
   2. Systemic conditions that are known to cause dementia
   3. Substance-induced conditions

E. Deficits do not occur during the course of a delirium.

F. The disturbance is not better accounted for by another Axis I disorder (major depression, schizophrenia).

Common Behavioral Problems

- Concealed memory losses (confabulation)
- Wandering
- Sleep disturbances
- Losing and hiding things
- Inappropriate sexual behavior
- Repeating questions and phrases (perserveration)

Criteria for Vascular Dementia

In contrast with AD, in which there are few identifiable physical findings, multiinfarct dementia is identified by the following characteristics (Hachinski et al., 1975)†:

- A history of high blood pressure
- Recurrent strokes or emboli, which may have affected other organs
- Rapid, as opposed to slow and insidious, onset

---

*Data from American Psychiatric Association: *Diagnostic and statistical manual of mental disorders (DSM IV)*, ed 4, Washington, DC, 1994, American Psychiatric Association.

†Source: National Institute of Neurological and Communicative Disorders and Stroke; Alzheimer's Disease and Related Disorders Association (NINCDS-ADRDA).

- A fluctuating course, with stepwise deterioration (a period of decline in cognitive functioning may be followed by some degree of improvement as compensatory brain function occurs)
- Relative preservation of personality
- Nocturnal confusion compared with relative lucidity during the day
- Distinctive neurologic signs such as weakness of arms or legs, defects in the visual fields, or diminished reflexes (these vary from case to case, depending on the areas of the brain that have been affected)
- Same as A, B, and E under Diagnostic Criteria, plus focal neurologic signs and symptoms or laboratory evidence of cerebrovascular disease (multiple infarctions involving cortex and underlying white matter) that is judged to be etiologically related to the disturbance

Inclusion Criteria

- Dementia established by clinical examination and documented by standardized mental status examination or neuropsychologic tests
- Deficits in two or more areas of cognition
- Progressive worsening of memory and other cognitive functions
- No disturbance of consciousness
- Onset between 40 and 90 years of age
- Absence of systemic disorders or other brain diseases

Supporting Criteria (Probable Diagnosis of Alzheimer's Disease)

- Progressive deterioration of specific cognitive functions
- Impaired activities of daily living (ADL) and altered patterns of behavior
- Family history of similar disorders
- Normal lumbar puncture
- Normal-pattern electroencephalogram
- Evidence of progression of cerebral atrophy documented by computed tomography

Exclusion Criteria

- Sudden, apoplectic onset
- Focal neurologic findings
- Seizures or gait disturbance very early in course of disease

Diagnostic Workup

History and physical examination, preferably with provider who knows the patient well

Neurologic examination

Careful mental status examination, including brief standardized mental status tests

Laboratory: Complete blood count; electrolytes, including calcium; thyroid-stimulating hormone; vitamin B_{12}, Venereal Disease Research Laboratories (VDRL), and other laboratory tests warranted by examination findings

Lumbar puncture (not routinely recommended) may be useful to rule out metastatic disease or an unusual presentation; may be done to rule out normal pressure hydrocephalus

ADL assessment

Instrumental ADL (IADL) assessment

Depression screening (Mangino and Middlemiss, 1997)

Social assessment (home visit preferable)

Drug review
Nutritional evaluation
Neurologic imaging assessments

Magnetic resonance imaging/computerized tomography (MRI/CT) or structural imaging scans: Not recommended as routine by consensus groups; may demonstrate atrophy, which is not helpful in diagnosis; white matter changes, the significance of which has not been determined; space-occupying lesions; and vascular disease

Single photon emission computed tomography/positron emission tomography (SPECT/PET) or functional imaging: Provides information on neuronal functioning by measuring cerebral blood flow and glucose uptake; can help differentiate AD from other dementias by revealing parietotemporal hypometabolism and right/left asymmetry; can reveal evidence for vascular dementias by identifying focal asymmetric cortical and subcortical deficits; currently being used in *some* clinical settings to increase the likelihood of specifically diagnosing AD in mild to moderately impaired individuals (Small, 1998)

Differential Diagnoses

- Normal age-related forgetfulness
- Alcohol abuse
- Polypharmacy or drug-related
- Hypothyroidism
- Delirium
- Depression (pseudodementia)
- Sensory impairment(s)
- Compensatory actions by spouse/family delays diagnosis

Primary Care Issues

- Communicate to the family and patient that judgment and memory impairment are key features.
- Dementia increases mortality; AD is not a benign disease.
- Multiple illnesses are common in older patients and complicated by the presence of AD.
- Medication management is a priority.
- Address advance directives early on.
- Minimize excess disability by identifying and treating other disorders.
- Always refer atypical presentations to a specialist.
- Family members will have multiple needs during the progression of the illness. Treatment plans must consider the health of and resources available to the caregiver members.

Pharmacologic Disease Management

Cholinesterase inhibitors that increase the supply of acetylcholine to the brain effectively moderate some symptoms and postpone, but do not prevent, cognitive decline. They are purely palliative in nature. QD dosing of donepezil requires no monitoring of liver function tests; tacrine does require monitoring. Both medications have cholinergic side effects, including nausea, vomiting, and diarrhea.

Disease Process

The disease process is marked by slow progression and decline of social and cognitive skills.

Stage 1

Stage 1 is often indiscernible to all but spouses or those very close to the patient on a daily basis. Attempts to hide memory loss are very common; withdrawal and depression may be present. Judgment and intellectual and social functioning seem faulty (Sunderland, 1998).

Most Common Symptoms

- Short-term memory loss
- Difficulty learning and retaining new material, which leads to inability to follow directions
- Loss of thinking ability, judgment, and decision-making capacity
- Difficulty completing common tasks (cooking, driving)
- Disorientation; gets lost, can't find way home
- Loss of time sense
- Loss of physical coordination
- Awareness of memory changes
- Communication loss: Includes forgetting events such as birthdays and names of acquaintances; long pauses between words and sentences; losing track and rambling; repetition; decreasing attention span
- Wandering
- Changes in personality; may become self-centered or passive
- Refusal to give up driving
- Loss of social inhibition
- Changes in emotion, including agitation, depression, and suspiciousness

Managing Communication

- Get the patient's attention in a calm environment.
- Avoid multiple distractions.
- Speak clearly.
- Use one-step commands when giving directions.
- Be willing to repeat and rephrase.
- Avoid traditional reality orientation; orient to season/holidays.

Stage 2

In Stage 2 there is a decrease in recall and word recognition; attention span is even shorter; digressions increase. Closely related words are often substituted for forgotten words. The patient will have more difficulty understanding and following directions.

Most Common Symptoms

- Delusions and hallucinations
- Impatience
- Wandering and pacing
- Striking out, physically or verbally
- Hiding things
- Resistance to help
- Intimacy/sexuality issues
- Decreased tolerance for stress
- Catastrophic reactions
- Purposeless behavior
- Motor apraxias
- Compulsive repetitive behavior

Managing Delusions and Hallucinations

- Check eyesight and hearing.
- Use glasses and/or hearing aid if needed.
- Avoid confusing noises (e.g., pagers, background radios, TV).
- Ignore the delusion/hallucination if it isn't frightening.
- Avoid contradicting or arguing about the delusion or hallucination.
- Distraction sometimes helps.
- False accusations (e.g., of unfaithfulness) may represent a need for reassurance.
- Recognize the underlying emotions. Give comfort if you can.
- Find new ways to deal with the problem. Example: If the patient is anxiously awaiting the arrival of her mother (long dead), *do not tell her that her mother died 10 years ago. This type of reality is harmful* to a distressed person who has lost intellectual capacity. Deal with the anxiety in a caring manner. If you are comfortable with saying, "Mother called to say she isn't coming today," consider saying that. Otherwise reassure her as best you can by saying, "Your mother isn't here right now, but I can help."
- Remember that delusions/hallucinations may be the symptoms of infection or other disease. When they arise, evaluate for other illnesses.
- If delusions or hallucinations are persistent and severe, medication may be used to help control them. Short-acting benzodiazepines such as lorazepam in *low doses* or high-potency neuroleptics such as Haldol in *low doses* may be helpful.

Other Potential Stage 2 Management Situations

- Promote function; allow patient to do as much as he or she can safely do.
- Control social situations.
- Determine when patient is no longer able to competently manage finances and legal matters.
- To control agitation try white noise, music, nature sounds, dimmed lighting.

Stage 3

Almost all ability to communicate is lost. Patient becomes nonverbal. Many patients are bedridden or chairbound and have the lost the ability to walk, talk, and care for themselves.

Management

- Continue speaking quietly with eye contact.
- Pat or stroke the patient. Touch with love.

- Smile.
- Comfort care is appropriate for this stage. The patient is no longer aware of what is happening.
- Long-term care placement is often best for patients and caregivers at this time.
- Recognize that you have done all you can.
- Assist family members to recognize they have done the best they could. Help them to recall the positive memories of their relative or friend.

Day-to-Day Caregiving

General Principles

- Promote as much function and independence as patient and situation allow.
- Prevent as much excess disability as long as possible.
- Help, but do not *do*—as long as possible.

Bathing

- Keep it simple with regular routine. Bathing every day is not necessary.
- Patient may tolerate shower better than bath.
- If tub bathing, fill tub after patient is in the tub—about 6 inches of water.
- Don't use slippery oils or bubble bath.
- Provide support with handrails, tub bench, or chair.

Grooming

- *Hair:* Keep in easy to care for style. The barber shop or beauty parlor may be the best solution for regular hair care.
- *Shaving:* Electric razors are easier. Let patient shave self as long as possible. Female patients may need help with leg shaving and facial hair.
- *Make-up:* If a woman is used to make-up, it will enhance her self-image.
- *Nails:* Trim nails about once a month. It may help to distract patient with TV or music. Bunions and calluses may need care of a podiatrist. A visit every 6 months should be adequate.
- *Teeth:* Have patient brush own teeth as long as possible. Schedule visits to the dentist.

Toileting

- Simplify the process.
- If patient has trouble finding the bathroom, put a picture on the bathroom door.
- Have the patient wear loose-fitting, easy-to-remove clothing.
- Remind the patient after meals and before going out.
- Respect privacy.

Constipation

- Constipation can be caused by soft diet, inactivity, some medications, or inadequate fluid.

- Institute high-fiber diet, daily exercise, five to eight glasses of water daily.
- Consider need for laxatives.
- Be observant. Patient will not remember nor be able to identify constipation symptoms.

Urinary Incontinence

- First rule out infection.
- Schedule toileting times—prompted voiding. Watch for nonverbal clues.
- Encourage use of adult absorbency pads.

Bowel Incontinence

- Bowel incontinence usually develops at the later stages of the disease.
- Check for impaction, drug effect.
- Protective pads will be needed.
- Watch diet to avoid diarrhea-causing foods.
- Provide good skin care to perianal area.

Dressing

- Simplify clothing with Velcro, front fastenings, and loose-fitting elastic waistbands.
- Provide tube sox, lace-up, or Velcro shoes.
- Use comfortable fabrics such as cotton.
- If patient has favorite clothing items, buy duplicates.
- Sort and arrange all clothing by type.
- Put out-of-season clothing away.
- Put accessories with the matching item of clothing.
- Don't offer too many choices.

Glasses

- Keep more than one pair.
- Get plastic lenses.
- Keep a copy of the prescription.

Eating

Planning and Preparing Meals

- Let the patient assist with meal preparation tasks as much as possible (Baum and Edwards, 1993).
- Serve favorite foods often.
- Use contrasting colors of dishes and placemats.
- Add extra nutrients to the diet of a patient who is underweight.
- Serve portions to the patient who eats too much.
- Spoons are easier than forks.
- Finger foods are easiest of all.

- Eat together.
- Keep presentation of food simple.

Eating Out

- Avoid the peak hours to avoid too much stimulation.
- Order for the patient; offer choice of two things.
- Tell the waiter your companion is confused.
- Consider take out.

Recreation

- Recreation can be anything the patient can do and used to enjoy.
- Watching TV may confuse some patients with AD.
- Encourage listening to music, especially old favorites.

Suggested Activities

- Looking at family photo albums
- Reminiscing
- Music and free form dancing
- Art therapies
- Playing with pets
- Walking the dog
- Stationary bicycle
- Tasks like arranging flatware, piling newspapers, folding clothes

Sleeping

- Room temperature and bedding should be comfortable.
- Night lights are invaluable in hallways and bathrooms.
- Encourage a dark room for sleep.
- Limit daytime naps.

Sleep-Wake Cycle Disturbance

- Establish bedtime routine.
- Use bedroom only for sleep or sexual activity.
- Sexual intimacy depends entirely on agreement between parties. If one person does not want to continue intimacy, separate beds and bedrooms are a good idea.
- Sexual appetite usually wanes as disease progresses.

Home Safety

1. Accidents happen even in the home without an AD patient. A first aid kit is a requirement.
2. Basic concepts
   a. Don't change too much.
   b. Make changes over time, as they are needed.

   c. Make changes that simplify.
   d. Make changes that make life easier for the caregiver.
3. Kitchen and bathroom safety list
   a. Turn off stoves, unplug them, and remove knobs.
   b. Put away matches and lighters.
   c. Unplug electrical equipment in kitchen at night. Use timers or circuit breakers to keep power off.
   d. Turn hot water temperature down.
   e. Remove lock from inside bathroom door.
   f. Be sure that smoke detectors are in working order.
   g. Remove weapons.
   h. Lock up potentially dangerous cleaning supplies.
4. General safety
   a. Be sure there is adequate lighting, especially on stairs, entryways, and bathrooms.
   b. Clear the clutter off stairs. Put railings on both sides.
   c. Consider covering mirrors. Some patients are afraid of their images.
   d. Fasten small rugs securely to the floor; don't use high gloss.
   e. Lock windows.
   f. Arrange furniture with clear pathways; furniture should be firm, not wobbly.
   g. Place locks on doors very high or very low to deter patients from wandering out of the house.
   h. Lock the garage.
   i. Do not allow driving; the car may have to be disabled.

Community Supports and Resources

Family and friends
Support groups
- Alzheimer's association (for all types of dementia)
- Church groups
- Caregiver support groups (often sponsored by hospitals, nursing facilities)

Adult day care
Professional support
- Registered nurses (RNs)
- Social workers
- Home health aids
- Homemakers
- Geriatric case managers (usually RNs or social workers)
- Adult homes, group homes, or assisted living facilities
- Hospitals and nursing homes

Long-term care facilities
- Skilled nursing facility
- Long-term care facility (often combined with skilled care)
- Continuing care facility
- Assisted living facility (may provide some ADL and medication management)

Summary

Primary care providers have an expanded role in providing continuous care throughout the course of a dementia-type illness. Much can be done in the early and mild stages of this disease to improve quality of life for the patient and his or her family. As the disease progresses, more assistance will be called for from the health care system. It is important to remember all that can be done rather than emphasizing the decline. As the disease progresses in severity and as institutional placement becomes an option, acknowledging the difficulties is an important element in the provider's ability to continue to assist family members as they make decisions regarding provision of care.

Resources

Alzheimer's Association
919 N. Michigan Ave.
Suite 1000
Chicago, IL 60611-1676
www.Alz.org

Children of Aging Parents
1609 Woodbourne Rd.
Levittown, PA 19057
(215) 945-6900

National Citizens Coalition for Nursing Home Reform
1224 M St. NW
Suite 301
Washington, DC 20005
(202) 393-2018

National Council on the Aging
409 Third St.
Suite 200
Washington, DC 20024
(202) 479-1200

Senate Special Committee on Aging
Dirksen Senate Office Bldg.
Room 623
Washington, DC 20510

Web site of Department of Health and Human Services is an excellent site to link to many types of information.
http://www.aoa.dhhs.gov

References

Aguero-Torres H et al: Natural history of Alzheimer's disease and other dementias: review of the literature in the light of the findings from the Kungsholmen Project, *Int J Geriatric Psychiatry* 13(11):755-766, 1998.

AHCPR: *Early Alzheimer's disease,* Clinical Practice Guideline No. 19. AHCPR Publication No. 96-0704. Washington, DC, September 1996, US Department of Health and Human Services.

American Psychiatric Association: *Diagnostic and statistical manual of mental disorders,* ed 4, Washington, DC, 1994, American Psychiatric Association.

Baum C, Edwards D: Cognitive performance in senile dementia of the Alzheimer's type: the kitchen task assessment, *Am J Occup Ther* 47(5):431-436, 1993.

Brookmeyer R Gray S, Kawas C: Projections of Alzheimer's disease in the United States and the public health impact of delaying disease onset, *Am J Public Health* 88(9):1337-1342, 1998.

Buckwalter K, Buckwalter J: Chronic cognitive dysfunction (dementia), *Arch Am Acad Orthop Surg* 2(1):20-32, 1998.

de la Torre JC: Cerebromicrovascular pathology in Alzheimer's disease compared to normal aging, *Gerontology* 43:1-2, 26-43, 1997.

Fox PJ: Service use and cost outcomes for persons with Alzheimer disease, *Alzheimer Disease Association Disorder* 11(suppl):s125-s134, 1997.

Grossberg C: Advance directives, competency evaluation, and surrogate management in elderly patients, *Am J Geriatr Psychiatry* 6(2)(suppl 1):s79-s84, 1998.

Hendrie H: Epidemiology of dementia and Alzheimer's disease, *Am J Geriatr Psychiatry,* 6(2)(suppl 1):s3-s17, 1998.

Hachinski VC et al: Cerebral blood flow in dementia, *Arch Neurol* 32(9):632-637, 1975.

Hux MJ, et al: Relation between severity of Alzheimer's disease and cost of caring, *Can Med Assoc J* 159(5):957-965, 1998.

Jorm AF: Alzheimer's disease risk and protection, *Med J Aust* 167(8):443-446, 1997.

Kirby L, Lehmann P, Majeed A: Dementia in people aged 65 years and older: a growing problem? *Population Trends* 92:23-28, 1998.

Lanska DJ: Dementia mortality in the United States: results of the 1986 National Mortality Followback Survey, *Neurology* 50(2):362-367, 1998.

Larson E: Management of Alzheimer's disease in a primary care setting, *Am J Geriatr Psychiatry* 6(2)(suppl 1):s34-s40, 1998.

Livingston G, Manela M, Katona C: Cost of community care for older people, *Br J Psychiatry* 171:56-59, 1997.

Lopez OL et al: Apolipoprotein E polymorphism in Alzheimer's disease: a comparative study of two research populations from Spain and the United States, *Eur Neurol* 39(4):229-233, 1998.

Mangino M, Middlemiss C: Alzheimer's disease: preventing and recognizing a misdiagnosis, *Nurse Pract* 22(10):58-75, 1997.

O'Connell JE et al: Atrial fibrillation and cognitive function: case-control study, *J Neurol Neurosurg Psychiatry* 65(3):386-389, 1998.

Seshadri S et al: Lifetime risk of dementia and Alzheimer's: the impact of mortality on risk estimates in the Framingham Study, *Neurology* 49(6):1498-1504, 1997.

Small G: Differential diagnoses and early detection of dementia, *Am J Geriatr Psychiatry* 6(2)(suppl 1):s26-s33, 1998.

Sunderland T: Alzheimer's disease: cholinergic therapy and beyond, *Am J Geriatr Psychiatry* 6(2)(suppl 1):s56-63, 1998.

Wu WS et al: Genetic studies on chromosome 12 in late onset Alzheimer's disease, *JAMA* 280(7):619-622, 1998.

18

Neurologic: Depression/Suicide

Depression is an affective illness characterized by disturbances in mood, cognition, and behavior. It is often associated with functional impairment and a reduced capacity for pleasure and enjoyment. Too often underdiagnosed and undertreated in the elderly population, depression can cause significant morbidity. In addition, several studies have demonstrated a higher mortality rate among depressed elderly patients and those suffering severe grief responses (Yoshikawa, Cobbs, and Brummel-Smith, 1993).

Depression is estimated to affect 5% to 10% of the elderly population in the community and up to 25% of elderly residents in long-term care facilities (Reynolds, 1995). The financial cost of mood disorders in the United States is estimated to be $44 billion per year.

The consequences of the failure to recognize and treat depression in this population are significant, including increased rates of institutional placement, physical illness, and suicide. Approximately two thirds of suicides in the older population are associated with depression, and 25% of all U.S. suicide victims are over 60. The attempted:completed ratio of suicide is 4:1 in older persons, compared with 200:1 in the younger population. One researcher found that approximately 75% of successful elderly suicide victims had visited their primary care clinic within 1 month of death (Rothschild, 1996). Elderly people typically use more lethal and reliable means of suicide such as guns, asphyxiation, and hanging.

The leading theory to explain the biologic basis of depression is the monoamine hypothesis. This theory proposes that depression is due to a deficiency in one or more of three monoamines, namely, serotonin, norepinephrine, and dopamine (Stahl, 1998). It is clear, however, that social and emotional factors affect brain chemistry and must be addressed in designing an effective treatment plan.

Risk Factors

Several factors increase the risk of depression in the older adult: being single or widowed; the presence of chronic illness; financial strain; lack of social supports; a personal or family history of affective illness; recent admission to a long-term care facility; loss of a body part (i.e., amputation); and loss of autonomy, privacy, or functional status. Alcohol or other substance abuse can play an important role, as can the use of other (often prescription) medications, as is discussed later in the chapter.

Comorbid medical illnesses, including Parkinson's, Alzheimer's, and stroke, as well as certain medications, are also associated with an increased risk of depression (Table 18-1 and Box 18-1). It is important to appropriately evaluate whether any of these associated factors may be contributing to the depressive presentation and to treat them if possible. Remember that the presence of these illnesses or conditions does not preclude treatment of the depressive syndrome.

Several factors increase the risk of suicide for an older person: personal or family history of mood disorders, living alone, recent death of a spouse or friend, alcohol use or abuse, physical illness and pain, and the feeling of being a burden. Others include recent

TABLE 18-1 Medical Conditions Associated with Depression

Body System	Condition
Neurologic	Alzheimer's disease
	Acquired immunodeficiency syndrome dementia complex
	Brain mass or tumor
	Multiple sclerosis
	Stroke
	Parkinson's disease
Cardiovascular	Congestive heart failure
	Myocardial infarction
	Hypertension
Autoimmune	Rheumatoid arthritis
	Systemic lupus erythematosus
Metabolic	Addison's disease
	Cushing's disease
	Diabetes mellitus
	Hypothyroidism
	Hyperthyroidism
	Hyperparathyroidism
Others	Malignancies (especially pancreatic, lung, colorectal, ovarian, lymphoma)
	Infectious disease
	Malnutrition
	Pancreatic disease
	Metabolic abnormalities
	Pernicious anemia
	Chronic pain syndrome
	Chronic obstructive pulmonary disease
	Rheumatoid arthritis
	Renal dialysis
	Hearing loss

Adapted from Butler RN, Lewis MI: Late-life depression: when and how to intervene, *Geriatrics* 50(8):44-55, 1995.

Box 18-1

Examples of Medications Associated with Depression

- Carbidopa-levodopa
- Antihypertensives
- Beta blockers
- Calcium channel blockers
- Reserpine
- Clonidine
- Barbiturates
- Anticonvulsants
- H_2 blockers
- Corticosteroids

Data from Reynolds CF: Recognition and differentiation of elderly depression in the clinical setting, *Geriatrics* 50(1):S6-S15, 1995.

admission to a long-term care facility; loss of autonomy, privacy, or functional status; expectation of death from some cause; and being a white male (higher rate of suicide than any other group) (Butler and Lewis, 1995). See Box 18-2 for risk factors associated with suicide.

Assessment

Depression must always be differentiated from other underlying medical conditions, including dementia. However, as mentioned before, another condition may not preclude the need to treat the depression as a separate but important entity.

The Diagnostic and Statistical Manual of Mental Disorders, fourth edition (DSM-IV, 1994) provides specific diagnostic criteria for a major depressive disorder (Box 18-3). Key signs of depression include being discouraged or sad; frequently complaining; and being anxious, irritable, agitated or slow, and self-effacing or demanding. There are several mnemonics for remembering the symptoms and behavior changes associated with depression. One of these is SIGECAPS:

S = Sleep disturbance (insomnia or hypersomnia)
I = lack of **I**nterest
G = feelings of **G**uilt
E = decreased **E**nergy
C = decreased **C**oncentration
A = change in **A**ppetite (increased or decreased)
P = **P**sychomotor retardation or agitation
S = **S**uicidal ideation

The presentation of the older person with depression may differ somewhat from that of the younger individual. Older people seem to have more somatic complaints (although some disagree with this) and an increase in psychotic or delusional symptoms, especially if the onset is after age 60. Frequently these delusions are of a somatic (cancer), persecutory, or nihilistic nature. Older patients are more likely to present with weight

Box 18-2

Risk Factors Associated with Suicide

Sociodemographic Risk Factors

Male sex
Age 60 or older
Widowed or divorced
Caucasian or Native American
Living alone
Unemployed or having financial problems
Recent adverse events, such as job loss or death of someone close

Clinical Risk Factors

Clinical depression or schizophrenia
Substance abuse
History of suicide attempts or ideation
Feeling of hopelessness
Panic attacks
Severe anxiety, particularly if combined with depression
Severe anhedonia

Data from Hirschfeld RMA, Russell JM: Assessment and treatment of suicidal patients, *N Engl J Med* 337(13):910-915, 1997.

Box 18-3

DSM-IV Criteria for Major Depressive Disorder

A. Five or more of the following symptoms for 2 weeks.
   Must include 1 or 2.
   1. Depressed mood
   2. Loss of interest or pleasure
   3. Weight loss or gain
   4. Insomnia or hypersomnia
   5. Psychomotor agitation or retardation
   6. Fatigue
   7. Worthlessness or inappropriate guilt
   8. Decreased concentration or indecisiveness
   9. Thoughts of death or suicidal ideation
B. Not a mixed episode
C. Impaired social, occupational, or other important area of functioning
D. Not secondary to substance abuse or a medical condition
E. Not better accounted for by bereavement

Source: *Diagnostic and statistical manual of mental disorders,* ed 4, Washington, DC, 1994, American Psychiatric Association.

loss, but they may tend to minimize their depressed mood (Blazer, 1997). Other prominent symptoms such as decreased appetite, sleep, energy, and pleasure may be attributed to physical illness or to social or economic problems by both the patient and the practitioner. On obtaining the history, the practitioner often discovers that older patients have had a previous episode of depression at some time in their earlier years.

Box 18-4

Diagnostic Studies for the Evaluation of Depression

- Complete blood count
- Chemistry profile (electrolytes, blood urea nitrogen, creatinine, glucose)
- Serologic test for syphilis (rapid plasma reagin)
- Thyroid studies (thyroid stimulating hormone, T_3, T_4)
- Vitamin B_{12} level (methylmalonic acid/homocysteine if low)
- Folate level
- Human immunodeficiency virus testing
- Urinalysis
- Chest x-ray
- Electrocardiogram

Primary anxiety disorders are uncommon in later life, and onset in late life is very rare. Therefore the newly anxious older patient with a diminished self-attitude, vague "vital sense changes" ("I'm sick, something's wrong"), and a low mood should be suspected of having depression (Rabins, 1998).

Older people may also present with a dementia-like syndrome of depression known as pseudodementia. One distinguishing factor is that, unlike true dementia, poor performance is usually neither global nor consistent. Attention and concentration are markedly affected, and the patient usually presents with less confabulation. For example, when asked a date, a demented person might say with confidence that it is 1942, whereas a patient with pseudodementia classically answers, "I don't know." Other distinguishing characteristics of dementia vs. pseudodementia follow (Raskind, 1998):

Dementia	Pseudodementia
Cognitive changes happen first.	Mood changes occur first.
Mood is labile.	Mood is consistently dysphoric.
Cooperative but inaccurate on Mini-Mental State Examination (MMSE).	Uncooperative or does not try on MMSE.
Aphasia is present.	Aphasia absent.
Can enjoy things.	Cannot enjoy things.

Simply questioning a patient regarding mood may be adequate to reveal symptoms of depression. Often, however, it is helpful to use a standardized screening tool such as the Geriatric Depression Scale (short form) to elicit information (see Chapter 1). The presence of other medical conditions besides dementia must be determined, as well as the impact of the presenting symptoms on the patient's ability to function on a daily basis. Diagnostic studies for the evaluation of depression are listed in Box 18-4.

Treatment

Several therapies are known to be effective, either alone or in combination, for the treatment of depression. They include psychotherapy, medications, and electroconvulsive therapy (ECT) (Rothschild, 1996). Usually the primary care provider can initiate treatment in an outpatient setting. People who do not respond to initial therapy or who have complicated needs such as psychotic or delusional symptoms should be referred to a psychiatrist, preferably one with experience working with the older population.

If the risk of suicide seems imminent, immediate hospitalization is usually required. If the risk of suicide is high but not imminent, Hirschfeld and Russell (1997) recommend certain steps that should be taken. First, try to involve a family member or another person who is close to the patient. With the patient's permission, advise this person of the problem. Suggest increased vigilance and a collaborative approach to dealing with the problem. Second, ask about (and document) the availability of firearms and ammunition, potentially lethal medications, and other means of suicide. Third, increase contact with the patient, including phone calls and visits. Communication of one's commitment to help the patient may be lifesaving. Fourth, if a psychiatric disorder is present, refer for treatment. If there is alcohol or other substance abuse, refer the patient to a comprehensive treatment program.

Psychotherapy

For many years it was thought that older patients did not benefit from psychotherapy because they were, as Freud stated in 1904, "no longer educable and, on the other hand, the mass of material to be dealt with would prolong the duration of the treatment indefinitely." However, recent studies have shown that older people do benefit from psychotherapy, either alone or in combination with medications, especially for patients with specific stressors or maladaptive personality factors (DasGupta, 1998). Unfortunately, because of the social stigma (and sometimes financial issues), many older patients may be unwilling to accept this treatment modality.

Pharmacotherapy

Practitioners must remember that the response to antidepressant therapy may be delayed in this population, so any treatment regimen must be given an adequate trial (4 to 6 weeks). Life-long treatment at full therapeutic doses may be necessary because of the high risk of relapse, recurrence, and suicide in this population (Reynolds, 1995).

The decision regarding an initial pharmacotherapeutic agent depends on the following factors:

- The patient's presenting symptoms (e.g., one of the more sedating medications at bedtime might be appropriate for a patient with associated insomnia)
- Coexisting illnesses
- Concurrent medications
- Alterations of pharmacokinetics in older persons
- Side-effect profile of the antidepressant being considered
- Response to prior treatment

If a patient had a positive response in the past to a particular antidepressant, generally that drug should be the initial therapy for subsequent depressive episodes. However, in the case of an older person who has been successfully treated with a tricyclic antidepressant (TCA), consider that increased age and the concomitant prescription of other medications will increase the risk for adverse effects from a TCA. A newer agent may be preferable. If the patient did not respond to a particular antidepressant in the past, an antidepressant from another class should be prescribed initially for subsequent episodes (Rothschild, 1996). Whichever drug is used, remember that the average geriatric patient is taking between six and eight medications already, which increases the risk of drug-drug interactions. The geriatric medicine adage of "start low, go slow" should be the rule for dosage.

Every known antidepressant increases neurotransmission of serotonin, norepinephrine, or dopamine, either alone or in combination. Six classes of antidepressants accomplish this effect by blocking one or more of the reuptake pumps or receptors for these three monoamines. One inhibits an enzyme, namely, monoamine oxidase (MAO) (Stahl, 1998), and the remaining class acts as monoamine-releasing agents (central nervous system stimulants). See Table 18-2 for classes and examples of antidepressants.

In treating patients who have anxiety secondary to major depression, antidepressants, not anxiolytics, are the treatment of choice. Remember, however, that patients who may have been taking benzodiazepines for "anxiety" for several weeks to months are psychologically and physiologically dependent. To successfully treat depression, add an antidepressant without changing the benzodiazepine dose initially. Once the antidepressant has had the opportunity to become effective, the patient will be feeling better, and the benzodiazepine can then be tapered and stopped (Rabins, 1998).

TABLE 18-2 Classes of Antidepressants

Class	Antidepressant Medication
Tricyclics (TCA)	Amitriptyline (Elavil) Desipramine (Norpramin) Doxepin (Sinequan) Imipramine (Tofranil) Nortriptyline (Pamelor)
Monoamine oxidase inhibitors	Phenelzine (Nardil) Tranylcypromine (Parnate)
Selective serotonin reuptake inhibitors	Fluoxetine (Prozac) Paroxetine (Paxil) Sertraline (Zoloft)
Dual serotonin and norepinephrine reuptake inhibitor (SNRI)	Venlafaxine (Effexor)
Serotonin-2 antagonist/reuptake inhibitors	Nefazodone (Serzone) Trazodone (Desyrel)
Norepinephrine and dopamine reuptake inhibitor	Bupropion (Wellbutrin)
Noradrenergic and specific serotonergic antidepressants	Mirtazepine (Remeron)
Psychostimulants	Dextroamphetamine (Dexedrine) Methylphenidate (Ritalin) Methamphetamine (Desoxyn) Pemoline (Cylert)

Source: Richardson JP, Gallo JJ: Geriatrics for the clinician: treatment of depression in the elderly, *Md Med J* 45(7), 1996; Stahl SM: Basic psychopharmacology of antidepressants, part 1: antidepressants have seven distinct mechanisms of action, *J Clin Psychiatry* 59(4), 1998; Hay DP, Rodriguez MM, Franson KL: Treatment of depression in late life, *Clin Geriatr Med* 14(1), 1998.

Serotonin syndrome is a potentially life-threatening complication of psychopharmacologic drug therapy. The syndrome is produced most often by the concurrent use of two or more drugs that increase brainstem serotonin activity, and it is often unrecognized because of the varied and nonspecific nature of its symptomatology. Serotonin syndrome is characterized by alterations in cognition, behavior, autonomic nervous system function, and neuromuscular activity. Patients with serotonin syndrome usually respond to discontinuation of drug therapy and supportive care alone, but they may require treatment with a specific antiserotonergic drug. Table 18-3 discusses several common antidepressants, their dosages, reuptake activity, and adverse effect profiles.

Electroconvulsive Therapy

ECT can be a safe and effective treatment modality for the psychiatrist to use for older patients with severe depression, those who have psychotic features, those who cannot tolerate or do not have a response to antidepressant medications, or those who have medical conditions that contraindicate such treatment (Hirschfeld and Russell, 1997). It is usually performed two or three times per week for a total course of 6 to 12 treatments, once a complete evaluation and anesthesia consult have been performed. Maintenance treatments may continue as warranted by the history.

Contraindications to this treatment include the following:

- All those who cannot withstand general anesthesia
- Space-occupying intracerebral lesion
- Cardiovascular problems such as recent myocardial infarction, unstable aneurysm, or risk of bradyarrhythmia
- Recent cerebral vascular accident (increased risk of bleed for weeks to months)
- Seizure disorder (relative contraindication)
- Medication interactions (e.g., MAO inhibitors increase the risk of elevating blood pressure)

The possible adverse effects of this treatment include the following:

- Delirium (usually short-lived)
- Prolonged cardiac arrhythmia
- Prolonged apnea
- Oral trauma
- Retrograde amnesia

Evaluation and Follow-up

Response to treatment should be monitored with frequent telephone contact and visits. During follow-up calls and visits, family members may need special attention to any burden they may be experiencing, because living with a depressed person is a great challenge. In addition, a formal evaluation of the therapy and response should be conducted after approximately 6 weeks. It can be accomplished by subjective reports from the patient and family members regarding symptoms, evaluation of sleep patterns, or objective signs such as affect and weight gain or loss. The goal is to determine whether

TABLE 18-3 Antidepressant Medications by Class

Name	Usual Adult Dose	Reuptake Blockade		Adverse Effect Profile				Dosage Considerations for Elderly Persons
		5-HT	NE	Anticholinergic	Sedation	Orthostatic Hypotension	Sexual Dysfunction	
Tricyclics								
Amitriptyline	75-200 mg/d (300 mg/d rarely)	Y	Y	xxxx	xxxx	xxxx	xx	Reduced (50 mg in divided doses may be effective)
Clomipramine	100-250 mg/d	Y	Y	xxxx	xxxx	xxxx	xxxx	Limited studies
Desipramine	100-300 mg/d	N	Y	xx	xx	xxx	xx	25-100 mg/d
Doxepin	100-300 mg/d	Y	Y	xxxx	xxxx	xxxx	xx	Reduced
Imipramine	75-200 mg/d	Y	Y	xxx	xxx	xxxx	xx	Tofranil available in lower doses than Tofranil-PM for initiation of therapy
Nortriptyline	50-200 mg/d	Y	Y	xxx	xxx	xx	xx	30-50 mg/d
Protriptyline	20-60 mg/d	Y	Y	xxxx	xx	xxx	xx	Monitor cardiovascular system closely if daily doses exceed 20 mg
Trimipramine	100-300 mg/d	Y	Y	xxx	xxx	xxxx	xx	50-100 mg/d
Selective Serotonin Reuptake Inhibitors (SSRIs)								
Fluoxetine	10-80 mg/d	Y	N	x	x	x	xxxx	Long half-life Available in oral suspension Insufficient safety data
Fluvoxamine	100-300 mg/d	Y	N	x	xxx	x	xxxx	Reduce dosage Indicated for obsessive-compulsive disorder
Paroxetine	20-50 mg/d	Y	N	xx	xxx	x	xxxx	10-40 mg/d Available in oral suspension

Sertraline	25-50 mg/d (200 mg/d for obsessive-compulsive disorder)	Y	N	x	xx	x	xxxx	Side effect profile similar to younger patients
Monoamine Oxidase Inhibitors (MAOIs)								
Phenelzine	45-90 mg/d	N	N	xx	xxx	xxxx	xxx	Intended for atypical or "neurotic" depression
Tranylcypromine	20-50 mg/d	N	N	xx	x	xxxx	xxx	
Others								
Amoxapine	200-300 mg/d	Y	Y	xx	xx	xx	xx	50-150 mg/d Risk of extrapyramidal symptoms
Bupropion	200-450 mg/d	N	Y	x	x	x	x	Few studies
Maprotiline	75-225 mg/d	N	Y	xxx	xxx	xxx	xx	Initially 25 mg/d then 50-75 mg/d
Mirtazapine	15-45 mg/d	N	N	x	xxx	x	x	Reduced clearance
Nefazodone	200-600 mg/d	Y	Y	x	xx	x	x	Initially 100 mg/d in divided doses
Trazodone	200-400 mg/d	Y	N	x	xxxx	xxxx	xx	
Venlafaxine	75-375 mg/d	Y	Y	x	xx	x	xxxx	No significant considerations

Adverse effects profile key: *x*, very low; *xx*, low; *xxx*, moderate; *xxxx*, high; *xxxxx*, very high.

the original diagnosis is still appropriate and to evaluate the extent of success of the treatment modalities thus far. Decisions regarding change in dose or medication should be made at this time. Also, the possible need to augment the original therapy with an additional modality or to refer for further consultation and treatment will be evident at this time.

Because of the high incidence of recurrence and chronicity of depression in this population, continued follow-up and monitoring for persistent or recurrent episodes is as important as recognizing and treating the initial depression in the older patient.

Suicide

More than 32,000 people in the United States kill themselves every year. Suicide accounts for 1.4% of all U.S. deaths and is the ninth leading cause of death. A person commits suicide about every 15 minutes, but it is estimated that an attempt is made about once a minute. The highest rates of suicide are in men over age 50. This 10% of the population represents 33% of all suicides. For women the rate of suicide peaks between the ages of 40 and 54 and again after the age of 75 (American Foundation for Suicide Prevention, 1996).

The practitioner must recognize a patient who is at risk of committing suicide. There are a number of warning signs that should prompt the health care provider to ask whether the patient has ever considered suicide as an option. A "yes" answer should be taken seriously. Patients who are at risk may exhibit certain behaviors that offer clues to their intentions: talking about suicide; statements about hopelessness, helplessness, or worthlessness; preoccupation with death; becoming suddenly happier or calmer; loss of interest in things they cared about; visiting or calling people they care about; making arrangements and setting their affairs in order; and giving things away. A patient who is being treated for depression is actually at higher risk for suicide as the depression lifts. There is no need to be concerned that asking about suicide will "put the idea into someone's head" who previously had not considered it. It can be a great relief for the patient to bring the subject out in the open.

The San Francisco Suicide Prevention Crisis Team (1998) has developed a screening tool (P.L.A.I.D.P.A.L.S) to help determine the degree of suicide risk for a patient:

Plan: Do they have one?
Lethality: Is it lethal? Can they die?
Availability: Do they have the means to carry it out?
Illness: Do they have mental or physical illness?
Depression: Have there been chronic or specific incidents?
Previous Attempts: How many? How recent?
Alone: Are they alone? Do they have a support system?
Loss: Have they suffered a loss? Death, job, relationship, self-esteem?
Substance Abuse: Drugs, alcohol, medicine? Current or chronic?

If the patient is thought to be at imminent risk for suicide, immediate referral to a psychiatrist or inpatient hospitalization is warranted. If the patient is at moderate to high risk, certain measures should be put in place to minimize this risk. The patient should not be left alone; a supportive friend or family member should stay with the him or her. The home, hospital room, or nursing home room should be cleared of all potential means (pills, plastic bags, sharp implements), and close follow-up by the psychiatrist and primary care provider is important. It is advisable to be in daily contact with these patients either through office visits or by phone to monitor their response to therapy.

Summary

Depression is a condition that many times is either missed entirely or underdiagnosed. This chapter provides assessment tools that assist the practitioner in the diagnosis of depression and the person at risk for suicide. Depression is a treatable condition, not an acceptable result of advanced age.

Resources

American Association of Suicidology
(202)-237-2280
http://www.suicidology.com

American Foundation for Suicide Prevention
(888)-333-2377
http://www.AFSP.org

The National Alliance for the Mentally Ill (NAMI)
200 N. Glebe Road, Suite 1015
Arlington, VA 22203-3754
(800) 950-NAMI
http://www.NAMI.org

The National Crisis Helpline
(800) 999-9999

National Depression Screening Project
(800) 573-4433

National Institute of Mental Health
NIMH Clinical Center, Bldg. 103N234
Bethesda, MD 20892
(800) 647-2642

National Mental Health Association (NMHA)
1021 Prince St.
Alexandria, VA 22314-2971
(800) 969-NMHA
http://www.NMHA.org

The Samaritans
(212) 673-3000
(212) 532-2400

References

American Foundation for Suicide Prevention and Prediction web site (1996). http://www.afsp.org

Blazer DG: Depression in the elderly: myths and misconceptions, *Psychiatr Clin North Am* 20(1):111-119, 1997.

Butler RN, Lewis MI: Late-life depression: when and how to intervene, *Geriatrics* 50(8):44-55, 1995.

DasGupta K: Treatment of depression in elderly patients: recent advances, *Arch Fam Med* 7:274-280, 1998.

Diagnostic and Statistical Manual of Mental Disorders, ed 4, Washington, DC, 1994, American Psychiatric Association.

Hirschfeld RMA, Russell JM: Assessment and treatment of suicidal patients, *N Engl J Med* 337(13):910-915, 1997.

NIH Consensus Development Panel on Depression in Late Life: Diagnosis and treatment of depression, *JAMA* 268:1018-1024, 1992.

Rabins P: An anxious insomniac, Presentation at Current Topics in Geriatrics, Sponsored by Johns Hopkins Geriatric Center and the American Geriatrics Society, Baltimore, October, 1998.

Raskind MA: Interactions between depression and dementia, Presentation at the American Association of Geriatric Psychiatry meeting, San Diego, 1998.

Reynolds CF: Recognition and differentiation of elderly depression in the clinical setting, *Geriatrics* 50(1):S6-S15, 1995.

Richardson JP, Gallo JJ: Geriatrics for the clinician: treatment of depression in the elderly, *Md Med J* 45(7):553-556, 1996.

Rothschild AJ: The diagnosis and treatment of late life depression, *J Clin Psychiatry* 57(5), 1996.

San Francisco Suicide Prevention Community Crisis Line Web Site (1998): http://www.sirius.com

Stahl SM: Basic psychopharmacology of antidepressants, part 1: antidepressants have seven distinct mechanisms of action, *J Clin Psychiatry* 59(4):5-14, 1998.

Yoshikawa TT, Cobbs EL, Brummel-Smith K: *Ambulatory geriatric care*, St Louis, 1993, Mosby.

19 Sensory Impairment

Vision

Vision is an amazing process that happens so quickly and so easily that many take it for granted until it is threatened by the slow but predictable process of aging. It has been estimated that 1.3 million elderly people experience some loss of vision, with increasing age leading to higher percentages of people with vision loss. The leading causes of blindness in the United States are glaucoma, diabetic retinopathy, and macular degeneration. Almost 95% of people over age 65 wear glasses to improve their visual acuity, and more than 40% report that their vision is not completely corrected (Kovar, 1986). The primary care practitioner is in an excellent position to institute early intervention and rehabilitation, because many elderly people with vision impairment have conditions that are amenable to treatment.

Age-related Changes

External changes result from a loss of orbital fat, a loss of elastic tissue, and decreases in muscle tone. The primary result is lid laxity, which can lead to senile entropion (a condition in which the lid margin turns inward) or senile ectropion (a condition in which the eyelid margin turns outward). Other age-related changes of the eye include the following:

- Xanthomas, cutaneous deposits of lipid material, sometimes appear at the inner portion of the lid; they may indicate elevated blood lipid levels.
- Arcus senilis, a gray-yellow ring around the iris, may begin on the upper portion of the eye and develop until the entire iris is encircled. It is caused by a fatty invasion of the corneal margin, which blurs demarcation between the cornea and the sclera. It is common but has no known pathologic or functional implications.
- Tear viscosity and production decrease, which predisposes the eye to more infections of the conjunctiva.

- The cornea tends to flatten, which reduces its refractory power and limits its protective function.
- The sclera tends to take on a yellow coloration because of fatty deposits.
- The pupil becomes smaller, and the response to different levels of illumination is lessened because of the loss of range of pupil dilation and constriction.
- The retina receives only one third the amount of light, which necessitates a higher level of illumination for reading.
- The lens increases in density and elasticity, which leads to impairment in accommodation; therefore glare increases as a severe adaptive problem for elderly people.
- Decreased contrast sensitivity and increased sensitivity to glare increase impairments in driving and detailed near-vision tasks.
- Adaptation to dark occurs more slowly and to a lesser total extent.
- There is difficulty in color perception, especially the blue-green distinctions.
- Floaters, opacities occurring in the vitreous humor, may appear in the elderly person's field of vision. Although floaters can be considered a normal process of the aging eye, they may be a harbinger of a serious problem in some instances, such as retinal detachment. Therefore the patient should see an ophthalmologist if floaters are observed (Burke, 1997).

Conditions Affecting Vision

Refractive Errors

Blurred vision is a common problem for an elderly person who is experiencing visual problems. Many times this complaint is the result of ineffective glasses or contact lenses. At times the transient problem may be caused by erratic control of diabetes or an adverse response to a drug, such as a motion sickness patch of scopolamine. Treatment is focused on the causal agent and on referral to an ophthalmologist if appropriate (Riordan-Eva and Vaughan, 1997).

Keratoconjunctivitis Sicca (Dry Eyes)

Complaints of dryness, redness, or a scratchy feeling of the eyes are usual in mild cases of dry eyes; marked discomfort with photophobia and excessive secretions of mucus accompany severe cases. This condition occurs primarily in older adults because of the age-related loss of tear production and viscosity. Other causes to consider are systemic disease (autoimmune conditions), drugs, and environmental factors (hot climates or high winds). Treatment depends on cause. Tear deficiency can be treated with artificial tears. Most preparations have no side effects and can be used three or four times a day, or more often if the patient finds it helpful. If the condition worsens after treatment, it is prudent to refer to an ophthalmologist.

Cataracts

The development of cataracts is influenced by advanced age, ultraviolet exposure, congenital, toxic, metabolic, or traumatic factors (Michaels, 1994). Studies have demonstrated an association between the progression of cataracts and heavy alcohol drinking and smoking. There is a 2.4 times greater relative risk of cataract progression for

Box 19-1
Screening for Visual Problems

1. What is different now about your vision?
2. When did you last see an ophthalmologist about your vision?
3. When was the last time the prescription for your glasses was changed?
4. When did you last purchase glasses? (Providers need to consider that Medicare does not reimburse patients for their purchase of prescribed glasses.)
5. Are you experiencing any difficulty in driving or watching television?
6. Are you experiencing any difficulty in seeing at night?
7. Do you see rings around lights?
8. Is your vision blurred?
9. Have you changed any of your activities because of your vision?
10. Have you experienced loss of vision in one eye?
11. Have you experienced lack of tears or any minor irritations of your eyes?
12. Have you experienced eye pain?
13. Have you taken any medicines or other treatments to correct any eye problem you have experienced?
14. Are you concerned about your vision?
15. Is there anything else you can tell me about your vision?

smokers than for nonsmokers (West, 1995). The process of lens opacification develops over time, with the formation of the cataract beginning at the periphery of the eye.

History

- Diminished ability to see detail because of a reduction in the amount of light available to the retina
- Increased difficulty in adjusting to glare
- Significant problems in adjusting between light and dark environments, creating a major safety problem
- Blurred vision that is progressive over time
- No report of pain or redness
- Screening for all unusual problems, which includes asking the questions listed in Box 19-1

Focused Physical Examination

- As the cataract matures, the retina becomes increasingly difficult to visualize.

Treatment

Referral to Ophthalmologist. When cataracts interfere significantly with vision and with the individual's quality of life, surgery may be appropriate. Lens extraction surgery improves visual acuity in 95% of patients (Riordan-Eva and Vaughan, 1997).

Health Promotion

- Risk-reduction education
- Decision-making consultation, with the following factors for review:
  - Degree of correctable visual acuity in each eye
  - Physical and psychologic ability to withstand the stress of the surgery
  - Type of work or leisure activities
  - Social support system available to provide immediate monitoring and care, if necessary
- Dark sunglasses to protect from glare
- Visual rehabilitation (Box 19-2)

Box 19-2

Low-Vision Rehabilitation

Educate patient and family about visual loss and compensation.
Instruct in use of visual aids.
Reduce impact of peripheral visual field loss through prisms, mirrors, and reorientation of materials into functional visual field.
Reduce loss of central visual field loss by magnification.
Optimize lighting intensity in the living environment.
Improve contrast sensitivity (bright nonskid tape at top and foot of basement stairs).
Control glare.
Improve safety in home.
Refer to Lighthouse National Center for Vision and Aging: 800 Second Street, New York, NY 10017; (212) 808-0077

Glaucoma

Glaucoma is characterized by a significant increase in intraocular pressure, damage to the optic nerve, and a loss in the visual field. There are two major types of glaucoma: primary open-angle glaucoma, which occurs in people over age 40 and constitutes 90% of glaucoma cases; and acute (angle-closure) glaucoma.

Primary Open-angle Glaucoma

History

- Insidious onset without symptoms in early stages
- Peripheral visual loss in late stages
- Halo effect around lights
- Risk factors: increased age, first-degree family history, and steroid therapy

Focused Physical Examination

- Slight cupping of optic disc
- Gradual constriction of visual fields

Ophthalmologist Examination

- Testing for increase in intraocular pressure
- Visualization of optic nerve for damage
- Testing of central and visual field

Treatment

- Eyedrops

  Beta-blockers (e.g., timolol) should not be used for patients with heart failure or reactive airway disease.

Parasympathomimetics (pilocarpine) and epinephrine must be used carefully with cataracts because vision may be constricted.

- Laser surgery—usually reserved for difficult-to-control situations.

Health Promotion

- Recommendation of an annual examination by an ophthalmologist if the patient is at risk for glaucoma
- Follow-up on adherence to eyedrop schedule and monitoring for side effects
- Visual rehabilitation (see Box 19-2)

Acute (Angle-closure) Glaucoma

History

Acute glaucoma presents in older adults as follows:

- Rapid onset of severe pain and loss of vision
- Possible nausea and vomiting

Focused Physical Examination

- Eye is red.
- Cornea is steamy.
- Pupil may be dilated and nonreactive to light.

Treatment

- Medical emergency
- Referral to an ophthalmologist
- Possibility of severe vision loss in 2 to 5 days if left untreated

Senile Macular Degeneration

Senile macular degeneration is an age-related condition that occurs over time and leads to a loss of central vision. It is one of the most common causes of legal blindness in the elderly. The cause is unknown, but incidence increases with age. There are two types: atrophic (dry), which constitutes 90% of cases, and exudative (wet).

History

- Atrophic type: gradual progressive bilateral loss
- Exudative type: rapid onset of greater severity of loss, with eyes affected sequentially
- Distortion of the center of the visual field (the usual first symptom)
- Deficits in form recognition and light sensitivity

Treatment

- Referral to an ophthalmologist

Health Promotion

- Education on progression of disease
- Oral vitamins (particularly zinc), which have been recommended for treatment and prevention although their efficacy has not been substantiated (Riordan-Eva and Vaughan, 1997)
- Visual rehabilitation: central field magnification to minimize loss; peripheral vision remains intact

Diabetic Retinopathy

The leading cause of legal blindness in older adults and working adults is diabetic retinopathy (Heath and Hoepner, 1997; Infield and O'Shea, 1998). It occurs at a rate of 7% in individuals who have had diabetes for less than 10 years, 26% in individuals who have had diabetes for 10 to 14 years, and 63% in individuals who have had diabetes for at least 15 years.

History

- Transient blurring
- Significant shifts in vision

Focused Physical Examination

- Funduscopic examination: small, irregular hemorrhages and yellow-white exudates in retina

Treatment

- Optimal control of blood glucose
- Laser photocoagulation
- Surgical treatment

Health Promotion

- Annual ophthalmology examination
- Education by diabetic educator if possible
- Visual rehabilitation (see Box 19-2)
- Close follow-up

Vascular Disease and the Eye

Temporal Arteritis

Temporal arteritis occurs in people over age 50 and is associated with polymyalgia rheumatica. This disease can be easily missed and if untreated can lead to blindness.

History

- Headache
- Preauricular tenderness
- Enlarged temporal artery
- General malaise
- Elevated sedimentation rate

Diagnostic

- Positive temporal artery biopsy

Treatment

- High-dose corticosteroids

Health Promotion

- Follow-up on adherence and side effects of drug

Amaurosis Fugax (Fleeting Blindness)

Amaurosis fugax is usually caused by retinal emboli from carotid disease. A retinal vascular spasm or muscular sclerosis may be the cause in younger patients or in those without carotid disease (Box 19-3).

History

- Vision loss in one eye, which lasts a few minutes
- Vision loss described as a curtain effect
- Obtain in-depth medical history

Focused Physical Examination

- Snellen chart
- Funduscopic examination
- Complete physical examination

Box 19-3
Important Points to Remember

Monocular Field Loss

Loss of vision in one eye
Indicator of retinal disease or optic nerve involvement
Medical emergency
Possible causes:
- Retinal detachment
- Chronic glaucoma
- Retinal artery occlusion
- Ischemic optic neuropathy

Bilateral Field Loss

Medical emergency
Possible causes:
- Pituitary tumor
- Retinal detachment
  - Chronic glaucoma
  - Retinal artery occlusion
  - Ischemic optic neuropathy

Treatment

- Evaluate carotid stenosis by Doppler. Referral to specialist.
- Surgery may be indicated in high-grade stenosis to prevent possible stroke (Easton and Wilterdink, 1994). Low-grade stenosis is treated with aspirin and other antiplatelets (Riordan-Eva and Vaughan, 1997).

Health Promotion

- Education concerning risks
- Consultation in decision making
- Follow-up
- Visual rehabilitation

Visual Acuity Screening

Snellen Chart

Each line of the Snellen chart is marked with a fraction (i.e., 20/20, 20/30, 20/40, up to 20/200). Visual acuity is recorded as a fraction, with the numerator of 20 indicating the distance of the patient from the chart. The distance at which a person with normal vision would see the line is the number assigned to the denominator. This is the significant number because it indicates the degree of vision lost. The higher the denominator, the more impaired the vision.

In situations such as bedside evaluation in a nursing home, in which no Snellen chart is available or the patient is unable to cooperate, a suggested method to test gross vision is as follows:

Ask the patient to count the number of fingers held up within the patient's field of vision; test each eye separately. After checking the patient's literacy level, have the patient read from printed material such as a newspaper. This allows assessment of the ability to read different sizes of type, such as headlines, headings, and regular newspaper print. In addition, ask the patient to describe your appearance (what color is my shirt?). This assessment provides a rough estimate of visual acuity and is readily available at all times and in all settings (Burke, 1997).

Hearing

The prevalence of hearing impairments in the elderly population in the United States is significant but not universal:

People age 65 to 74 years: 25% have hearing loss
People age 75 to 84 years: 39% have hearing loss
People over age 85 years: 65% have hearing loss
Nursing home residents: 70% have hearing loss

For too many elderly people, a hearing loss goes unrecognized by the older person and undetected by primary care practitioners, which leads to an unnecessary loss of self-confidence and quality of life for the older patient. For a large majority of patients, the hearing loss can be corrected or at least ameliorated (Tolson, 1997). Not addressing the problem is an unethical professional practice.

Age-related Changes

As with many conditions ascribed to aging, age-related hearing loss is multifactorial in nature. Most cases are due in part to a loss of cochlear hair cell function; severe hearing loss is generally due to cochlear hair loss combined with age-related diseases (Gates and Rees, 1997). Two aspects of hearing are affected by biologic aging:

Loss of high-frequency sensitivity
Reduction in ability to understand speech

The loss is insidious. Most patients do not report hearing loss but instead complain of not being able to understand what was said. Contributing factors to hearing loss in older adults include the following:

- Cerumen impaction
- Otosclerosis, otitis media, head trauma
- Disease: Paget's, Ménière's, acoustic neuroma
- Intense noise exposure
- Certain ototoxic drugs
  - Salicylates
  - Aminoglycosides
  - Vancomycin

Furosemide
Cisplatin (Jackler and Kaplan, 1997)

Classification of Hearing Impairments

Presbycusis

Associated with normal aging, presbycusis includes the following:

Impairment for high-frequency tones
Impairment of frequency discrimination
Impairment of sound localization
Impairment of speech discrimination

Tinnitus

Tinnitus is a continuous or intermittent sound not due to external sources. It is a common symptom that accompanies hearing loss.

Conductive Hearing Loss

With conductive hearing loss, normal sound waves are not transmitted through the external auditory canal, the tympanic membrane, or the ossicles.

Sensorineural Hearing Loss

Dysfunction of the inner ear, the eighth cranial nerve, or the auditory pathway produces sensorineural hearing loss.

Mixed Hearing Loss

Mixed hearing loss is a combination of both conductive and sensorineural losses.

History

The symptoms of hearing loss include gradual loss of auditory sensitivity, with the perception of high-frequency sounds diminishing first. In addition, there is difficulty in localizing signals and a problem in understanding speech in unfavorable situations. This loss leads to a distortion of words, and sounds become jumbled. The resultant effect is poor speech discrimination, characterized by an often-heard remark of the hearing-impaired person: "I can hear you, but I can't understand what you are saying."

Hearing loss is not uniform; some sounds are heard, and others are not. For example, hearing loss is worse for high than for low frequencies and is greater for consonants than for vowels. This loss makes word discrimination extremely difficult. The sentence "The thinner cat is red" may be heard as "The dinner hat is red," leading to an inappropriate response, ensuing embarrassment, and perhaps social withdrawal for the elderly person who is hard-of-hearing.

Box 19-4
Screening for Hearing Loss

1. Is there any specific problem you are experiencing that is related to your hearing loss?
2. Have you changed in any way your communications with family or friends?
3. Are you having difficulties listening on the telephone or listening to the radio, television, or movies?
4. At times, does your hearing problem cause you to avoid groups of people?
5. Do you feel a loss of self-confidence because of your hearing problem?
6. At times, does your hearing problem cause you to feel depressed?
7. Is there any information you need to help you live with your hearing problem?
8. Is there anything that I have not covered that you would like to tell me about concerning your hearing?

One form of hearing loss is referred to as "loudness recruitment." With this type of hearing loss, the sounds of normal speech cannot be understood and must be made more intense to be heard; however, the sounds are heard with disturbing loudness if they exceed the individual's hearing threshold.

Psychosocial complications that need to be assessed for during the history include the following:

Depression
Isolation
Fatigue
Irritability
Loss of confidence in abilities
Negativism
Paranoia
Diminished quality of life

Social reasons for the increased denial of hearing loss may be attributed to the negative stereotypes of older people not hearing well, a loss of social status, and an inability to compensate for hearing problems. This image persists in spite of the many successful individuals who are hard of hearing. The elderly patient who experiences a hearing loss has lost a significant sensory ability that often goes unrecognized by both the patient and the patient's family. There is an opportunity to make a contribution to the quality of life for many elders by providing screening and early detection of hearing loss. Suggested screening questions are listed in Box 19-4.

Hearing Assessment

Examination

The first step in the hearing assessment is to examine each ear for cerumen impaction, which is very common and often overlooked.

Spoken Word Test. Test both ears by simply standing behind the patient and saying, once at close range and then at arm's length, two series of numbers in a normal and then in a whispered voice. Patients who are unable to decipher whispered numbers from 2 feet will benefit from formal audiometric evaluation.

Weber's Test. People with sensorineural hearing loss hear the sound in the better ear, those with conductive loss hear the sound in the impaired ear, and those with normal hearing hear the sound equally in both ears.

Rinne's Test. With conductive hearing loss, the sound of the vibrating tuning fork is heard louder and longer at the mastoid process.

Screening Audiometer Housed Within an Otoscope. This test can identify hearing impairment with 80% accuracy (Rees, Duckert, and Milczuk, 1994).

Treatment

A referral to an audiologist is appropriate. Hearing aid fitting, instruction in use, hearing tactics, and lip reading are components of a successful auditory rehabilitation program for individuals using a hearing aid for the first time (Beynon, Poole, and Thornton, 1997). Contemporary hearing aids have improved remarkably in the last decade, but many people still need further reevaluation, support, or instruction. The main drop-out point in hearing aid use occurs within the first year (Schumacher and Carruth, 1997). The economic status of the elder patient has a significant impact on the ability to purchase and maintain a hearing aid because the current Medicare program does not cover hearing aids.

Advances in hearing aid technology hold great promise for improving ease of adaptability and increased efficiency in correcting for each individual's hearing loss.

Other Assistive Listening Devices

Some elderly people are unable to use a hearing aid successfully because of physical, cognitive, or social conditions. Common reasons for not purchasing or using hearing aids include an inability to manipulate the hearing aid successfully because of arthritis, an inability to understand instructions because of dementia, an inability to afford the high cost of the hearing aid, or even an unwillingness to accept the necessity of wearing a hearing aid. Another reason may be that the hearing aid is not effective in particular situations, such as listening to the television or listening in noisy environments.

Assistive listening devices (ALDs) can be used either in addition or as an alternative to hearing aids (Jerger et al., 1995). These devices enhance the ability of the elderly person to understand speech in difficult situations. An inexpensive and easy-to-use ALD is a hardwire system that includes (a) a microphone that is held close to the sound source, (b) an amplifier, (c) a transducer, and (d) a headphone. The ALD (hardwire) system can be used to facilitate interviews and history taking for hearing-impaired elders who may have chosen not to use a conventional hearing aid. The low cost and the commercial availability of these devices make them an attractive alternative for some elderly people.

Follow-up

The efficacy and use of the hearing aid should be assessed during all subsequent visits.

Summary

Vision and hearing are senses taken for granted, with little attention given to them until they begin to fade. For the most part, older adults experience some sensory loss and make a successful accommodation. This chapter alerts the practitioner to the vigilance necessary for the recognition of signs and symptoms, methods of treatment, and risk factors of common disorders that affect these senses.

Resources

Better Hearing Institute
http://www.betterhearing.org

Self-Help for Hard of Hearing People
http://www.shhh.org

Macular Degeneration Foundation
http://www.eyesight.org/index.html

American Academy of Ophthalmology
http://www.eyenet.org

References

Beynon GL, Thornton FL, Poole C: A randomized controlled trial of the efficacy of a communication course for first time hearing aid users, *Br J Audiol* 31(5):345-351, 1997.

Burke M: Sensation. In Burke M, Walsh M, editors: *Gerontologic nursing: wholistic care of the older adult,* ed 2, St Louis, 1997, Mosby.

Easton JD, Wilterdink JL: Carotid endarterectomy: trials and tribulations, *Ann Neurol* 35:5, 1994.

Gates GA, Rees TS: Hear ye? Hear ye! Successful auditory aging, *West J Med* 16(4):247-252, 1997.

Heath J, Hoepner J: Vision. In Ham RJ, Sloane PD, editors: *Primary care geriatrics: a case-based approach,* ed 3, St Louis, 1997, Mosby.

Infield DA, O'Shea JG: Diabetic retinopathy, *Postgrad Med J* 74(869):129-133, 1998.

Jackler R, Kaplan M: Ear, nose, and throat. In Tierney LM, McPhee SJ, Papadakis MA, editors: *Current medical diagnosis and treatment 1997,* ed 36, Stamford, Conn, 1997, Appleton & Lange.

Jerger J et al: Hearing impairment in older adults: new concepts, *J Am Geriatr Soc* 43(80):928-935, 1995.

Kovar MG: Aging in the 80's: preliminary data from the supplement on aging to the national health interview survey, United States, Jan-June, 1984 (Advance data from the Vital and Health Statistics of the National Center for Health Statistics 115, DHHS Pub No 86-1250), Hyattsville, Md, 1986, Public Health Service.

Michaels D: The eye. In Hazzard WM et al, editors: *Principles of geriatric medicine and gerontology,* ed 3, New York, 1994, McGraw-Hill.

Rees TS, Duckert LG, Milczuk HA: Auditory and vestibular dysfunction. In Hazzard WM et al, editors: *Principles of geriatric medicine and gerontology,* ed 3, New York, 1994, McGraw-Hill.

Riordan-Eva P, Vaughan DG: Eye. In Tierney LM, McPhee SJ, Papadakis MA, editors: *Current medical diagnosis and treatment 1997,* ed 36, Stamford, Conn, 1997, Appleton & Lange.

Schumacher DU, Carruth JA: Long-term use of hearing aids in patients with presbyacusis, *Clin Otolaryngol* 22(5):430-433, 1997.

Tolson D: Age-related hearing loss: a case for nursing intervention, *J Adv Nurs* 26(6):1150-1157, 1997.

West S: Cigarette smoking and the risk of progression of nuclear opacities, *Arch Ophthalmol* 113:1377-1380, 1995.

20

Sleep Disorders

Insomnia is reported by 60 million Americans (Chilcott and Shapiro, 1996). Occasional poor sleep is reported by 35% of adults, and 15% consider it a chronic problem (Buysse and Reynolds, 1990). Complaints of sleeping difficulties increase with age. More than 50% of people age 65 and older report regular problems with sleep (Ancoli-Israel, 1997). Older people complain about getting less sleep, of waking up too frequently at night, of waking up too early in the morning, and of being sleepy during the day (Miles and Dement, 1980).

Stedman's Medical Dictionary, 25th edition, defines *insomnia* as "the inability to sleep, in the absence of external impediments . . . during the period when sleep should normally occur; may vary in degree from restlessness or disturbed slumber to a curtailment of the normal length of sleep or to absolute wakefulness." It implies a deterioration of sleep quantity or quality associated with complaints of daytime fatigue or changes in mood or level of concentration (Thorpy, 1990).

Insomnia is associated with increased use of medical services, functional impairment, and reduced productivity (Simon and VonKorff, 1997). Impaired sleep not only represents a quality-of-life issue but also may be associated with increased morbidity and mortality.

People reporting a change in sleep that is not associated with excessive daytime sleepiness, concentration deficits, mood changes, or other signs of deterioration in daytime functioning may require only assurance that the change is part of normal aging. Sleep complaints indicating true sleep disorders are associated with the emergence of bizarre or dangerous behavior during sleep or the deterioration of function during the period of normal wakefulness (McCall, 1995). (See Table 20-1 for a glossary of sleep-related terms.)

Normal Age-related Changes

There are three types of sleep that occur during a typical night: rapid eye movement (REM) sleep (dream sleep), non–rapid eye movement (NREM) light sleep, and NREM deep sleep (Lee, 1997). Box 20-1 describes the characteristics of the various stages of sleep.

TABLE 20-1 Glossary of Sleep-Related Terms

Term	Definition
Actigraph	A biomedical instrument used to measure body movement.
Apnea	Cessation of airflow at the nostrils and mouth lasting at least 10 seconds. The three types of apnea are obstructive, central, and mixed. Obstructive apnea is secondary to upper-airway obstruction; central apnea is associated with a cessation of all respiratory movements; mixed apnea has both central and obstructive components.
Arousal	An abrupt change from a "deeper" stage of sleep to a "lighter" stage of sleep. Multiple arousals occurring during the night in association with sleep disorders can cause severe daytime sleepiness.
Central Sleep Apnea Syndrome (CSAS)	A disorder characterized by a cessation or decrease of ventilatory effort during sleep usually associated with oxygen desaturation. May be associated with nocturnal arousals and daytime sleepiness.
Deep Sleep	A common term for NREM stages 3 and 4 sleep (also called delta or slow wave sleep).
Excessive Daytime Sleepiness (EDS)	A subjective report of difficulty in maintaining the alert awake state.
Insomnia	Difficulty in initiating or maintaining sleep. This term is employed ubiquitously to indicate any and all gradations and types of sleep loss.
NREM Sleep	Non–rapid eye movement sleep; divided into four stages, 1 through 4, based on EEG wave forms.
Multiple Sleep Latency Test (MSLT)	A series of measurements of the interval from "lights out" to sleep onset that is used in the assessment of excessive sleepiness. Subjects are allowed a fixed number of opportunities (typically four or five) to fall asleep during their customary awake period. Excessive sleepiness is characterized by sleep short latencies (<10 minutes).
Obstructive Sleep Apnea Syndrome (OSAS)	A disorder characterized by repetitive episodes of upper airway obstruction that occur during sleep usually associated with a reduction in blood oxygen desaturation. May be associated with nocturnal arousal and daytime sleepiness.
Periodic Leg Movement (PLM)	A rapid partial flexion of the foot at the ankle, extension of the big toe, and partial flexion of the knee and hip that occurs during sleep. May be associated with nocturnal arousals and daytime sleepiness.
Periodic Leg Movement Disorder (PLMD)	A disorder characterized by periodic episodes of repetitive and highly stereotyped limb movements that occur during sleep.
Polysomnogram	The continuous and simultaneous recording of multiple physiologic variables during sleep (i.e., electroencephalogram, electrooculogram, electromyogram, electrocardiogram, respiratory air flow, respiratory movements, leg movements, and other electrophysiologic variables).
REM Sleep	Rapid eye movement sleep.
Restless Legs Syndrome (RLS)	A disorder characterized by disagreeable leg sensations that usually occur prior to sleep onset and that cause an almost irresistible urge to move the legs.
Sleep Architecture	The NREM-REM sleep-stage and cycle infrastructure.
Sleep Cycle	Synonymous with the NREM-REM cycle.
Sleep Efficiency (SE)	The proportion of sleep in the episode potentially filled by sleep (the ratio of total sleep time to time in bed).
Sleep Latency (SL)	The duration of time from "lights out" or bedtime to the onset of sleep.
Sleep Maintenance	The maintenance of sleep after sleep onset is achieved.
Total Sleep Time (TST)	The amount of actual sleep time in a sleep episode; this time is equal to the total sleep episode less the awake time.

From American Sleep Disorders Association: *The international classification of sleep disorders,* Rochester, Minn, 1997, The Association.

Box 20-1
Sleep Stage Characteristics

Stage I (NREM)

Lightest sleep stage
Presence of theta waves on the EEG
Transitional state between wakefulness and deeper sleep
Lasts only a few minutes in normal persons
Person very easily awakened by sensory stimulation such as touch or noise
Slow, rolling eye movements
Sensation of drowsiness and relaxation
Vital signs (pulse, blood pressure, and respirations) gradually decrease
Body temperature and metabolism declining
Constitutes about 5% of normal sleep time
Increases in those with chronic illness and in the elderly

Stage 2 (NREM)

Light sleep stage
Presence of sleep spindles and K complexes on the EEG
Person not as easily awakened
Vital signs (pulse, blood pressure, and respirations) decreased
Body temperature and metabolism continue to decline
Constitutes about 50%-55% of normal sleep time

Stage 3 (NREM)

Deep sleep stage
Presence of some delta waves on the EEG
Person is difficult to arouse
Vital signs (pulse, blood pressure, and respirations) decreased
Body temperature and metabolism low
Constitutes about 10%-15% of normal sleep time in young adults
Reduced or absent in chronic illness and in the elderly

Stage 4 (NREM)

Deepest sleep stage
Delta waves predominant on the EEG
Person very difficult to arouse
Vital signs (pulse, blood pressure, and respirations) lowest
Body temperature very low
Constitutes about 5%-10% of normal sleep time in young adults
Reduced or absent in chronic illness and in the elderly

REM

Fast, low-amplitude random EEG waves, similar to the awake state
Normally first occurs about 90 minutes after falling asleep
Occurs earlier than 90 minutes in the elderly and in those with major depression
Occurs at onset of sleep in persons with narcolepsy
REM periods normally get longer and closer together as the night progresses
Rapidly darting eye movements visible
Visible twitching of small facial muscles
Skeletal muscle paralysis
Periods of oxygen desaturation in persons with diminished respiratory muscle function (i.e., chronic obstructive pulmonary disease)
Vivid dreaming reported if awakened from this stage
Vital signs increase and widely fluctuate
Hypothalamus unable to regulate body temperature (cannot thermoregulate)
Probably responsible for mental alertness and memory recall
Constitutes about 20%-25% of normal sleep time in adults
Constitutes more than 50% of normal sleep time in newborns and infants

---

Adapted from Lee KA: Rest and sleep. In CA Lindeman, M McAthie, editors: *Fundamentals of contemporary nursing practice*, Philadelphia, 1998, WB Saunders.

Several aspects of the physiology of sleep appear to undergo change as part of what is presumed to be the normal process of aging. These alterations occur in various measures of sleep architecture, in circadian rhythm, and possibly in the sleep requirements of elderly individuals (Brown, 1997). Studies have suggested that it is not the *need* for sleep but the *ability* to sleep that is reduced with age (Ancoli-Israel, 1997).

Box 20-2
The International Classification of Sleep Disorders

Dyssomnias

Intrinsic Sleep Disorders

Psychophysiologic insomnia
Sleep state misperception
Idiopathic insomnia
Narcolepsy
Recurrent hypersomnia
Idiopathic hypersomnia
Posttraumatic hypersomnia
Obstructive sleep apnea syndrome
Central sleep apnea syndrome
Central alveolar hypoventilation syndrome
Periodic limb movement disorder
Restless legs syndrome
Intrinsic sleep disorder NOS

Extrinsic Sleep Disorders

Inadequate sleep hygiene
Environmental sleep disorder
Altitude insomnia
Adjustment sleep disorder
Insufficient sleep syndrome
Limit-setting sleep disorder
Sleep-onset association disorder
Food allergy insomnia
Nocturnal-dependent sleep disorder

Extrinsic Sleep Disorders—cont'd

Stimulant-dependent sleep disorder
Alcohol-dependent sleep disorder
Toxin-induced sleep disorder
Extrinsic sleep disorder NOS

Circadian Rhythm Sleep Disorders

Time-zone change (jet lag) syndrome
Shift work sleep disorder
Irregular sleep-wake pattern
Delayed sleep phase syndrome
Advanced sleep phase syndrome
Non–24-hour sleep-wake disorder
Circadian rhythm sleep disorder NOS

Parasomnias

Arousal Disorders

Confusional arousals
Sleepwalking
Sleep terrors

Sleep-Wake Transition Disorders

Rhythmic movement disorder
Sleep starts
Sleepwalking
Nocturnal leg cramps

From American Sleep Disorders Association: *International classification of sleep disorders: diagnostic and coding manual,* Rochester, Minn, 1990, The Association.
NOS, Not otherwise specified.

In general, nocturnal sleep becomes lighter, more commonly disrupted, and shorter in the elderly (Bliwise, 1993). Sleep efficiency (the amount of time asleep, given the amount of time in bed) decreases to approximately 70% to 80% compared with more than 95% for younger individuals. In part this change is due to a higher number of arousals and awakenings and to increases in sleep latency (the time from "lights out" to the onset of sleep) (Brown, 1997). Because of this, there is a shift toward lighter stages of sleep with older people and a greater proportion of stage 1 sleep at the expense of the deeper stages of NREM sleep. A study by Gigli et al. (1996) demonstrated these changes as a normal consequence of aging, even in a healthy older population.

The sleep-wake cycle is controlled by circadian rhythm, which also shows changes in older people. The average younger adult gets sleepy at around 10 or 11 PM, sleeps for approximately 8 to 9 hours, and wakes between 6 and 8 AM. The circadian clock advances with age, causing advanced sleep phase syndrome. This is one of the primary reasons that older adults wake early in the morning. People with an advanced sleep cycle get sleepy early in the evening (8 or 9 PM). If they go to bed at that time and sleep for 8 hours, they wake at 4 or 5 AM. However, when people with advanced sleep phase stay up until their

Box 20-2
The International Classification of Sleep Disorders—cont'd

Parasomnias Usually Associated with REM Sleep
Nightmares
Sleep paralysis
Impaired sleep-related penile erections
Sleep-related painful erections
REM sleep-related sinus arrest
REM sleep behavior disorder

Other Parasomnias
Sleep bruxism
Sleep enuresis
Sleep-related abnormal swallowing syndrome
Nocturnal paroxysmal dystonia
Primary snoring
Congenital central hypoventilation syndrome
Benign neonatal sleep myoclonus
Other parasomnia NOS

Sleep Disorders Associated with Medical or Psychiatric Disorders

Associated with Mental Disorders
Psychoses
Mood disorders
Anxiety disorders
Panic disorder
Alcoholism

Associated with Neurologic Disorders
Cerebral degenerative disorders
Dementia
Parkinsonism
Fatal familial insomnia
Sleep-related epilepsy
Electrical status epilepticus of sleep
Sleep-related headaches

Associated with Other Medical Disorders
Sleeping sickness
Nocturnal cardiac ischemia
Chronic obstructive pulmonary disease
Sleep-related asthma
Sleep-related gastroesophageal reflux
Peptic ulcer disease
Fibrositis syndrome

Proposed Sleep Disorders
Short sleeper
Long sleeper
Subwakefulness syndrome
Fragmentary myoclonus
Sleep hyperhidrosis
Menstrual-associated sleep disorder
Pregnancy-associated sleep disorder
Terrifying hypnagogic hallucinations
Sleep-related neurogenic tachypnea
Sleep-related laryngospasm
Sleep choking syndrome

customary 10 or 11 PM, their bodies still wake up at 4 or 5 AM. Therefore they get only 5 to 6 hours of sleep before their advanced sleep-wake cycle wakes them up (Ancoli-Israel, 1997). Other factors associated with aging are also thought to interfere with the circadian mechanism: insufficient exercise, less exposure to sunlight (particularly nursing home residents), and irregular mealtimes.

Common Sleep Disorders in the Elderly

Of the many sleep disorders that are recognized (Box 20-2), several are more common in the elderly: dyssomnias such as periodic limb movement disorder and sleep apnea, medical disorders, psychiatric disorders (especially depression and anxiety). For medications used to treat these disorders see Table 20-2. Patients who have a dyssomnia should be referred to a specialist in sleep disorders.

A variety of medical conditions are known to adversely affect sleep patterns: rheumatologic disorders (pain, inability to change position), Parkinson's disease

TABLE 20-2 Patient Complaint, Assessment, and Interventions for Sleep Disorders Prevalent in the Elderly

Possible Underlying Pathology	Client Symptom	Assessment	Interventions
Dyssomnias			
Obstructive sleep apnea syndrome	Waking frequently to urinate; snoring; morning headache; unusual daytime sleepiness; frequent daytime naps	24-hour sleep diary Interview of bed partner Polysomnography	Continuous positive airway pressure; surgery; weight loss
Periodic limb movement disorder	Frequent awakenings; muscle soreness; nocturnal restlessness; daytime fatigue	Interview of bed partner Polysomnography Medication history	Clonazepam, trazodone hydrochloride, benzodiazepines
Restless legs syndrome	Prolonged sleep latency; crawling or pulling in the legs, especially the calves after lying down or sitting	Sleep history Medication history	Vitamin E; quinine; low-dose narcotic analgesics
Medical Disorders			
Cardiovascular disease	Frequent awakenings; excessive urination at night	Medical history Sleep history	Sustained-release nitroglycerin; nitroglycerin at the bedside; diuretics in morning; restriction of fluids after supper
Diabetes	Early morning awakening secondary to hypoglycemia; unpleasant dreams or nightmares	Medical history Sleep history Fasting blood glucose levels	Carbohydrate bedtime snack; reevaluation of insulin or oral hypoglycemic agent

From Beck-Little R, Weinrich SP: Assessment and management of sleep disorders in the elderly, *J Gerontol Nurs* 24(4):21-29, 1998.

(inability to change position), congestive heart failure (orthopnea, paroxysmal nocturnal dyspnea), chronic obstructive lung disease (dyspnea, cough, wheezing), prostatism (nocturia), and diabetes mellitus (nocturia, nightmares) (Brown, 1997).

A variety of medications are also known to disrupt sleep by various mechanisms: theophylline, beta-adrenergic antagonists, hypolipidemic agents, levodopa, anticonvulsants, diuretics (Brown, 1997), alcohol, decongestants, and caffeine.

Sleep-disordered Breathing

Also known as *sleep apnea,* sleep-disordered breathing is the primary dyssomnia that affects elderly people (Beck-Little and Weinrich, 1998). A study of 427 elderly people living in the community, 436 elderly hospital patients, and 235 nursing home residents found that 24% to 42% had five or more episodes of sleep apneas in an hour

TABLE 20-2 Patient Complaint, Assessment, and Interventions for Sleep Disorders Prevalent in the Elderly—cont'd

Possible Underlying Pathology	Client Symptom	Assessment	Interventions
Medical Disorders—cont'd			
Gastrointestinal reflux	Prolonged sleep latency or frequent awakening secondary to abdominal or chest discomfort related to gastric secretions	Medical history Sleep history	Restricted intake after supper; antacid medication 2 hours before bedtime; elevation of the head and shoulders for sleeping
Arthritis	Early morning awakening secondary to pain/muscle stiffness	Medical history Sleep history	Sustained-release analgesic 30 minutes before sleep
Psychiatric Disorders			
Anxiety disorder	A feeling of dread or doom; pacing, irritability, or fidgeting; stomach or nerve trouble; feelings of uneasiness	Psychosocial history Hamilton's Anxiety Rating Scale 24-hour sleep diary	Supportive care; explanation of new routines and treatments; encouragement of decision making; support of previous lifestyle
Depression	Early morning awakenings; feelings of helplessness, hopelessness, or sadness; decreased energy; low self-esteem; withdrawal; confusion or disorientation; history of recent loss	Psychosocial history Hamilton's Depression Rating Scale 24-hour sleep diary	Counseling; low-dose tricyclic antidepressants; socialization; reminiscence
Cognitive deficits	Agitation at bedtime; nocturnal wanderings	Folstein Mini Mental Examination Psychosocial history	Antipsychotic medication; structured environment

(Ancoli-Israel and Kripke, 1991). The prevalence among elderly people in the community is thought to be 9% of men and 4% of women (Ancoli-Israel, 1997).

Obstructive sleep apnea (OSA) is caused by muscular relaxation of the throat or oral structures during sleep and results in a period of apnea that awakens the person. This awakening period may last only a few seconds and is usually not remembered. Sleep apnea is classified as "obstructive" if there is functional closure of the upper airway, "central" if there is a decrease in central respiratory drive, or "mixed" when both processes occur simultaneously (Mendelson and Aikens, 1998). (See Table 20-3 for the types of sleep apnea and their treatments.)

Obstructive sleep apnea is more common in males than in females and typically emerges between the ages of 30 and 55. In adults, OSA is associated with snoring, obesity, and hypertension. Snoring is less typical with central sleep apnea.

The most common and effective treatment of OSA is continuous positive airway

TABLE 20-3 Differential Diagnosis of Sleep Apnea: Obstructive vs. Central Types

Type	Causes	Symptoms	Treatments
Obstructive	Obesity and short neck Hypognathia or jaw deformity Large tonsils, tongue, uvula Narrow airway Neurologic deficits Central or peripheral	Excessive daytime sleepiness Loud snoring, gasping, or choking during sleep Nocturnal hypertension and arrhythmias Morning headache Nocturnal confusion Intellectual deterioration	Continuous positive airway pressure (CPAP) Tongue retaining device (TRD) and other mouth pieces Tricyclic antidepressants Weight loss Body position during sleep
Central	COPD Pickwickian syndrome High altitude Stroke Heart failure	Insomnia Mild and intermittent snoring Depression	Antidepressants Theophylline Acetazolamide

From Ancoli-Israel S, Kripke DF: Prevalent sleep disorders in the aged, *Biofeedback Self Regul* 16(4):349-359, 1991.

pressure (CPAP), in which room air is blown into the nose via a nasal mask or cushioned cannula. CPAP requires ongoing monitoring for effectiveness and tolerance by the patient and must be performed by a specialist well trained in such therapy.

The major surgical treatment for OSA is uvulopalatopharyngoplasty. Pharmacologic treatments are generally of less benefit. General interventions include educating the patient to avoid sleeping on his or her back, weight loss, and avoidance of alcohol and other respiratory depressants (Mendelson and Aikens, 1998).

Periodic Limb Movement Disorder

Periodic limb movement (PLM) disorder consists of rhythmic and stereotypic movements of the legs or arms that occur only during sleep. The problem emerges primarily during middle and older ages and has an equal sex distribution (Mendelson and Aikens, 1998). Incidence increases with age and is estimated to occur in 44% of people older than 65 (Montplaisir et al., 1994). Typically patients have a normal neurologic examination while awake, with no evidence of seizure disorder on the electroencephalogram. However, while asleep these patients demonstrate characteristic PLM that involves the anterior tibialis and lasts 0.5 to 5 seconds every 20 to 40 seconds, usually in clusters and without the person awaking (Mendelson and Aikens, 1998). However, the person experiencing PLM perceives sleep as restless and unrestorative. The usual management for PLM involves low-dose clonazepam (Klonopin), or temazepam (Restoril).

Rapid Eye Movement Sleep Behavior Disorder

Rapid eye movement sleep behavior disorder (RBD) is characterized by violent behaviors that occur during REM sleep, usually in the context of a dream with violent content (e.g., fleeing from an attacker). Although a rare disorder, most of the reported cases of RBD have been in the elderly population. The disorder may be idiopathic or may be associated with central nervous system (CNS) disease, including dementia and subarachnoid hemorrhage (Brown, 1997). Treatment is usually with clonazepam; however, patients with RBD often have coexisting sleep-disordered breathing; treatment should also be started for this condition because clonazepam can worsen sleep apnea (Brown, 1997). In addition, safety measures such as padding furniture and removing sharp objects from the bedroom may be indicated.

Circadian Rhythm Disorders

Circadian rhythm disorders are also known as *delayed sleep phase syndrome* (DSPS). The endogenous CNS sleep-wake cycle regulatory mechanisms operate in a stable but delayed phase relationship to socially conventional waking and sleeping times. This disorder is due to the inability of the endogenous pacemaker to respond adequately to environmental time cues such as sunlight (Mendelson and Aikens, 1998). These patients may present with a complaint of initial insomnia or difficulty awakening in the morning. It often begins in adolescence and almost always occurs before age 30, with approximately equal distribution between the sexes.

Interventions for DSPS include chronotherapy (moving the patient's bedtime forward gradually) or light therapy (exposing the patient to bright artificial sunlight for 2 hours in the morning to phase advance the sleep-wake rhythm) (Mendelson and Aikens, 1998).

Intensive Care Delirium

Also known as *ICU psychosis*, intensive care delirium is commonly seen in patients who have been on intensive care units (ICUs) for 3 to 5 days. It is worth mentioning because of the susceptibility of the older population to this disorder. Although its cause is unknown, it has been correlated with sleep deprivation, sensory deprivation, age, severity of illness, duration of surgery, and time spent on the heart-lung bypass machine (Lee, 1997). Symptoms can include those of sleep deprivation as well as hallucinations, psychosis, and paranoia. Regardless of the underlying etiology, this condition typically resolves with the patient's return to a more conducive sleep environment and a full night's sleep.

Dementia

The changes in sleep architecture are largely related to Alzheimer's type dementia and include lower sleep efficiency, more stage 1 sleep, and a greater number of awakenings and arousals than occur in nondemented elderly (Brown, 1997). Nocturnal delirium, or sundowning, is one of the most important causes of institutionalization in demented people and is thought to occur in 12% to 14% of nursing home residents. *Sundowning* is defined as the recurrent appearance or exacerbation of behavioral disturbances at night. These behaviors may include agitation, pacing, restlessness, confusion, aggression, and paranoid ideation (Brown, 1997).

Treatment involves the elimination of metabolic, toxic, pharmacologic, and infectious factors that may exacerbate delirium (Bliwise, 1993). Attempts to correct the circadian rhythm, maintain a relaxing bedtime ritual, and minimize sleep disturbances (i.e., bed checks) may be helpful. Antipsychotic medications in *small* doses may be necessary to prevent harm or minimize fright for the patient.

Box 20-3

Areas to Be Assessed

1. *Presenting (Chief) Complaint*
   A. What does the patient think is wrong with his sleep?
   B. Why is the patient concerned about his problem?
2. *History of Current Problem*
   A. Nature and duration of problem
   B. Severity of sleep problem
      1. Frequency of occurrence
      2. Interference with usual activities
      3. What the patient has done to remedy the problem
   C. Habits
      1. Usual sleep times; since recall may be inaccurate, ask about specific days (e.g., yesterday, over the weekend)
      2. Use of caffeine, tobacco, alcohol, and other recreational drugs; have patient estimate the amount used each day and describe time of day when used
      3. Changes in weight and collar size in males, very important if patient snores loudly
3. *Health History*
   A. HEENT
   B. Cardiovascular system
   C. Pulmonary system
   D. Gastrointestinal system
   E. Genital-urinary system
   F. Endocrine system
   G. Musculoskeletal system
   H. Neurologic system
   I. Psychiatric history
4. *Medication History*
   A. Need to ask about both prescription and nonprescription drugs
   B. Current and past use of sedative/hypnotics and stimulants
5. *Family and Social History*
   A. Social history
      1. Demographic data, including educational level and occupation; check for shift work
      2. Living arrangements (e.g., with spouse, roommates, in a dormitory)
      3. Any unusual stressors and/or the presence of an infant or other family member requiring care during the night
   B. Family history of sleep problems
      1. Insomnia
      2. Obstructive sleep apnea
      3. Narcolepsy
      4. Restless legs/periodic leg movements

From Lee KA: An overview of sleep and common sleep problems, *ANNA J* 24(6):614-623, 1997.

Assessment

Assessment of sleep complaints requires delineation of total sleep amounts, timing of sleep, and impact of the complaint on waking function. However, not all patients can provide an accurate account of the complaint from memory. Patients have a tendency to focus on their most recent night or their worst night, but these experiences may not be representative of their usual sleep patterns. For a detailed assessment of the complaint, the clinician may request that patients keep diaries of their sleep experiences for at least

Box 20-4
Physical Findings Often Associated with Obstructive Sleep Apnea

- Mandibular hypoplasia, craniosynostosis, and retrognathia
- Boggy, edematous nasal mucosa (seen in patients with allergies)
- Deviated nasal septum
- Elongated soft palate and uvula
- Edema and erythema of peritonsillar pillars, uvula, soft palate, or posterior oropharynx
- Redundant pharyngeal mucosa
- Enlarged tongue
- Enlarged tonsilar tissue
- Enlarged thyroid or prominent fatty infiltration suggesting the likelihood of excess retropharyngeal adipose tissue
- Signs of right-sided heart failure such as hepatomegaly, ascites, and ankle edema

From Lee KA: An overview of sleep and common sleep problems. *ANNA J* 24(6):614-623, 1997.

2 weeks and bring in this information during a separate office visit (McCall, 1995). Often an interview of the bed partner proves invaluable in obtaining sleep information about which the patient is not even aware.

A complete medical history, as well as the current and past medication list, needs to be obtained. It is important to know if the patient has used medications for sleep or anxiety in the past, especially if she or he is or has been habituated to these medications. A social history should include the living situation, occupation and work schedule (even if retired), and stressors that may be interfering with sleep. Data should be obtained about napping, snoring, bedtime routine, diet and eating patterns, use of alcohol and tobacco, medications, and bedroom activities not related to sleep (e.g., watching TV, reading). (See Box 20-3 for a complete list of historical information that should be assessed.)

Physical examination is guided by history and may include the following:

- General information such as body habitus and vital signs
- A complete oral and facial examination (especially if apnea is suspected)
- Neck, including thyroid
- Pulmonary examination
- Cardiovascular examination, including the abdomen and extremities to evaluate signs of heart failure
- Musculoskeletal-neurologic examination to evaluate ability to reposition self in bed
- Prostate (if nocturia is present)
- Urogynecologic examination (if appropriate to address incontinence)

Box 20-4 describes the physical findings often associated with obstructive sleep apnea.

A laboratory evaluation is usually not indicated and should be guided by the history and physical examination.

Treatment

Treatment of any medical conditions that are contributing to sleep disturbance is obviously warranted.

Behavioral Interventions

In general, older patients benefit from education regarding the normal changes in sleep patterns in older age. Changing their expectation of maintaining a sleep pattern similar to previous years helps to qualm fears that something is wrong.

With many patients, sleep can be improved by behavioral interventions that establish a functional, routine approach to sleep. If nocturnal sleep is fragmented and the patient is napping frequently, sleep restriction therapy can be very effective (Rogers, 1997a). Limiting time in bed creates a degree of partial sleep deprivation and is believed to result in deeper, more continuous sleep. The following approach can be used (Rogers, 1997b):

1. Have the patient determine a time to get up each morning.
2. Once this time is set, stress that the patient should get out of bed at that time every day, even if he or she has not slept well the night before.
3. Ask the patient how much sleep he or she needs at night to function during the day. Subtract 30 to 60 minutes from this to determine how much time the patient is allowed to be in bed each night.
4. Set the patient's bedtime by counting back the required number of hours from the designated arising time. Instruct the patient not to go to bed before that time, even if he or she is sleepy.
5. Limit napping during the day to 60 minutes or less for older patients; no napping is allowed for younger people. Encourage a substitution of physical activity for napping.
6. Remind the patient that sleep will improve within a few days if this routine if followed correctly.
7. Once the patient's sleep is consolidated, add 15 to 30 minutes of sleep at a time until the desired number of hours is reached or the patient's sleep fragments again.

The following practical "sleep hygiene" tips should be provided to patients:

- Establish a relaxing routine and follow it every night before bed.
- Go to bed and get up at the same time every day.
- Avoid alcoholic beverages before bedtime (can cause awakenings).
- Avoid tobacco, caffeine, and decongestants within 8 hours of bedtime.
- Maximize exposure to bright light, preferably sunlight, every day.
- Exercise daily (but not right before bedtime).
- Use the bed only for sleep and sexual activities. Do not watch TV, read, or talk on the phone in bed.
- Keep the bedroom quiet and dark and the temperature in a comfortable range.
- If unable to fall asleep in 30 minutes, get up, do something else, and return to bed when drowsy.
- A small snack such as warm milk or cheese may help to promote sleep.
- Avoid daytime naps.
- Evaluate snoring for possible sleep apnea.

If behavioral approaches are not effective after a reasonable time and if the sleep disorder is disruptive to the patient's health or functional status, medications may be considered for *short-term* management of the problem. However, no sedative medica-

TABLE 20-4 Sedative/Hypnotics for Short-Term Treatment of Insomnia

Drug	Half-Life (Hours)	Recommended Dosage
Estazolam (ProSom)	10 to 24	1 to 2 mg at bedtime
Flurazepam (Dalmane)	50 to 100	7.5 to 30 mg before bedtime
Quazepam (Doral)	25 to 41	Start with 7.5 to 15 mg at bedtime; after 1 to 2 nights, attempt to reduce to 7.5 mg as tolerated
Temazepam (Restoril)	10 to 17	7.5 to 30 mg before bedtime
Triazolam (Halcion)	1.5 to 5.5	0.125 to 0.25 mg before bedtime
Zolpidem tartrate (Ambien)	≈2.5	5 to 10 mg immediately before bedtime

From Ancoli-Israel S, Kripke DF: Prevalent sleep disorders in the aged. *Biofeedback Self Regul* 16(4):349-359, 1991.

tion, even over-the-counter preparations, should be considered completely safe for this population. The patient's particular needs must be considered when deciding on the choice of drug. For instance, does the patient require help to fall asleep initially or need coverage later in the night for frequent awakenings?

The most commonly used over-the-counter preparations to induce sleep are antihistamines, especially diphenhydramine (Benadryl). Although they cause drowsiness, there are no scientific data to show that antihistamines either improve insomnia or prolong sleep (Ancoli-Israel, 1997). Their anticholinergic effects warrant caution for use in this population because they can lead to falls and delirium. In addition, they can cause daytime sleepiness ("hangover") and produce tolerance effects.

Melatonin has been receiving a great deal of media attention as a sleep aid. However, studies are insufficient to demonstrate its effectiveness or determine its safety at this time.

A number of prescription sedatives and hypnotics are available, and most of these are in the benzodiazepine class. Although they may be effective for short-term therapy (7 to 10 days), the high incidence of physical and psychologic dependence precludes long-term use. In addition, their side effect profile must be carefully considered, especially in the susceptible older population. Side effects include "hangover" (next-day drowsiness), rebound insomnia with discontinuation, and temporary memory loss of events immediately following administration of the drug. (See Table 20-4 for a list of available sedatives and hypnotics.) *Triazolam (Halcion) should NOT be used in the elderly population because of the increased risk of the side effect mental status changes. Flurazepam (Dalmane) should be avoided because of its extensive half-life.*

A newer medication now available, zolpidem tartrate (Ambien), is the first member of the imidazopyridine class. It is intended for short-term use.

Summary

It is important to assess and treat disordered sleep in the older individual to avoid associated morbidity and mortality and to improve the quality-of-life issues surrounding this common problem. Often sleep can be improved simply by addressing behavioral issues and minimizing the insult from comorbidities and medications. Occasionally, however, it may be necessary to treat older patients with sedative-hypnotic medications for limited periods. It is critical that the practitioner be familiar with these medications to ensure the safety and efficacy of the prescribed treatment and monitoring and to minimize untoward outcomes.

Resources

National Sleep Foundation
1367 Connecticut Ave. NW
Suite 200
Washington, DC 20036

Doctor's Guide to Insomnia
http://www.pslgroup.com/insomnia.htm

Open Directory Project
http://dmoz.org/health/conditions_and_diseases/s/sleep_disorders/

References

Ancoli-Israel S: Sleep problems in older adults: putting myths to bed, *Geriatrics* 52(1):20-30, 1997.

Ancoli-Israel S, Kripke DF: Prevalent sleep problems in the aged, *Biofeedback Self Regul* 16(4):349-359, 1991.

Beck-Little R, Weinrich SP: Assessment and management of sleep disorders in the elderly, *J Gerontol Nurs* 24(4):21-29, 1998.

Bliwise DL: Sleep in normal aging and dementia, *Sleep* 16:40-81, 1993.

Brown LK: Sleep and sleep disorders in the elderly, *Nurs Home Med* 5(10):346-353, 1997.

Buysse DJ, Reynolds CF: Insomnia. In Thorpy MJ, editor: *Handbook of sleep disorders*, New York, 1990, Marcel Dekker.

Chilcott LA, Shapiro CM: The socioeconomic impact of insomnia: an overview, *Pharmacoeconomics* 10(suppl 1):1-14, 1996.

Gigli GL et al: Sleep in healthy elderly subjects: A 24-hour ambulatory polysomnographic study, *Int J Neurosci* 85:263-271, 1996.

Lee KA: An overview of sleep and common sleep problems, *ANNA J* 24(6):614-623, 1997.

McCall WV: Management of primary sleep disorders among elderly persons, *Psychiatr Serv* 46(1):49-55, 1995.

Mendelson WB, Aikens JE: Insomnia: exploring underlying processes and treatment, *Med Behav* October, pp 1-11, 1998.

Miles L, Dement WC: Sleep and aging, *Sleep* 3:119-120, 1980.

Montplaisir J et al: Restless legs syndrome and periodic limb movements during sleep. In Kryger MH, Roth T, Dement WC, editors: *Principles and practice of sleep medicine*, Philadelphia, 1994, WB Saunders.

Rogers A: Nursing management of sleep disorders: part 1, assessment, *ANNA J* 24(6):666-671, 1997a.

Rogers A: Nursing management of sleep disorders: part 2, behavioral interventions, *ANNA J* 24(6):672-675, 1997b.

Simon GE, VonKorff M: Prevalence, burden and treatment of insomnia in primary care, *Am J Psychiatry* 154(10):45-56, 1997.

Thorpy MJ: *Handbook of sleep disorders*, New York, 1990, Marcel Dekker.

21

Pressure Ulcers

Pressure ulcers in the elderly are costly complications of many illnesses. Each pressure ulcer can cost as much as $15,000 in health care costs and add more than 16 days to a hospital stay. Estimated annual cost reached $1.5 billion in the United States. More alarming is the rise of mortality associated with pressure ulcers (Jahnigen, 1993).

Pressure ulcers, the result when ischemic damage and subsequent necrosis affect the skin, subcutaneous tissue, and often muscle, are primarily caused by intense pressure exerted for a short time or pressure exerted for a longer time.

When tissues are compressed, usually over a bony prominence, the average pressure of the vascular bed may be exceeded. The blood supply to the affected area and its lymphatic drainage is then reduced. The normal capillary blood pressure at the arteriole end of vascular bed averages 32 mm Hg. At times in a sitting position, pressures >300 mm Hg can be measured at the ischial tuberosities, a common site for skin breakdown in individuals who sit for long periods or who are confined to a wheelchair (Panel for the Prediction and Prevention of Pressure Ulcers in Adults, 1992).

The most common sites for pressure ulcers are the sacrum, greater trochanters, ischium, medial and lateral condyles, malleoli, and heels. Less common sites are the elbows, scapulae, vertebrae, ribs, ears, and the back of the head (Panel for the Prediction and Prevention of Pressure Ulcers in Adults, 1992).

Age-related Changes

Normal age-related changes that increase an older person's risk for pressure ulcers include the following:

- Thinning and flattening of the epidermis, which increases skin permeability and reduces the effectiveness of barrier functions
- Decreases in cell replacement to less than half that of a young adult (Nissen, 1997)
- Decreases in vascularity and elasticity
- Decreases in subcutaneous tissue, particularly over joints and bony prominences
- Decreases in sebaceous and sweat gland activity (Seidel et al., 1995)

Assessment and Prevention of Risk

Two validated assessment tools are available for identifying patients at risk for developing pressure ulcers: the Braden Scale and the Norton Scale. These tools allow the clinician to evaluate accurately the potential risk of pressure ulcer development and then take appropriate steps to decrease the risks. The risk factors contained in these scales are

TABLE 21-1 Braden Scale for Predicting Pressure Ulcer Risk

Patient's Name ____________________

Sensory Perception Ability to respond meaningfully to pressure-related discomfort	1. Completely Limited: Unresponsive (does not moan, flinch, or grasp) to painful stimuli, due to diminished level of consciousness or sedation, OR limited ability to feel pain over most of body surface.	2. Very Limited: Responds only to painful stimuli. Cannot communicate discomfort except by moaning or restlessness, OR has a sensory impairment which limits the ability to feel pain or discomfort over ½ of body.
Moisture Degree to which skin exposed to moisture	1. Constantly Moist: Skin is kept moist almost constantly by perspiration, urine, etc. Dampness is detected every time patient is moved or turned.	2. Moist: Skin is often but not always moist. Linen must be changed at least once a shift.
Activity Degree of physical activity	1. Bedfast: Confined to bed	2. Chairfast: Ability to walk severely limited or nonexistent. Cannot bear own weight and/or must be assisted into chair or wheelchair.
Mobility Ability to change and control body position	1. Completely Immobile: Does not make even slight changes in body or extremity position without assistance.	2. Very Limited: Makes occasional slight changes in body or extremity position but unable to make frequent or significant changes independently.
Nutrition Usual food intake pattern	1. Very Poor: Never eats a complete meal. Rarely eats more than ⅓ of any food offered. Eats 2 servings or less of protein (meat or dairy products) per day. Takes fluids poorly. Does not take a liquid dietary supplement, OR is NPO and/or maintained on clear liquids or IVs for more than 5 days.	2. Probably Inadequate: Rarely eats a complete meal and generally eats only about ½ of any food offered. Protein intake includes only 3 servings of meat or dairy products per day. Occasionally will take a dietary supplement, OR receives less than optimum amount of liquid diet or tube feeding.
Friction and Smear	1. Problem: Requires moderate to maximum assistance in moving. Complete lifting without sliding against sheets is impossible. Frequently slides down in bed or chair, requiring frequent repositioning with maximum assistance. Spasticity, contractures, or agitation leads to almost constant friction.	2. Potential Problem: Moves feebly or requires minimum assistance. During a move skin probably slides to some extent against sheets, chair, restraints, or other devices. Maintains relatively good position in chair or bed most of the time but occasionally slides down.

measures of physical and mental condition, nutrition, mobility, and continence. Patients with scores of 16 or less on the Braden Scale and 14 or less on the Norton Scale are considered to be at high risk (Tables 21-1 and 21-2). Peiper and Sugrue (1998) report in their review of the literature that patients with pressure ulcers demonstrate scores on the Braden Scale that are significantly lower than those of ulcer-free patients.

Evaluator's Name ______________________	**Date of Assessment**				
3. Slightly Limited: Responds to verbal commands but cannot always communicate discomfort or need to be turned, OR has some sensory impairment which limits ability to feel pain or discomfort in 1 or 2 extremities.	4. No Impairment: Responds to verbal commands. Has no sensory deficit which would limit ability to feel or voice pain or discomfort.				
3. Occasionally Moist: Skin is occasionally moist, requiring an extra linen change approximately once a day.	4. Rarely Moist: Skin is usually dry; linen requires changing only at routine intervals.				
3. Walks Occasionally: Walks occasionally during day but for very short distances, with or without assistance. Spends majority of each shift in bed or chair.	4. Walks Frequently: Walks outside the room at least twice a day and inside room at least once every 2 hours during waking hours.				
3. Slightly Limited: Makes frequent though slight changes in body or extremity position independently.	4. No Limitations: Makes major and frequent changes in position without assistance.				
3. Adequate: Eats over half of most meals. Eats a total of 4 servings of protein (meat, dairy products) each day. Occasionally will refuse a meal, but will usually take a supplement if offered, OR is on a tube feeding or TPN regimen, which probably meets most of nutritional needs.	4. Excellent: Eats most of every meal. Never refuses a meal. Usually eats a total of 4 or more servings of meat and dairy products. Occasionally eats between meals. Does not require supplementation.				
3. No Apparent Problem: Moves in bed and in chair independently and has sufficient muscle strength to lift up completely during move. Maintains good position in bed or chair at all times.					
	Total Score				

TABLE 21-2 Norton Risk Assessment Scale

		Physical Condition	Mental Condition	Activity	Mobility	Incontinent	
		Good 4 Fair 3 Poor 2 Very Bad 1	Alert 4 Apathetic 3 Confused 2 Stupor 1	Ambulant 4 Walk/help 3 Chairbound 2 Bed 1	Full 4 Sl. limited 3 V. limited 2 Immobile 1	Not 4 Occasional 3 Usually/Urine 2 Doubly 1	TOTAL SCORE
Name	Date						

From Norton D, McLaren R, Exton-Smith AN: *An investigation of geriatric nursing problems in hospital,* Edinburgh, 1962, reissue 1975, Churchill Livingstone.

Nutritional Assessment

It is estimated that 25% of older Americans are malnourished (Wellman, 1997). Low levels of protein, hemoglobin, and total lymphocyte count (TLC) contribute to skin breakdown and prevent healing. A nutritional assessment should include height, weight, biochemical data, dietary habits, and preferences. Patients who are not properly nourished are at high risk for skin breakdown, and wounds that occur are extremely difficult to heal (Bergstrom et al., 1994; Salcido, 1997).

Laboratory Tests

A serum albumin measurement of 3.3 g/dl or less is associated with protein malnourishment and increased morbidity and mortality. Hypoproteinemia leads to edema because of changes in osmotic pressures, which in turn decreases oxygenation of tissue and creates an environment for tissue breakdown. Adequate protein is necessary for healing (Peiper and Sugrue, 1998).

Levels of hemoglobin below 11.1 g/dl increase the risk for the development of pressure ulcers and greatly increase the healing time of existing ulcers (Saunders and Grezesk, 1996). A TLC of 800 or below is considered severe malnutrition. Levels from 800 to 1200 suggest moderate malnutrition. TLC can be calculated by multiplying the percent of lymphocytes by the total white blood count and dividing by 100. Nursing home patients with serum cholesterol levels below 120 to 150 mg/ml demonstrate a higher mortality rate (Saunders and Grezesek, 1996).

There is strong evidence that low levels in any or all of these areas are predictive of increased risk for pressure ulcer development and decreased healing ability. The cost of obtaining these laboratory values should be taken into consideration when using these tools in an assessment (Bergstrom et al., 1994; Haas, 1995; Salcido, 1997; Tallon, 1995; Xakellis and Frantz, 1997).

Hydration Assessment

Hydration is an important factor in the prevention and healing of pressure ulcers. The skin of an older person often appears to hang loosely on bony frames as a result of the loss of elasticity, underlying adipose tissue, and years of gravitational pull. Tenting is often the result when testing for skin turgor; thus turgor may not be a reliable or valid estimate of the hydration status of an elderly individual (Seidel et al., 1995). The most reliable assessment of hydration is blood urea nitrogen and creatinine studies.

Prevention

The very best line of treatment for at-risk patients is the prevention of pressure to body surfaces that could result in ulceration. Prevention intervention options include the following (Panel for the Prediction and Prevention of Pressure Ulcers in Adults, 1992):

- Support surfaces: pressure-relief or pressure-reduction surfaces
- A turning and positioning schedule
- Protective films or real sheepskins
- Maintenance of range of motion and ambulation
- Maintenance of clean and appropriately dry skin
- Maintenance of good nutrition

Support Surfaces

Pillows and rubber rings (donuts) should not be used, because they cause compression and decrease further blood supply to the area. Two types of support surfaces can be used: pressure-relief surfaces and pressure-reduction surfaces. Pressure-relief surfaces are the various mattresses designed to reduce interface pressures below 25 mm Hg (i.e., below capillary closure). Pressure-reduction surfaces are less expensive and are designed to lower pressure but not below the 25 to 35 mm Hg threshold. These devices include alternating pressure pads, foam, and gel pads.

Convoluted Polyurethane Egg Crate Foam Mattress. This high-density foam is made of plastic or silicone and has the advantage of being inexpensive, lightweight, and comfortable. Its disadvantages are that it provides minimal pressure relief and causes retention of body heat, which potentiates perspiration and maceration. This product is considered a fire hazard by many. Although the popular 2-inch Egg Crate pads do not provide any real pressure reduction, they do provide a comfortable surface.

Alternating Pressure Mattress. This vinyl, air-filled mattress is designed to inflate and deflate small air cells at regular intervals by means of an electric pump. Some models also have vents that allow the air to circulate between the mattress and the patient. This type of mattress should be placed on top of a bed mattress. Its advantages are that it mechanically alters the points of pressure against the body, provides a moderate degree of protection against pressure, can decrease maceration (when the model with the air vents is used), is lightweight, and is easy to clean if soiled. Its disadvantages are that it minimizes but does not completely reduce pressure, may be uncomfortable because it feels lumpy, and is more costly because an electric pump is needed. The indications for use are patients who are at high risk for skin breakdown or patients who have stage I or II pressure ulcers (Bergstrom et al., 1994; van Rijswijk and Barr, 1995).

Water Mattress. A heavy vinyl mattress filled with water can be placed on top of a bed mattress. Its advantages are that it evenly distributes the patient's weight over the greatest possible surface, it provides a moderately high degree of protection against pressure, and it is comfortable, easy to maintain, and easy to clean if soiled. Its disadvantages are that it minimizes but does not prevent pressure, it is heavy when filled, and it costs about the same as an air mattress. The indications are for patients who are at high risk or who already have stage I, II, or III pressure ulcers (Bergstrom et al., 1994; van Rijswijk and Barr, 1995).

Air-fluidized Bed. This type of bed consists of a mattress filled with ultrafine silicone-coated beads and warm air flowing through a compressor. A loose polyester sheet separates the patient from the beads, which allows the air to circulate and body fluids to drain into the bed. When the compressor is turned off, the beads firmly mold around the patient to facilitate positioning for dressing changes, transfers, or cardiopulmonary resuscitation.

Its advantages are the support of the patient at a subcapillary closing pressure (<15 to 33 mm Hg) and provision of a high degree of protection against pressure, friction, shearing, and maceration. Its disadvantages are the physical size and weight of the bed, and the circulating warm air may have a dehydrating effect on the patient and the wounds. In addition, patient repositioning (unless the bed does it automatically) is difficult because of the motion and molding. The rental fee is very expensive, and new Medicare rules may make reimbursement more problematic for certain nursing home residents. Indications for use include patients with any stage of skin breakdown (particularly stages III and IV pressure ulcers), patients undergoing graft or flap surgery, patients with intractable pain, and patients who fail to improve with pressure-reduction surface treatment (Bergstrom et al., 1994; van Rijswijk and Barr, 1995).

Turning and Positioning

The patient's position should be changed every 2 hours, but turning may need to be more frequent for some patients. When positioning, use multiple pillows, positioning wedges, or towels or other rolls to prevent a patient's bony prominences from rubbing together (Peiper and Sugrue, 1998).

Techniques for Positioning

- Keeping the head of the bed elevated less than 30 degrees prevents shearing forces and reduces pressure on the greater trochanter.
- When positioning patients in the supine position, place pillows at the lateral aspect of each buttock to decrease pressure on the sacrum.
- Heels should never rest on the surface of the bed. A pillow placed under the patient's legs or a towel roll superior to the patient's heel eliminates this source of risk.
- For bed-bound patients or patients with pressure ulcers on their feet or lower legs, use of a bed cradle prevents the bedclothes from exerting pressure on these sensitive areas.
- Placing pillows at the end of the bed gives the feet something to rest or push against and decreases the incidence of footdrop.

- Change of position in the wheelchair or gerichair: Pressure on the sacrum is at its highest when a person is sitting above a 45-degree angle. Many patients are unable to change position by themselves, and therefore turning schedules and pressure-relieving devices are imperative. Consult a physical or occupational therapist to ensure that each person is using proper wheelchair and pressure-relieving devices.

Use of Protective Films or Real Sheepskin

Protective films are effective because they reduce both friction and injury. They are also effective protection against incontinence. This type of dressing may be used to protect against friction can be used on the heels and elbows. Lubricants can be used to protect unbroken skin from friction (Nissen, 1997; Regan, 1995).

Real sheepskin can be useful to reduce friction and shear. Real skins work well and are good for controlling perspiration. Polyesters should not be used except for comfort (Nissen, 1997; Panel for the Prediction and Prevention of Pressure Ulcers in Adults, 1992; Regan, 1995).

Maintaining Range of Motion and Ambulation

Improving mobility and patient activity helps to keep the pressure off areas at risk. The use of exercise bars or a trapeze over the bed may reduce the risk for bedfast patients. Range-of-motion exercises and ambulation are important to prevent contractions and improve circulation (Panel for the Prediction and Prevention of Pressure Ulcers in Adults, 1992).

Maintaining Clean and Appropriately Dry Skin

The suggested procedure for cleaning an elderly patient is to gently cleanse the affected area with a skin cleaner, plain water, or a minimal amount of mild soap and water. After cleaning, apply a thin layer of moisturizing lotion, taking care to massage gently around rather than over the reddened area. Vigorous massage increases tissue damage by creating shearing forces. This treatment should be followed by the application of a thin layer of a petroleum-based product. Petroleum products are water resistant, provide a protective barrier against urine and feces, and protect denuded skin. A mixture of 30% petroleum jelly with zinc oxide provides protection for fecal incontinence or episodes of diarrhea (Nissen, 1997).

The placement of indwelling catheters is not necessary to protect the skin of an incontinent patient. A catheter puts a patient at increased risk for developing a urinary tract infection and sepsis (Cooney, 1997).

Pressure Ulcer Staging

Once a pressure ulcer has developed, it must be staged to classify the degree of tissue damage. Staging is used as a tool for assessment and communication between health care professionals. The stagings were devised by National Pressure Ulcer Advisory Panel

Consensus Development Conference (NPUAP, 1995) after consultation with the Wound Ostomy and Continence Nurses Society (WOCN). Ulcers are staged as follows:

Stage I: Nonblanchable erythema of *intact* skin, the herald lesion of skin ulceration. In individuals with darker skin, skin discoloration, increased warmth, edema, induration, and hardness may also be indicators.

Stage II: Partial-thickness skin loss involving the epidermis, dermis, or both. The ulcer is superficial and presents clinically as an abrasion, blister, or shallow crater. The wound base is moist, pink, and free of necrotic tissue. An intact blister over a bony prominence is a stage II ulcer. Keep the blister intact, if possible, to promote healing. This stage is reversible with appropriate treatment and care.

Stage III: Full-thickness skin loss that involves damage to or necrosis of subcutaneous tissue and may extend down to, but not through, underlying fascia. The ulcer presents clinically as a deep crater with or without undermining of adjacent tissue. Serous or purulent drainage is usually present. This stage may be life-threatening without appropriate treatment and care.

Stage IV: Full-thickness skin and subcutaneous tissue loss with extensive destruction or necrosis of tissue, which exposes muscle, bone, or supporting structures (e.g., tendon, joint capsule). Serous or purulent drainage is usually present. Sinus tracts and widely undermined areas may be present. The wound base itself is not painful, but the sides of the wound may be. Osteomyelitis or septic arthritis in adjoining joints that results from an infection of this wound type may be fatal without appropriate treatment and care (Bergstrom et al., 1994).

The following limitations are inherent in these definitions:

Because the skin remains intact in stage I pressure ulcers, these lesions are not ulcers in the usual sense. In addition, stage I pressure ulcers are not always reliably assessed, especially in patients with darkly pigmented skin. Despite these limitations, identification of a stage I pressure ulcer is critical for indicating the need for more vigilant assessment and preventive care.

Assessing stage I ulcers in individuals with darker skin tones requires careful observation for (1) any change in the feel of the tissue; (2) any change in the appearance of the skin in a high-risk area, such as the orange peel look; (3) a subtle purplish hue; and (4) extremely dry, crustlike areas that, on close examination, are found to cover a break in the tissue (Henderson et al., 1997).

An ulcer cannot be accurately staged until the eschar, if present, is removed. Eschar is a black, leatherlike layer of dry necrotic cells and debris in the wound. It is either level with the epidermis or somewhat concave. By comparison, a scab sits on top of the skin and feels rough and slightly flaky (Maklebust, 1997).

Pressure ulcers should be staged to classify the degree of tissue damage observed. It may be difficult to assess pressure ulcers in patients with casts, other orthopedic devices, or support stockings. Routine assessment to check for adequate circulation, movement, and sensation may fail to detect pressure ulcers beneath casts. Be sure to (1) assess the skin under the edges of casts, (2) be alert to patient complaints of pressure-induced pain, (3) determine whether casts need to be altered or replaced to relieve pressure, and (4) remove support stockings to assess the skin.

Documentation

Accurate assessment and documentation are essential to proper staging of a pressure ulcer. At a minimum, pressure ulcer assessment should include the location; the stage or grade of the wound; the quality of the circulation; the dimensions (size); the presence or absence and estimated amount of necrotic tissue; the condition of the wound base; the condition of the periwound skin; the amount, quality, and nature and the presence or absence of exudate; an estimate of the presence or absence of infection; and the presence of healed pressure ulcers.

A Polaroid picture is excellent for documentation purposes. Put the pictures in the patient chart with the date of the pictures written on the back. Draw a simple diagram of the wound with areas of tunneling, undermining, or sinus tracts. Staging, showing progression of the ulcer, can go from I to II to III to IV; however, a healing ulcer should be referred to as "healing stage III" (with measurements) rather than upstaging (i.e., "now Stage II"). The only exception to this type of staging is the minimum data set, the federally mandated reporting system in use in nursing homes. Because of reimbursement issues, healing ulcers are coded in the healed stage. Slough and eschar prevent accurate staging and should be documented as such. Consistency in documentation is of great importance for any health care situation but especially in wound care because of the number of staff and caregivers who are observing and treating the wound.

Elements of a Wound

Wound Size

Measurement of the wound includes length, width, and depth. Depth can be measured by observing how far a saline-moistened sterile cotton tip can be inserted into the wound; a double-gloved finger can also be used. To a great extent, the staging of a wound is an estimate of its depth (Plassmann, 1995).

Wound Edges

Wound edges are good indicators of the healing process. A sloped edge with epithelium around the wound is a good sign. Rolled under or punched out edges may be a sign that the wound is deteriorating or enlarging. Wounds with rolled edges will not heal, and it is wise to debride them. Rolled edges can be a sign of undermining that was not detected or documented (Tallon, 1995).

Necrotic Tissue

The presence of necrotic tissue in a wound indicates that it is at least a full-thickness wound (stage III or IV). Documentation includes the percent of the wound covered with necrotic tissue and the color and consistency of the tissue. The removal of necrotic tissue does not often cause bleeding. If bleeding occurs, the tissue being removed is most likely a scab of dried blood (Nissen, 1997; Tallon, 1995; Xakellis and Frantz, 1997).

Wound Base

A description of the wound base includes any tunneling or undermined edges. The base of the wound should be probed to assess it completely. Granulation tissue should be evident in the wound bed, and the percentage of the wound covered with red granulation tissue should be documented (Nissen, 1997).

Wound Exudate

Wound exudate contains growth factors that actively promote healing. Problems occur when there is too much or too little exudate. Too little exudate creates a desiccated wound; too much overwhelms the dressing and can flood the surrounding skin, causing maceration of the periwound tissues (Xakellis and Frantz, 1997).

Contamination or Infection

A wound will not heal until any infection is resolved. Infected wounds have the same types of organisms that are present in chronic open wounds, but they are present in much larger numbers. Infection may be signaled by the presence of one or more of the following: induration, fever or a feeling of general malaise, erythema, edema, and purulent, foul-smelling drainage, particularly when accompanied by an elevated white blood count. Infected wounds are usually painful to the patient (Melchor-MacDougal and Lander, 1995).

Wound Cultures

Routine wound culturing of pressure ulcers in the absence of clinical symptoms and signs of infection is of questionable value. The growth of common pathogens (e.g., *Staphylococcus* organisms, *Escherichia coli*) in such cultures does not necessarily imply the presence of infection that requires antibiotic therapy. If there are signs and symptoms of bacterial or systemic infection or if the healing of the pressure ulcer is delayed, a wound culture and a sensitivity test are indicated (Bergstrom et al., 1994).

The guidelines of the Centers for Disease Control and Prevention and the Agency for Health Care Policy and Research (AHCPR) recommend needle aspiration culture or tissue biopsy cultures because swab cultures are seen to have no diagnostic value. Bacterial counts of 100,000 organisms/g of tissue (determined by biopsy) represent the critical value for wound infection and correlate with the inability of the wound to heal normally (Bergstrom et al., 1994).

All chronic wounds are contaminated. They will heal, they do not need to be sterilized, and they cannot be sterilized. Adequate cleaning and debridement usually prevent colonization from progressing to infection (Bergstrom et al., 1994).

Wound Healing

Healing of a pressure ulcer usually involves three phases: granulation, contraction, and reepithelialization (Haas, 1995; Nissen, 1997).

First Phase

The first phase of healing takes place for the first 4 days after a break in skin integrity. During this time the body prepares the wound bed by removing dead tissue. The presence of foreign material or necrotic tissue prevents the wound from progressing. Observation of the wound at this time shows warm, reddened skin and increased serosanguineous fluid and exudate. The exudate is composed of phagocytized bacteria, neutrophils, and living bacteria. During this phase, the exudate or wound drainage is at a peak (Haas, 1995; Salcido, 1997).

Second Phase

The second phase of healing occurs from day 4 through day 21. Healing activities involve the formation of granulation tissue, contraction of the wound, and the final epithelialization. A new vascular bed is formed, and granulation tissue fills the wound bed to provide the base for the migration of the epithelial cells. The process is a contraction of the wound edges, with a filling in from the bottom. The wound is rough and red; this is the area that must be kept moist to facilitate the mobility of granulation tissue cells. These cells are very fragile and can be easily damaged by dressings. The second phase ends when the edges of the wound are white with epithelialization cells. As might be anticipated for elderly individuals, this phase can take longer; it may take double the usual time (Haas, 1995; Salcido, 1997).

Third Phase

The third and last phase of healing can be as short as 3 weeks or as long as 2 to 3 years. The tensile strength of the scar tissue begins to increase. The wound now consists of scar tissue covered by new epithelium from the wound edges. The scar consists of granulation tissue covered by thin epithelial tissue. Ultimately all healed pressure ulcers have only 70% to 75% of their original strength. Further injury is problematic, and these skin areas are at high risk.

• • •

The three phases of healing overlap, and various parts of the wound are at different phases at different times. At any specific point in time it is sometimes difficult to determine what is occurring in the wound in terms of healing phases (Nissen, 1997; Salcido, 1997).

Factors That Affect Wound Healing

Wound healing depends on a normal blood supply; anything that impedes circulation influences healing of the wound.

Intrinsic factors include the following:

- Advanced age
- Nutritional and hydration status
- Diabetes mellitus
- Other comorbidity

Extrinsic factors include the following:

- Mechanical stress (pressure, friction, and shear)
- Medications
- Nonsteroidal antiinflammatory drugs, long-term steroid use
- Debris in the wound
- Infection
- Temperature
- Desiccation (lack of moisture in the wound bed)
- Maceration (abundance of fluid in the wound bed)
- Chemical stress (Xakellis and Frantz, 1997)

Temperature. Frequent dressing can alter the temperature of a wound enough to interfere with healing. High fevers, diapers that trap body heat, and high ambient temperature in the patient's environment can alter wound temperature. Applications of ice packs or heating pads for any reason may cause damage to the local circulation and thus affect wound healing (Bergstrom et al., 1994; Haas, 1995; Nissen, 1997).

Chemical Stress. Chemical stress results from the use of many traditional treatments, such as Dakin's solution, peroxide, acetic acid, povidone iodine (Betadine), iodine, hexachlorophene, alcohol, or hypochlorites. These agents are cytotoxic and delay wound healing. They are excellent bacteriostatic agents, but they also kill maturing endothelial cells in a healing wound (Bergstrom et al., 1994; Xakellis and Frantz, 1997).

Treatment

Stage I

Assess and modify the risk factors. Cleaning the wound with normal saline solution alone is safe and effective. The selection of a dressing may be determined by the location of the wound. Either a transparent vapor-permeable dressing, a liquid barrier, or an opaque hydrocolloidal occlusive barrier may be used. All decrease friction, shearing, and maceration (Krasner et al., 1993; Nissen, 1997; van Rijswijk and Barr, 1995).

Heat lamps are not recommended for this or any other stage of skin breakdown. In addition to being a source of potential injury to the patient, heat lamps dry and dehydrate wounds and inhibit the healing process (Krasner et al., 1993; Nissen, 1997; van Rijswijk and Barr, 1995).

The use of tincture of benzoin on reddened areas is discouraged because it has a high alcohol content and becomes sticky when dry and thus can pull and damage fragile skin (Krasner et al., 1993; Nissen, 1997; van Rijswijk and Barr, 1995).

Stage II

Assess and modify the risk factors. Cleansing is the same as in stage I. The dressing may be a transparent vapor-permeable dressing, an opaque hydrocolloidal occlusive barrier, or enzymatic spray, which has a mild debriding action and improves epithelialization by stimulating the vascular bed. Wet-to-dry dressings may also be used but require more frequent changes, tend to be less comfortable, and inhibit inspection of the wound. Dry sterile dressings are not recommended because they dry out a wound at this stage and inhibit healing (Krasner et al., 1993; Nissen, 1997; van Rijswijk and Barr, 1995).

Stage III

Assess and modify the risk factors. At this stage, it is easy to become so focused on local care that the risk factors are overlooked. For healing to occur, the wound must be free of infection and necrotic tissue. Wound debridement is necessary if necrotic tissue is present. Culture and sensitivity studies should be performed if there are signs of infection (elevated temperature, malodorous exudate, inflamed tissue surrounding the wound). In addition, wound and skin precautions should be taken until the results are known (Krasner et al., 1993; Nissen, 1997; van Rijswijk and Barr, 1995).

Local care of a wound that is free of necrotic material consists of three basic components: irrigation, packing, and outer dressings. For irrigation, normal saline is recommended in clean wounds. With aseptic technique, a catheter-tipped syringe may be used to direct the flow of the irrigant into the wound. Packing material should be appropriate to the depth and size of the wound. If wet-to-dry techniques are used, the dressing should be plain gauze without cotton filling because it is more absorbent. Using aseptic technique, the dressing should be gently packed to conform to the wound without extending onto the intact skin, which may cause tissue irritation or maceration. Care must be taken not to pack the wound too tightly, which inhibits the absorption capability of the dressing and applies pressure to the area (Krasner et al., 1993; Nissen, 1997; van Rijswijk and Barr, 1995).

Other absorption dressings may be used. The outer dressing should be applied over the packed wound to prevent contamination from the external environment. The dry sterile dressing should be of a size appropriate for the wound and secured with hypoallergenic tape or other methods (e.g., Montgomery straps or a stockinette). Care must be taken to protect the surrounding skin. Care of a stage III ulcer is costly and labor intensive (Krasner et al., 1993; Nissen, 1997; van Rijswijk and Barr, 1995).

Stage IV

Assess and modify the risk factors. The procedures for care are similar to those for stage III. Variations may be indicated by the presence of sinus tracts or exposed bone. Irrigation should be performed with aseptic technique. If sinus tracts are present, the flow of the irrigant needs to be appropriately directed. All exudate and necrotic debris must be removed from these narrow pathways. The wound should be packed. Packing should be loosely directed into all crevices and sinuses, with no dead or empty spaces. If used, rolled gauze (available in various widths) should be kept in one piece to permit easy removal and prevent the possibility of dressing material being left in the wound. If more than one roll is used, the rolls should be tied together. Exposed bone should be covered with a wet, normal saline dressing and changed every 4 hours to avoid drying and to maintain viability of the bone tissue. An outer dressing should be applied, as in stage III (Krasner et al., 1993; Nissen, 1997; van Rijswijk and Barr, 1995).

Pressure Ulcer Treatment: Debridement of Necrotic Tissue

The three methods of debridement are mechanical, surgical, and chemical. Chemical is best used in conjunction with one of the other two methods. All three are intended to assist the natural process of autolytic debridement (Bergstrom et al., 1994; Nissen, 1997; van Rijswijk and Barr, 1995).

For mechanical debridement, normal saline is used to irrigate a wound that has purulent drainage or necrotic debris. A whirlpool bath is often used as well. A wet-to-moist dressing consisting of plain gauze moistened with normal saline is then gently packed into the wound. Loose necrotic tissue and wound drainage are absorbed into the dressing and removed with each dressing change. These dressings are usually changed every 8 hours. Wet-to-moist gauze dressings changed three or four times daily remove necrotic debris, but mechanical debridement is minimally effective on eschar. It is slower, time-consuming, and uncomfortable for the patient. There is also the problem of removing viable tissue along with the necrotic tissue. Care must be taken when removing a dry dressing to avoid damaging new cell growth and destroying viable tissue (Bergstrom et al., 1994; Nissen, 1997; van Rijswijk and Barr, 1995).

Surgical debridement is the fastest way to remove necrotic tissue and the only effective method of removing eschar. Although effective surgical debridement may add the risks of hemorrhage, infection, increased wound size, and pain, the advantages of surgical debridement are speed and completeness for patients who have large, thick, necrotic debris. When sepsis threatens, the best method is to surgically remove the necrotic tissue. Removal can be performed with laser surgery, which reduces some risks. Surgical debridement for thorough excision of infected or necrotic tissue usually is followed by a musculocutaneous flap procedure. Postoperative care includes monitoring the patient for infection and keeping pressure off the flap (Bergstrom et al., 1994; Nissen, 1997; van Rijswijk and Barr, 1995).

Chemical debridement is accomplished with enzymatic agents. Debriding enzymes are proteolytic or fibrinolytic agents that act against devitalized tissue. They are most useful on superficial wound layers because they must be in contact with the substrata of the wound. They are ineffective on dense, dry eschar. These agents should be used as an adjunct to mechanical or surgical debridement (Bergstrom et al., 1994; Nissen, 1997; van Rijswijk and Barr, 1995).

Enzymatic Agents. Enzymes are recommended in the AHCPR pressure ulcer treatment guidelines as an effective method of debriding pressure ulcers. Enzymes are useful when a patient's inflammatory response is suppressed. The manufacturer's written recommendations should be followed carefully and fully. The enzymes are designed to liquefy necrotic tissue and can be somewhat unpleasant when used. The use of enzymes should be discontinued as soon as the wound is free of necrotic tissue. These products are generally available to Medicaid beneficiaries under the prescription drug benefit but are not covered under Medicare Part B (Bergstrom et al., 1994; Nissen, 1997; van Rijswijk and Barr, 1995).

Autolytic debridement is the process by which the normal enzymes contained in the wound exudate are retained in the wound. The collected moisture and enzymes act to liquefy and rehydrate the eschar and slough. Creating a moist environment by using films, hydrocolloids, or gels has been shown to effectively remove necrotic debris in 7 to 10 days. The advantage is that only necrotic debris is removed. It is relatively inexpensive compared with other debriding modalities, and it is easy for the patient because there is less pain. The wound must be cleaned with each dressing change. Daily dressing changes are usually required when the wound undergoes autolytic debridement because the liquefied debris should be irrigated from the wound. The daily use of hydrogel covered with transparent film is recommended for yellow, stringy slough (Bergstrom et al., 1994; Nissen, 1997; van Rijswijk and Barr, 1995).

Important Considerations. All hardened or dry eschar should be removed or cross-hatched so the enzyme can come in contact with the wound. The use of antibacterials and antiseptics (povidone-iodine, hexachlorophene, silver nitrate, hydrogen peroxide, benzalkonium chloride) is discouraged because they may inhibit the action of some enzymes. Because some preparations become inactive in 24 hours, they must be freshly reconstituted so that each use is optimally effective. They may also require refrigeration. Enzymatic sprays are easy-to-use, economical products for home use or on superficial wounds (Doughty, 1994; Krasner et al., 1993; Melchor-MacDougal and Lander, 1995; Nissen, 1997; van Rijswijk and Barr, 1995).

When necessary, silver nitrate can be used to debride rolled wound edges. Wounds with rolled edges are slow to heal (Nissen, 1997).

Pressure Ulcer Treatment: Commonly Used Dressings and Topical Agents

There are at least 3000 products on the market for wound care. The care products used for long-term care residents are often based on corporate decisions having nothing to do with the individual but everything to do with cost savings through contracts (Krasner et al., 1993; Melchor-MacDougal and Lander, 1995; Nissen, 1997; van Rijswijk and Barr, 1995).

Remember that no single product meets all needs and situations; the location of the wound influences the type of dressing chosen, and dressing choices may change from week to week (Krasner et al., 1993; Nissen, 1997; van Rijswijk and Barr, 1995).

The goal is a wound that is neither too dry nor too wet. The choice of dressing should meet this goal. When wounds are moist, there is less pain, faster healing, a cleaner appearance, and the dressing changes are faster (Krasner et al., 1993; Nissen, 1997; van Rijswijk and Barr, 1995).

The recommendations from AHCPR are that the best choice of a wound dressing is one that will keep the wound bed moist and the periwound skin dry. There is a rule of thumb regarding dressing a wound: If it is wet, absorb it; if it is dry, moisten it (Bergstrom et al., 1994; Krasner et al., 1993; Nissen, 1997; van Rijswijk and Barr, 1995).

Traditional gauze dressings are still in use for chronic wound care. Although the cost may be less, they are more time consuming in many instances, and the frequent dressing changes cause the patient additional pain and discomfort. In contrast, modern dressings can often be changed every 2 to 3 days vs. two or three times each day for gauze. Moist dressings cost more per piece than gauze, but less personnel time is involved because the dressing is not changed as frequently (Krasner et al., 1993; Nissen, 1997; van Rijswijk & Barr, 1995).

Dressing choices are films, hydrocolloids, gels and gel sheets, foams, alginates, and exudate absorbers. Films, hydrocolloids, and gels and gel sheets are excellent for autolytic debridement. Foams, alginates, and exudate absorbers are excellent for exudate management (Krasner et al., 1993; Melchor-MacDougal and Lander, 1995; Nissen, 1997; Tallon, 1995; van Rijswijk and Barr, 1995).

Films. Liquid barrier film dressings contain plasticity agents that provide a protective waterproof coating over affected areas to reduce maceration and shearing. Application is by spray, wipes, or a roll-on method. These dressings are generally nonirritating and not affected by urine, perspiration, or digestive acids. Although insoluble in water, they can be dissolved by a soap solution (Krasner et al., 1993; Nissen, 1997; van Rijswijk and Barr, 1995).

Transparent vapor-permeable dressings are made from polyurethane that is permeable to oxygen and moisture vapor but not to fluids. These dressings allow oxygen to reach the healing tissues while preventing the entrance of fluids that would contaminate the wound. The dressing stays in place for 3 to 5 days, creates a moist environment that keeps the wound exudate against the wound surface, and promotes migration of epithelial cells across the wound. The exudate that collects under the dressing varies in color and consistency from thin, clear, and serous to thick, cloudy, and brown. This range is considered normal, and the exudate should not be drained. The dressing may need to be changed if the exudate leaks from its edges. If a wound infection is suspected, the dressing should be changed daily. As the amount of exudate decreases, the wound becomes darker and begins to dry. When healing is complete, the dressing may be removed or left on to protect the new skin by reducing shearing, friction, and maceration (Krasner et al., 1993; Nissen, 1997; van Rijswijk and Barr, 1995).

Important Considerations. The wound should be cleaned, and the surrounding skin must be completely dry for the dressing to adhere. This dressing should cover at least a 1-inch margin around the wound and should not be tightly stretched over the wound, which causes shearing forces against the tissues. Dressings may be cut or overlapped without reducing their effectiveness (Krasner et al., 1993; Nissen, 1997; van Rijswijk and Barr, 1995).

Films cannot absorb wound exudate and cause a collection of fluid under the dressing if used to dress a draining wound. *They are not considered a good choice for draining a wound.* If excessive exudate threatens to loosen and pull the dressing off the drainage, the exudate may be aspirated through the dressing with a small-bore needle. The dressing may seal itself or may need to be patched with another piece of dressing. A film is an excellent dressing for wounds in the later stages of healing when there is little drainage because it will not stick to moist wound tissue. It is now widely used as a secondary dressing for gauze, alginates, and gels (Krasner et al., 1993; Nissen, 1997; van Rijswijk and Barr, 1995).

Films are also used as protective dressings over skin that is at risk for breakdown. These are removed with care with the lateral pull technique: Support the dressing with one hand while pulling the edges laterally away from the center and parallel to the skin surface with the other hand, thus removing it slowly from the sides (Krasner et al., 1993; Nissen, 1997; van Rijswijk and Barr, 1995).

Hydrocolloids. Hydrocolloids are the most popular group of moist wound-healing dressings. Like films, they are also waterproof and bacteria-proof, but they have the advantage of being able to absorb moderate amounts of wound exudate. Hydrocolloids are easy to apply and are very versatile (Krasner et al., 1993; Nissen, 1997; van Rijswijk and Barr, 1995).

Opaque hydrocolloid occlusive barriers are occlusive dressings made of inert hydrophobic polymers containing fluid-absorbent hydrocolloid particles. When these particles come in contact with the wound exudate, they swell to form a moist gel that promotes debridement, granulation, and cell migration. The product works on the principle that optimal wound healing occurs in a closed, moist environment. The lack of atmospheric oxygen is not thought to prevent healing when the wound is superficial (Krasner et al., 1993; Nissen, 1997; van Rijswijk and Barr, 1995).

Important Considerations. Hydrocolloids can be used on most wound types but are best on a light to moderately exuding wound. This dressing is only really good with small to moderate amounts of exudate. It is a good idea to warm the dressing in your hands before putting it on because it adheres better if warmed. It is also a good idea to tape it in place as if placing it in a picture frame (Krasner et al., 1993; Nissen, 1997; van Rijswijk and Barr, 1995).

The wound and surrounding skin should be cleaned before to application. The surrounding skin should be completely dry so the dressing can adhere. This dressing should completely cover the wound and extend at least 1 to 2 inches beyond the wound edges. Care must be taken because it is easy to get macerated skin around the wound with this type of dressing. The dressing may be left in place up to 7 days unless leakage of exudate necessitates a change. If the wound becomes infected, the dressing must be changed more frequently. *This dressing is not recommended for wounds that show clinical signs of infection;* an infected wound must be looked at daily (Krasner et al., 1993; Nissen, 1997; van Rijswijk and Barr, 1995).

Hydrocolloids are almost totally occlusive. When this dressing is removed from the wound, there is some gelled residue to clean up, and the odor is often unpleasant (Krasner et al., 1993; Nissen, 1997; van Rijswijk and Barr, 1995).

Gels and Gel Sheets. Gels are absorption dressings that use hydrophilic beads, grains, or flakes designed to absorb excess wound exudate and necrotic debris that may inhibit tissue regeneration. At the same time, they keep the wound moist enough to encourage healing, and they hydrate eschar and necrotic tissue. Wound gels high in water content can donate water from the gel to desiccated eschar and slough and thus help to liquefy necrotic tissue. These dressings also deodorize the wound (Krasner et al., 1993; Nissen, 1997; van Rijswijk and Barr, 1995).

Gels and gel sheets are amorphous hydrogels and create a hydrophilic environment over the wound. The gel sheets are transparent and conformable, similar to a soft contact lens. They are soothing when initially applied because of the cool nature of the dressing. The gel can absorb a small amount of exudate and permit evaporation from the upper surface of the gel. In this way, the gels wick watery exudate from the wound surface through the hydrophilic gel. The moisture is then allowed to evaporate without drying the wound surface. However, gels can also run out of the wound and allow it to dry out if exposed (Krasner et al., 1993; Nissen, 1997; van Rijswijk and Barr, 1995).

Important Considerations. These types of dressings usually require changing once or twice a day. The products should be reconstituted according to the manufacturer's instructions and then gently packed into the wound and covered with a dry outer dressing (Krasner et al., 1993; Nissen, 1997; van Rijswijk and Barr, 1995).

Hydrogel sheets are best for dressing lightly to moderately draining wounds because the gel sheets do not absorb a large amount of drainage. Gels require a secondary dressing, and gauze and nonwoven tape are the best combinations for such a dressing. The gel sheet may be cut to the shape of the wound, which assists in returning moisture to dry wounds. However, there is a tendency for fluid to collect under the gel sheets, which leads to maceration (Krasner et al., 1993; Nissen, 1997; van Rijswijk and Barr, 1995).

Foams. Foams are made from polyurethane and are ideal for more heavily draining wounds. Some are now available in easy-to-apply adhesive versions, which make the foam more versatile. Foams do not leave any dressing residue in the wound and generally provide clean, moist healing environments (Krasner et al., 1993; Nissen, 1997; van Rijswijk and Barr, 1995).

Important Considerations. Foams are best used for moderately to heavily draining wounds and for those with friable skin surrounding the wound. The nonadhesive foams do not damage this fragile periwound skin. A roller bandage such as Kerlex is a good covering for these dressings (Krasner et al., 1993; Nissen, 1997; van Rijswijk and Barr, 1995).

Alginates. Alginates are nonwoven absorbent dressings derived from seaweed. They are placed into the wound dry, absorb exudate, and form a gel over the wound, thus maintaining a moist healing environment. The gel is hydrophilic and permits evaporation of excess exudate. This combination of absorption and evaporation allows alginates to handle more exudate than absorption alone. *A wound with little exudate is not a good candidate for alginate dressing* because alginates desiccate wounds with a low volume of exudate, and the dressing then tends to stick to the dried wound edges. Medicare Part B has covered these products in the past, but with new regulations it is wise to check with the fiscal intermediary regarding coverage (Krasner et al., 1993; Nissen, 1997; van Rijswijk and Barr, 1995).

Important Considerations. Alginates are not good for wounds with sinus tracts or undermining and tunneling because they are difficult to remove. They should not be used on a dry wound (Krasner et al., 1993; Nissen, 1997; van Rijswijk and Barr, 1995).

An alginate goes in dry and comes out like mucus. It should not be wet before use. The dressing should be dated, and the time applied should be included on the dressing. There can be copious drainage through the alginate. It must be monitored regularly or the drainage may soil clothing and bedding. All alginates require secondary dressings. Secondary dressings should be highly permeable to moisture vapor so that the evaporation of exudate from the top surface of the gelled alginate is not inhibited. Gauze, nonwoven tapes, and highly moisture vapor–permeable film dressings are excellent for covering alginates. When the drainage lessens, it is time to change to another product (Krasner et al., 1993; Nissen, 1997; van Rijswijk and Barr, 1995).

Exudate Absorbers. Exudate absorbers are copolymer starch dressings that maintain a moist environment while absorbing exudate from the wound. They are messy to apply but easily removed from the wound by irrigation. All exudate absorbers require a secondary dressing to keep them in place. *The copolymer starches are best used in heavily draining, cavity-type wounds* (Krasner et al., 1993; Nissen, 1997; van Rijswijk and Barr, 1995).

Important Considerations. It is wise to use a skin preparation before applying an adhesive for the secondary dressing. This practice allows the removal of the dressing but leaves the first level of the skin intact. Do not fill the wound to the top because the dressing swells a great deal (Krasner et al., 1993; Nissen, 1997; van Rijswijk and Barr, 1995).

Cost consideration is an essential component in planning the management of pressure ulcers. The stage of the ulcer determines the need for more aggressive and thus more expensive treatment. Costly specialty beds, such as the Mediscus and Clinitron, are reserved for extreme cases such as multiple stage III or stage IV nonhealing ulcers.

Nutritional Considerations

It is important to maximize nutritional and hydration status by maximizing protein and fluid intake. A prescription of 500 mg of vitamin C and 220 mg of zinc sulfate daily has been widely recognized as effective in promoting wound healing.

Pain

For many years it was thought that pressure ulcers did not cause pain, but this belief has been disproved. In their study of pressure ulcer pain, Dallam et al. (1995) concluded that most patients with pressure ulcers experience pain and that most patients never receive analgesia. Many patients studied were unable to respond; therefore clinicians failed to consider whether these wounds were painful.

According to Krasner (1996), chronic wound pain is a complex subjective phenomenon of extreme discomfort experienced by a person in response to skin or tissue injury. Pain assessment for pressure ulcers should be no different. The clinician should question the patient about the quality, quantity, onset, duration, and type of pain. If a patient is unable to respond, the clinician should look for nonverbal signs and symptoms of pain, including restlessness, grimacing, and agitation. When pain is assessed, the wound is treated with analgesics. The clinician should ensure that the analgesic has been given before changing the dressing. As with any chronic pain, an around-the-clock pain control regimen should be considered.

Summary

The importance of a true team approach to the care of a patient with a pressure ulcer cannot be stressed enough. Education of all staff and family, especially if they are caregivers, is essential to providing even minimal effective care. Consultation with knowledgeable clinicians in nutrition and physical and occupational therapy, plus the involvement of all paraprofessional staff, is critical. It is a challenge to prevent tissue damage to the debilitated patient for whom adequate nutrition and hydration are no longer possible. In spite of the difficulty, these patients deserve no less than the best effort to heal the ulcer and provide quality of life that is pain-free. For all other patients, pressure ulcers are preventable with proper assessment and care.

Resources

Wound Care Community Network
http://www.woundcarenet.com

Tissue Viability Society
http://www.tvs.org.uk

References

Bergstrom N et al: *Treatment of pressure ulcers,* Clinical practice guideline 15, Agency for Health Care Policy and Research, Pub No 95-0652, Rockville, Md, 1994, US Department of Health and Human Services, Public Health Service.

Cooney Jr LM: Pressure sores and urinary incontinence, *J Am Geriatr Soc* 45(10):1278-1279, 1997.

Dallam L et al: Pressure ulcer pain: assessment and quantification, *J Wound Ostomy Continence Nurs* 22(5):211-215, 1995.

Doughty D: A rational approach to the use of topical antiseptics, *J Wound Ostomy Continence Nurs* 21(6):224-231, 1994.

Haas AF: Wound healing, *Dermatol Nurs* 7(1):28-34, 1995.

Henderson CT et al: Draft definition of stage I pressure ulcers: inclusion of persons with darkly pigmented skin, *Adv Wound Care* 10(5):16-19, 1997.

Jahnigen D: Pressure ulcers. In Yoshikawa TT, Cobbs EL, Brummel-Smith K: *Ambulatory geriatric care,* St Louis, 1993, Mosby.

Krasner D: Using a gentler hand: reflections of patients with pressure ulcers who experience pain, *Ostomy Wound Manage* 42:20-29, 1996.

Krasner D et al: The ABCs of wound care dressings, *Ostomy Wound Manage* 39(8):66-86, 1993.

Maklebust J: Policy implications of using reverse staging to monitor pressure ulcer status, *Adv Wound Care* 10(5):32-35, 1997.

Melchor-MacDougal F, Lander J: Evaluation of a decision tree for management of chronic wounds, *J Wound Ostomy Continence Nurs* 22(2):81-87, 1995.

National Pressure Ulcer Advisory Panel Consensus Development Conference: Position on reverse staging of pressure ulcers, *Adv Wound Care* 8(6):32-33, 1995.

Nissen C: *Options for wound and skin care management* (seminar workbook), Largo, Fla, 1997, Smith & Nephew.

Panel for the Prediction and Prevention of Pressure Ulcers in Adults: *Pressure ulcers in adults: prediction and prevention* (Clinical practice guideline 3, Agency for Health Care Policy and Research, Pub No 92-0047), Rockville, Md, 1992, US Department of Health and Human Services, Public Health Service.

Peiper B, Sugrue M: Risk factors, prevention methods and wound care for patients with pressure ulcers, *Clin Nurse Spec* 12(1):7-12, 1998.

Plassmann P: Measuring wounds, *J Wound Care* 4(6):262-269, 1995.

Regan MB: Efficacy of a comprehensive pressure ulcer prevention program in an extended care facility, *Adv Wound Care* 8(3):49-55, 1995.

Salcido R: Will all pressure ulcers heal? *Adv Wound Care* 10(5):28-30, 1997.

Saunders SL, Grezesek KA: Meeting the challenge of pressure ulcers: promoting prevention and appropriate management, *Adv Nurse Pract* 4(12):23-29, 1996.

Seidel HM et al: *Mosby's guide to physical examination,* ed 3, St Louis, 1995, Mosby.

Tallon R: Critical paths for wound care, *Adv Wound Care* 8(1):26-34, 1995.

van Rijswijk L, Barr JE: *The principles of wound cleaning* (training module), Charleston, SC, 1995, Hill-Rom.

Wellman NS: A case manager's guide to nutrition screening and intervention, *J Care Manage* (3):12-26, 1997.

Xakellis GC, Frantz RA: Pressure ulcer healing: What is it? What influences it? How is it measured? *Adv Wound Care* 10(5):20-26, 1997.

22

Foot Problems

Foot problems in older adults are extremely common. Approximately 75% to 80% of the older population exhibits pathologic conditions of the foot (Beiser and Shuman, 1998). Diminished opportunities for walking because of social factors and health conditions, increased foot neglect, and deterioration of vascular, neurologic, skeletal, and dermatologic structures all contribute to foot problems in the elderly.

Walking is a low-impact, relatively safe form of aerobic exercise for the older adult and is essential to a person's overall health, including foot health. Walking with proper footwear tones and strengthens foot and leg muscles, maintains joint flexibility and motion, increases arterial blood flow, and helps evacuate venous blood flow (Figure 22-1). Unfortunately, many older adults become isolated, less active, and less ambulatory because of a variety of social and health conditions. Social factors that commonly affect the older person's desire to walk include a fear of falling, a loss of driving privileges, and a loss of friends and family. Health conditions such as vision deterioration, arthritic pain, chronic heart or lung disease, and foot and leg pain and weakness also limit an older person's ability to walk.

Foot neglect also contributes to problems in the older person. Visual impairment, an inability to reach the feet, unmanageable hypertrophic toenails, and transportation limitations to health care providers all contribute to foot neglect and the development of foot problems.

In addition, both natural and pathologic deterioration of vascular, neurologic, skeletal, and dermatologic structures contribute to foot problems. Peripheral vascular disease is often diagnosed in older patients and can be detrimental to ambulation capability and healing potential. Disease or neuropathy in lower extremity nerves accompanies many systemic diseases and nervous system traumas.

Neuropathic pain, weakness, and sensory loss can cause a variety of foot problems. Skeletal or orthopedic foot changes in the older patient are responsible for a great percentage of foot problems. Causes for the foot's mechanical and functional deterioration and its adaptive orthopedic changes include increased weight gain, decreased muscle strength, inadequate or ill-fitting shoes, decades of ambulation, limited exercise, and systemic diseases. Dermatologic changes such as dystrophic nails and painful corns and calluses are responsible for the majority of foot complaints in older adults.

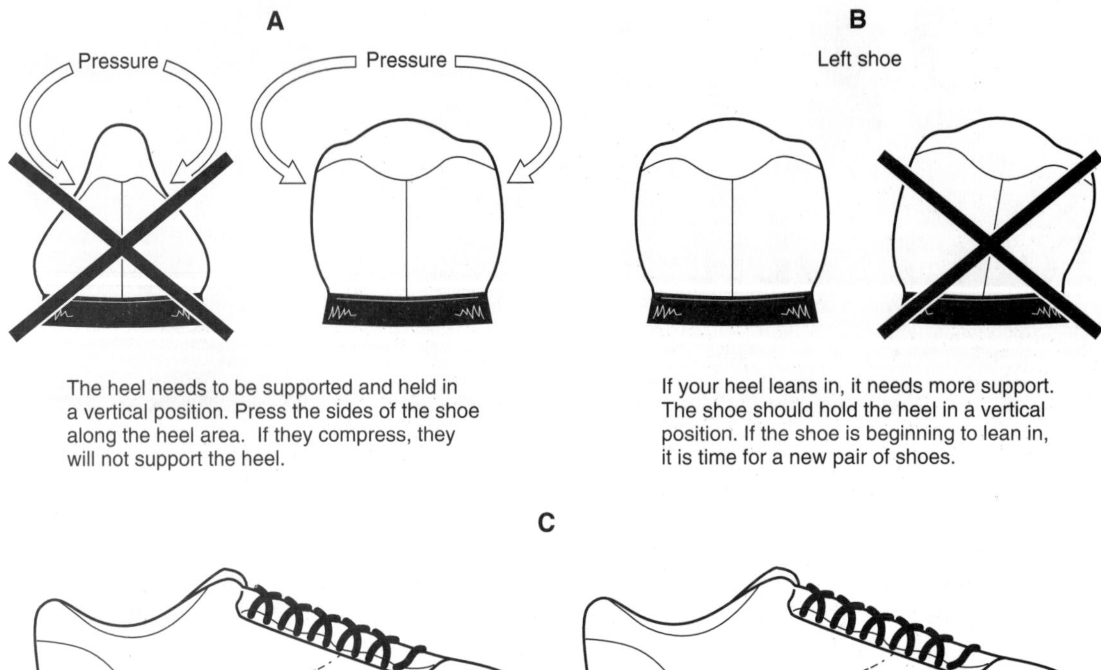

A
Pressure
Pressure
B
Left shoe
The heel needs to be supported and held in a vertical position. Press the sides of the shoe along the heel area. If they compress, they will not support the heel.
If your heel leans in, it needs more support. The shoe should hold the heel in a vertical position. If the shoe is beginning to lean in, it is time for a new pair of shoes.
C
The midsole and outer-sole (in black) play an important role in absorbing shock. Unfortunately, this part of the shoe is the heaviest. However, since the foot only bears weight on the heel and forefoot, contouring the middle and ends of this area (left picture) results in a lighter shoe without disturbing the shock absorption under the heel and forefoot. It is a positive feature.

Figure 22-1 Choosing a proper walking shoe.

Common Foot Problems and Treatments

Orthopedic, mechanically induced, and dermatologic changes are common reasons for foot complaints in the older patient. Understanding what causes these changes helps the primary care provider recognize and treat current problems and foresee as well as prevent future problems.

Maintaining a normal gait requires the foot to accomplish four major functions: (1) adapt to an uneven surface (ground topography adaptation), (2) become a rigid lever for propulsion, (3) translate rotary forces generated by the hip, and (4) absorb shock (Beiser and Shuman, 1998). Shock absorption and ground topography adaptation are achieved with foot flexibility caused by subtalar joint pronation (foot abduction and eversion). Pushing off the ground requires foot rigidity and stability, which is achieved with subtalar joint supination (foot adduction and inversion). With age, the subtalar joint

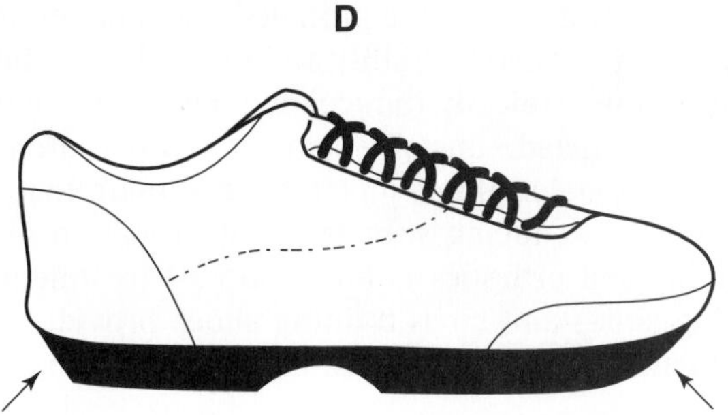

Contouring of the midsole and outer-sole on the ends of the shoe has an advantage in addition to making the shoe lighter. Look below.

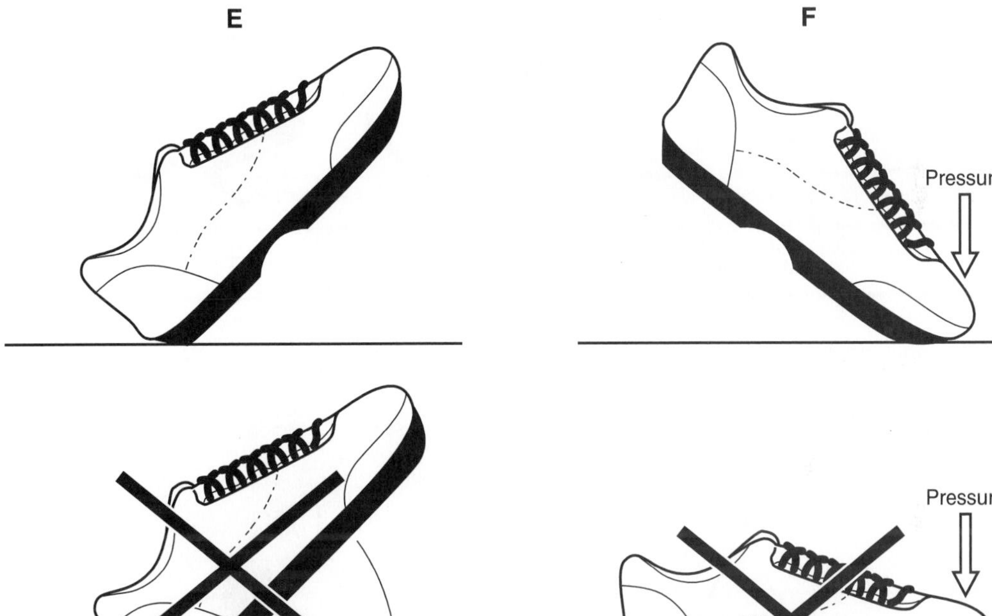

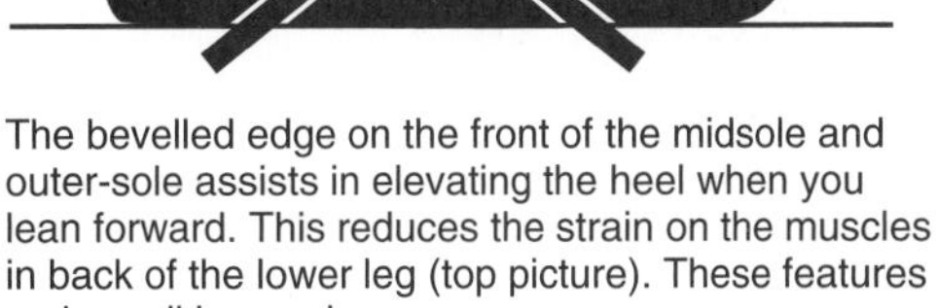

When a step is taken, the bevelled edge on the back (top picture) allows the foot to be balanced on the heel until it is ready to come down. A sharp angle (bottom picture) forces the foot down when the heel hits the ground, and this puts strain on the muscles in front of the lower leg.

The bevelled edge on the front of the midsole and outer-sole assists in elevating the heel when you lean forward. This reduces the strain on the muscles in back of the lower leg (top picture). These features make walking easier.

Figure 22-1, cont'd For legend see opposite page. *Continued*

of the foot progresses to function in the pronated position and loses supination capacity. This adaptation causes excessive flexibility and instability during foot propulsion, which can lead to significant mechanically induced foot changes and problems.

Ambulation on a pronated, unstable foot can cause arch and heel pain, bunion deformities, hammer toe deformities, metatarsalgia, neuroma pain, tendinitis, arthritis, and an apropulsive gait. Reducing subtalar joint pronation via adequate shoe gear or generic or custom-molded orthotics is an important treatment consideration for these conditions. Running shoes and cross-training shoes provide the best foot support and usually help mild to moderate cases of tendinitis, heel pain, arch pain, neuroma pain, and

G

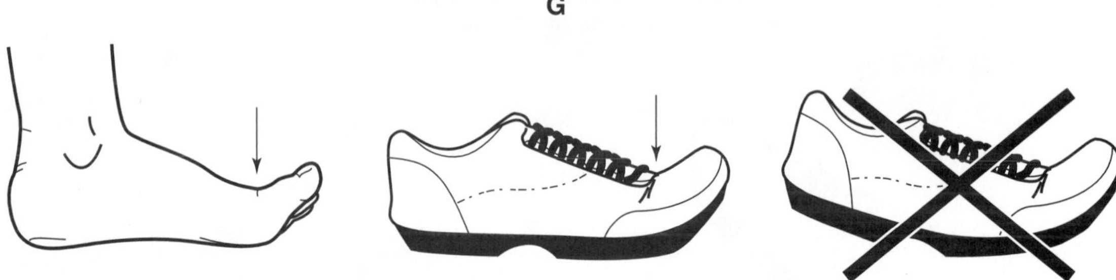

The foot only bends in one place (see arrow). Therefore the shoe should only bend in that one place. If the shoe bends in areas that the foot does not, the shoe will not support the foot well.

H

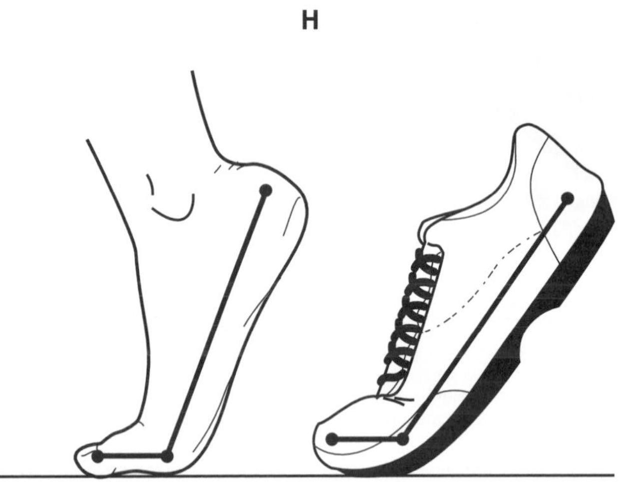

It is important that the shoe be as flexible as the foot in the area where the foot bends. If the shoe can not bend as much as the foot, the heel of your foot will pull put of the shoe when walking. This will result in excessive movement and rubbing between your heel and shoe and result in blistering, soreness, or infection.

Figure 22-1, cont'd For legend see p. 488.

metatarsalgia. Moderate to severe cases should be treated with some degree of arch support. Moderate cases can be treated with generic arch supports, which can be purchased in most pharmacies. Severely pronated feet should receive custom-molded arch supports made by a podiatrist.

Subtalar Joint Pronation

Subtle increases in subtalar joint pronation are responsible for painful conditions but may be difficult to recognize. Recognition of the signs of pronation requires both a non–weight-bearing and a weight-bearing foot examination. While not bearing weight, the patient will exhibit excessive flexibility of the subtalar joint with passive range of motion, and there will be some degree of bunion and hammertoe deformity. While bearing weight, the patient will show a noticeable arch reduction, and there will be an increase in the degree of bunion and hammertoe deformity. The foot will be in some degree of abduction, and there may be some degree of detectable rearfoot valgus. During walking, the heel may demonstrate an abductory twist as it elevates off the ground during propulsion.

The most applicable use of arch support and pronation reduction is for the treatment of heel pain and plantar fasciitis (Figure 22-2). Pronation reduction and arch elevation relaxes the plantar fascia and reduces tension at its calcaneal attachment. A combination of arch support, mild heel elevation, ice, and antiinflammatory medication in the form of oral nonsteroidal antiinflammatory drugs (NSAIDs) or injected cortisone successfully treats most heel and arch pain.

Bunion and Hammertoe Formations

Bunion and hammertoe formations are mechanically induced and are often painful (Figure 22-3). Excessive pronation and increased weight bearing on the inside of the foot cause bunions and lead to dorsiflexion, adduction, and hypermobility of the first

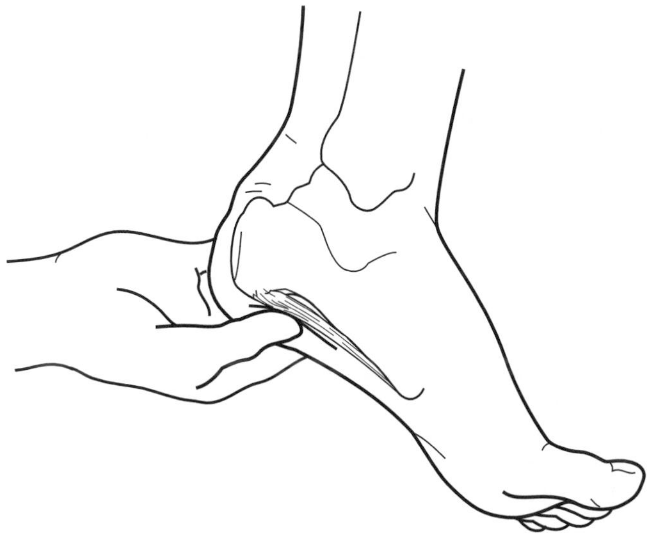

Figure 22-2 Painful plantar fasciitis with an associated heel spur. (From Holman J, Poehling C, Martin D: Common foot problems. In Hazzard WR et al, editors: *Principles of geriatric medicine and gerontology,* ed 3, New York, 1994, McGraw-Hill.)

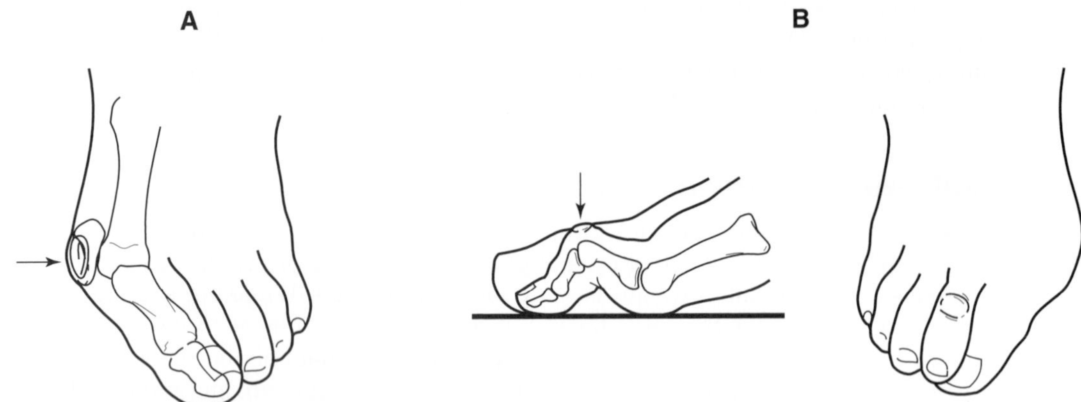

Figure 22-3 A, Bunion with painful callosity and bursitis. B, Hammering of the second toe with dorsal proximal interphalangeal callosity secondary to bunion. (From Holman J, Poehling C, Martin D: Common foot problems. In Hazzard WR et al, editors: *Principles of geriatric medicine and gerontology,* ed 3, New York, 1994, McGraw-Hill.)

metatarsal. The hallux abducts as the first metatarsal adducts, and the joint becomes malaligned. Bunion pain presents as either "bump" pain or joint pain. A distinction between these two types of pain is important. "Bump" pain is superficial pain or irritation caused by shoe pressure; it is treated with shoe modification or padding to reduce local pressure. Joint pain is associated with inflammation within the first metatarsal-phalangeal joint; this inflammation is created by the malalignment. Joint pain is improved with pronation reduction and antiinflammatory medication.

Hammertoe formation is generally the product of high-heeled shoes. Toes assist in balance. When a person leans back, the toes elevate. When a person leans forward, the toes grip the ground. When a person stands erect, the toes should be relaxed. High-heeled shoes push weight forward onto the forefoot, and as a result the toes grip the ground in hammertoe formation, which involves hyperextension of the metatarsal-phalangeal joint (MPJ), hyperflexion of the proximal interphalangeal joint (PIPJ), and hyperextension of the distal interphalangeal joint (DIPJ). Hammertoes can create joint inflammation at the hyperextended MPJ and shoe pressure irritation at the dorsally prominent PIPJ.

Treatment of hammertoe formation is based on the degree of rigidity. Flexible hammertoes will reduce and realign with significant heel reduction and adequate arch support. Rigid hammertoe treatment depends on the location of the pain. Dorsal shoe irritation can be accommodated by extra-depth shoes that have a higher toe box. Inflamed, hyperextended metatarsal-phalangeal joints require antiinflammatory medication and adequate arch support.

Severely hyperextended MPJs cause plantar-flexed and plantarly prominent metatarsal bones. This condition, in association with fat-pad atrophy of the plantar forefoot, causes a painful condition that the patient describes as a feeling of "walking on my bones." Treatment for this painful, chronic condition involves application of a cushioned pad beneath the metatarsal heads and proximal to the metatarsal heads so that pressure is redistributed to the metatarsal necks and away from the prominent metatarsal heads.

Dermatologic Changes

An examination of the dermatologic status of the older person's foot provides information about the foot's circulation, function, and shoe fit. Corns and calluses are areas of thickened epidermis caused by intermittent pressure on a broad area (callus) or focal area (corn). Pressure pushes the local circulation away from the skin, causing blanching and pallor. A rebound hyperemic response occurs when pressure is removed. Over time this repetitious, intermittent, hyperemic response causes epidermal thickening.

A thickened epidermis can cause two potential problems. As the epidermis thickens, it loses softness and flexibility. As a result, it can crack, causing a painful fissure and a potential infection risk. Focal epidermal thickening (e.g., a corn) causes focal, painful pressure to the underlying tissue. Advanced corns can cause subepidermal bleeding or ulceration.

Because rebound hyperemia in response to ischemic pressure is responsible for thickening of the skin, well-formed corns and calluses suggest the presence of good skin circulation. A poorly formed callus or the absence of a callus on a pressure area is a sign of limited skin circulation because an adequate hyperemic response to pressure does not occur. This explains why patients with poor arterial circulation cannot tolerate firm, supportive shoes. The pressure from a shoe holding the foot in a mechanically proper position causes ischemic pain, and therefore these patients need soft, accommodating shoes.

The treatment of painful corns and calluses requires debridement and pressure removal. Debridement can be accomplished by mechanical or chemical means. Mechanical debridement by a skilled health care provider should be performed with a sharp blade or scalpel. Patients can perform routine mechanical debridement with a pumice stone. Chemical debridement can be accomplished with over-the-counter corn remover pads that contain salicylic acid. The primary care provider should monitor this treatment, and it should not be used on patients with diabetes or peripheral vascular disease. Pressure removal can be accomplished by shoe modification, padding, or surgical intervention.

Nail Problems

Nail problems account for most foot problems in older adults. With age, the toenails undergo predictable changes to varying degrees—they thicken, incurvate, and become more susceptible to nail fungus. Various digital deformities cause added shoe, floor, and adjacent toe pressures that further deform the nails and cause them to become dystrophic and difficult to manage. Often people either injure their feet by attempting to cut their nails with scissors or wirecutters or neglect their nails until they cause a problem. Common nail problems include painful hypertrophic nails, mycotic nails, periungual calluses, and ingrowing nails.

Onychomycosis. Onychomycosis, or nail fungus, is often encountered in older patients. Fungus thrives in a dark, warm, wet environment. Shoes cause darkness; socks keep feet warm; and foot perspiration, foot soaks, showers, baths, and closely positioned toes all contribute to chronic foot moisture. These factors create a favorable environment for fungal growth. Peripheral vascular disease and age-related, slowed nail growth maintain nail tissue on the toes for a longer time, increasing the chances of infection.

Onychomycosis has four common presentations: superficial white, distal subungual, proximal, and candidal (Beiser and Shuman, 1998). It causes nail discoloration, hypertrophy, and dystrophy, which often results in painful conditions. The extent of treatment for onychomycosis depends on a person's symptoms, degree of pedal circulation, and overall health. Treatment options include routine nail debridement, temporary or permanent nail removal, topically applied antifungal medication, oral antifungal medication, or a combination of these options. Routine nail debridement is the sole treatment for patients with extensive peripheral vascular disease and multiple medical problems. Permanent nail removal is used for patients who have an isolated chronic problematic nail and who have the circulation to heal a matrixectomy. Temporary nail removal is used for patients who have chronic or acute problematic nails and lack the circulation to heal a matrixectomy. Topical antifungal medications are effective for superficial nail fungal infections such as white superficial onychomycosis.

Oral antifungal therapy, which is used for more extensive mycotic nails, is becoming commonplace because of the introduction of newer and safer oral antifungal medications. However, oral treatment for older patients should be reserved for painful nail conditions—not for cosmetic reasons. It should also be reserved for healthy patients with no history of liver disease. Mild to moderately infected toenails require 3 months of therapy, whereas severely infected toenails often need 5 to 6 months of therapy. Temporary nail removal should be combined with oral antifungal therapy for the most infected nails. With oral therapy, the proximal aspect of the nail grows in thin and clear, compared with the distal, hypertrophic, infected, fungal nail tissue. Occasionally the fungal infection can spread from a distally infected nail to an uninfected proximal nail while the patient is undergoing oral therapy. Removing severely infected nails before initiating oral therapy eliminates this problem.

Ingrown Nails. Ingrown nails are a problem for both younger and older populations (Figure 22-4). Ingrown nails occur when the nail groove skin is pushed into the way of the normal growing nail because of confining shoes or when the nail plate is deformed and grows errantly into the skin. In general, older patients suffer from the second scenario. Incurvated, mycotic, dystrophic nails are usually the cause of the ingrown nail. Incurvated, dystrophic, ingrown nails may or may not puncture the skin. Chronic nail pressure often creates significant callus buildup in the nail groove, which causes pain and the feeling of an ingrown nail. Patients may relate gaining some relief from soaking their feet because the macerated callus softens and produces less pressure. Debridement of the

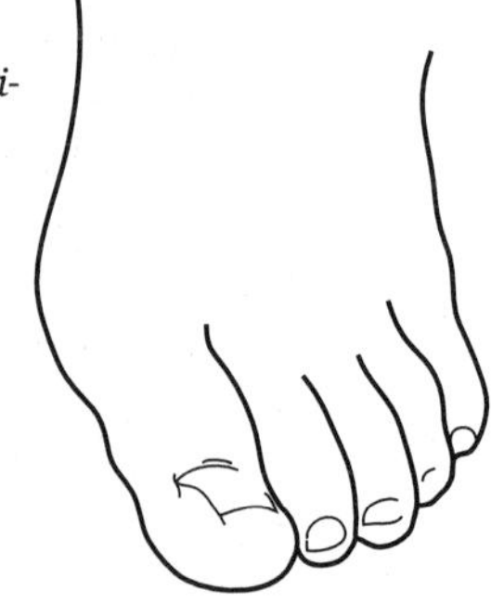

Figure 22-4 Great toe ingrown toenail. (From Holman J, Poehling C, Martin D: Common foot problems. In Hazzard WR et al, editors: *Principles of geriatric medicine and gerontology,* ed 3, New York, 1994, McGraw-Hill.)

nail groove callus and the offending nail edge brings instant relief. Excision of an ingrown nail should be referred to a podiatrist or a health care provider with expertise, training, and experience in the procedure.

Diabetes and the Foot

A significant percentage of patients over the age of 55 have diabetes. Diabetes is responsible for the majority of nontraumatic lower extremity amputations, a feared complication of diabetes that in many cases is preventable. Prevention begins with a careful foot assessment and patient education.

Assessment

Assessment of the foot of a patient with diabetes involves evaluation of the foot's circulation, bony prominences, corn and callus formation, skin condition, nail dystrophy, shoe gear fit, and sensation loss. Any abnormal finding or combination of abnormal findings can cause a skin break and infection risk. Diminished circulation can cause skin atrophy, breakdown, and ulceration. A bony prominence from a bunion or hammertoe can cause shoe irritation and blister formation. Thick calluses can crack, and thick corns can create subepidermal ulcers. Chronic wet or dry skin can result in skin cracks. Dry skin can develop a fissure, whereas wet skin can promote a fungal infection that can cause blistering or fissuring. Dystrophic nails can cause infected, ingrown nails. Poorly fitting footwear can create dangerous pressure sores.

The loss of sensation can result in delayed detection and the escalation of any of these problems. For example, severe circulation impairment, which typically causes extreme ischemic pain, goes unnoticed in the presence of significant numbness. The first sign of poor circulation to a diabetic patient with numbness may be gangrene and subsequent amputation. Sensation loss should be evaluated and classified as superficial pressure sensation loss, deep pressure sensation loss, or bone sensation loss by using a 10-g Semmes-Weinstein monofilament, a 75-g Semmes-Weinstein monofilament, and a tuning fork, respectively.

Prevention

Preventive treatment addresses any abnormal findings. Diminished circulation needs to be carefully monitored. Corns, calluses, and dystrophic nails should be regularly debrided by a podiatrist. The patient needs to wear footwear that provides support and accommodates bony prominences. Excessively wet or dry skin should be treated. Dry skin is best treated with 20% urea or 10% to 12% lactic acid cream or lotion. Excessive skin moisture, often found between the toes, can be "acutely" treated with povidone-iodine (Betadine) solution, a drying agent that reduces the risk of bacterial infection. It should be used for only a short period and for an acute episode. Chronic treatment includes interdigital powder, topical antifungal medication, and toe spacers.

Knowing the depth of sensation loss helps the primary care provider make treatment decisions and educate patients about their condition. Loss of superficial pressure sensation predisposes the patient to unrecognized shoe irritation and superficial skin ulceration. This degree of sensory loss also prevents recognition of the "itch" sensation caused by a developing fungal infection. Corns and calluses may thicken to a dangerous level, and skin cracks go unnoticed. Patients should be educated to wear less stylish shoes and pay daily attention to the skin condition of their feet.

A loss of deep pressure sensation puts the patient at risk for not noticing objects in their shoes, ingrown nails, deeper ulcers, and excessive hot or cold temperatures. This degree of numbness warrants special footwear. For nondystrophic feet, an orthopedic shoe with a Plastizote lining is indicated; a custom-molded shoe with a Plastizote lining is indicated for dystrophic feet. Patients should be told to check inside their shoes and socks before putting them on, avoid going barefooted, inspect their feet daily, and have their toenails treated by a podiatrist.

With a loss of bone sensation, the patient can develop an undetected ulceration down to the bone, causing osteomyelitis. The patient is also at risk for developing a Charcot joint that can create a limb-threatening skeletal breakdown of the foot. This condition occurs in the presence of profound numbness and excessive pedal blood flow and is initiated by undetected chronic microtrauma or acute foot or ankle macrotrauma. In either case, the uneducated patient feels no pain and will probably continue to ambulate on the injured foot until a joint in the foot literally dislocates. Prevention of chronic microtrauma requires prescription footwear and firm arch support. Prevention of a Charcot joint after acute trauma requires immediate immobilization and no weight bearing, as well as appropriate diagnostic imaging studies to determine the extent of injury. The patient should be instructed to look daily for signs of discoloration, warmth, and swelling in the feet, using a mirror if necessary, and to seek medical attention for these changes.

The keys to preventing diabetic amputations in patients with diabetes are understanding, recognition, and treatment of the multiple amputation risks by the provider, as well as daily foot inspections by the informed patient, spouse, or friend.

Summary

Foot problems in older adults are common; these problems develop for several reasons, and the appropriate footwear and treatments are important. An understanding of how common problems develop gives the provider foresight, which increases clinical acumen and enables the practice of preventive health care. For example, understanding that a diabetic foot callus is prone to crack compels the primary care provider to treat the callus instead of treating the forthcoming fissure or foot infection. Knowing that a patient with diabetes has superficial pressure loss around the toes and cannot feel an "itch" persuades the provider to look between the patient's toes for fungal infections. A patient who presents with an area of chronic shoe pressure and pain and has no corn or callus formation should be evaluated for peripheral vascular disease. If a patient presents with developing bunions and hammertoes, the patient should be evaluated for excessive foot pronation, and arch support should be considered.

With the exception of routine nail debridement, preventive foot care practices are rare. The immense number of mechanically induced foot problems in older adults justifies the use of custom-molded orthotics more frequently and sooner. The excessive number of amputations among the diabetic population demands more aggressive implementation of preventive treatment. Preventive foot care practices will keep older adults on their feet longer and, as a result, they will be healthier.

Resources

Foot and Ankle Link Library
http://www.footandankle.com/podmed

Foot Care 4 U
http://www.footcare4u.com

Reference

Beiser IH, Shuman CJ: Foot care. In Yoshikawa TT, Cobbs EL, Brummel-Smith K, editors: *Practical ambulatory geriatrics,* ed 2, St Louis, 1998, Mosby.

23

Falls

Prevalent, dangerous, and often difficult to predict, falls are a major cause of death and a significant source of morbidity for people over age 65. In the United States, accidents represent the sixth leading cause of death in this age-group, with falls being a major component of this category. Falls also produce annual medical costs that are estimated to be $3.7 billion (Herndon et al., 1997). Multiple falls are associated with an increased risk of death (Dunn et al., 1992). Seventy percent of all fall-related deaths occur in the over-75 age-group. Even if falls have not occurred or have not resulted in injury, the fear of falling is a serious detriment to the functioning of the older person and may severely reduce quality of life.

Falls occur in all settings—home, hospital, and long-term care facility. Up to one third of community-dwelling older Americans suffer from falls, often without explanation (Weiner et al., 1998). Of the estimated 1.7 million nursing home residents in the United States, approximately half fall each year—twice the rate for people dwelling in the community—and 11% sustain a serious fall-related injury (Ray et al., 1997).

Age-related Risk Factors

The causes of falls in the elderly are multifactorial, and there are many contributing factors—both intrinsic and extrinsic. Intrinsic factors include any problems that affect the person's functional status (e.g., strength and conditioning, mobility, and sensory impairments). Chronic medical problems such as Parkinson's disease, stroke, arthritis, and anemia are associated with a higher risk of falls. Extrinsic factors include the effects of medications, which have been studied extensively; although not all findings are identical, there is general agreement regarding an increased fall risk for patients who are taking psychotropic medications, antidepressants, diuretics, and laxatives. Environmental causes may include floor surfaces, clutter, lighting, accessibility of objects, bathroom equipment, and appropriateness and integrity of assistive devices. Box 23-1 lists the identified risk factors for falls in all settings (Yoshikawa, 1998).

Box 23-1
Risk Factors for Falls

Intrinsic

Advanced age
Female sex
Caucasian race
Chronic medical conditions
Neuromuscular dysfunction
Cognitive impairment
ADL dependence
Impaired vision and hearing

Extrinsic

Medications
Environmental hazards
Improper assistive devices
Gait and balance disorders

Source: Herndon JG et al: Chronic medical conditions and risk of fall injury events at home in older adults; *J Am Geriatr Soc* 45:739-743, 1997; and Ray WA et al: A randomized trial of a consultation service to reduce falls in nursing homes, *JAMA* 278(7):557-562, 1997.

Assessment

History

If a fall has occurred, the details of events surrounding the fall should be ascertained as much as possible. Questions to be asked include the following:

- What was the patient doing when he or she fell?
- Was there an aura (suggesting seizure)?
- Was there a loss of vision (suggesting syncope)?
- Did the patient experience any dizziness (sensation of movement)?
- Was there a loss of consciousness?
- In what direction did the patient fall (e.g., forward or backward)?
- Did the patient break the fall (suggests alertness vs. syncope)?
- Was he or she using any prescribed assistive devices appropriately?
- Did witnesses notice any seizure activity?

It is important to determine if falls are recurrent or if they have recently increased, which might suggest a more acute underlying cause, such as an infection. A thorough history should be obtained regarding any history of falls, medical problems, medications (including any recent changes), and the use of alcohol or medications for pain. It is also important to ask about the patient's fear of falling, even if there have been no previous falls. Patients often do not volunteer information about previous falls, and this history might be obtained only if the practitioner asks the question. This history is especially important when assessing a patient who is frail or has impaired balance or mobility. Table 23-1 outlines the possible differential diagnoses for various findings.

TABLE 23-1 Possible Differential Diagnoses Based on Findings

Historical Factors and Symptoms	Possible Differential Diagnoses
Historical Factors	
Change in position	Orthostatic hypotension
"Trip or slip"	Gait instability Balance problems Visual disturbance Environmental hazard
"Drop attack" with loss of consciousness	Vertebrobasilar insufficiency
Looking up or sideways	Arterial or carotid sinus compression
Loss of consciousness	Syncope or seizure
Symptoms Near Time of Fall	
Dizziness or giddiness	Orthostatic hypotension Vestibular problems Hypoglycemia Arrhythmia Drug side effect
Palpitation	Arrhythmia
Incontinence	Seizure
Tongue biting	Seizure
Asymmetric weakness	Cerebrovascular disease
Chest pain	Myocardial infarction Coronary insufficiency
Loss of consciousness	Any cause of syncope

It is very important to assess the patient's environment. Whether the patient is at home or in a health care facility, assessment of the surroundings for risk factors such as clutter, poor lighting, and throw rugs can prove critical in preventing falls. If the provider is not able to make a visit to the home, a visiting nurse or social worker can perform the assessment. If none of these options is feasible, the patient, a family member, or a caregiver can perform the assessment with a tool such as the Home Safety Checklist, developed by the National Safety Council (1982) (Fig. 23-1). The patient can bring this information to the next appointment for review and discussion, and the practitioner can make recommendations based on the findings.

Physical Examination

The physical examination should be comprehensive, with a special focus placed on the following aspects:

1. Orthostasis: blood pressure and pulse checks with the patient in the supine, sitting, and standing positions; systolic or diastolic changes of 20 mm Hg or more indicate orthostasis, especially if the patient is symptomatic
2. Cardiovascular system: arrhythmia, murmurs, carotid bruits
3. Sensory system: visual or hearing impairments

This checklist is used to identify fall hazards in the home. After identification, hazards should be eliminated or reduced. One point is allowed for every *NO* answer. A score of 1 to 7 is excellent, 8 to 14 is good, 15 or higher is hazardous.

	YES	NO
Housekeeping		
1. Do you clean up spills as soon as they occur?	____	____
2. Do you keep floors and stairways clean and free of clutter?	____	____
3. Do you put away magazines, sewing supplies, and other objects as soon as you are through with them and never leave them on floors or stairways?	____	____
4. Do you store frequently used items on shelves that are within easy reach?	____	____
Floors		
5. Do you keep everyone from walking on freshly washed floors before they are dry?	____	____
6. If you wax floors, do you apply 2 thin coats and buff each thoroughly or else use self-polishing, nonskid wax?	____	____
7. Do all small rugs have nonskid backings?	____	____
8. Have you eliminated small rugs at the tops and bottoms of stairways?	____	____
9. Are all carpet edges tacked down?	____	____
10. Are rugs and carpets free of curled edges, worn spots, and rips?	____	____
11. Have you chosen rugs and carpets with short, dense pile?	____	____
12. Are rugs and carpets installed over good-quality, medium-thick pads?	____	____
Bathroom		
13. Do you use a rubber mat or nonslip decals in the tub or shower?	____	____
14. Do you have a grab bar securely anchored over the tub or on the shower wall?	____	____
15. Do you have a nonskid rug on the bathroom floor?	____	____
16. Do you keep soap in an easy-to-reach receptacle?	____	____
Traffic Lanes		
17. Can you walk across every room in your home, and from one room to another, without detouring around furniture?	____	____
18. Is the traffic lane from your bedroom to the bathroom free of obstacles?	____	____
19. Are telephone and appliance cords kept away from areas where people walk?	____	____
Lighting		
20. Do you have light switches near every doorway?	____	____
21. Do you have enough good lighting to eliminate shadowy areas?	____	____
22. Do you have a lamp or light switch within easy reach from your bed?	____	____
23. Do you have night lights in your bathroom and in the hallway leading from your bedroom to the bathroom?	____	____
24. Are all stairways well lighted?	____	____
25. Do you have light switches at both the tops and bottoms of stairways?	____	____
Stairways		
26. Do securely fastened handrails extend the full length of the stairs on each side of stairways?	____	____
27. Do rails stand out from the walls so you can get a good grip?	____	____
28. Are rails distinctly shaped so you are alerted when you reach the end of a stairway?	____	____
29. Are all stairways in good condition, with no broken, sagging, or sloping steps?	____	____
30. Are all stairway carpeting and metal edges securely fastened and in good condition?	____	____
31. Have you replaced any single-level steps with gradually rising ramps or made sure such steps are well lit?	____	____
Ladders and Step Stools		
32. Do you have a sturdy step stool that you use to reach high cupboard and closet shelves?	____	____
33. Are all ladders and step stools in good condition?	____	____
34. Do you always use a step stool or ladder that is tall enough for the job?	____	____

Figure 23-1 Home safety checklist. (From National Safety Council: *Falling—the unexpected trip. A safety program for older adults,* Program Leader's Guide, 1982.)

Continued

Ladders and Step Stools—cont'd

35. Do you always set up your ladder or step stool on a firm, level base that is free of clutter? _____ _____
36. Before you climb a ladder or step stool, do you always make sure it is fully open and that the stepladder spreaders are locked? _____ _____
37. When you use a ladder or step stool, do you face the steps and keep your body between the side rails? _____ _____
38. Do you avoid standing on top of a step stool or climbing beyond the second step from the top on a stepladder? _____ _____

Outdoor Areas

39. Are walks and driveways in your yard and other areas free of breaks? _____ _____
40. Are lawns and gardens free of holes? _____ _____
41. Do you put away garden tools and hoses when they are not in use? _____ _____
42. Are outdoor areas kept free of rocks, loose boards, and other tripping hazards? _____ _____
43. Do you keep outdoor walkways, steps, and porches free of wet leaves and snow? _____ _____
44. Do you sprinkle icy outdoor areas with de-icers as soon as possible after a snowfall or freeze? _____ _____
45. Do you have mats at doorways for people to wipe their feet on? _____ _____
46. Do you know the safest way of walking when you cannot avoid walking on a slippery surface? _____ _____

Footwear

47. Do your shoes have soles and heels that provide good traction? _____ _____
48. Do you wear house slippers that fit well and do not fall off? _____ _____
49. Do you avoid walking in stocking feet? _____ _____
50. Do you wear low-heeled oxfords, loafers, or good-quality sneakers when you work in your house or yard? _____ _____
51. Do you replace boots or galoshes when their soles or heels are worn too smooth to keep you from slipping on wet or icy surfaces? _____ _____

Personal Precautions

52. Are you always alert for unexpected hazards, such as out-of-place furniture? _____ _____
53. If young grandchildren visit, are you alert for children playing on the floor and toys left in your path? _____ _____
54. If you have pets, are you alert for sudden movements across your path and pets getting underfoot? _____ _____
55. When you carry bulky packages, do you make sure they do not obstruct your vision? _____ _____
56. Do you divide large loads into smaller loads whenever possible? _____ _____
57. When you reach or bend, do you hold onto a firm support and avoid throwing your head back or turning it too far? _____ _____
58. Do you always use a ladder or step stool to reach high places and never stand on a chair? _____ _____
59. Do you always move deliberately and avoid rushing to answer the phone or doorbell? _____ _____
60. Do you take time to get your balance when you change position from lying down to sitting and from sitting to standing? _____ _____
61. Do you hold on to grab bars when you change position in the tub or shower? _____ _____
62. Do you keep yourself in good condition with moderate exercise, good diet, adequate rest, and regular medical checkups? _____ _____
63. If you wear glasses, is your prescription up-to-date? _____ _____
64. Do you know how to reduce injury in a fall? _____ _____
65. If you live alone, do you have daily contact with a friend or neighbor? _____ _____

SCORE: _____

Figure 23-1, cont'd For legend see p. 501.

4. Musculoskeletal system: arthritic changes, limitations in joint motion, deformities, fractures, foot problems, strength of lower extremities
5. Neurologic: nystagmus, neuropathy, tremors, rigidity, focal deficits, weakness
6. Cognitive status: Mini-Mental State Examination
7. Mood: Geriatric Depression Scale

Special attention must be given to the individual's gait and balance by simply observing ambulation with and without any assistive devices (e.g., canes, walkers) that may normally be used (Edwards, 1998). Footwear must be assessed for stability, fit, and appropriateness. Assistive devices should be checked for size, fit, integrity, and the patient's knowledge of its correct use. A more formal assessment is Tinetti's (1986) Performance-Oriented Assessment of Balance (Table 23-2).

Diagnostic studies to consider are listed in Box 23-2. As always, the decision to perform a test is based on the presenting symptoms and the anticipated benefits for the individual patient.

Interventions

Interventions are focused on correcting reversible causes, preventing future falls and injury, and alleviating the patient's fear of falling. A patient's risk for falling should be assessed annually (if not more often), and approaches must be tailored for the patient's individual needs on the basis of underlying risk factors. It is important to include family members or caregivers in education and intervention planning. Physical therapy often provides excellent benefits through balance training, gait training, and strengthening. The benefits of weight training for older individuals are now widely recognized, and such exercise is becoming widely practiced in a variety of settings (Evans, 1996). Assistive devices such as a cane or walker may provide additional stability for patients while they ambulate or transfer. Table 23-3 outlines issues in prescribing assistive devices for the elderly person (Wasson, et al., 1990).

General steps to be taken include the following:

1. Minimize medications and dosages; eliminate high-risk drugs if possible.
2. Prevent and treat osteoporosis.
3. Recommend proper footwear.
4. Recommend an obstacle-free, glare-free, and well-lit environment.
5. If necessary, raise toilet seats and chair heights and provide armrests.
6. Remove home hazards.
7. Install grab bars in bathrooms and other appropriate sites.
8. Provide physical therapy for flexibility, strength, gait, and balance training.
9. Add assistive devices as appropriate.
10. Avoid quick changes in position, especially if orthostatic changes are present.
11. Install motion alarms to alert staff or family members when a person with cognitive impairment has risen from a chair or bed.

Even with close supervision and minimized risk factors, some patients may continue to experience falls. For these patients, perhaps the best outcome is the prevention of injury related to falls. In such instances, innovative approaches (e.g., mattresses placed

Table 23-2 Performance-oriented Assessment of Balance*

Maneuver	Response: Normal	Response: Adaptive	Response: Abnormal
Sitting balance	Steady, stable	Holds on to chair to keep upright	Leans, slides down in chair
Arising from chair	Able to arise in a single movement without using arms	Uses arms (on chair or walking aid) to pull or push up; and/or moves forward in chair before attempting to arise	Multiple attempts required or unable without human assistance
Immediate standing balance (first 3-5 seconds)	Steady without holding on to walking aid or other object for support	Steady, but uses walking aid or other object for support	Any sign of unsteadiness†
Standing balance	Steady, able to stand with feet together without holding object for support	Steady, but cannot put feet together	Any sign of unsteadiness regardless of stance or holds on to object
Balance with eyes closed (with feet as close together as possible)	Steady without holding on to any object with feet together	Steady with feet apart	Any sign of unsteadiness or needs to hold on to an object
Turning balance (360°)	No grabbing or staggering; no need to hold on to any objects; steps are continuous (turn is a flowing movement)	Steps are discontinuous (patient puts one foot completely on floor before raising other foot)	Any sign of unsteadiness or holds on to an object
Nudge on sternum (patient standing with feet as close together as possible, examiner pushes with light even pressure over sternum 3 times; reflects ability to withstand displacement)	Steady, able to withstand pressure	Needs to move feet, but able to maintain balance	Begins to fall, or examiner has to help maintain balance

Neck turning (patient asked to turn head side to side and look up while standing with feet as close together as possible)	Able to turn head at least halfway side to side and able to bend head back to look at ceiling; no staggering, grabbing, or symptoms of lightheadedness, unsteadiness, or pain	Decreased ability to turn side to side to extend neck, but no staggering, grabbing, or symptoms of light-headedness, unsteadiness, or pain	Any sign of unsteadiness or symptoms when turning head or extending neck
One leg standing balance	Able to stand on one leg for 5 seconds without holding object for support		Unable
Back extension (ask patient to lean back as far as possible, without holding on to object if possible)	Good extension without holding object or staggering	Tries to extend, but decreased ROM (compared with other patients of same age) or needs to hold object to attempt extension	Will not attempt extension, no extension seen, or staggers
Reaching up (have patient attempt to remove an object from a shelf high enough to require stretching or standing on toes)	Able to take down object without needing to hold on to other object for support and without becoming unsteady	Able to get object but needs to steady self by holding on to something for support	Unable or unsteady
Bending down (patient is asked to pick up small objects, such as pen, from the floor)	Able to bend down and pick up the object and is able to get up easily in single attempt without needing to pull self up with arms	Able to get object and get upright in single attempt but needs to pull self up with arms or hold on to something for support	Unable to bend down or unable to get upright after bending down or takes multiple attempts to upright
Sitting down	Able to sit down in one smooth movement	Needs to use arms to guide self into chair or does not have a smooth movement	Falls into chair, misjudges distances (lands off center)

From Tinetti ME: Performance-oriented assessment of mobility in elderly patients, *J Am Geriatr Soc* 34:119-126, 1986.
ROM, Range of motion.
*The patient begins this assessment seated in a hard, straight-backed, armless chair.
†Unsteadiness is defined as grabbing at objects for support, staggering, moving feet, or having more than minimal trunk sway.

Box 23-2

Diagnostic Studies in the Evaluation of Falls

CBC: rules out anemia or infection
Urinalysis: rules out infection
Serum chemistry screen: rules out electrolyte imbalance
TSH
Vitamin B_{12}
Sedimentation rate
Drug levels as indicated
ECG
Chest x-ray examination
Holter monitor: if transient arrhythmia is suspected
Head CT scan: if mental status or neurologic changes are present

CBC, Complete blood count; *CT,* computed tomography; *ECG,* electrocardiogram; *TSH,* thyroid-stimulating hormone.

on the floor for patients who fall out of bed) may help to prevent harm while maximizing freedom of movement. Plans for such situations should be created by a multidisciplinary team of nurses, physicians, and therapists, with input and agreement from family members, caregivers, and the patient, if appropriate. These plans can be tailored for any setting, including the hospital, long-term care facility, or home. Establishment of a primary goal of maximum mobility and independence, with acceptance of the inevitability of the risks and dangers of falls, may need to be negotiated with the family.

Restraints must be avoided at all costs. Restraints can cause both physical and psychologic harm to patients and thus have been highly regulated and monitored in hospitals and long-term care facilities. Restraints include any equipment, medication, or intervention designed to prevent or limit movement. This definition goes beyond Posey vests and wrist restraints to include such devices as seatbelts and wedge pillows in wheelchairs, locked tray tables on recliners, and even raised bed rails.

Summary

Falls by the elderly are prevalent and costly, not only financially but also in terms of quality of life. Many falls are preventable, and they should never be assumed to be a natural outcome of the aging process. The cause of a fall is often multifactorial, and every effort must be made to address as many of these causes as possible. A multidisciplinary approach is often necessary to successfully accomplish this task. The practitioner may need to treat medical problems and adjust medications. Physical and occupational therapists can provide strengthening exercises as well as education regarding the proper use of assistive devices and adaptive equipment. Weight training for older people has proven to be very beneficial in enhancing strength and mobility. Social work can assist patients in obtaining support and resources for personal care and homemaking services. A coordinated management plan is often successful in preventing costly and dangerous falls in all settings.

TABLE 23-3 Assistive Devices for Common Disabilities of the Elderly

Device	Indications	Limitations	Comments
Upper Extremity			
"Soap on a rope," long-handle back sponge, tub seat, shower bench, toothbrush grip, electric razor with rotary edges, and reaching devices (see also lower extremity)	Bathing, oral care, and grooming	Some grip or thumb opposition and range of motion required	
Splints	Wrist pain or instability, carpal metacarpal arthritis	Patient compliance	
Balance/Back/Lower Extremities			
Reaching device(s), long shoehorns, back sponges, elastic shoelaces, Velcro straps	Dressing and grooming	Dexterity necessary	
Canes†	Articular pain, mild weakness	Upper extremity weakness	Four-legged canes can be cumbersome
Crutches†	Significant weakness or pain of one or both lower extremities	Upper extremity weakness or incoordination	Forearm crutches preferable for chronic use; platform attachment for elbow, wrist, or hand disease
Walkers†	Significant imbalance or weakness	Cumbersome	Wheel and platform attachments available
Braces*†	Isolated severe joint or muscle dysfunction	Difficult to put on	
Wheelchair*†	Limited endurance or inability to walk	Poor access to house, weight of chair	Prescription should be individualized
Bathroom grab bars, raised toilet seat, tub seat, commode	Transferring; weak or limited hip or knee motion; imbalance	Installation problems	

From Wasson JH et al: The prescription of assistive devices for the elderly: practical considerations, *J Gen Intern Med* 5:48-49, 1990.
*Consultation is usually indicated.
†Medicare coverage when prescribed by a physician as medically necessary.

Resources

AGENET Falls Prevention
http://www.agenet.com/fall_prevention.html

American Academy of Orthopaedic Surgeons
http://www.aaos.org/wordhtml/pat_educ/fallsbro.htm

References

Dunn JE et al: Mortality, disability, and falls in older persons: the role of underlying disease and disability, *Am J Public Health* 82:395-400, 1992.

Edwards BJ, Lee S: Gait disorders and falls in a retirement home: a pilot study, *Annals of Long Term Care* 6(4), 1998.

Evans WJ: Reversing sarcopenia: how weight training can build strength and vitality, *Geriatrics* 51(5): 46-53, 1996.

Herndon JG et al: Chronic medical conditions and risk of fall injury events at home in older adults, *J Am Geriatr Soc* 45:739-743, 1997.

National Safety Council: *Falling—the unexpected trip: a safety program for older adults,* Itaska, Ill., 1992, Program Leader's Guide.

Ray WA et al: A randomized trial of a consultation service to reduce falls in nursing homes, *JAMA* 278(7):557-562, 1997.

Tinetti ME: Performance-oriented assessment of mobility in elderly patients, *J Am Geriatr Soc* 34:119-126, 1986.

Wasson JH et al: The prescription of assistive devices for the elderly: practical considerations, *J Gen Intern Med* 5(1):46-54, 1990.

Weiner OK, Hanlon JT, Studenski SA: Effects of central nervous system polypharmacy on falls liability in community-dwelling elderly, *Gerontology* 44:217-221, 1998.

Yoshikawa TT, Cobbs El, Brummel-Smith K: *Practical ambulatory geriatrics,* ed 2, St Louis, 1998, Mosby.

24

Incontinence

Urinary incontinence (UI), the involuntary loss of urine, is a significant health problem—*not* a normal consequence of aging. Urinary incontinence affects 15% to 30% of community-dwelling older individuals, up to one third of elderly patients in acute care settings, and approximately 50% of residents in long-term care facilities. In total, this problem affects approximately 13 million Americans and costs $15 billion per year (Ouslander et al., 1996; Jay and Staskin, 1998). Urinary incontinence is a treatable and, at times, a preventable condition. The consequences of UI are formidable and can have an impact on the physical, psychologic, social, and financial realms, not only for the patient but also for the caregiver.

Physically, UI can cause skin breakdown, lead to recurrent urinary tract infections (UTIs), and inhibit the healing of any existing skin conditions. Psychologically, an older person who is incontinent may experience isolation, a loss of self-esteem, and even depression as he or she withdraws from social settings and becomes more reliant on caregivers to maintain continence and hygiene. Socially, incontinence is likely to lead to the older person's restriction of social engagements to avoid the embarrassment associated with UI. Incontinence is also burdensome because of the expense of incontinence supplies and the management of laundry and other cleaning costs.

Providing care for an incontinent older person can be both physically and emotionally demanding. The amount of time needed to provide appropriate assistance to an older person with UI may be more than most people can easily manage. Toileting is a 24-hour-a-day need. Many older people with UI need aid in transferring to a commode or in taking care of personal hygiene, and they require assistance throughout the day and night. Laundry and cleaning responsibilities are likely to fall on the caregiver. When the assistance needed by an incontinent elder is more than the caregiver alone can provide, caregivers often must hire home health aides or similar staff to assist them in providing care. Caregivers often cite UI as one of the reasons for placing an older loved one in a nursing home. This problem is significant for older adults, and primary health care providers need to offer assistance in managing it.

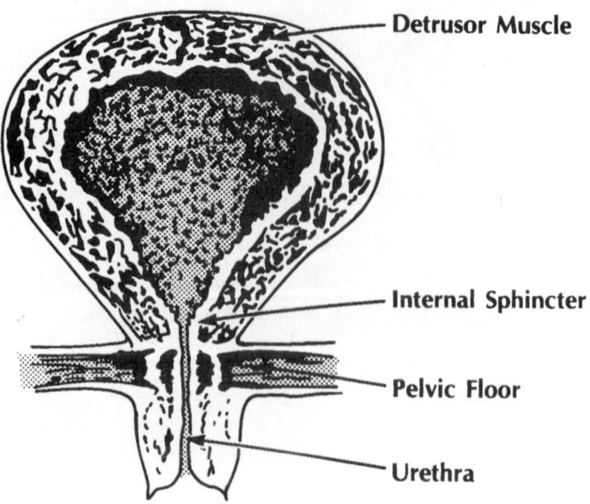

Figure 24-1 The urinary bladder. (From Burke MM, Walsh MB: *Gerontologic nursing: wholistic care of the older adult,* ed 2, St Louis, 1997, Mosby.)

Genitourinary Anatomy and Physiology

Anatomically, the lower urinary tract is composed of the bladder; the detrusor muscle, which is best thought of as a large, trainable muscle; and the sphincter mechanism (Figure 24-1). There are two parts to the urinary sphincter: the internal urethral sphincter, which is composed of both smooth and striated muscle and surrounds the urethra, and the external striated muscle sphincter, which is part of the pelvic floor. The bladder and the sphincters need to be intact to maintain urine control. Strengthening the external sphincter may compensate for damage to the sphincter mechanism.

Bladder function is primarily a spinal reflex mediated at S2 to S4. If central nervous system centers are not intact, the bladder empties as a spinal reflex. Stretch receptors are triggered as the bladder fills, and messages are sent to the sacral micturition center and the brain via autonomic pathways. The supraspinal centers either inhibit or facilitate voiding. The micturition center in the brainstem coordinates detrusor contraction and sphincter relaxation. Centers in the cerebral cortex inhibit detrusor contractions to delay voiding. Voiding occurs when detrusor contraction and sphincter relaxation are coordinated. As increasing amounts of urine collect in the bladder, the sphincters increase their resistance and the cortex inhibits detrusor contractions. Micturition occurs when the inhibition is released, the sphincters relax, and parasympathetic stimulation causes detrusor contractions.

Normal Age-related Changes

Normal age-related changes in the genitourinary system make maintaining control of urine more challenging for the elderly. The changes in themselves do not cause incontinence, but incontinence can develop in association with other problems, particularly problems with mobility or cognitive ability (Table 24-1). The normal adult bladder has a capacity of about 400 to 600 ml, whereas the bladder capacity of an older person is decreased to approximately 250 ml. The functional capacity of the older person is further decreased because the bladder is no longer completely emptied during micturition; 50 ml

Table 24-1 Normal Age-related Changes in the Genitourinary System

Change	Effect
Decreased bladder capacity	Limited functional volume
Residual urine	Limited functional volume
Increased uninhibited detrusor contractions	Feelings of urgency
Late onset of urge to void	Feelings of urgency
Postmenopausal tissue changes	Less competent sphincter
Prostatic enlargement	Hesitancy

of residual urine is normal for an aging bladder. Residual urine contributes to the high incidence of urinary tract infections.

Older people also experience a delayed onset of the desire to void when their bladder capacity has been reached. For men, some degree of prostatic hypertrophy occurs as a normal part of aging, which, depending on the degree of enlargement, can influence bladder patterns (such as hesitancy in starting their stream). For women, urethral tissues are affected by the estrogen changes associated with menopause and become less robust with aging, making the external sphincter less competent. The many changes of normal aging result in smaller, more irritable bladders that do not alert older people to the need to void in a timely fashion. Although all of these changes increase the older person's vulnerability to incontinence, none of these causes incontinence without the presence of other contributing factors. *Incontinence is not the result of age-related changes.*

Types of Incontinence

Transient Incontinence

Transient or reversible incontinence is caused by a temporary condition that, when corrected, resolves the incontinence. The causative factors for transient incontinence are usually associated with acute changes in cognition, limited mobility, undue stress on the bladder, or a temporary condition that causes temporary genitourinary dysfunction (Table 24-2). Many times the older person first experiences incontinence while hospitalized. *The treatment is not to insert a catheter.* Finding the causative condition and treating the underlying problem will resolve the incontinence.

Altered mobility is another common factor in transient incontinence. A person who is unable to get to a bathroom or commode in sufficient time will experience episodes of incontinence. Impaired mobility may result from arthritis, pain, clutter, side rails, or other mechanical or pharmacologic restraints.

Common contributing causes to transient incontinence include delirium, infection, limited mobility, fecal impaction, vaginitis, medications, and emotional causes (Palmer, 1996). UI is often cited as a side effect of several medications (Box 24-1). Particular attention should be given to any newly prescribed medications. Medications that can cause urinary retention and overflow incontinence include anticholinergics, antidepressants, antipsychotics, alpha-adrenergic agonists, beta-adrenergic agonists, and calcium channel blockers. Diuretics cause polyuria, which can overwhelm an elderly bladder.

TABLE 24-2 Risk Factors Associated with the Development of Transient Incontinence

Risk Category	Risk Factor
Problems with cognition	Temporary confusion Delirium Confusion from side effects of medication or environmental changes
Immobility	Artificial restriction of movement
Undue stress on bladder	Environmental barriers to toileting Conditions causing polyuria Caffeine Diuretic therapy
Temporary genitourinary dysfunction	Bladder infection Fecal impaction Medications Fluid restriction

Box 24-1

Drug Side Effects Related to Urine Control

Alcohol: polyuria
Alpha-adrenergic blockers: urethral relaxation
Alpha-adrenergic agonists: urinary retention
Anticholinergics: urinary retention with overflow incontinence
Antidepressants: anticholinergic effects
Antipsychotics: anticholinergic effects
Beta-adrenergic agonists: urinary retention
Caffeine: polyuria
Calcium channel blockers: urinary retention
Diuretics: polyuria, frequency, urgency
Narcotic analgesics: urinary retention
Over-the-counter cold and diet preparations: contain alpha-adrenergic agonists

Bladder infections, which are common in older people, are often associated with incontinence. Fecal impaction can be the causative factor in the development of an overflow incontinence; this problem can be relieved by removal of the impaction.

An adequate amount of fluid must be consumed for the bladder to function correctly. Chronic fluid restriction results in the formation of concentrated urine, which irritates bladder tissue and does not provide adequate stimulus for normal bladder functioning. Older adults should drink at least six glasses of noncaffeinated liquid in a 24-hour period. Older people sometimes restrict fluids to control their incontinence, but this actually tends to increase UI, and can lead to a UTI—in itself a common cause of UI.

Urinary Tract Infections

In an older person, incontinence is often one of the first symptoms of a UTI, the prevalence of which increases with age. Residual urine provides a breeding ground for the development of infections. Restriction of fluids in an attempt to prevent urine loss leads to a decreased urine flow, and thereby the urinary tract is not washed out as frequently. Another cause of UTI in an older person is an indwelling catheter; indwelling catheters should be avoided or at least removed as soon as possible.

UTIs may present as urinary frequency with incontinence, urgency, and dysuria. Hematuria and fever may be present but often are not. *Infections in older people are often atypical;* any change in behavior from baseline, including lethargy, agitation, flulike symptoms, and delirium, may result from a UTI and warrants evaluation. Pyuria revealed by urinalysis should be treated with a full course of an appropriate antibiotic. However, bacteriuria without symptoms is probably colonization and should not be treated, lest the risk of antibiotic resistance be increased. Patient teaching regarding taking the full course of the antibiotic and increasing fluid intake is very important. Symptoms *often* subside shortly after the patient begins the medication, and an older person may try to save money by hoarding some of the pills for a future infection.

Chronic Incontinence

Chronic incontinence is a more persistent type of UI and is not related to acute illness. In most types of chronic incontinence the pathologic condition occurs in the genitourinary system and disrupts the normal control of urine. The primary types of chronic incontinence are stress, urge, overflow, and functional urinary incontinence (FUI). In addition, the various chronic UI conditions can occur in combination in a condition referred to as a mixed incontinence.

Stress Incontinence

Stress urinary incontinence involves the leakage of small amounts of urine when pressure inside the abdomen increases. The leakage is related to congenital or acquired incompetence of the urinary sphincter. The acquired urethral deficiency may be related to surgical damage, trauma, radiation therapy, or a sacral cord lesion (Fantl et al., 1996). In women it is commonly associated with postmenopausal tissue changes and previous child bearing, in combination with the wear and tear of living and the years of the general pull of gravity (Fantl et al., 1996). Laughing, coughing, and sneezing, all of which increase intraabdominal pressure, are often precipitating factors in stress incontinence. Continuous leakage, even during resting or with minimal exertion, can occur in more severe cases.

Urge Incontinence

Urge incontinence is the inability to inhibit bladder contractions until a toilet is reached. Pathologic conditions associated with urge incontinence include involuntary detrusor (bladder) contractions, detrusor hyperactivity with impaired bladder contractility, and an involuntary sphincter. Detrusor hyperreflexia is associated with stroke, supraspinal lesions, and multiple sclerosis. Detrusor hyperactivity with impaired bladder contractility is also seen in frail elderly, whose involuntary detrusor contractions occur in conjunction with the need to strain in order to empty the bladder. The usual symptoms are loss of urine with an abrupt and strong desire to void; loss of urine on the way to the bathroom, and high postvoid residual urine (Fantl et al., 1996).

Overflow Incontinence

Overflow incontinence is the loss of small amounts of urine at times when the bladder is excessively full. In this condition the outflow of urine is disrupted by mechanical or neurologic causes. The most common mechanical disruption is associated with prostatic enlargement, but it can also result from a urethral stricture or from mechanical pressure caused by an organ prolapse or fecal impaction. It can occur as a consequence of an underactive or a contractile detrusor muscle that may develop secondary to medications, neurologic conditions such as diabetic neuropathy, surgical damage to nerves, a spinal cord injury low in the cord, or idiopathic causes (Fantl et al., 1996). In overflow incontinence the pressure in an overdistended bladder builds until it is sufficient to overcome the outflow resistance and allow the passage of urine.

Functional Incontinence

Functional incontinence is caused by factors outside the genitourinary system that result in an inability to reach the toilet before urine is lost. Functional problems that prevent normal toileting behaviors include environmental restraints, mobility restriction, cognitive difficulties, and psychiatric disorders. Symptoms are mixed and can include frequent leakage and symptoms of urge or stress incontinence.

Mixed Incontinence

Mixed incontinence is a combination of urge and stress incontinence and is most common in older women. See Table 24-3 for a summary of chronic incontinence.

Primary Care Evaluation of Urinary Incontinence

The purpose of the initial evaluation is to objectively confirm the presence of UI, rule out potentially reversible conditions, distinguish between patients in need of further evaluation and patients appropriate for initial behavioral intervention, and identify the presumptive cause of the UI if possible (Fantl et al., 1996).

History

The history of UI begins with a focused medical, neurologic, and genitourinary history that includes an assessment of risk factors and a review of medications. A detailed exploration of the symptoms of the UI and associated symptoms and factors includes the following:

Number of wetting episodes
Usual times of wetting episodes

TABLE 24-3 Symptoms and Subtypes of Urinary Incontinence

Type of UI	Definition	Pathophysiology	Symptoms and Signs
Urge	Involuntary loss of urine associated with a strong sensation of urinary urgency	Involuntary detrusor (bladder) contractions (detrusor instability [DI])	Loss of urine with an abrupt and strong desire to void; usually loss of urine on way to bathroom
		Detrusor hyperactivity with impaired bladder contractility (DHIC)	DHIC-elevated post void residual (PVR) volume
		Involuntary sphincter relaxation	Involuntary loss of urine (without symptoms)
Stress	Urethral sphincter failure usually associated with increased intraabdominal pressure	Urethral hypermobility due to anatomic changes or defects such as fascial detachments (hypermobility)	Small amount of urine loss during coughing, sneezing, laughing, or other physical activities
		Intrinsic urethral sphincter deficiency (ISD) failure of the sphincter at rest	Continuous leak at rest or with minimal exertion (postural changes)
Mixed	Combination of urge and stress UI	Combination of urge and stress features as above Common in women, especially older women	Combinations of urge and stress UI symptoms as above; one symptom (urge or stress) often more bothersome to the patient than the other

From Fantl JA et al: *Quick reference guide for clinicians: managing acute and chronic urinary incontinence,* AHCPR Pub 96-0686, Rockville, Md, 1996, US Department of Health and Human Services, Public Health Service, Agency for Health Care Policy and Research.

Continued

TABLE 24-3 Symptoms and Subtypes of Urinary Incontinence—cont'd

Type of UI	Definition	Pathophysiology	Symptoms and Signs
Overflow	Bladder overdistention	Acontractile detrusor Hypotonic or underactive detrusor secondary to drugs, fecal impaction, diabetes, lower spinal cord injury, or disruption of the motor innervation of the detrusor muscle In men, secondary obstruction due to prostatic hyperplasia, prostatic carcinoma, or urethral stricture In women, obstruction due to severe genital prolapse or surgical overcorrection of urethral detachment	Variety of symptoms, including frequent or constant dribbling or urge or stress incontinence symptoms, as well as urgency and frequent urination
Other			
Functional	Chronic impairments of physical and/or cognitive functioning	Chronic functional and mental disabilities	Urge incontinence or functional limitations
Unconscious or reflex	Neurologic dysfunction	Decreased bladder compliance with risk of vesicoureteral reflux and hydronephrosis Secondary to radiation cystitis, inflammatory bladder conditions, radical pelvic surgery, or myelomeningocele In many nonneurogenic cases, no demonstrable DI	Postmicturitional or continual incontinence; severe urgency with bladder hypersensitivity (sensory urgency)

From Fantl JA et al: *Quick reference guide for clinicians: managing acute and chronic urinary incontinence,* AHCPR Pub 96-0686, Rockville, Md, 1996, US Department of Health and Human Services, Public Health Service, Agency for Health Care Policy and Research.

Amounts of urine lost each time
Activities before and after wetting episodes
Presence of leakage
Number of continent episodes
Amounts and types of fluids consumed
Times fluids are consumed
Home environment toileting conditions
Effects on family and social activities (most bothersome symptom to the patient)
Precipitants of incontinence (e.g., situational antecedents such as coughing, laughing, or exercising; "on way to the bathroom")
Surgery, trauma or injury, radiation therapy, recent illness
Medications: prescriptions and over-the-counter (new and old)
Other urinary tract symptoms (e.g., nocturia, dysuria, hesitancy, enuresis, straining, poor or interrupted stream, pain)
Bowel habits
Alteration in sexual function
Amount and type of perineal pads or protective devices
Previous self-care treatments and effects on UI
Previous treatments from formal health care providers and effects on UI
Expectations of treatment

The mental status assessment should include the following:

Cognition
Motivation to self-toilet
Depressive symptoms

The functional assessment should evaluate the following:

Transfer ability
Manual dexterity
Mobility
Balance
Arm strength and torso flexibility
Toileting (hygiene, pulling up clothes, changing pads)
Vision

The environmental assessment should include the following:

Access (to include obstacles) and distance to toilets or commode
Chair or bed that allows ease when rising
Lighting in bathroom

The social factors to be evaluated include the following:

Relationship of UI to work or social life
Living arrangements (e.g., home, apartment, alone, family)
Identified caregiver and degree of involvement (Fantl et al., 1996)

Bladder records are extremely helpful in identifying a pattern and potential contributing factors to the urine loss. Figure 24-2 is a record that tracks frequency, timing, and amount of voids and incontinent episodes; activities associated with UI; and fluid intake. If possible, the patient should bring the completed record to each visit.

NAME: ______________________________

DATE: ______________________________

INSTRUCTIONS: Place a check in the appropriate column next to the time you urinated in the toilet or when an incontinence episode occurred. Note the reason for the incontinence and describe your liquid intake (for example, coffee, water) and estimate the amount (for example, one cup).

Time interval	Urinated in toilet	Had a small incontinence episode	Had a large incontinence episode	Reason for incontinence episode	Type/amount of liquid intake
6–8 AM					
8–10 AM					
10–noon					
Noon–2 PM					
2–4 PM					
4–6 PM					
6–8 PM					
8–10 PM					
10–midnight					
Overnight					

No. of pads used today: ______________ No. of episodes: ______________

Comments: ______________________________

Figure 24-2 Sample bladder record. (From Fantl JA et al: *Quick reference guide for clinicians: managing acute and chronic urinary incontinence,* AHCPR Pub 96-0686, Rockville, Md, 1996, US Department of Health and Human Services, Public Health Service, Agency for Health Care Policy and Research.)

Physical Examination

General examination (edema, neurologic abnormalities, mobility)
Abdominal examination
- Diastasis recti
- Organomegaly
- Masses
- Bladder size
- Peritoneal irritation
- Fluid collections

Rectal examination
- Perineal sensation
- Sphincter tone
- Fecal impaction
- Masses

Genital examination in men
- Skin condition
- Abnormalities of the foreskin, penis, and perineum
- Consistency and contour of the prostate

Pelvic examination in women
- Skin condition
- Genital atrophy
- Pelvic organ prolapse
- Pelvic masses
- Perivaginal muscle tone
- Other abnormalities

Direct observation of urine loss
- Urine loss with full bladder, using cough stress test
- Estimation of postvoid residual (PVR) volume; a straight catheterization or, if a noninvasive test is called for, a portable ultrasound may be reliably used to estimate PVR (Ireton et al., 1990)

Laboratory tests
- Urinalysis
- Blood urea nitrogen, creatinine, calcium, glucose

Office Testing of Lower Urinary Tract Function

Sometimes the basic evaluation reveals neither transient causes nor indications for specialized testing, and the history and physical do not permit a distinction between urge and stress incontinence. In this situation simple tests of lower urinary tract function may be helpful and can easily be performed in the primary care office (Weiss, 1998).

Simple office cystometry is a test for urge incontinence and can be performed at the same time that PVR urine is measured. In this test, as described by Weiss (1998), a French nonballooned urinary catheter (No. 12-14) is inserted into the bladder. After the bladder empties, the plunger is removed from a bayonet-tipped 50-ml syringe, and the tip is inserted into the end of the catheter (Figure 24-3). With the practitioner holding the center of the syringe approximately 15 cm above the urethra, 50 ml of sterile water

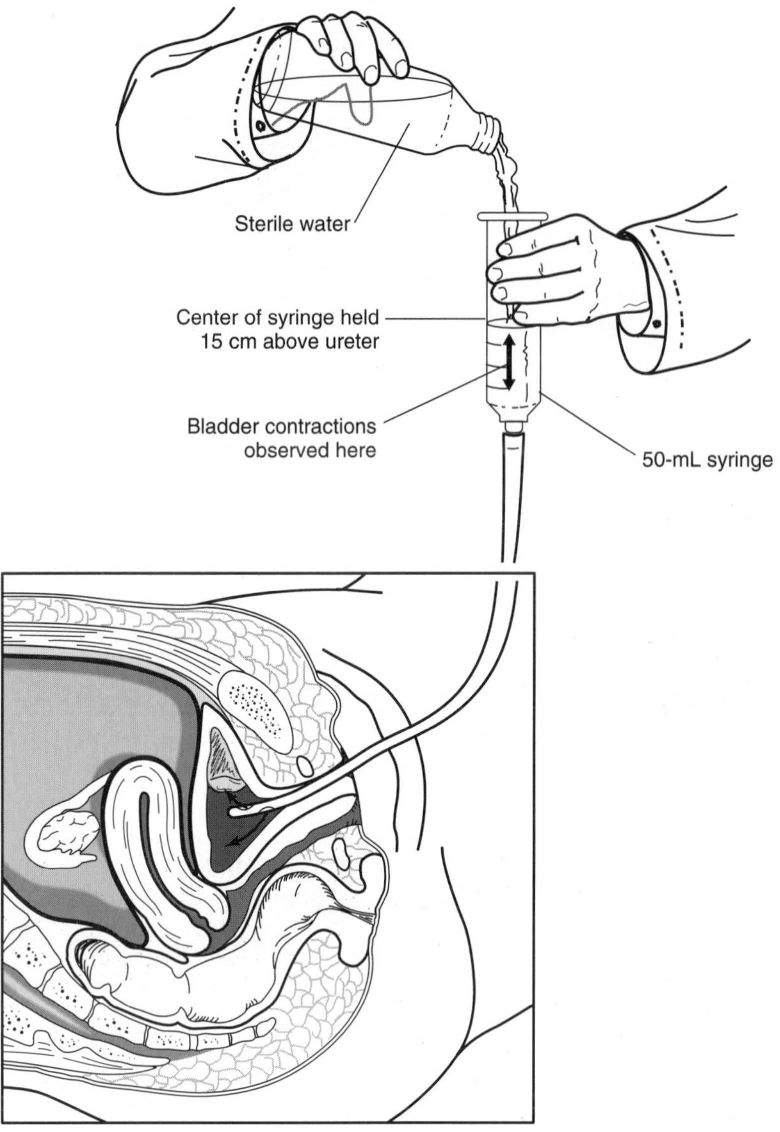

Figure 24-3 Simple office cystometry. (From Weiss BD: Diagnostic evaluation of urinary incontinence in geriatric patients, *Am Fam Physician* 57(11):2675-2684, 2688-2690, 1998.)

is poured into the open end of the syringe and allowed to flow into the bladder. Keeping track of the total amount of water used, the practitioner continues to instill water in 50-ml increments until the patient experiences the urge to urinate. At this point water instillation is continued in 25-ml increments until the patient experiences severe urgency ("I can't hold it anymore") or until bladder contractions occur. Contractions are detected by monitoring the fluid level that appears in the syringe after

Box 24-2
Relaxation Techniques

Divert attention away from bladder.
Use quick, rapid contractions of pelvic muscles.
Avoid strenuous activities.
Keep self busy with sedentary activities.
Take some deep breaths and concentrate on diversional music.
Avoid stimuli such as running water or putting hands in water.
Use absorbent padding in clothes to help relaxation.
Avoid any stimuli that increase bladder contraction.

several aliquots of water have been instilled. A rise and fall of fluid level indicates pressure changes (i.e., contractions) within the bladder. Severe urgency or bladder contractions at less than 300 ml of bladder volume constitute a presumptive diagnosis of urge incontinence.

Treatment Options

Treatment options for chronic incontinence include behavioral, pharmacologic, and surgical interventions depending on the type of incontinence and the patient's ability and desire to pursue certain options. Most experts suggest that if the patient has stress, urge, or mixed UI, low-risk behavioral treatments should be attempted first (if there are no contraindications).

Behavior Treatments

Bladder Training. Bladder training is noninvasive, relatively inexpensive, and easy to administer. With bladder training the patient works to achieve a certain amount of time between voidings. After the goal is reached, the interval is lengthened; each incremental time change takes approximately 1 week. Relaxation techniques to divert attention from the older person's full bladder are helpful (Box 24-2). It should be emphasized that the bladder is a large muscle that can be trained to hold more urine in the same way that frequent voidings have resulted in a bladder that holds less urine.

Toileting Program. Most often FUI is best approached with some type of toileting program. The problem is usually related to cognitive impairment or mobility problems, and in both instances the older person requires assistance to maintain continence. Individualized scheduled toileting (IST) involves identifying the person's usual bladder patterns and developing a toileting schedule based on these patterns (Jirovec, 1991). An IST program provides reminders to toilet in a timely fashion. When appropriate, encouragement and praise should be given while the patient is toileting. An adequate amount of fluid must be taken on a regular basis to maintain bladder patterns. The key to a successful IST program is the consistency with which it is provided. Routine scheduled toileting (RST) is similar to an IST program but differs in that the schedule is not individualized to the person's usual bladder patterns. RST is often adopted in nursing homes where staffing and ward routines prevent individualization of toileting schedules. The success of these programs usually depends on the consistency of the caregiver.

Containment Strategies

Absorbent products should be used for chronic UI or in combination with other treatments to provide protection (Fantl et al., 1996). Most older people with UI already use these products, but the primary care provider should address the issue in a way that prevents undue embarrassment to the older person. The discussion should center on product differences in availability, ease of use, and cost.

When feasible, intermittent catheterization is the preferred alternative to indwelling catheters. Indwelling urethral catheters (IUCs) are recommended for containment in elders whose UI results from obstruction or when other interventions are not feasible (Fantl et al., 1996). *IUCs should be the treatment of last resort;* all other approaches, including the use of absorbent products and toileting programs, should be considered before an IUC is used. It is inappropriate to use an IUC as a convenient way to contain the urine loss. IUC may be the appropriate treatment choice in a patient for whom

Box 24-3
Kegel Exercises

Purpose

Designed to strengthen and give voluntary control of the pubococcygeus (PC) muscle, which stretches from the pubic bone in front to the tailbone in back and encircles the urinary opening.

Identifying the PC Muscle

While urinating on the toilet, stop the flow of urine without moving the legs.

The Exercises

Can be done anywhere, anytime.

Slow Kegel

Tighten the PC muscle and hold for a slow count of three, then relax.

Quick Kegel

Tighten and relax the PC muscle as rapidly as you can.

Pull in, Push out

Pull up the entire pelvic floor as though trying to suck water into your vagina. Then push out or bear down as if trying to push the imaginary water out. (This uses a number of abdominal muscles as well as the PC muscle).

At first do each of these exercises (one "set") five times every day. Each week, increase the number of times you do each exercise by five (15, 20, 25, etc.).

changing absorbent padding is painful, a patient whose urinary output needs to be strictly measured.

Pelvic Muscle Exercise

Pelvic muscle exercises can be used with most types of UI to strengthen muscles to delay voiding. A common intervention for women with pubococcygeus muscle weakness is education regarding Kegel exercises. Box 24-3 provides an approach to educating women on the proper way to perform this maneuver. If used in conjunction with exercises, biofeedback enhances a person's ability to identify the muscles that need to be exercised. It is important that the person be able to distinguish between abdominal, gluteal, and pelvic floor muscles in order to exercise the right muscles.

Weighted vaginal cones have also been used to strengthen pelvic muscles. The person is given a set of vaginal cones of increasing weight and taught how to insert the cones. She is then asked to insert the cone twice a day and try to keep it from falling out for up to 15 minutes. When she can easily keep a particular weight from falling, she is encouraged to try retaining a heavier weight. Both PME and vaginal cones exercise the pelvic musculature.

Pharmacologic Treatment

Pharmacologic intervention has been shown to be effective in treating some types of UI. For urge UI an anticholinergic agent (e.g., oxybutynin, dicyclomine hydrochloride, and propantheline) is the first medication selected. Of these, oxybutynin is thought to be most effective and is recommended first in treating urge UI (Fantl et al., 1996). Side effects related to the anticholinergic action often make compliance an issue. Tricyclic antidepressants have also been used to treat urge UI and are associated with cardiac and anticholinergic adverse effects. For stress UI, phenylpropanolamine or pseudoephedrine is useful in strengthening the bladder outlet resistance. Oral or vaginal estrogen may also be used as an adjunct therapy in postmenopausal women. When a behavioral intervention fails or does not produce the desired degree of urine control, pharmacologic treatment may be considered, but each person must be individually assessed as an appropriate candidate for whichever therapy is chosen. See Table 24-4 for an expanded discussion of the various classes of, and precautions regarding, the various medications used to treat UI.

Referral

Referral is appropriate under the following conditions:

- Uncertain diagnosis and inability to develop a reasonable management plan
- Failure to respond to the patient's satisfaction to an adequate therapeutic trial, with the patient interested in pursuing further therapy
- Consideration of surgical intervention, particularly if previous surgery failed or if the patient is a high surgical risk
- Hematuria without infection

TABLE 24-4 Pharmacotherapy of Urinary Incontinence

Incontinence Type	Drug Class	Drug Therapy	Adverse Effects and Precautions	Comments
Urge incontinence	Anticholinergic agents	Oxybutynin (2.5-5 mg bid-qid), propantheline (7.5-30 mg at least tid), dicyclomine (10-20 mg tid)	Dry mouth, visual disturbances, constipation, dry skin, confusion	Anticholinergics are the first-line drug therapy (oxybutynin is preferred); propantheline is a second-line therapy
	Tricyclic antidepressants (TCAs)	Imipramine, desipramine, nortriptyline (25-100 mg/day)	Anticholinergic effects (as above), orthostatic hypotension and cardiac dysrhythmia	TCAs are generally reserved for patients with an additional indication (e.g., depression, neuralgia) at an initial dose of 10-25 mg 1-3 times/day
Stress incontinence	Alpha-adrenergic agonists	Phenylpropanolamine (PPA) in sustained-release form (25-100 mg bid), pseudoephedrine (15-60 mg tid)	Anxiety, insomnia, agitation, respiratory difficulty sweating, cardiac dysrhythmia, hypertension, tremor; should not be used in obstructive syndromes and/or hypertension	PPA (preferred) or pseudoephedrine are first-line therapies for women with no contraindication (notably hypertension)
Stress or combined urge/stress incontinence	Estrogen replacement agents	Conjugated estrogens (0.3-0.625 mg/day orally or 1 g vaginal cream at bedtime)	Should not be used if suspected or confirmed breast or endometrial cancer, active or past thromboembolism with past oral contraceptive, estrogen, or pregnancy; headache, spotting, edema, breast tenderness, possible depression	Estrogen (oral or vaginal) is an adjunctive therapy for postmenopausal women as it augments alpha-agonists such as PPA or pseudoephedrine

			Give progesterone with estrogen if uterus is present; pretreatment/periodic mammogram, gynecologic, breast examination advised	Progestin (e.g., medroxyprogesterone 2.5-10 mg/day) continuously or intermittently
	Imipramine (10-25 mg tid)		May worsen cardiac conduction abnormalities, postural hypotension, anticholinergic effects	Combined oral or vaginal estrogen and PPA in postmenopausal women if single drug is inadequate; imipramine is an alternative therapy when first-line therapy is inadequate
Overflow incontinence	Alpha-adrenergic antagonists	Terazosin (1 mg at bedtime with first dose in supine position and increase by 1 mg every 4 days to 5 mg/day)	Postural hypotension, dizziness, vertigo, heart palpitations, edema, headache, anticholinergic effects	Possible benefit in men with obstructive symptoms of benign prostatic hyperplasia; monitor postural vital signs with first dose/each dose increase; may worsen female stress incontinence
		Doxazosin (1 mg at bedtime with first dose in supine position and increase by 1 mg every 7-14 days to 5 mg/day)	Same as terazosin (may be smaller incidence of hypotension)	Same as terazosin

From Ouslander J et al: *Urinary incontinence clinical practice guidelines,* Columbia, Maryland, 1996, American Medical Directors Association.

TABLE 24-5 Urodynamic Diagnostic Tests to Evaluate UI

Test	Uses
Simple cystometry	Detects detrusor contractions and abnormalities in bladder compliance, and determines postvoid residual and bladder capacity
Cystometry	Assesses bladder sensation, capacity, and compliance and estimates voluntary and involuntary detrusor contractions
Cystometrogram (CMG), multichannel or subtracted	Determines total bladder, intraabdominal, and true detrusor pressures; distinguishes source of pressure (detrusor, intraabdominal)
Voiding CMG	Measures detrusor and urethral pressures during voiding
Uroflowmetry	Identifies abnormal voiding patterns
Urethral pressure profilemetry	Measures resting and dynamic urethral pressures
Electromyography	Measures integrity and function of urethral innervation

- The presence of other comorbid conditions, such as the following:
  Incontinence associated with recurrent symptomatic UTI
  Persistent symptoms of difficult bladder emptying
  History of previous antiincontinence surgery or radical pelvic surgery
  Pelvic prolapse
  Prostate nodule, asymmetry, or other suspicion of prostate cancer
  Abnormal PVR urine
  Neurologic condition such as multiple sclerosis and spinal cord lesions or injury (Fantl et al., 1996)

A variety of surgical procedures may be appropriate for a particular incontinent older person. If urine control has not been achieved with behavioral intervention, the patient should be referred for additional evaluation of the incontinence and, if appropriate, to a urologist. Urodynamic tests, which are summarized in Table 24-5, require referral to a practitioner with specialized training in urine control problems. Table 24-6 outlines the various therapeutic techniques for each type of incontinence, including recommendations for and against various treatments. Box 24-4 suggests some helpful interventions for noninstitutionalized older people in controlling incontinence; many of these principles are also applicable in hospital and long-term care settings.

Summary

Urinary incontinence is not a normal consequence of aging and can be the cause of much embarrassment, expense, comorbidity, and loss of function for the older adult. Knowledge of the genitourinary anatomy and physiology is necessary to understand the pathophysiology of the various types of incontinence. A patient history, including bladder records, and a physical examination help the practitioner determine which type of

TABLE 24-6 Summary of Therapeutic Interventions

	Recommendation For	Recommendation Against
Behavioral Interventions		
Routine/scheduled toileting	Routine/scheduled toileting on a consistent schedule for patients who cannot participate in independent toileting.	
Habit training	Habit training for patients for whom a natural voiding pattern can be determined.	
Prompted voiding	Prompted voiding in patients who can learn to recognize some degree of bladder fullness or the need to void, or who can ask for assistance or respond when prompted to toilet. Patients who are appropriate for prompted voiding may not have sufficient cognitive ability to participate in other, more complex behavioral therapies.	
Bladder training	Bladder training strongly recommended for management of urge and mixed incontinence. Also recommended for management of stress urinary incontinence (SUI).	
Pelvic muscle rehabilitation	PMEs strongly recommended for women with SUI. PMEs recommended in men and women in conjunction with bladder training for urge incontinence. PMEs may also benefit men who develop UI following prostatectomy. Pelvic muscle rehabilitation and bladder inhibition using biofeedback therapy for patients with stress UI, urge UI, and mixed UI. Vaginal weight training for SUI in premenopausal women. Pelvic floor electrical stimulation has been shown to decrease incontinence in women with SUI and may be useful for urge and mixed incontinence.	

From Fantl JA et al: *Quick reference guide for clinicians: managing acute and chronic urinary incontinence,* AHCPR Pub 96-0686, Rockville, Md, 1996, US Department of Health and Human Services, Public Health Service, Agency for Health Care Policy and Research.

Continued

TABLE 24-6 Summary of Therapeutic Interventions—cont'd

	Recommendation For	Recommendation Against
Long-Term Management of Chronic Intractable UI		
Physical and environmental alterations	Caregiver assessment of the environment in which the elderly or disabled patient resides. Simple alterations or the addition of toileting or ambulation devices to eliminate or reduce episodes of involuntary urine loss. Strategies that maintain or improve mobility to prevent or reduce incontinent episodes in the frail elderly.	
Fluid and dietary management	A bowel regimen based on adequate fiber and fluid intake. Elimination of bowel impaction and consequent pressure on the bladder and urethra as necessary first steps in the treatment of chronic UI.	
Management of nocturia	Preventive measures to decrease nighttime voids. Simple electronic urine detection devices for more efficient and effective patient monitoring of nighttime urine loss.	
Interventions for protection and comfort	Most absorbent and skin-friendly products. However, no scientific literature was found to guide in selection of the most effective product. Intermittent catheterization preferable to indwelling catheters for the management of urinary retention and overflow incontinence. Suprapubic catheters as alternative for indwelling urethral catheters when patient choice or circumstances require the use of a bladder drainage device.	
Skin care	Standard measures of cleansing the skin immediately before and after urine loss. Most absorbent and skin-friendly pads and garments for protection from skin damage.	

Public and Professional Education		
	Comprehensive and multidisciplinary patient education about incontinence and all management alternatives. More research to test the effectiveness of patient education activities. Inclusion of education about UI evaluation and treatment in the basic curricula of undergraduate and graduate training programs of all health care providers. Continuing education programs on UI for health care providers.	
Other Measures and Supportive Devices		
Intermittent catheterization	Intermittent catheterization (IC) as a supportive measure for patients with spinal cord injury, persistent UI, or with chronic urinary retention secondary to underactive or partially obstructed bladder. Clean technique for IC in young, male neurologically impaired individuals. Sterile technique for IC for elderly patients and patients with compromised immune system.	Routine use of long-term suppressive therapy with antibiotics in patients with chronic, clean IC. In high-risk populations (e.g., those with internal prosthesis or those who are immunosuppressed due to age or disease), the use of antibiotic therapy for asymptomatic bacteriuria must be individually reviewed.
Indwelling catheters	As a supportive measure for patients whose incontinence is caused by obstruction and for whom other interventions are not feasible. Incontinent patients who are terminally ill or for patients with pressure ulcers as short-term treatment. In severely impaired individuals in whom alternative interventions are not an option and when a patient lives alone and a caregiver is unavailable to provide other supportive measures.	
Suprapubic catheters	For short-term use following gynecologic, urologic, and other surgery, or as an alternative to long-term catheter use.	In persons with chronic unstable bladder (DI, DH) and ISD.

From Fantl JA et al: *Quick reference guide for clinicians: managing acute and chronic urinary incontinence,* AHCPR Pub 96-0686, Rockville, Md, 1996, US Department of Health and Human Services, Public Health Service, Agency for Health Care Policy and Research.

Continued

Table 24-6 Summary of Therapeutic Interventions—cont'd

	Recommendation For	Recommendation Against
Other Measures and Supportive Devices—cont'd		
External collection systems	For incontinent men and women who have adequate bladder emptying. who have intact genital skin. in whom other therapies have failed or are not appropriate.	
Penile compression devices	Penile compression devices are known to be used in clinical practice in the treatment of UI. No scientific literature was found to support the use of these devices. The panel recognizes the temporary use of penile compression devices in males in selected circumstances under the supervision of a health care provider.	
Pelvic organ support devices	Pessaries for women who have symptomatic pelvic organ prolapse.	Data are not available to recommend or discourage the use of pessaries for the treatment of UI in women.
Absorbent products	During evaluation. As an adjunct to other therapy. For long-term care of patients with chronic, intractable UI.	
Surgical Treatment		
Stress incontinence	Surgery is recommended for treatment of stress incontinence in men and women and may be recommended as first-line treatment for appropriately selected patients and those who are unable to comply with other nonsurgical therapies.	
Hypermobility in women	Retropubic or needle suspension for women with hypermobility when SUI is the primary indication for surgery. On the basis of greater efficacy, these procedures are recommended over anterior vaginal repair for hypermobility.	

Intrinsic sphincter deficiency (ISD) in women	Sling procedures for women who have ISD with coexisting hypermobility or as first-line treatment for ISD. Periurethral bulking injections as first-line treatment for women with ISD who do not have coexisting hypermobility. Artificial sphincter for ISD patients who are unable to perform intermittent catheterization and have severe SUI that is unresponsive to other surgical treatments. Because of the high complication rate, this treatment is rarely used as primary therapy.	
ISD in men	Periurethral bulking injections as a first-line surgical treatment for men with ISD. Artificial sphincter for ISD during the 6 months after prostatectomy. Behavioral intervention should also be tried during this period.	
Urge incontinence: detrusor instability	Augmentation intestinocystoplasty for those with intractable, severe bladder instability or for those with bladders that have poor compliance when the patient is unresponsive to other nonsurgical therapies. Urinary diversion is recommended in severe intractable cases of detrusor instability that is unresponsive to other therapies.	
Overflow incontinence: bladder neck or urethral obstruction	Symptoms of overflow or incontinence secondary to obstruction should be addressed with a surgical procedure to relieve the obstruction. Intermittent catheterization or an indwelling catheter in patients who are not candidates for surgery.	The panel found no evidence to support the use of urethral dilation for treating incontinence in women, although it may be useful in the extremely rare cases of primary obstruction. Internal urethrotomy for treating urethral obstruction in women.

From Fantl JA et al: *Quick reference guide for clinicians: managing acute and chronic urinary incontinence,* AHCPR Pub 96-0686, Rockville, Md, 1996, US Department of Health and Human Services, Public Health Service, Agency for Health Care Policy and Research.

Box 24-4

Helpful Interventions for Noninstitutionalized Elders to Control or Eliminate Incontinence

Empty bladder completely before and after meals and at bedtime.

Urinate whenever the urge arises; never ignore it.

A schedule of urinating every 2 hours during the day and every 4 hours at night is often helpful in retraining the bladder. An alarm clock may be necessary.

Drink 1½ to 2 quarts of fluid a day before 8 PM. This helps the kidneys to function properly. Limit fluids after supper to ½ to 1 cup (except in very hot weather).

Drink cranberry juice or take vitamin C to help acidify the urine and lower the chances of bladder infection.

Eliminate or reduce the use of coffee, tea, cola, and alcohol, which have a diuretic effect.

Take prescription diuretics in the morning upon rising.

Limit the use of sleeping pills, sedatives, and alcohol, which decrease sensation to urinate and can increase incontinence, especially at night.

If overweight, lose weight.

Exercises to strengthen pelvic muscles that help support the bladder are often helpful for women.

Make sure the toilet is nearby with a clear path and good lighting, especially at night. Grab bars or a raised toilet seat may be needed.

Dress protectively with cotton underwear, sanitary pads for women, and protective pants or incontinent pads if necessary.

From Ebersole P, Hess P: *Toward healthy aging: human needs and nursing response,* ed 5, St. Louis, 1998, Mosby.

incontinence the patient is exhibiting (stress, urge, overflow, functional, or mixed) and therefore help to guide the treatment plan. Although much of the evaluation and intervention can be carried out in the primary care setting, a referral to a urologist may be necessary to explore certain causes and modalities.

Resources

Bladder Health Foundation
c/o American Foundation for Urologic Disease
300 West Pratt Street, Suite 401
Baltimore, MD 21201
(800) 242-2383
(410) 727-2908

National Association for Continence
P.O. Box 8310
Spartanburg, SC 29305
(800) BLADDER

Simon Foundation for Continence
P.O. Box 835
Wilmette, IL 60091
(800) 23-SIMON

References

Fantl JA et al: *Urinary incontinence in adults: acute and chronic management. Clinical practice guideline 2,* 1996 update, AHCPR pub 96-0682, Rockville, Md, 1996, US Department of Health and Human Services, Public Health Service, Agency for Health Care Policy and Research.

Ireton RC et al: Bladder volume determination using a dedicated, portable ultrasound scanner, *J Urol* 143:909-911, 1990.

Jay J, Staskin D: Urinary incontinence in women: strategies for effective diagnosis and treatment, *Adv Nurse Pract* 6(10):32-37, 1998.

Jirovec M: Effect of individualized prompted toileting on incontinence in nursing home residents, *Appl Nurs Res* 4:188-191, 1991.

Ouslander J et al: *Urinary incontinence: clinical practice guideline,* Silver Spring, Md, 1996, American Medical Directors Association.

Palmer MH: Incontinence: a major problem for patients, a major concern for OBRA, *Nurs Home Med* 4(9):260-267, 1996.

Weiss BD: Diagnostic evaluation of urinary incontinence in geriatric patients, *Am Fam Physician* 57(11):2675-2684, 2688-2690, 1998.

25

Constipation

Constipation is a frequently cited problem in the elderly population, with more than 2.5 million annual visits to physicians made because of this complaint. This figure does not include the millions of self-treated people who use laxatives either routinely or during an acute occurrence. Studies have found that more than 30% of 60-year-old community-dwelling people are regular laxative users and that close to 30% of men and women over age 65 consider themselves to be constipated (Pettigrew, Watt, and Sheldon, 1997).

However, the definition of constipation is misunderstood and misinterpreted by both health care providers and patients. Although constipation in medical terms has been defined as a frequency of fewer than three bowel movements a week, a patient may define constipation as one or more of the following: straining at stool, painful bowel movements, perceived infrequent bowel movements, feelings of incomplete bowel movements, or loss of ability to recognize the urge to defecate. What is a normal pattern of bowel elimination for one person may constitute constipation for another.

Age-related Changes

Many age-related changes and other causes contribute to reports of constipation in older adults. A decreased motility of the colon, which leads to chronic slowing of transit time, may contribute to constipation. Decreased motility results in the diminished capacity of the muscles controlling bowel elimination to coordinate properly; which leads to pain, incomplete evacuation, and failure to defecate in spite of effort and urge (Wieman, 1997). Other causes are diseases that affect motility such as hypothyroidism, neurologic disorders such as Parkinson's disease or stroke, drugs, laxative habituation, psychologic disorders, and colorectal conditions (Box 25-1).

History

It is important to clarify what the patient is defining as constipation. Patients should be guided to include all dimensions of their constipation. A complete medical history, with particular emphasis on rectal bleeding and abdominal pain, must be carefully obtained from the patient during the review of systems. If the presentation is acute onset of constipation in a healthy elderly person, the practitioner should suspect a colonic obstruction (Barloon and Lu, 1997). A review of all of the patient's current medications, including all laxatives and over-the-counter (OTC) drugs, is an important consideration because many drugs can cause or contribute to constipation (Box 25-2).

Lifestyle factors, including diet, functional ability, cognitive status, exercise patterns, bowel hygiene, and living conditions need to be assessed (Fig. 25-1).

Box 25-1
Causes of Constipation

Acute-onset Constipation

Bowel obstruction
Colonic cancer
Cancers of gastrointestinal tract
Diverticulitis

Chronic Constipation

Age-related Changes

Slowed transit time
Decreased agility and mobility
Loss of muscle tone

Response to Diseases

Stroke
Parkinson's disease
Thyroid conditions
Irritable bowel syndrome

Response to Mental Health Conditions

Depression
Obsessive behaviors

Response to Medications

Laxative habituation

Environmental Factors

Institutional living
Lack of privacy
Lifestyle factors
Diet and hydration
Lack of exercise

Box 25-2
Drugs That Contribute to Constipation

- Antacids
  - Aluminum hydroxide
  - Calcium carbonate
- Anticholinergics
- Antidepressants (tricyclic)
- Antihistamines
- Barium
- Iron preparations
- Narcotics
- Verapamil
  - Pseudoephedrine

DIET

1. What high-fiber foods do you eat on a daily basis?
2. How many glasses of water do you drink during a normal day?
3. What fluids and how many glasses or cups of each do you drink in a normal day (e.g., 2 cups of coffee and 1 small glass of juice)?
4. What did you eat yesterday? Please list all meals and anything between meals.
5. Are you now or have you been in the last 6 months on any type of a diet?

EXERCISE

1. On a scale of 1 to 10, with 10 being the highest, how active do you consider yourself?
2. What physical activities do you participate in?
3. How often do you participate?
4. What hinders your participation in physical activities?

BOWEL HYGIENE

1. How long have you had problems moving your bowels?
2. Do you have a particular time that you usually move your bowels?
3. What do you do when you feel constipated?
4. Have you taken any laxatives or enemas during the past 7 days?
5. Do you take or use laxatives or enemas on most days?
6. What helps the most when you are constipated?

Figure 25-1 Lifestyle Assessment Tool. (Patient should complete before appointment.)

LIVING CONDITIONS

1. Do you live alone?

2. If not, with whom do you live?

3. Do you have free access to a bathroom?

4. Do you have enough privacy and time in the bathroom?

5. Are the conditions in the bathroom comfortable and pleasant?

FUNCTIONAL STATUS

1. Do you have any problems getting to the bathroom when you feel the urge to move your bowels?

2. Do you always realize you have the urge to move your bowels?

3. Do your bowels ever move when you are not expecting it?

Figure 25-1, cont'd For legend see opposite page.

Physical Examination and Diagnostic Testing

A focused examination centers on detecting a localized abdominal mass and local anorectal lesions such as internal or external hemorrhoids, an anal fistula, or a tumor. Confirmation of bowel sounds by auscultation is essential. Digital examination of the rectum and anal canal assesses the tone and strength of the internal and external sphincter and the puborectalis muscles. A patient with a fecal impaction often presents with a complaint of diarrhea. In these cases the digital examination finds hard, dry, rocklike stool in the rectal vault.

Flexible sigmoidoscopy may be appropriate for newly diagnosed patients, even if there is no report of rectal bleeding or pain (Cheskin and Schuster, 1994). Stool testing for occult blood (guaiac) should be part of the rectal examination in spite of the many false-positive results that occur.

In chronic constipation, abdominal radiographs can determine the extent of a fecal impaction (Barloon and Lu, 1997). In half of 98 study patients with severe constipation, physiologic testing (defecography and transit time studies) added significant information; surprisingly, the pretest history and symptoms did not predict which patients were likely to benefit from the studies (Halverson and Orkin, 1998).

Acute onset of constipation may suggest colonic obstruction, and abdominal radiographs are sufficient to determine the level and, at times, the cause of the obstruction. To rule out more serious conditions, constipated patients with occult or gross rectal bleeding, patients with complaints of a change in bowel habits, and patients who complain of abdominal pain should be referred for barium enemas and colonoscopy.

Conditions to Consider

- Fecal impaction
- Diverticulitis
- Anal stricture
- Hemorrhoids
- Bowel obstruction
- Colon cancer

Treatment

1. If causal, treat the underlying disease such as hypothyroidism.
2. If medication is suspected, change or stop medication.
3. For nonpathologic constipation, first try a lifestyle modification (step 1):
   Diet and fluid
   Exercise
   Fiber supplements (e.g., Metamucil)
   Relaxed, unhurried toilet time after breakfast or dinner
4. If the first attempt at lifestyle changes fails or does not produce improvement, try step 2: add Milk of Magnesia at bedtime, which is to be used *only* during the beginning phase of the modification program. The goal is to continue the education and support needed to assist in the lifestyle change.
5. If the patient is found to have an impaction, the following treatments are appropriate:
   Digital disimpaction
   Suppositories
     Glycerin
   Enemas
     Oil retention
6. Education, support, and follow-up

Laxatives

Unless the constipation complaint is acute and of fairly sudden onset, the patient most likely has been self-medicating for a significant period of time. In a nonthreatening and nonaccusatory manner, obtain an accurate history to include all alternative treatments. It is usually safe to start with the premise that most patients whose complaint is constipation are already using laxatives. Trying to get the patient to stop or change to a less harmful laxative is actually more common than prescribing a laxative. It is essential to respect the patient's self-care practices by providing information that assists in decision making.

Five types of laxatives are now available to the general public in OTC medications. A review of 36 randomized trials of laxative or fiber therapies with a treatment duration of at least 1 week concluded that both fiber and laxatives modestly improved bowel movement frequency in adults with chronic constipation. There was inadequate evidence to establish whether fiber was more effective than laxatives, and no one laxative class was superior (Tramonte et al., 1997). Interestingly, lifestyle modification was never included or combined with any of the treatment modalities.

Bulk-forming products (bran and psyllium mucilloid [Metamucil]) are the first choice for treatment of constipation. They tend to increase stool mass and soften its consistency. The dose needs to be adjusted to 15 g fiber, and each dose has to be taken with 8 oz of fluids. The side effects of bulk laxatives include flatus, cramping, bloating and, in extreme cases, obstruction related to inadequate fluid intake (Ferlotti, 1997). The normal American diet is deficient in fiber, and foods high in fiber should be stressed, such as bran cereal, beans (baked, kidney, lima, and navy), fruits (prunes and prune juice), and vegetables.

Emollients or stool softeners are usually considered the second step in treatment to relieve idiopathic constipation (Cheskin and Schuster, 1994). Docusate or dioctyl sodium sulfosuccinate (Colace) works by lowering surface tension and allowing water to enter the stool. These preparations are safe, well tolerated, and quite useful for even bed-bound elderly patients. By contrast, mineral oil is not safe and is not generally recommended; it may impede the absorption of fat-soluble vitamins and increase the risk of pneumonia by aspiration, especially in the elderly impaired population.

Saline and electrolyte laxatives and enemas are OTC treatments and used by the public as Milk of Magnesia and Fleet Enema. These preparations are contraindicated for people with impaired renal function (Wieman, 1997).

Stimulant laxatives are common and habituating. Senna (Senokot) and bisacodyl (Dulcolax) are effective but carry the risk of electrolyte imbalance and long-term toxicity. Bisacodyl has less toxicity than other stimulant laxatives.

GoLYTELY and Colyte are lavage laxatives; these relatively new types of preparations, are used mainly as bowel preparation before procedures.

Summary

Complaints of constipation should be treated with respect and with an understanding of the possible dangers of not attending to this concern. Follow-up either by telephone or during the next visit will acknowledge concern for a problem that has the potential to be a frequent irritant for the elderly person or, at the other extreme, may pose a serious yet unrecognized health threat.

Resources

Henry Ford Health System
Patient Information Web Site
http://www.henryfordhealth.org/cancer/constipation.htm

American Gastroenterological Association
http://www.gastro.org

References

Barloon TJ, Lu CC: Diagnostic imaging in the evaluation, *Am Fam Physician* 56(2):513-520, 1997.

Cheskin L, Schuster M: Constipation. In Hazzard WM et al, editors: *Principles of geriatric medicine and gerontology,* New York, 1994, McGraw-Hill.

Ferlotti T: Bowel elimination. In Burke M, Walsh M, editors: *Gerontologic nursing: wholistic care of the older adult,* ed 2, St Louis, 1997, Mosby.

Halverson AL, Orkin BA: Which physiologic tests are useful in patients with constipation? *Dis Colon Rectum* 41(6):735-739, 1998.

Pettigrew M, Watt I, Sheldon T: Systematic review of the effectiveness of laxatives in the elderly, *Health Technol Assess* 1(13):1-52, 1997.

Tramonte SM et al: The treatment of chronic constipation in adults: a systematic review, *J Gen Intern Med* 12(1):13-24, 1997.

Wieman HM: Constipation. In Ham R, Sloane P, editors: *Primary care geriatrics: a case-based approach,* ed 3, St Louis, 1997, Mosby.

Unit IV

26

Driving

The number of older drivers in the United States is increasing. As with people of all ages, older people prefer to travel by car, reserving public transportation for only about 3% of their trips (Eberhard, 1998). Individuals over age 65 account for approximately 13% of both the population (33 million older people) and the number of licensed drivers (22 million older drivers). By 2020 approximately 22 million people over age 75 will be eligible for a driver's license, and 7 million of these individuals will be age 85 or older (American Association of Motor Vehicle Administrators, 1998).

The absolute number of crashes involving older drivers is lower than the crash rate for the entire population of drivers. However, when adjusted for the relatively low mileage driven by older people the number of crashes per mile driven is comparatively high (Marottoli et al., 1998). The roadways most often used by older drivers involve lower speeds but have more intersections and more opportunities for vehicle-to-vehicle conflict. Thus older drivers are exposed to more potential crash situations per mile than the average driver, who more often uses interstate highways and other major roadways (Janke, 1991). In the absence of certain medical conditions, age alone has not been shown to correlate with poor driving performance, but there is evidence to suggest that the skills needed for safe driving begin to deteriorate in later years (Adler, 1997).

Of great concern is the increased likelihood of injury, hospitalization, and death among older individuals following a crash (Evans, 1988). Drivers over age 80 who are involved in a crash are four to eight times more likely to be seriously injured or killed than are younger persons (Eberhard, 1998).

Although 16 states and the District of Columbia have established legal restrictions or policies for drivers once they have reached a certain age (Adler, 1997), the standard licensing and renewal procedures in most states do not adequately assess the ability of an older person to operate a motor vehicle safely. Unless an individual has been involved in an at-fault accident, the Department of Motor Vehicles (DMV) in most states will probably never be prompted to investigate an older person's capabilities behind the wheel. At that point (if not before), the primary care provider may be asked by the state's DMV or even family members to perform an assessment and make recommendations regarding the patient's ability to drive. Most providers have never received training in how best to assess a patient's ability to perform this complicated task. There are no standardized testing procedures, and very few resources provide helpful information. The practitioner needs to be aware of the required skills and potential impact of various factors on a person's ability to operate a motor vehicle safely. It is important to know who should be assessed, how to assess them, and how to proceed appropriately, on the basis of findings. Many people at risk can benefit from interventions to improve their driving safety and thus maintain their driving privileges. Others may be deemed unsafe behind the wheel. Just as a young person views a driver's license as a rite of passage into the adult world of independence, when elderly drivers are deprived of their license, it is viewed as a loss of independence and even identity.

Age-related Risk Factors

A complex interaction of both human (personal) and situational (contextual) factors may affect safety (Galski, Ehle, and Williams, 1998). When examining the risk of adverse outcomes from the operation of a motor vehicle, an epidemiologic approach should be considered. Epidemiologists consider three "players" in the evaluation of the risk of any accident or injury: the agent, the host, and the environment.

In this case, the agent is the car: its motion and maneuverability, its mechanical reliability, and all of the skills required for its successful operation. The host is the elderly driver, with all of his or her capabilities and limitations in mastering and maintaining the necessary skills, both in a general sense and at any given moment while driving the car. The environment includes such factors as weather and road conditions. Less than ideal circumstances in any one of these players makes the operation of the vehicle more difficult, with less chance of a desirable outcome (i.e., the driver arriving at the chosen destination safely and without incident). Complications in any combination of these factors will cumulatively increase the risk of an adverse outcome (e.g., a crash).

Studies of older drivers have focused on the host (the older driver) and the environment and have found that several factors affect the outcomes within these areas.

The Host

A driver must possess a variety of physical and cognitive functions in order to successfully perform the complicated task of operating a motor vehicle. Motor difficulties such as a loss of strength, coordination, and reaction speed can have serious effects on a person's ability to operate a motor vehicle. Steering, braking, shifting, and monitoring surrounding traffic require certain physical skills such as mobility and strength in the neck, torso, and extremities. Brisk reaction is required to brake urgently or to swerve to avoid an obstacle or collision. Recent and recurrent falls have proven to be a reliable predictor of driving difficulty (Sims et al., 1998). Table 26-1 lists the common physical limitations of elderly drivers and some intervention options.

In many studies sensory deficits, such as those of visual or auditory acuity, have been demonstrated to be a factor in driving performance. Besides near and distance vision, other aspects of vision such as glare and contrast sensitivity, motion perception, and visual field perception play important roles (Galski, Ehle, and Williams, 1998). Drivers with greater than 40% reduction in the visual field are five times more likely to have an accident (Walston, 1998). Hearing loss impairs the driver's awareness of surrounding traffic and ability to respond to the horns of other cars that are sounded in warning.

TABLE 26-1 Common Physical Limitations of Elderly Drivers

Problem	Impact on Driving	Options
Limited neck ROM	Decreased ability to turn head for visual checks; impairments in seeing cars, traffic signs, and pedestrians	OTR/RPT to increase ROM and strength; driving program or vendor for special mirrors
Limited shoulder ROM	Difficulty or inability to fasten seat belt; difficulty turning the steering wheel	OTR/RPT to increase ROM and strength; OTR to modify seat belt for independent use
Arthritic changes in hand	Difficulty opening car door and grasping/turning keys	OTR key holder, door opener devices; driving program or vendor for steering device, built-up steering wheel, modified dashboard knobs
Impaired or nonfunctional upper limb	Unsafe steering with one hand, especially in turns or emergencies; unsafe operation of transmission shift lever or turn signals	Driving program or vendor for steering device, cross-over transmission, or turn signal lever
Lower back syndrome or orthopedic changes	Impaired visual checks; limited driving; decreased concentration	OTR/RPT to increase strength, flexibility, and positioning; driving program or vendor for lumbar supports, rearview mirror
Lower extremity impairment	Difficulty lifting legs in and out of car; difficulty lifting foot up from low accelerator pedal to high brake pedal	OTR/RPT to increase ROM and strength, modify transfer technique; driving program or vendor for foot pedal extensions, left foot accelerator
Cognitive	Slow information processing and delayed or impaired judgments; impaired recognition of unsafe driving practices	OTR for cognitive evaluation and training; driving program or motor vehicles department to road test for a minimum of 30 min

From Yoshikawa TT, Cobbs EL, Brummel-Smith K: *Ambulatory geriatric care,* St Louis, 1997, Mosby.
OTR, Occupational therapist, registered; *ROM,* range of motion; *RPT,* registered physical therapist.

Driving is a demanding task that requires a person to possess and use many cognitive-perceptual skills and abilities at generally higher levels of intensity in all conditions. Cognitive impairments—for example, problems with attention, scanning, speed in information processing, visuospatial perception, and decision making—have an impact on a person's ability to recognize and react appropriately to the many stimuli received at each moment when driving.

Personality and behavioral disturbances that may cause anxiety or impulsivity can also affect a person's ability to make safe and accurate judgments when driving a car (Galski, Ehle, and Williams, 1998). Boxes 26-1 and 26-2 outline the medical conditions and medications that may affect driving ability.

Box 26-1

Medical Conditions That May Affect Driving Ability

- Cardiac disease
- Memory loss or dementia
- Diabetes
- Parkinson's disease
- Seizure disorder
- Stroke
- Glaucoma and macular degeneration
- Sleep apnea

Source: Marottoli RA et al: Development of a test battery to identify older drivers at risk for self-reported adverse driving events, *J Am Geriatr Soc* 46:562-568, 1998; Eberhard JW: Driving is transportation for most older adults, *Geriatrics* 53 (suppl 1):S53-55, 1998.

Box 26-2

Drugs That May Affect Driving Ability

- Antidepressants
- Benzodiazepines
- Antihistamines
- Alcohol
- Any other drug that can cause sedation or drowsiness

The Environment

Driving is regarded as more demanding in some situations than in others, depending on contextual determinants such as type of driving (e.g., highway, city, residential), density of traffic (Galski, Ehle, and Williams, 1998), weather, and road conditions. Research has centered on the situational determinants of accidents, such as the effects of road designs and highway surfaces (i.e., the environment). Results of this research have shown that accidents in all populations of drivers tend to occur in specific locations (e.g., intersections), and under specific conditions (e.g., glare). In addition, certain operations such as left-turning and right-of-way decisions tend to lead to more accidents (Galski, Ehle, and Williams, 1998). These findings, especially in regard to the negotiation of intersections, have also proven true in studies of older drivers.

When assessing a patient's ability to drive, the provider should determine the type of driving the patient does most often. Studies have shown that driving on the highway demands significantly greater speed and accuracy in information-processing and passing skills, whereas city driving demands greater stopping and braking skills (Galski, Ehle, and Williams, 1998). This information helps to guide the assessment of the patient's ability to drive. Box 26-3 lists the errors commonly made by older drivers.

An awareness of the type of behavior that prompted an evaluation will enable the practitioner to appropriately evaluate the situation. Referrals are often prompted by a

Box 26-3

Common Driving Errors in Older Drivers

Difficulty backing up and making turns
Not seeing traffic signs or other cars quickly enough
Difficulty in locating and retrieving information from dashboard displays and traffic signs
Delayed glare recovery when driving at night
Not checking rearview mirrors and blind spots
Bumping into curbs and objects
Not yielding to oncoming traffic or right-of-way vehicles
Irregular or slow vehicle speeds
Difficulty with situations requiring quick decision making

From Yoshikawa TT, Cobbs EL, Brummel-Smith K: *Ambulatory geriatric care,* St Louis, 1997, Mosby.

police officer who has observed the older driver in behaviors or situations that cause concern, such as the following:

Driving the wrong way or on the wrong side of the road
Driving off the road
Rear-ending another vehicle
Failing to yield the right of way or come to a complete stop at a stop sign
Infringing on the rights of a pedestrian or cyclist
Turning across the path of oncoming vehicles
Crossing lane markings
Operating at a low speed
Backing improperly

Once the police officer has made contact with the driver, the following behaviors suggest the need for further evaluation:

Aberrant behavior (e.g., taking too long to pull over or difficulty in producing identification)
Attention deficit (unawareness of what he or she did that resulted in a violation or crash)
Cognitive deficit (lack of recall, inability to comprehend or to follow the rules of the road)
Medical problems (e.g., black outs, diabetes, Parkinson's disease, seizure, stroke)
Mental problems (e.g., slow reflexes, inappropriate manipulation of controls such as brake and accelerator)
Sensory deficits (impaired vision or hearing, poor depth perception, degraded night vision, recent eye surgery, cataracts)

Assessment

History

A thorough medical history is important to ascertain risk factors as well as any medical conditions or medications that may affect a driver's capabilities behind the wheel. Functional status provides important information regarding the patient's general abilities. Information regarding recent or recurrent falls is very significant.

A driving history inquires about driving habits and problems. Driving habits may include frequency, distance, and circumstances of travel; the use of a copilot; and familiarity with roadways used. Problems may include getting lost, becoming angry or confused while driving, or a history of accidents, traffic violations, and near misses. The observations and concerns of family members may provide additional information, especially if the patient is unaware of or denying the deficits (Adler, 1997). It is also helpful to elicit details about any prior accidents in which the patient was involved (if he or she is forthcoming with this information). This background may reveal impairments in physical function or judgment that were previously undetected (e.g., a failure to see traffic approaching from the side or to recognize road signs).

Physical Examination

The physical examination should assess overall function as well as the presence of any medical conditions that may affect driving abilities. In one study by Marottoli et al. (1998), three factors were associated with the occurrence of an adverse event: an inability to copy a design from a brief mental status test, walking fewer blocks, and the presence of foot abnormalities. The study also showed that the factors most closely associated with a self-reported history of adverse driving events were poor near visual acuity, poor visual attention, and limited neck rotation. Neck rotation is important in detecting cars or objects to the side of or behind a vehicle, particularly at intersections or when merging, areas in which older people typically have problems. Box 26-4 shows elements of the physical examination, including tools used in the assessment of driving ability.

Assessment Tools

One helpful screening tool is the number cancellation test to measure visual attention, an important skill for scanning the visual field for road hazards while driving (Marottoli et al., 1998). The Mini-Mental State Examination is an excellent screening tool for memory and attention. The clock-drawing test elicits information regarding executive functioning. The geriatric depression scale helps to determine the presence of a mood disorder, which may affect judgment and cognitive function.

Some occupational therapists are skilled in performing driving assessments and can provide additional information. Where available, a driving evaluator (e.g., veteran's association, private, or DMV) can also make recommendations.

Interventions

Often an assessment of driving skills does not lead to a clear-cut decision about a person's ability to operate a motor vehicle. There may be appropriate "between ground" of unrestricted driving vs. no driving at all. The practitioner's evaluation may be used to determine that a person has ubiquitous driving capacity (i.e., fit to drive in any situation) or only situation-specific driving capacity (i.e., fit to drive in certain situations). Recommendations may range from unconditional motor vehicle operation to stipulated driving to complete abstinence from driving (Galski, Ehle, and Williams, 1998). In stipulated driving, a person is restricted to situations for which he or she has the requisite

Box 26-4

Elements of Physical Examination in Assessing Driving Ability

General

Appearance
Affect (Geriatric Depression Scale)
Thought content

Sensory

Hearing
Vision
  Near and far vision
  Field of vision

Cardiac

Murmurs, carotid bruits, etc.

Musculoskeletal

Range of motion (neck, torso, extremities)
Strength
Gait
Time Distance Walking Test

Neurologic

Including the number cancellation test, Mini-Mental State Examination, and clock-drawing test

abilities: within his or her familiar community, in good weather, only daytime, and in areas with no four-way intersections. Whether the provider's findings must be reported to motor vehicle authorities depends on state-determined reporting guidelines. Fourteen states and Canadian provinces currently require health care providers to report to licensing agencies any medical conditions hazardous to driving: California, Delaware (epilepsy), Georgia, Nevada (epilepsy), New Jersey, Oregon, Pennsylvania, Manitoba, New Brunswick, Northwest Territories, Ontario, Prince Edward Island, Saskatchewan, and the Yukon Territory. All grant the practitioner immunity from legal action by the driver (American Association of Motor Vehicle Administrators, 1998).

Specific interventions may be instituted on the basis of the individual's needs. For example, drivers with a field of view in the range of 45 to 70 degrees to either side can install special mirrors to partially compensate for the loss of peripheral vision. Referral to physical and occupational therapy often helps to improve strength, mobility, and motor functioning, thereby preserving driving ability. A few programs are available to assist older drivers to stay on the road safely for as long as possible. One of these is the AARP "55 Alive" program, which provides education that attempts to refine existing skills and to develop defensive techniques for the older driver. This 8-hour course is taught in two 4-hour sessions spanning 2 days; the cost is $8. Drivers completing the course may be eligible for discounts on their auto insurance premiums.

Recommendations should be reviewed with patients and family members. The older person who is still able to drive should be educated about risky driving times and patterns to be avoided. The evaluation should be repeated periodically. A person with advanced cognitive impairment who has been judged to be incapable of driving safely and who continues to have access to an automobile may require creative interventions to maintain this person's safety and dignity. The primary provider needs to work with family members to reach a successful solution to this dilemma.

The loss of a driver's license can seriously affect an older person's ability to take care of day-to-day needs. It can lead to social isolation and depression (Adler, 1997). Information about public or private transportation may help the higher risk driver find acceptable alternatives. The involvement of available family members and friends may also provide an alternative transportation system for the older person. A consultation with an experienced social worker may help to address the objections and frustrations associated with the loss of a driver's license and locate alternative transportation resources (Adler, 1997). Table 26-2 lists resources for older drivers.

Summary

Evaluation of the older person's ability to drive a car safely is a skill for which most providers have not received adequate training. The decision to limit or revoke a license to drive can be devastating to the older person who relies on a car for social, professional, and medical contact, as well as routine functioning. However, it is crucial to the health and well-being of the patient, family, and other drivers on the road to prevent unsafe drivers from placing themselves and others in hazardous situations. Several specific aspects of function have been shown to play a role in the ability to drive safely. Most of these can be assessed effectively in the office of the primary care provider so that appropriate recommendations can be made regarding the person's ability to continue driving.

Resources

American Association of Motor Vehicle Administrators
4301 Wilson Blvd., Suite 400
Arlington, VA 22203
(703) 908-5774

American Association of Retired Persons
AARP 55 Alive
601 E Street NW
Washington, DC 20049
(202) 434-2277
http://www.aarp.org

National Safety Council
1121 Spring Lake Drive
Itasca, IL 60143-3201
Phone: (630) 285-1121
Fax: (630) 285-1315
http://safety.webfirst.com

TABLE 26-2 Resources for Older Drivers

Resource	Service
The Handicapped Driver's Mobility Guide American Automobile Association Traffic Safety Department 1000 AAA Drive Heathrow, FL 32746 Approximately $5.95	Provides state-by-state listing of driver evaluation programs, including those with an occupational therapist, driver instructors, vehicle modification vendors, and basic guidelines for vehicle modification
A Flexibility Fitness Training Package for Improving Older Driver Performance (pamphlet) American Automobile Association Foundation for Traffic Safety 1730 M Street, N.W., Suite 401 Washington, DC 20036	Provides written directions and diagrams for flexibility exercises for the neck, shoulder, trunk, and back specific to driving
Reporting Alzheimer's Disease and Related Disorders: Guidelines for Physicians State of California Health and Welfare Agency Department of Health Services PO Box 942732 Sacramento, CA 94234	Provides reporting guidelines and legal information for patients with dementia; although specific to California law, it is generally useful for determining interventions
Perceptual Motor Evaluation for Head Injured and Other Neurological Impaired Adults Santa Clara Valley Medical Center Occupational Therapy Department 751 South Bascom Avenue San Jose, CA 95128 Approximately $15.00	Provides directions for administering gross visual screenings and other perceptual motor tests and includes an established scoring system
Drivers 55 Plus: Test Your Own Performance (booklet) *55 Alive/Mature Driving* (pamphlet) Publication No. PF3798(791). D934 American Association of Retired Persons 601 E Street, N.W. Washington, DC 20049	Provides self-test booklet for older drivers, materials on the 55 Alive/Mature Driving Program for both participants and prospective instructors, and other miscellaneous materials
U.S. Department of Transportation National Highway Traffic Safety Administration 400 Seventh Street, N.W. Washington, DC 20590	Provides consumer information in brochures or newsletters about traffic safety for older drivers; gathers data; conducts research; institutes plans for national highway traffic safety of older drivers
Older Driver Resource Directory Circular #385 National Research Council 2101 Constitution Ave., N.W. Washington, DC 20418	Provides domestic and international listing of persons and agencies involved with older drivers

From Yoshikawa TT, Cobbs EL, Brummel-Smith K: *Ambulatory geriatric care,* St Louis, 1997, Mosby.

References

Adler G: Driving and dementia: dilemmas and decisions, *Geriatrics* 52(suppl 2):S26-29, 1997.

American Association of Motor Vehicle Administrators: *Transportation in an Aging Society*, Arlington, Va., 1998, The Association.

Eberhard JW: Driving is transportation for most older adults, *Geriatrics* 53(suppl 1):S53-55, 1998.

Evans L: Older driver involvement in fatal and severe traffic crashes, *J Gerontol* 43:S186-193, 1988.

Galski T, Ehle HT, Williams B: Estimates of driving abilities and skills in different conditions, *Am J Occup Ther* 52(4):268-275, 1998.

Janke MK: Accidents, mileage, and the exaggeration of risk, *Accid Anal Prev* 23(2-3):183-188, 1991.

Marottoli RA et al: Development of a test battery to identify older drivers at risk for self-reported adverse driving events, *J Am Geriatr Soc* 46:562-568, 1998.

Sims R, Owsley C et al: A preliminary assessment of the medical and functional factors associated with vehicle crashes by older adults, *J Am Geriatr Soc* 46:556-561, 1998.

Walston J: *The elderly driver*, presentation at Current Topics in Gerontology, Johns Hopkins Geriatrics Center, Baltimore, October 1998.

27

Alcohol Abuse

Of the 26 to 30 million people in the United States over age 65, 4% to 8% are estimated to abuse alcohol; and approximately one third of these people began to problem drink after age 65. Alcoholism is the third most prevalent psychiatric disorder among elderly men, following dementia and anxiety disorders (Campbell, 1997). Health-related consequences of alcohol abuse include functional decline, dependency, and cognitive impairments that lead to excessive emergency department visits and hospitalization (Solomon et al., 1993). In one study hospitalizations related to alcohol accounted for 87,147 admissions (1.1% of total admissions); alcohol was the primary diagnosis in 33,039 of these hospitalizations, resulting in a total cost of more than $200 million in Medicare money (Adams et al., 1993). Other studies demonstrate that medical staff make the diagnosis of alcohol abuse in fewer than 25% of elderly patients who are abusing alcohol and refer to treatment fewer than half of those who are diagnosed (McInnes and Powell, 1994). Other factors contributing to low reporting rates are listed in Box 27-1.

Metabolism of Ethanol

Ethanol (the chemical component of consumable alcohol) has direct toxic effects on the gastrointestinal system, heart, kidney, brain, and liver. Oxidation of ethanol through the alcohol dehydrogenase pathway produces acetaldehyde, which is converted to acetate. Hydrogen is transferred from ethanol to a cofactor, nicotinamide adenine dinucleotide (NAD), which in turn is reduced to NADH. NADH is responsible for many of the metabolic problems associated with alcohol abuse: hyperlactacidemia, hyperuricemia, hypoglycemia, and hyperlipidemia (Nelson, 1998). Ethnic differences are an important consideration; 40% of Japanese—and perhaps other groups not yet studied—have aldehyde dehydrogenase deficiency and thereby are more susceptible to the effects of alcohol (Eisendrath, 1997).

Box 27-1
Factors Leading to Low Reporting of Alcohol Abuse in Older Adults

Underdiagnosis by health care providers
Denial of condition by patient
Unwillingness of family to report
Increased biologic sensitivity
Less interaction with social institutions
Less pressure to initiate treatment

Age-related Changes and Relationship to Alcohol Consumption

Gastrointestinal System

1. Atrophy of the gastric mucosa
2. Alteration of prostaglandin synthesis (which increases the risk for gastritis)
3. Decreased absorption of calcium, iron, lactose, and vitamin D
4. Increased absorption of fat-soluble compounds such as vitamins A and K and cholesterol
5. Decreasing liver mass
6. Decreased blood flow to the liver (approximately 10% per decade)
7. Blood concentration of alcohol that is increased disproportionately to the amount consumed because *the volume of distribution for alcohol is decreased* in the elderly

Cardiovascular System

1. Left ventricular muscle mass increases, and maximum heart rate declines.
2. Systolic and diastolic blood pressure increase with age (Reuben et al., 1996).
3. Incidence of atherosclerosis and atherosclerotic heart disease increases.
4. Alcohol consumption increases plasma triglyceride levels and elevates blood pressure.

Nervous System

1. Weight of the brain decreases.
2. Blood supply to the brain decreases.
3. The blood-brain barrier becomes more penetrable, increasing the sensitivity of elders to the central effects of alcohol.
4. The incidence of short-term memory loss and dementia increases with age.
5. Long-term alcoholism can produce dementia secondary to the nutritional deficit resulting from the alcoholism. Estimates are that 10% of dementia cases in the elderly are alcohol related (Campbell, 1997). Increasing blood alcohol levels have shown to be associated with progressively decreasing perception, and older subjects perform less well at all blood alcohol levels (Lieber, 1995).

Muscular and Skeletal Systems

1. Gait and balance impairments increase.
2. The incidence of falls in the elderly is high. Accidents are the sixth leading cause of death in the elderly, and two thirds of these deaths are related to falls.
3. In all age-groups alcohol plays a significant role in accidents, especially falls. Alcohol-related cognitive and physical effects contribute to gait and balance impairments and increase the risk of falls.
4. Alcohol is identified as a significant risk factor for the development of osteoporosis (Kimble, 1997).

Diagnostic Criteria

Substance dependence is defined as a maladaptive pattern of use in the presence of three of the seven elements of dependence within a 12-month period. The seven elements of dependence are tolerance, withdrawal, use of the substance in larger amounts and for a longer time than intended, a persistent desire to use and unsuccessful efforts to cut down, spending a great deal of time in obtaining the substance, giving up or reducing activities because of use, and continued use despite recurrent physical or psychologic problems caused by use (American Psychiatric Association, 1994).

Criteria for Alcohol Abuse

According to the *Diagnostic and Statistical Manual of Mental Disorders,* fourth edition (DSM-IV) (American Psychiatric Association, 1994), the following are the criteria for alcohol abuse:

A. A maladaptive pattern of substance use leading to clinically significant impairment or distress, as manifested by one (or more) of the following, occurring within a 12-month period:
   1. Recurrent alcohol use resulting in a failure to fulfill major role obligations at work, school, or home
   2. Recurrent alcohol use in situations in which it is physically hazardous
   3. Recurrent alcohol-related legal problems
   4. Continued alcohol use despite having persistent or recurrent social or interpersonal problems caused or exacerbated by the effects of alcohol

B. The symptoms have never met the criteria for alcohol dependence for this class of substance.

Elderly abusers of alcohol do not always meet the preceding criteria for alcohol abuse. It is difficult to apply these criteria to the elderly because most are no longer working or in school settings. A decline in social interactions due to retirement and the loss of friends and family to death may make many older people prone to social isolation. Social isolation, grief, and boredom are often precursors for alcohol abuse and subsequent dependency.

According to the DSM-IV, the criteria for alcohol dependency include a definition of *tolerance:* a need for markedly increased amounts of alcohol to achieve intoxication or markedly diminished effects with continued use of the same amount of alcohol

(American Psychiatric Association, 1994). As a person ages, the quantity of alcohol consumed generally decreases; however, as mentioned previously, an elderly person is more sensitive to the effects of alcohol. The decrease in the amount of alcohol consumed may cause the patient and practitioner to minimize the problem.

Alcohol use disorders can be categorized into six groupings that are not mutually exclusive: dependence, abuse, harmful, hazardous, heavy, and binge drinking (see Box 27-2 for definitions) (Nelson, 1998; Saunders et al., 1993; USDHHS, 1996).

A helpful distinction for older drinkers may be early-onset vs. late-onset drinkers. In spite of the widely held view by clinicians that alcoholics die at a young age, two thirds of older drinkers began drinking in their youth. Those who have survived to old age have multiple medical and psychologic problems related to their long pattern of alcohol ingestion. By contrast, late-onset use of alcohol is usually related to the stress associated with age, such as death of a spouse, retirement, and financial strains. This group of older adults has fewer health problems and contains more women than men (Nelson, 1998).

Box 27-2
Definitions of Terms

Dependence

Maladaptive pattern of use to include three of the following seven elements of dependence within a 12-month period (American Psychiatric Association, 1994):
- Tolerance
- Withdrawal
- Use of larger amounts and for longer time periods than intended
- Persistent desire to use and unsuccessful efforts to cut down
- Giving up activities because of use
- Spending a great deal of time in obtaining the substance
- Continued use despite adverse problems related to use (DSM-IV)

Abuse

Maladaptive pattern of use to include one or more of the following four elements of abuse within a 12-month period (American Psychiatric Association, 1994):
- Failure to fulfill obligations because of use
- Use in situations that are physically hazardous
- Legal problems related to use
- Persistent use despite social and interpersonal problems

Harmful Drinking

Evidence of adverse physical and psychologic problems related to use

Hazardous Drinking

Use that places user at risk for adverse consequences

Heavy Drinking

Consuming 5 or more drinks* on the same occasion on at least 5 different days in the past month

Binge Drinking

Ingesting 5 or more drinks* on the same occasion once in the past month

*A drink is 12 oz of beer, 5 oz of wine, or 1.5 oz of 80-proof distilled spirits (US Department of Health and Human Services, 1995).

"Ageism" can interfere with the diagnosis and treatment of alcohol abuse: *"He is 85 years old. His wife is dead. He suffers from cataracts, arthritis, hypertension, and diabetes. It is no wonder that he is depressed. Let him drink!"* There are alternatives to alcohol in this situation. Many patients use alcohol as self-medication for emotional and physical pain and for insomnia because of myths about the effects of alcohol.

History

Diagnosing alcohol abuse in the elderly requires a high index of suspicion. Clinicians need to be aware of their tendency to overlook many of the presenting symptoms of alcohol abuse in the older person because of *the typical atypical presentation* and because of the stigma attached to the older alcoholic. Clues may include missed appointments, personality changes, irritability, uncontrolled hypertension, uncontrolled diabetes, poor personal hygiene, sleep disturbances, recurrent falls, weight loss, and memory loss (immediate, recent, or remote) (Box 27-3). The concurrent use of cigarettes and a family history of alcohol problems are associated with an increased risk of alcohol abuse. These problems are often brought to the attention of the practitioner by family members or friends. Most patients generally deny that there is a problem, whereas others may defend their drinking and become angry when confronted.

At times, enabling behavior by the patient's spouse, adult children, or formal caregivers may make the differential diagnosis extremely difficult. For whatever reason, many caregivers use denial to deal with an older person's alcoholism. The primary care provider needs the assistance of caregivers to successfully treat most older people who are abusing alcohol.

A review of prescription and over-the-counter medications is normal procedure in the history taking for any older adult, but it is especially critical if there is a suspicion of alcohol abuse. Alcohol is a drug that places the older person at unrecognized risk for adverse drug interactions. Alcohol has the potential to adversely affect medications and can lead to injury, acute illness or, at times, even death. A referral to current drug

Box 27-3

Symptoms of Alcohol Abuse Missed by Many Health Care Providers and Ascribed to the Aging Process

New symptoms of confusion
Increased short-term memory loss
Weight loss
Apathy
Falls
Bruises
Polypharmacy
Sleep disturbance
Functional decline
Self-neglect
Chronic fatigue
Poorly managed disease (diabetes, hypertension)

Solution: Maintain a high degree of suspicion and assess for the problem.

Box 27-4
The CAGE Questionnaire

1. Have you ever felt you ought to *C*ut down?
2. Have you ever been *A*nnoyed by criticism of your drinking?
3. Have you ever felt *G*uilty about your drinking?
4. Have you ever felt the need for an *E*ye opener?

manuals is necessary to check the potential risk for interactions with the patient's prescription and over-the-counter drugs.

Many older women may be at risk for the development of late-onset alcohol problems. The practitioner needs to maintain an awareness of the person's individual risk and consider that women tend to outlive their partners and have higher poverty rates and different patterns of intake than men. Women are more apt to drink at home and alone, which makes detection by friends, family, and neighbors quite difficult (Gomberg, 1995).

Many tests are available to screen for alcohol abuse. The CAGE questionnaire and the MAST-G (Michigan Alcoholism Screening Test—Geriatric Version) have been studied in older people (Blow et al., 1992; Buchsbaum et al., 1992; Jones et al., 1993). The advantages of the four-question CAGE questionnaire are that it is brief and inoffensive and may be given in written or oral form. The CAGE questionnaire does not make a distinction between current and past problems, but the sensitivity and specificity are 70% and 91%, respectively (cutoff two or more yes responses). The MAST-G, a 24-item tool, is age appropriate and very useful (Box 27-4 and Figure 27-1).

Physical Examination

A physical examination or the patient can be helpful in diagnosing alcoholism. Signs to look for include a disheveled appearance, a smell of alcohol or urine, pale conjunctivae, icteric sclerae, a coated tongue, multiple caries, a hyperactive gag reflex, epigastric tenderness, a palpable liver, tremors, and ataxia. Although these signs are inconclusive by themselves, a positive diagnosis can be made in conjunction with a good history and supportive laboratory data.

Diagnostic Tests

Diagnostic tests may include blood tests and radiologic evaluation of the liver, pancreas, and heart. Abnormal laboratory results suggestive of alcohol abuse include elevated mean corpuscular cell volume; decreased vitamin B_{12}, folate, and albumin; elevated gamma-glutamyl transferase; and an aspartate aminotransferase and alanine aminotransferase ratio greater than 2:1. A normal blood alcohol level does not rule out a diagnosis of chronic alcohol abuse. Radiographic studies demonstrating cardiomegaly, hepatomegaly, or pancreatitis also warrant consideration of a diagnosis of alcohol abuse.

	Yes (1)	No (0)
1. After drinking have you ever noticed an increase in your heart rate or beating in your chest?	1. ___	___
2. When talking with others do you ever underestimate how much you actually drink?	2. ___	___
3. Does alcohol make you sleepy so that you often fall asleep in your chair?	3. ___	___
4. After a few drinks have you sometimes not eaten or been able to skip a meal because you didn't feel hungry?	4. ___	___
5. Does having a few drinks help decrease your shakiness or tremors?	5. ___	___
6. Does alcohol sometimes make it hard for you to remember parts of the day or night?	6. ___	___
7. Do you have rules for yourself that you won't drink before a certain time of the day?	7. ___	___
8. Have you lost interest in hobbies or activities you used to enjoy?	8. ___	___
9. When you wake up in the morning do you ever have trouble remembering part of the night before?	9. ___	___
10. Does having a drink help you sleep?	10. ___	___
11. Do you hide your alcohol bottles from family members?	11. ___	___
12. After a social gathering have you ever felt embarrassed because you drank too much?	12. ___	___
13. Have you ever been concerned that drinking might be harmful to your health?	13. ___	___
14. Do you like to end an evening with a night cap?	14. ___	___
15. Did you find your drinking increased after someone close to you died?	15. ___	___
16. In general, would you prefer to have a few drinks at home rather than go out to social events?	16. ___	___
17. Are you drinking more now than in the past?	17. ___	___
18. Do you usually take a drink to relax or calm your nerves?	18. ___	___
19. Do you drink to take your mind off your problems?	19. ___	___
20. Have you ever increased your drinking after experiencing a loss in your life?	20. ___	___
21. Do you sometimes drive when you have had too much to drink?	21. ___	___
22. Has a doctor or nurse ever said they were worried or concerned about your drinking?	22. ___	___
23. Have you ever made rules to manage your drinking?	23. ___	___
24. When you feel lonely does having a drink help?	24. ___	___

Scoring: 5 or more "yes" responses is indicative of alcohol problem.

Figure 27-1 Michigan Alcoholism Screening Test–Geriatric Version (MAST-G). (From Blow FC et al: The Michigan Alcoholism Test–Geriatric Version (MAST-G): a new elderly-specific screening instrument, *Alcohol Clin Exp Res* 16(2):372, 1991. Copyright of The Regents of the University of Michigan.)

Management and Treatment

The general principles of treatment of alcohol abuse emphasize things that can be done and emphasize building a relationship that allows the patient and caregivers to realize that there is a caring environment and that recovery is a strong possibility. For many elderly patients the inclusion of family or the caregiver becomes essential to the ability to successfully participate in treatment and recovery.

Care needs to be individualized on the basis of the extent and type of alcohol disorder. Patients with more acute dependence are referred (Reid and Anderson, 1997), and hospitalization should be considered for the withdrawal period. Therapy for less acute patients needs to deal with their particular age-related stresses and how their coping mechanism of alcohol use is harmful. When discussing treatment options, the practitioner must be knowledgeable about local programs and community resources available to the patient. Alcoholics Anonymous (AA) members are excellent resources, and the older patient should be informed that AA is certainly appropriate for older adults—more than one third of its members are over age 50. The treatment plan should begin the day the patient is confronted with the diagnosis (Campbell, 1997).

One way to approach the treatment of alcohol abuse in the elderly is to use a staging process and relate the treatment to the stage that applies to the patient (Table 27-1) (Haugland, 1989).

The following paragraphs provide an example of the progression of the staging process:

Mr. Recent Widower is an elderly man who usually has one drink a day after dinner. Since his wife died 3 months ago, he spends his evenings drinking beer while watching television. He has passed out on the couch three times in the last month. This is stage I: nonsocial drinking pattern, and a nonconfrontational approach is recommended. It is important for the patient to hear from the practitioner that his *pattern* of drinking is *problematic*. Appropriate evaluation and treatment for grief and depression are necessary. A 90-day abstinence trial may be effective with weekly AA meetings. Patients should be encouraged to schedule group activities to avoid social isolation. Suggestions may include weekly meals with family members and friends and participation in senior or recreational center activities.

As Mr. Recent Widower enters stage II, his drinking takes precedence over his eating. His daughter finds his home in disarray. The patient is unshaven, and his clothes are dirty. When confronted by his daughter, the patient states, "Stop nagging and leave me alone." The daughter reluctantly complies. The psychologic dependency and social problems begin. Temporary inpatient treatment may be necessary; Medicare will cover some of the inpatient days. AA can offer support and guidance to the patient and family members.

Without treatment the patient progresses to stage III. The physiologic dependency begins, and health problems become evident. There are frequent emergency department visits and hospitalizations for trauma, loss of consciousness, and recurrent infections. Diagnoses include peripheral neuropathy, pneumonia, urinary tract infections, gastrointestinal bleeding, seizure disorders, cardiomyopathy, and congestive heart failure. Treatment at this stage generally requires benzodiazepines to prevent withdrawal seizures; therefore hospitalization is normally advised. Follow-up should include an outpatient program, AA, and 1 to 2 years of continuing care.

Elderly patients in stages IV and V are easy to identify. Treatment includes an inpatient program followed by a lifelong outpatient program. Outpatient programs are most effective when tailored to the individual. Treatment with individuals in the same age-group as the patient also yields a better response.

TABLE 27-1 Staging of Problem Drinking in the Elderly

Stage	Features	Dependency	Prognosis	Intervention
I	Nonsocial drinking pattern	Minimal	Good	Nonconfrontational
II	Social problem	Psychologic	Good	Confrontational
III	Health problems	Physiologic	Fair	Group intervention
IV	Laboratory evidence	Severe	Poor	Multidisciplinary intervention
V	Minimal social functioning	Terminal	Poor	Involuntary

Guidelines for Intervention

1. Avoid being judgmental.
2. Persuade the patient to have an evaluation for possible treatment.
3. Do something today.
4. Have the telephone number of an AA person who can talk to the patient.
5. Have a plan.
6. Make use of family and friends.
7. If all else fails, consider legal commitment.

Prevention

Older adults should be counseled about the risks and the age-related changes that increase the dangers of alcohol-related problems, and the harmful interactions of alcohol and many medications, both prescription and over the counter, need to be clarified. Information regarding the physical changes that accompany aging and the effects on alcohol metabolism needs to be readily available in all forms—verbal, visual, and written. Abstinence or at least moderation of intake should be strongly encouraged for all older patients.

Summary

Alcohol abuse is a prevalent but commonly overlooked problem in the elderly. The economic, social, psychologic, and medical consequences of alcohol abuse lead to increased functional impairment and increased risk for dependency in the elderly. Alcohol abuse in the elderly should be diagnosed and effectively treated to decrease mortality and morbidity. Overall medical costs will be reduced by the decreased need for hospitalization and treatment for alcohol-related medical conditions.

Resources

Alcohol Abuse USA Information Page
http://www.drug-abuse.com

National Institute on Alcohol Abuse and Alcoholism
http://www.niaaa.nih.gov

Alcoholism Net
http://www.alcoholism.net

References

Adams W et al: Alcohol-related hospitalizations of elderly people: prevalence and geographic variation in the United States, *JAMA* 270(10):1222-1225, 1993.

American Psychiatric Association: *Diagnostic and statistical manual of mental disorders,* ed 4, Washington, DC, 1994, American Psychiatric Association.

Blow FC et al: The Michigan Alcoholism Test–Geriatric Version (MAST-G): a new elderly-specific screening instrument, *Alcohol Clin Exp Res* 16(2):372, 1992.

Buchsbaum DG et al: Screening for drinking disorders in the elderly using the CAGE questionnaire, *J Am Geriatr Soc* 40(7):662-665, 1992.

Campbell JW: Alcoholism. In Ham R, Sloane P: *Primary care geriatrics: a case-based approach,* ed 3, St Louis, 1997, Mosby.

Eisendrath E: Psychiatric disorders. In Tierney LM, McPhee SJ, Papadakis MA: *Current medical diagnosis and treatment,* ed 38, Stamford, Conn, 1997, Appleton & Lange.

Gomberg ES: Older women and alcohol use and abuse, *Recent Dev Alcohol* 12:61-79, 1995.

Haugland S: Alcoholism and other drug dependencies, *Prim Care* 16(2):411-428, 1989.

Jones TV et al: Alcoholism screening questionnaires: are they valued in elderly medical outpatients? *J Gen Intern Med* 8: 674-678, 1993.

Kimble RB: Alcohol, cytokines and estrogen in the control of bone remodeling, *Alcohol Clin Exp Res* 21(3):385-391, 1997.

Lieber CS: Medical disorders of alcoholism, *N Engl J Med* 333(16):1058-1065, 1995.

McInnes E, Powell J: Drug and alcohol referrals: are elderly substance abuse diagnoses and referrals being missed? *BMJ* 308:444-446, 1994.

Nelson M: Alcohol use in the older adult, *Am J Nurse Pract* 2(6):24-32, 1998.

Reid MC, Anderson PA: Geriatric substance use disorders, *Med Clin North Am* 81(4):999-1016, 1997.

Reuben D et al: *Geriatrics review syllabus,* ed 3, New York, 1996.

Saunders JB et al: Alcohol consumption and related problems among primary health care: WHO collaborative project on early detection of persons with harmful alcohol consumption, *Addiction* 88:349-362, 1993.

Solomon K et al: Alcoholism and prescription drug abuse in the elderly: Saint Louis University Grand Rounds, *J Am Geriatr Soc* 41:57-69, 1993.

US Department of Health and Human Services: National household survey on drug abuse, 1996. From World Wide Web: http://wwwnalusda.gov/finc/dga/dguide95.html.

28

Abuse and Neglect

Mistreatment of older persons in the United States occurs across all social, racial, and class strata. Each year approximately 1 million older Americans are physically injured, emotionally debilitated, or neglected by a caregiver (Murray and DeVos, 1997). It is estimated that only 1 in 14 incidents of domestic elder abuse is ever reported or detected. Whatever the estimate, it is generally agreed that the number of elder abuse incidents will increase over the next 30 years. The projected increase in abuse cases is the result of the following factors: (1) people living longer, which increases the need for more long-term care; (2) increased demands on family caregivers; and (3) increased legal obligations to report suspected elder abuse (Murray and DeVos, 1997).

To determine the boundaries of elder abuse or neglect, the California penal code is an excellent standard; however, providers need to be cognizant of the legal standards of their particular state. *Abuse* is defined in the California Welfare and Institution code as "Physical abuse, neglect, intimidation, cruel punishment, financial abuse, abandonment, isolation, abduction or other treatment with resulting physical harm, pain, or mental suffering, or the deprivation by a care custodian of goods or services which are necessary to avoid physical harm or mental suffering" (California Welfare and Institution Code).

Types of Abuse and Neglect

Physical abuse and neglect produce a wide range of bodily injuries such as bruising, scratches, broken areas on the skin, undetected and untreated pressure ulcers, and neglected personal grooming. Physical abuse may take the form of striking, shoving, shaking, restraining, or physical coercion. Sexual assault refers to any form of sexual intimacy that occurs without consent or by force or threat of force.

Psychologic abuse and neglect encompass behaviors that cause emotional anguish to the older person. This type of abuse includes verbal mistreatment such as threats, insults, or harsh commands, as well as silence and ignoring the person.

Material or financial abuse is the misuse or exploitation of, or inattention to, an older person's possessions, funds, or resources. It includes irresponsible management of the person's money, pressuring of the victim to distribute assets, and outright theft (Box 28-1).

Box 28-1

Clues to Financial or Material Abuse

- Having an inability to pay bills or to purchase prescriptions or food
- Withdrawing money (especially in large sums) from accounts
- Giving away large sums of money
- Turning over property rights
- Having an inability to account for living expenses
- Having a disparity between assets and satisfactory living conditions

Active neglect refers to the refusal or failure to undertake a caregiving obligation (including a conscious and intentional attempt to inflict physical or emotional stress on the elder). Passive neglect is a refusal or failure to fulfill a caretaking obligation (excluding a conscious and intentional attempt to inflict physical or emotional distress on the elder) (Penhale and Kingston, 1997). Interestingly, the most commonly reported type of neglect is self-neglect, which is defined as "an adult's inability, due to physical and/or mental impairments or diminished capacity, to perform self-care tasks . . . to maintain physical health . . . general safety, and/or manage financial affairs" (Capezuti, Brush, and Lawson, 1997). Most self-neglecting elders have functional or mental impairments as well as a poor social network. Interventions in this situation present many practical and ethical challenges.

The circumstances that surround an elderly abusive situation are composed of three elements: the abuser, the abused elderly person, and the context of the social situation that leads to and supports the act of abuse. There is no typical abusive scenario that is valid. In fact, the diversity of situations that lead to abuse makes it crucial that providers assess all three elements of an abusive situation before making a diagnosis.

The Abuser

Factors that may indicate that a caregiver is at risk of becoming an abuser include substance abuse; poor physical health; mental confusion or cognitive impairment; emotional or mental illness; inexperience in caregiving; emotional or financial dependence on the care recipient; having been abused as a child, especially if the older person was the abuser; social isolation and lack of a support system; and being involved in conflict either with the older person or with an outside relationship, which may increase stress. Caregivers who have a history of alcoholism, drug use, or gambling addiction may resort to financial abuse of an elder to support these habits or to escape financial crisis. Many caregivers are older themselves and may have physical or medical problems. The behavior traits of the older person, the daily tasks to be performed, and isolation and frustration can lead to stress (Pritchard, 1996). Unintentional abuse, or *neglect,* can be the result of ignorance, inexperience, overburdened caregivers, or a lack of desire or ability to provide proper care (Murray and DeVos, 1997).

The Abused Elderly Person

Common characteristics of abused elderly people include being older, female, dependent, alcoholic, isolated, or impaired; having a history of abuse; engaging in provocative (e.g., overdemanding, unappreciative) or aggressive and combative behavior; and having unrealistic expectations (Reis and Nahmiash, 1998; Mendonca, Velamoor, and Sauve, 1996). Although victims of elder abuse have long been characterized as being frail, dependent women, it is important to remember that any older person—male or female, cognitively impaired or intact—can be a victim.

The Social Context

The history of the relationship between the caregiver and the care recipient must also be considered. A parent-child (or other) relationship that was always strained or abusive cannot be expected to improve when the stresses of caregiving and dependence are added. Dependence of the caregiver on the older person for financial support or housing can also lead to or sustain an abusive relationship.

Subjective Findings

The abuse or neglect of seniors by their caregivers is not always readily visible or obvious to providers. Unfortunately, there are few validated screening measures to assist providers in identifying cases of abuse. One tool that is based on abuse indicators and is designed to be completed by the practitioner is the Indicators of Abuse Screen in Box 28-2. A score of 16 or above, the "abuse alert" score, is considered to be indicative of abuse; however, the need for more research into the use of this tool has been recognized (Reis and Nahmiash, 1998).

The practitioner cannot rely solely on interviews with, or reports from, abusers or victims (Reis and Nahmiash, 1998). Communication barriers such as dementia, aphasia, or delusions may render a victim incapable of alerting a practitioner to an abusive situation. In rare cases a victim who is able will talk openly about ongoing abuse. More often, however, victims do not want to report abuse because of embarrassment, shame, intimidation, or fear. Some victims even blame themselves for the abuse and believe it is somehow deserved. They may be unwilling to talk openly and may respond to questions with implausible stories, anger, or denial.

Despite the importance of avoiding confrontation with the victim and the caregiver, it is possible to elicit reports of abuse with direct questions: "Do you feel safe where you live?" "Do you ever have disagreements with your caregiver?" "Have you ever been treated roughly or intimidated?" The responses to such questions are often revealing. Conversations with the caregiver usually rely on opened-ended types of questions worded in a nonthreatening, nonjudgmental way: "Can you tell me what a normal day providing care for [the patient] is like for you?" "It must be difficult. Do you ever lose control?"

These types of questions allow the abuser to perceive the practitioner as empathic and create a nonjudgmental environment that is helpful in obtaining necessary information. Victims fear reporting abuse for a number of reasons. They may want to protect their loved one from criminal action. The older person may have a long history of "saving" the abuser, who is often an alcoholic, drug-dependent, or mentally ill adult child (Capezuti, Brush, and Lawson, 1997). It is important to interview the patient and suspected abuser together *and* individually. Observe interactions between them and be aware of disparities in their accounts regarding care routines, history and, especially, injuries. Behavioral indications of an abusive relationship are identified in Box 28-3.

Box 28-2

Indicators of Abuse (IOA) Screen

Indicators of abuse are listed below, numbered in order of importance.* After a two- to three-hour home assessment (or other intensive assessment) please rate each of the following items on a scale of 0 to 4. Do not omit any items. Rate according to your current opinion.

Scale: Estimated extent of problem:
0 = nonexistent
1 = slight
2 = moderate
3 = probably/moderately severe
4 = yes/severe
00 = not applicable
000 = don't know

Caregiver Age _____ years
Caregiver and Care Receiver Kinship ____ spouse
____ nonspouse

Caregiver

____ 1. Has behavior problems
____ 2. Is financially dependent
____ 3. Has mental/emotional difficulties
____ 6. Has alcohol/substance abuse problem
____ 7. Has unrealistic expectations
____ 9. Lacks understanding of medical condition
____ 10. Caregiving reluctancy
____ 12. Has marital/family conflict
____ 13. Has poor current relationship
____ 14. Caregiving inexperience
____ 17. Is a blamer
____ 24. Had poor past relationship

Care Receiver

____ 4. Has been abused in the past
____ 5. Has marital/family conflict
____ 8. Lacks understanding of medical condition
____ 11. Is socially isolated
____ 15. Lacks social support
____ 16. Has behavior problems
____ 18. Is financially dependent
____ 19. Has unrealistic expectations
____ 20. Has alcohol/medication problem
____ 21. Has poor current relationship
____ 22. Has suspicious falls/injuries
____ 23. Has mental/emotional difficulties
____ 25. Is a blamer
____ 26. Is emotionally dependent
____ 27. No regular doctor

From Reis M, Nahmiash D: Validation of the indicators of abuse screen, *Gerontologist* 38(4):471-480, 1998.
*The majority of the most important indicators are the caregiver ones.

Box 28-3

Behavioral Clues to an Abusive Relationship

- The patient is not given the opportunity to speak for himself or herself or to see others except in the presence of the caregiver.
- The caregiver exhibits an attitude of indifference or anger toward the dependent person.
- The caregiver blames the patient for his or her condition, for example, by claiming that the patient's incontinence is a deliberate act.
- The caregiver exhibits aggressive behavior toward the patient or toward health care providers, including threats, insults, or harassment.
- The caregiver and the patient present conflicting accounts of incidents.
- The caregiver shows an unwillingness or reluctance to comply with planning for care.

Data from Murray L, DeVos D: The escalating problem of elder abuse, *Radiol Technol* 68(4):351-353, 1997.

Box 28-4
Indications of an Abusive Relationship

- Pattern of physician or hospital "hopping"
- An injury that has not been properly treated
- Any injury that is not compatible with the given history
- Recurrent injuries due to "accidents"
- Frequent trips to the emergency department for injuries
- Pain on touching (requires further assessment)
- Cuts, lacerations, or puncture wounds
- Bruises, welts, and discolorations (especially those in a suspicious pattern)
- The presence of new and old bruises together
- Dehydration or malnutrition without illness or related cause
- Sunken eyes or cheeks
- Evidence of inadequate care, such as pressure ulcers, weight loss, unfilled prescriptions, unscheduled or unkept appointments
- Poor hygiene or soiled clothing or bed linens
- Burns (especially those that appear due to cigarettes, ropes, etc.)
- Signs of confinement
- Lack of bandages on injuries, unset fractures, lack of sutures if needed
- Signs of sleep disruption (e.g., complaints of insomnia, excessive sleepiness)
- Absence of assistive devices (e.g., cane, hearing aids, dentures)

Objective Findings

Physical examination of the abused or neglected elder may reveal the following findings:

General appearance: poor hygiene, inappropriate dress
Skin: poor turgor, skin lesions, bruises, pressure ulcers
Head and neck: trauma (hematomas, lacerations, abrasions), alopecia
Trunk: bruises, welts
Genitourinary tract: rectal or vaginal bleeding, infestations
Extremities: wrist or ankle bruising, immersion (or other) burns
Musculoskeletal: fractures, pain (observe gait)
Neurologic: cognitive deficits

Signs that indicate abuse or neglect are listed in Box 28-4.

Discernment Before Intervention

Once a diagnosis is made, a review of the data obtained during the assessment phase is essential before any intervention can be implemented. Interventions must be based on the identified underlying causes. Successful interventions are those that are multidisciplinary in nature.

The review of data includes the following (Abrams and Berkow, 1990):

1. Is access to the victim a problem? Victims and abusers are often reluctant to allow contact by health care professionals. Practitioners may need to be creative in their approach to the situation and must always be aware of safety and other risks to themselves.

2. How serious is the abuse? If the pattern of abuse has escalated, the victim may be in serious danger, which may increase the urgency for intervention.
3. Is the victim aware of the problem? The victim's awareness of and reaction to the abuse will affect the practitioner's options in the situation.
4. Who is inflicting the abuse? Is it a family member or an outside caregiver? Does the victim have access to other family or friends? It is also important to remember that more than one person may be involved.
5. What is the victim's cognitive status? Does the victim have the capacity to make decisions regarding her or his care? Is the victim capable of following a plan of action should the situation become dangerous? It is very important to determine if any apparent cognitive deficits are actually pseudodementia caused by dehydration, improper medication management, or other acute disease that has been neglected or caused by the abuse itself.
6. What is the victim's health and functional status? Does the victim have a medical condition or mobility problem that will modify management?
7. What are the victim's resources? What are the financial resources? Are there supportive family members, concerned neighbors, and friends?
8. What community resources are available? Are respite care options available (e.g., temporary shelters, day care, or foster care)?
9. Has any intervention been made in the past? Information about previous interventions (e.g., court orders of protection) and why they failed should be obtained to avoid embarking on the same approach.

Intervention

The Abuser

The counseling of abusers must start with an assessment of their abilities and knowledge level so that deficits can be corrected. This step is especially important in attempting to discern between intentional and unintentional neglect.

Counseling can include the following:

1. Assess the caregiver's understanding of the illness and knowledge of the patient's care needs (e.g., medication schedules, tube feeding administration, pressure relief).
2. Assess the caregiver's physical capabilities in caring for a dependent older person. The caregiver's physical health, emotional stability, social support system, and other responsibilities must also be taken into consideration.
3. Educate the caregiver regarding the patient's illness, follow-up care, medications, behavior management, and hands-on caregiving; this can reduce confusion and alleviate stress.
4. Explore insurance benefits, financial relief programs, free medication programs offered by some pharmaceutical companies, and other resources, which may help ease the burden of paying for medication and supplies. A social work consultation may help to provide this information.
5. Arrange respite time for the caregiver to provide a "break" from responsibilities.
6. Seek alternative or assistant caregivers if a caregiver is thought to have mental

or psychologic impairments that affect his or her ability to provide care. If the impairment is related to substance abuse, the provider can attempt to assist the caregiver in seeking treatment, including provision of care for the older person while the caregiver is undergoing rehabilitation.

The Abused Elderly Person. Victims often require education and time before the decision is made to change the situation. The provider must develop a trusting and therapeutic alliance with the abused elder. Allowing the victim the opportunity to recognize the danger inherent in the situation and the benefits of alternatives can take time.

Counseling of the victim should consist of the following (Paris et al., 1995):

1. Educating the victim regarding options (e.g., making other living arrangements, obtaining an order of protection, having the abuser evicted, having the locks changed, or pressing formal charges). Legal options can be discussed with the office of the local district attorney.
2. Examining the positive and negative aspects of each option.
3. Allowing the victim to talk about feelings in a nonjudgmental atmosphere.
4. Enabling the victim to express his or her angers or fears.
5. Assuring the victim that these feelings are normal.
6. Helping the victim understand that choosing an option different from the caregiver's wishes would not necessarily sever the relationship, if the patient wants to retain it.

The Social Context. If possible, every effort should be made to correct situations so that the older person can remain in as independent a setting as possible. Occasionally the abused elder will not allow intervention. Although victims who have been determined to have capacity may refuse help, they cannot prevent the practitioner from reporting the problem as required by law. Most states require health care professionals to report suspected cases of abuse or neglect to the state's adult protective services (APS) agency. These mandatory reporting laws require the disclosure of suspected elder mistreatment regardless of the wishes of the adult victim. The APS agencies must then investigate reports by interviewing victims and others who may be knowledgeable about the situation (Capezuti, Brush, and Lawson, 1997). See Table 28-1 for information regarding elder mistreatment statutes by state. "At-risk" older persons who refuse needed help are of great concern to health care providers, who often must grapple with difficult ethical and legal issues concerning when to intervene against a person's will and when to respect his or her right to self-determination.

People for whom self-neglect is an issue present a variety of practical and ethical challenges. The person's capacity to make decisions must often be assessed to determine that he or she understands the potential risks in deciding to decline intervention. A surrogate or guardian is often assigned until an evaluation and determination can be completed. When working with a judgmentally impaired individual, it is necessary to consider the person's lifestyle choices and try to make decisions consistent with those choices. Individuals must not be judged incapable if their choices are consistent with those made over the course of their lives, even if they seem eccentric or outlandish to others. Regardless of the individual aspects of a situation, the least restrictive choice should be made—as long as it ensures safe and appropriate care for the elder.

TABLE 28-1 Elder Mistreatment Statutes*

State	APS Low	Minimum Year of Age	Reporting Requirement
Alabama	1977	18	M-O
Alaska	1988	18	M-O
Arkansas	1977	18	M-N
Arizona	1980	18	M
California	1986	18	M-N
Colorado	1991	18	V
Connecticut	1977	60	M-N
Delaware	1982	18	M-O
District of Columbia	1985	18	M-O
Florida	1974	18	M-N
Georgia	1981	18	M-N
Hawaii	1989	Adult	M-N
Idaho	1991	18	M-N
Illinois	1988	60	V
Indiana	1985	18	M-O
Iowa	1983	18	M-O
Kansas	1985	18	M-N
Kentucky	1976	18	M-N
Louisiana	1982	18	M-O
Maine	1981	18	M-N
Maryland	1977	65	M-O
Massachusetts	1983	60	M-N
Michigan	1982	18	M-O
Minnesota	1980	18	M-O
Mississippi	1986	18	M-O
Missouri	1980	18	M-N
Montana	1975, 1983	60, 18	M-N
Nebraska	1988	18	M-N
Nevada	1981	60	M-N
New Hampshire	1978	18	M-O
New Jersey	1993	18	V
New Mexico	1989	18	M
New York	1975	18	V
North Carolina	1973	18	M-O
North Dakota	1989	18	V
Ohio	1981	60	M-N
Oklahoma	1977	18	M-O
Oregon	1975, 1981	18, 65	M-N
Pennsylvania	1987	60	V

From Capezuti E, Brush BL, Lawson WT: Reporting elder mistreatment, *Journal of Gerontological Nursing* 23(7):24-32, 1997.

M, Mandatory reporting; *V,* voluntary reporting; *N,* law specifically names nurses as mandated reporters; *O,* law does not name nurses specifically but names health care professionals or anyone with knowledge.

Continued

29

Grief

The Role of Spirituality in Coping with Loss

One of the essential elements of the grieving process is finding meaning in the loss and suffering (Doka and Davidson, 1997). Most people have something in their life that gives them meaning. To many this meaning may be defined in terms of their careers, their relationships, or their social status. But once a person experiences a loss such as a death of a loved one or the loss of health or previous level of functioning, the previous way of looking at the world and at defining meaning may not suffice. Illness or death of a loved one is a major life event that causes people to question themselves, their purpose, and the meaning in life. Grief and loss disrupt career, family life, and ability to enjoy life, three areas essential to a healthy mind. These losses inevitably raise profound questions as to who we are and what is the purpose of our lives. The process of dealing with these questions is really one of finding new meaning in life. This is the essence of a spiritual journey. Victor Frankl (1993) wrote, "Man is not destroyed by suffering; he is destroyed by suffering without meaning." When he wrote about concentration camp victims, he noted that survival itself may depend on seeking and finding meaning. People can cope with their suffering by seeking and finding meaning in it. Thus spirituality plays such a critical role.

Spirituality can be defined as the transcendent relationship that gives meaning and purpose to people's lives, joys, and sufferings. Downey (1997) defines spirituality as "an awareness that there are levels of reality not immediately apparent and that there is a quest for personal integration in the face of forces of fragmentation and depersonalization." It is the aspect of human beings that seeks to heal. Often spirituality is expressed as religion. Foglio and Brody (1981) write:

> For many people religion forms a basis of meaning and purpose in life. The profoundly disturbing effects of illness can call into question a person's purpose in life and work, responsibilities to spouse, children, and parents and motivations and fidelity priorities. Healing, the restoration of wholeness (as opposed to merely technical healing) requires answers to these questions (p. 473).

The healing of grief involves an acceptance of the loss, be it of a loved one or of one's health. Spirituality offers people hope and helps them understand their grief in the context of a deeper reality.

Spirituality and Religion

There is often confusion about the differences between spirituality and religion. As we work with patients, it is important to recognize that spirituality is universal. Individual patients may or may not be religious, but spirituality is inherent in everyone. Religion is the expression of one's spirituality in a particular, organized community with a set of doctrines accepted by the community. Historically, spirituality was referenced only in the context of religion. The current use of the term *spirituality* as separate from religion is thought to originate from the rise of secularism in this century and from a growing disillusionment with religious institutions in western society. In the 1960s and 1970s, spirituality began to acquire distinct meanings separate from religion (Turner et al., 1995). As spirituality has become differentiated from religion, spirituality has become the broader, more inclusive term (Pargament, 1997). Nonetheless, it is important to recognize that, according to a Gallop survey, Americans are very religious, with over 90% or the population believing in God and a large segment of the population attending religious services regularly (Gallop, 1990). Spirituality, defined as a universal concept of search for meaning, can appeal and provide solace to a large segment of the population served by the health care system. This definition allows for the diversity in beliefs and backgrounds. The search for meaning through a relationship with the transcendent or divine can be expressed in many ways: religion, nature, music, art, and relationship with others. There is no one expression of spirituality: everyone has a personal understanding and expression of his or her beliefs. What is uniform is that it is these beliefs that help people cope with their grief, loss, and suffering.

Patient Need

Several national surveys have documented patients' desire to have spiritual concerns addressed by health care professionals who are providing their care. A 1990 Gallop poll showed that religion, one expression of spirituality, plays a central role in the lives of many Americans. When asked, 95% of Americans surveyed espouse a belief in God, 57% report praying daily, and 42% report attending a worship service in the prior week. The need for attentiveness to the spiritual concerns of dying patients has been well recognized by many authors (Conrad, 1985; Moberg, 1982; Moberg, 1965). The recent survey by George Gallop showed that people overwhelmingly want their spiritual needs addressed when they are close to death. Gallop (1997) writes, "the overarching message that emerges from this study is that the American people want to reclaim and reassert the spiritual dimensions in dying." Other surveys found that 75% of Americans say that religion is central to their lives; a majority feel that their spiritual faith can help them recover from their illness. More than 50% to 75% of hospital patients believed that their physicians should address spiritual issues and pray with them (King and Bushwick, 1994). To prepare physicians to respond to this growing need, spirituality and medicine courses are being incorporated into medical school curricula (Puchalski and Larson, 1998; Levin, Larson, and Puchalski, 1997). Historically, nursing schools have always emphasized the role of spirituality in health care.

Research Demonstrating the Role of Spirituality in Health and in Coping with Illness and Loss

There is a growing body of evidence documenting the relationship between patients' religious and spiritual lives and their experiences of illness and disease (Levin and Schiller, 1987). In addition to surveys that demonstrate that spirituality is important to people and that a significant percentage of our patients would like their health care providers to discuss their spiritual beliefs with them, there are a number of studies that show that spirituality is beneficial to patients, particularly those with serious illness. Reviews of the literature demonstrated a statistically significant relationship between measures of religious commitment and health measures, including morbidity and mortality, in studies of many diseases (Levin, Larson, and Puchalski, 1997; Larson and Larson, 1994; Craige et al., 1990). A number of studies suggest that mortality is reduced among those who attend worship services more frequently compared to those who do not attend worship services (Strawbridge et al., 1997). Research suggests that there is reduced mortality following cardiac surgery among those who receive comfort and support from religion (Oxman, Freeman, and Manheimer, 1995).

There are also data demonstrating the importance of spirituality for people experiencing grief secondary to loss of a loved one or secondary to chronic or serious illness. Parents whose children died found much support following their child's death in their faith and church life (Cook and Wimberly, 1983). Patients with advanced cancer who also found comfort from their religious and spiritual beliefs were more satisfied with their lives, were happier, and also had diminished pain (Yates et al., 1981). One of the key steps in the Twelve Step Program of Alcoholics Anonymous, one of the most well known programs in the treatment of addiction, is, "came to believe that a power greater than ourselves could restore us to sanity." (Strachan, 1982). Addicts see their drug of choice as central in their lives; recovery hinges on the ability to find a meaning and purpose outside of oneself. People tend to become more religious as they get older. Studies have shown that the elderly see health and illness as being partly attributable to God and, to some extent, God's interventions (Bearon and Koenig, 1990). In these studies prayer appeared to complement medical care rather than compete with it. Meditation has been found to be a useful adjunct to conventional medical therapy for chronic problems such as headaches, anxiety, depression, acquired immunodeficiency syndrome, and cancer (Benson, 1996). How these modalities work is unclear. Pargament (1990) and his colleagues found the use of religious variables, especially items seeing and seeking for God as help, extends the individual's coping resources and is associated with improvement in health care outcomes. Spirituality and religion offer people hope and help give meaning to their suffering.

Putting Spirituality in the Practice of Medicine and the Art of Healing

Cassell (1991) writes, "Since in suffering, disruption of the whole person is the dominant theme, we know the losses and their losses and their meaning by what we know of others out of compassion for their suffering." It should be the obligation of all health care providers to respond to all types of suffering, as well as to relieve all physical suffering.

We have seen from the survey data that patients would like to discuss their spiritual beliefs with health care providers and incorporate those beliefs into the therapeutic plan. Data also demonstrate the beneficial effects of spirituality in health, particularly in chronic and serious illness and bereavement. Therefore health care providers should be able to communicate with patients about spirituality as integral to health and as an aid in coping with suffering.

Spiritual issues can be explored effectively with patients of all ages, including children and older, demented adults (Maugins, 1996; Frankel, 1993). The depth and focus of the discussion will vary, depending on the cognitive and developmental ability of the patient. The goals of a spiritual history are to recognize the spiritual belief of the patient and to make the appropriate referral if necessary. One way to obtain a patient's spiritual history is to talk with a patient and listen to that patient's story about what is central and important to him or her (i.e., who the patient is at his or her deepest core). Kuhn (1988) identified 14 items one might ask in a spiritual history: questions about what a person believes in, who a person loves, whether patients pray or enjoy being alone, and whether patients can forgive. Another approach to a spiritual history is suggested by Maugins (1996), who describes an assessment using the mnemonic SPIRIT, which lists several questions for each of six categories: (1) spiritual belief system; (2) personal spirituality; (3) integration in a spiritual community; (4) ritualized practices and restriction; (5) implications for medical care; and (6) terminal events planning.

FICA is yet another effective spiritual assessment tool (Puchalski et al., 1999) that is currently being used in both academic and practice settings. The use of this tool, like all such tools, must be used with a deep respect for each patient's beliefs, strengths, and needs. FICA is outlined briefly below.

F: Faith and Beliefs

The provider asks the patient about the faith or beliefs that are important to the patient. It seeks to understand what gives meaning to the person's life. The provider should use language that is familiar and comfortable for the provider. Some open-ended questions that can be used are:

"Do you consider yourself spiritual or religious?" *or*
"What gives your life meaning and purpose?" *or*
"What types of beliefs help you cope?"

I: Importance and Influence

One needs to know what role these beliefs play in the person's life. Are they important and what role do they play in how the patient takes care of his or her health? For example, a patient may be very religious, attending services regularly and seeing God as central in his or her life. For that person, any "bad news" may eventually be viewed as God's will, and such views may enable a person to cope better with his illness. On the other hand, patients may have left their church and be searching for something broader. Patients may want the provider to give them referrals to chaplains or other spiritual resources. How a provider responds to patients regarding their spirituality varies, depending on the role that spiritual belief has in a patient's life.

It is important to recognize that not all spiritual beliefs are helpful. In fact, some may interfere with the patient's ability to heal. For example, in many cases a patient's relationship with God is positive and supportive. But patients may see God in ways that can interfere with care. For example, patients may view God as punitive and may refuse medical treatment because they believe the illness is deserved. Others may refuse to take any tests or medication because they believe that any outcome is in God's hands. Therefore it is important for providers to refer to professionals such as chaplains trained as clinical pastoral educators, spiritual directors, and pastoral counselors to help patients differentiate between healthy and unhealthy beliefs.

C: Community

One needs to know if the patient expresses his spiritual beliefs in the context of a religious or spiritual community. This could be a church, temple, or mosque, or it could be a group of like-minded friends who could provide social support and assistance when the patient is facing serious or chronic illness. Many people, particularly the elderly who are often alone, may be supported by and even brought to their provider's offices by their faith community members.

A: Address and Application

The provider needs to know how the patient would like the provider to address the patient's beliefs in the context of the patient-provider relationship. Some patients may want to discuss their spiritual issues briefly and routinely at each visit. Some may simply want them noted in the event of some serious life-threatening event in the future. In addition, it is important to know what actions the patient would like the provider to take with respect to the patient's responses stemming from the initial spiritual history-taking discussion. For example, patients may need or want a referral to a chaplain, they may want clergy involved, or they may want advice regarding community resources such as meditation classes. Most patients want their beliefs to be respected and advocated for by their provider.

The health care provider should use FICA as a guide, not a checklist. Many times a patient is so pleased to have the issue of spirituality addressed that the conversation flows naturally after the first question regarding the patient's beliefs. Others may not be willing to discuss spirituality. If a patient is not interested in talking about his or her beliefs, the conversation should not be pursued further. It is critical that these conversations should never appear to be coercive. No health care provider should let these conversations seem to proselytize or ridicule a patient for his or her beliefs. Respect for the patient's privacy regarding these issues is paramount.

Resources Available in the Community

It is also important to know what spiritual resources are available in the community. Chaplains with training in clinical pastoral education (CPE) are very skilled at helping patients resolve spiritual crises or questions. A CPE-certified chaplain is trained to work with patients of any religious denomination or spiritual belief system. Many hospitals have CPE-certified chaplains. In addition, there is a growing movement to include chaplains in outpatient settings. Referrals to chaplains are as appropriate as referrals to any other specialty. Because the spirituality of patients is so important to patients and to potential outcomes, chaplains should be integral to health care teams.

The patient may also want to discuss issues with a member of the clergy (i.e., his or her own minister, priest, rabbi, or Imam). Clergy are not trained in the same way as chaplains and therefore usually do not work with patients of religious beliefs different from their own. Some religious denominations also have spiritual directors who are trained specifically to work with people on spiritual issues. They are not counselors; they work specifically on a person's spiritual journey.

Many other resources are available that may be appropriate for particular patients (e.g., music therapy, art therapy, guided imagery, meditation, and Yoga).

Summary

In working with geriatric patients, practitioners will encounter many cases of bereavement, ranging from grief following the loss of a loved one to grief associated with serious illness. Grief associated with depression may need to be treated with medications and/or psychotherapy. Many people who grieve become stressed and consequently are more susceptible to colds, headaches, and other maladies, which may be stress related. In all cases of grief, however, spirituality plays a central role in how people cope with loss. Substantial data exist from both surveys and other studies to support the beneficial role spirituality plays in health care. Therefore it is important for all health care providers to be able to recognize this important factor in patient's lives and to be able to communicate with patients about their spiritual beliefs and incorporate those beliefs into the patient's therapeutic plan. In patient care spirituality is an ongoing issue and one that frequently is discussed at subsequent visits, particularly with patients who are experiencing suffering and loss. Health care providers who can speak and listen to patients discuss their beliefs, fears, and concerns in terms of spirituality have an opportunity to bring a form of healing from pain, loss, and suffering into a patient's life.

Resources

Family Caregiving Alliance
http://www.caregiver.org/factsheets/grief.html

References

Bearon LB, Koenig HG: Religious cognition and use of prayer in health and illness, *Gerontologist* 30(2):249-253, 1990.

Benson H: *Timeless healing: the power and biology of belief,* New York, 1996, Scribner.

Cassell EJ: *The nature of suffering and the goals of medicine,* New York, 1991, Oxford University Press.

Conrad NL: Spiritual support of the dying, *Nurs Clin North Am* 20(2):415-426, 1985.

Cook JA, Wimberly DW: If I should die before I wake: religious commitment and adjustment to the death of a child, *J Scientific Study Religion* 22(3):222-238, 1983.

Craige FC et al: A systematic analyses of religious variables in The Journal of Family Practice, 1976-1986, *J Fam Pract* 2:509-513, 1990.

Doka KJ, Davidson JD, editors: *Living with grief: who we are, how we grieve,* Miami, 1997, Hospice Foundation of America.

Downey M: *Understanding Christian spirituality,* Machwah, NJ, 1997, Paulist Press.

Foglio JP, Brody H: Religion, faith and family medicine, *J Fam Pract* 27(5):473-474, 1981.

Frankl VE: *Man's search for meaning,* 1993, Buccaneer Books.

Gallop G: *Religion in America: 1990,* Princeton, NJ, 1990, Princeton Religion and Research Center.

Gallop G: *Spiritual beliefs and the dying process,* 1997, National Survey for the Nathans Cummings Foundation and the Fetzer Institute.

King DE, Bushwick B: Belief and attitudes of hospital patients about faith healing and prayer, *J Fam Pract* 39:349-352, 1994.

Kuhn CC: A spiritual inventory of the medically ill patient, *Psychiatr Med* 6(2):87-100, 1988.

Larson DB, Larson SS: *The forgotten factor in physical and mental health: what does the research show?* Rockville, Md, 1994, National Institute for Healthcare Research.

Levin JS, Schiller PL: Is there a religious factor in health? *J Religion Health* 26(1):9-36, 1987.

Levin JS, Larson DB, Puchalski DM: Religion and spirituality in medicine: research and education, *JAMA* 278(9):792-793, 1997.

Maugins TA: The SPIRITual history, *Arch Fam Med* 5:11-16, 1996.

Moberg DO: Religiosity in old age, *Gerontologist* 5:78-87, 1965.

Moberg DO: Spiritual well-being of the dying. In Lesnoff-Caravaglia G, editor: *Aging and the human condition,* New York, 1982, Human Science Press.

Oxman TE, Freeman DH, Manheimer ED: Lack of social participation of religious strength and comfort as risk factors for death after cardiac surgery in the elderly, *Psychosomatic Med* 57(1):5-15, 1995.

Pargament KI: The psychology of religion and spirituality? yes and no. Paper presented at the American Psychological Association Annual Conference, Chicago, 1997.

Pargament KI et al: Religious coping efforts as predictors of the outcomes to significant negative life events, *Am J Community Psychol* 18(6):793-824, 1990.

Puchalski CM, Larson DB. Developing curricula in spirituality and medicine, *Acad Med* 73(9):970-974, 1998.

Puchalski CM et al: FICA: a guide to spiritual assessment in the clinical setting. In press.

Strachan G. *Alcoholism: a treatable disease,* Center City, Minn, 1982, Hazelden Foundation.

Strawbridge WJ et al: Frequent attendance at religious services and mortality over twenty-eight years, *Am J Public Health* 87(6):9657-9661, 1997.

Turner RP et al: Religious or spiritual problems: a culturally sensitive diagnostic category in the DSM-IV, *J Nerv Ment Dis* 183(7):435-444, 1995.

Yates JW et al: Religion in patients with advanced cancer, *Med Pediatr Oncol* 9:121-128, 1981.

30

Caregivers

In past generations, family caregiving was not a social or health issue; it was simply the way people responded to a dependent family member. The expectation that women would quietly and efficiently care for both the children and dependent elders was so ingrained in our collective thinking that it was rarely questioned. As a result of the shifting of women's roles and the aging of our society, there are fewer women available to provide care for more older people. The role of caregiver is often compounded by conflicting responsibilities, including job, children, family, and friends. Such conflicts are easy to understand when considered in light of the fact that many caregivers spend 35 hours per week providing care in addition to working outside the home full-time (Petty and Friss, 1987).

Family caregiving problems are further complicated by a widespread lack of affordable services that could potentially ease these problems. In some parts of the country, adult day care rates exceed $60 per day, and it is typical for personal care aides to cost $15 per hour. When the family is facing a devastating and progressive disease such as Alzheimer's disease, the economic toll is even greater. The National Institute on Aging (1997) estimates that the total cost of caring for a family member with dementia at home is more than $47,000 per year, not counting loss of productivity or income. At times, it may be less expensive to stop working to care for an older relative than to hire formal supports.

Family caregiving also comes at a high physical and emotional cost. Caregivers have long been recognized as a group characterized by high levels of poor health, depression, burden, and stress (Zarit, 1996). Yet despite all these obstacles, family caring is widespread and accounts for the majority of the long-term care provided in the United States, estimated at 60% to 70% (Stone, Cafferata, and Sangl, 1987). This proportion is only expected to grow as diseases that are strongly associated with aging such as Alzheimer's disease drive the demand for both family and formal supports.

Health care providers are in a unique position to influence the health and well-being of family caregivers. Usually the issues associated with caring are not presented as a primary reason for seeking medical intervention, yet these issues may lie at the heart of medical problems for which the patient/caregiver is seeking treatment. When the functionally dependent family member is the patient, a prudent health care provider knows to inquire about the health of his or her caregiver(s). As Deimling (1994) says, "It is as necessary to care for the caregivers as it is to care for the older adult patient." Nurse practitioners, with their health promotion and family-based approach, are trained to identify and intervene in the spiral of interconnected medical, psychologic, and emotional issues that surround family caregiving. This chapter provides the background necessary to form health-promoting partnerships with family caregivers—including caregiver characteristics, role responsibilities, and needs—in relationship to their implications for assessment and intervention by health care providers.

Traditionally, when the need for direct care arises, families turn to the spouse, then a daughter, and finally a daughter-in-law. Caregiving is widely regarded as a female issue, largely due to the fact that the average caregiver is a middle-aged woman, usually the daughter or daughter-in-law of the person needing care (Stone, Cafferata, and Sangl, 1987). More recently and in response to lack of available caregivers, a greater number of sons have become involved in their aging parents' care, but this involvement mostly assumes the form of financial support for paid help in the home.

Caregiving has been called a cultural activity, reflecting a tendency for individuals to provide care consistent with culturally determined values and beliefs (Abel, 1991; Lyman, 1993). As such, there are notable gender and race differences in caregiving outcomes, although fewer differences in terms of the process of caregiving (Miller, 1995). For instance, among whites, 35% of caregivers are spouses, and most of the remainder are adult daughters (Stone, Cafferata, and Sangl, 1987). In contrast, far fewer spouses are caregivers in black families; caregivers are drawn from an extended network of individuals who may or may not be directly related to the care recipient. Spirituality and support by a religious organization are cited as important factors in caregiving more often by blacks than by whites (Haley et al., 1992; Fredman, Daly, and Lazur, 1995). Greater spirituality may be a factor in findings by Miller (1995) that black caregivers are less likely to report depression and role strain. Research with Asians and Latinos has only recently been initiated, but preliminary results suggest discernible patterns and preferences in caregiving patterns and outcomes among both groups.

Gender-specific responses to caregiving also influence how caregivers choose and carry out their care tasks. In one qualitative study of 26 caregiving spouses, husbands were observed to approach caregiving in a prioritized, linear fashion, completing care tasks one at a time in order of importance or efficiency (Corcoran, 1992a). On the other hand, the female caregivers in the study preferred "nesting" caregiving tasks, or attempting to perform several at one time (cooking dinner while looking at a photo album with Mom and writing a grocery list). Other findings from the gerontologic literature report higher levels of psychologic distress, more time spent in direct care tasks, and greater difficulty asking for help among women caregivers (Chang and White-Means, 1991; Jette, Tennstedt, and Crawford, 1995; Miller, 1987). These findings suggest that health-promoting strategies must reflect gender-related beliefs about care provision while helping caregivers modulate any unhealthy care practices.

To develop effective health interventions, it is useful to understand the range of disabilities addressed by caregivers. The most common physical ailments are arthritis (50%), hypertension and heart disease (33%), and diabetes (11%). Dementia is the most common source of disability related to psychiatric problems and may be attributed to a range of pathologies, including Alzheimer's disease, multi-infarct dementia, and Parkinson's disease. It is not uncommon for caregivers to be caring for an individual who has a number of physical and psychiatric disorders, which can make care tasks time consuming and nearly constant.

A special note is in order regarding care for an individual with Alzheimer's disease or a related dementia. Despite scientific advances in understanding the etiology and progression of Alzheimer's disease, there is concern that dementia care will place a tremendous burden on our health care system and the informal network of family caregivers who provide the bulk of care (Brookmeyer, Gray, and Kawas, 1998). Alzheimer's disease is a significant health policy issue of the coming millennium (NIA, 1997); it is projected that Alzheimer's disease prevalence in the United States will exceed 5 million by 2030 (Brookmeyer, Gray, Kawas, 1998). Most individuals with Alzheimer's disease will continue to be females without a living spouse, meaning that adult daughters will comprise the largest group of caregivers. One major effort in response to these projections is an attempt to delay onset of symptoms with medications. However, the effectiveness of medications introduced to this point is marginal. Thus it is clear that health care providers must expect to encounter in their daily practice a significant number of middle-aged women who are fatigued, depressed, and overwhelmed as a result of caregiving.

Caregivers of individuals with dementia, especially when the disease has progressed to the moderate and severe stages of impairment, are likely to be involved in caregiving tasks 24 hours per day. It is not uncommon for these overworked caregivers to be isolated from family and friends who are uncomfortable with the disease and have no understanding of how to help. Of all caregiving groups, individuals who live with and care for a loved one with dementia pay the highest toll in terms of emotional and physical well-being and should be the concern of health care providers in every clinical arena.

The Role of the Caregiver

It is widely accepted in the gerontologic literature that unpaid family caregivers provide the bulk of care required by a dependent older person who lives at home (Stone, Cafferata, and Sangl, 1987). Family caregivers as a group perform every care task, from activities of daily living to financial assistance, and are the primary resource preventing institutionalization (Colerick and George, 1986).

Literature suggests that caregivers work within a "style" of caregiving (Corcoran, 1992b; Le Navenec and Vonhof, 1996). Styles specific to dementia care are *thinking and action processes* by which spouses manage the daily care and difficult situations that arise in caring for their family member. In other words, caregivers develop and act on a set of beliefs about caregiving and disability to prioritize and perform care tasks. In a preliminary study of caregiving style in dementia, interviews with 26 spouse caregivers were analyzed to determine a caregiving style. Three distinct but overlapping styles emerged that were labeled and defined (Table 30-1).

The importance of ascertaining a caregiver style is that it may influence the type of suggestion a provider may make to a caregiver. For instance, if a caregiver who is predominately a preserver is encouraged to spend more time during the day engaging his wife in cognitively stimulating activities, he may reject the suggestion based on its potential for reducing time for himself. A more relevant recommendation for this caregiver would maintain his free time while finding other means to address his impaired

TABLE 30-1 Results of Preliminary Study of Caregiving Styles (N = 26)

Differences	Enforcer	Preserver	Enabler
Distribution	4	8	14
Average age	75	71	72
Gender	75% female	75% males	71% females
Length of care time	30 months	52 months	41 months
Focus of care concerns	Physical health of family member	Physical and emotional health of family member	Emotional health of family member
Use of tasks	Cognitive, solitary tasks (read book)	Simple, repetitive, familiar tasks (sweeping, dusting)	Social, meaningful tasks (work or recreation)
Reaction to family member's mistakes	Family member must correct mistakes	Ignores family member mistakes	Helps family member to feel OK about mistakes
Communication style	Complex, lecturing style	Simple, repetitive style	Complex, reasoning style
Interactions	Separate from family member	Parallel to family member	Cooperative with family member

From Corcoran MA: Spousal caregivers of elderly with dementia, Ann Arbor, 1992, University of Michigan.

wife's needs (such as emphasizing cognitive stimulation at adult day care or by other family members).

Caregiver Needs and Issues Related to Service Use

It is crucial for anyone interacting with the elderly to understand the network of aging services in their particular community. Sometimes, special projects or demonstrations may be available that cannot be accessed elsewhere. For instance, in Philadelphia County a home modification program is available through the local Area Agency on Aging (Philadelphia Corporation for Aging). This unique program provides adaptive equipment (e.g., bath benches, raised toilet seats) and home modifications (e.g., ramps, banisters) for elderly individuals who qualify. Other possibilities include professional programs at local universities who may wish to find unique clinical placements for their students. The best place to start may be a presentation by a social worker who specializes in community resources for the elderly in your area.

Programs may be available on either a county or regional basis. The Office on Aging in all counties is a valuable resource of information about county-wide services. Often the Office on Aging has programs that provide adult day care and transportation on a sliding fee basis. Also locally, many services are provided by the Area Agency on Aging (AAA), which is legislated by the Older Americans Act. The range of services among AAAs is broad, but each agency serves the primary function of coordinating aging services and providing case management. The vast majority of AAAs also provide the opportunity for meals (Meals on Wheels), recreation (Senior Citizen's Centers), and personal care assistance. Finally, for individuals caring for an elderly person with memory loss, the local chapter of the Alzheimer's Association is an invaluable resource. This nonprofit organization serves the public through support groups, educational programs, a lending library, telephone information and referral, and programs to assist the safe return of individuals who wander away from home. Recently a survey conducted by the Northern Virginia Chapter of the Alzheimer's Association indicated that caregivers are primarily concerned with accessing information about the disease process and management.

Despite the fact that caregiving research has been predominated by studies of stress and burden, substantial literature exists to suggest the types of services and supports that caregivers need and use. As suggested earlier, needs and service use are influenced by caregiver gender and ethnic background. For the purposes of discussion, in this chapter caregiving needs are organized into the following four categories: information, skills, supports, and services. Although only a few issues within each category are listed, the list provides a framework by which health practitioners can assess and address caregivers' needs:

Information about the pathology
Disease course
Etiology
Prognosis
Genetic disposition (when relevant)
Treatments
Research findings

Skills to manage symptoms related to the pathology
Effect of the environment on functional ability
How to promote independence in self care
Maintaining health
Adaptive equipment
Transfer and handling techniques
Methods for interacting with professionals and para-professionals

Supports
Support groups
Educational programs
Social service organizations
Self-help programs
Demonstration

Services
Financial and legal advice
Chore services
Respite
Adult day care
Transportation

Implications for Health Care Providers

Gwyther (1990) reasons that caregiving families are concerned with both the personal and knowledge or skill-based characteristics of health care professionals. The following discussion of implications for health care providers is organized around these two types of characteristics.

Personal Characteristics

Working with caregivers who are often stressed and isolated requires careful listening to understand the individual's mix of emotions. Caregivers can simultaneously experience a vast range of responses, including guilt, remorse, grief, resentment, and embarrassment. For instance, a wife caring for her husband may feel guilty at anything less than perfection in her own performance while resentful that she has to provide care during her "golden years." It is important to listen and acknowledge caregivers' feeling without judgment, while focusing on the disease as the culprit responsible for the family member's dependency or difficult behaviors. At times, wives in particular are embarrassed to disclose all their caregiving issues for fear that some situations will reflect badly on the caregiver herself. When a caregiver seems reticent to fully discuss the issues, listen and acknowledge the caregiver's feelings while assuring him or her that the disease has caused the family member to behave irrationally rather than a bad choice in a marriage partner.

Unfortunately, in today's health care industry, some encounters with caregivers are brief, infrequent, or one-time only. Caregivers require a level of sustained availability (Gwyther, 1990) to identify care problems and develop potential solutions. An effective schedule involves regular visits with the same health care provider over time and the opportunity for telephone contact if a serious issue arises or worsens. These visits and contacts do not have to be lengthy or frequent; often all that is needed is a few minutes for the caregiver to discuss how things are going. If this type of encounter is not possible in your clinical arena, attempt to refer the caregiver to a professional who can be available to specifically address the care issues.

If the health care provider is in a position to sustain availability with the caregiver, the next set of personal characteristics that caregivers request is a creative and flexible approach to problem solving. Caregiving problems are naturally complex, involving interactions among several family members, environmental demands, sociocultural constraints, financial resources, and functional abilities. Solutions rarely come easily or quickly and often involve several refinements to find a workable approach.

Health care providers should be willing to familiarize themselves with the family's idiosyncrasies. Caregiving is a cultural activity, and no two families are alike. Rich sources of information about the family are found in responses to questions about caregiving goals and methods, as well as daily routines. Particular attention should be paid to how the caregiver describes acceptable uses of time. Conflicts often arise when a resting or fatigued family member is regarded by the caregiver as lazy, unwilling to help out, or unconcerned with the caregiver's needs. In this case, education about the typical effects of the disease on activity levels may reduce this source of conflict. Education may be followed up with suggestions as to how the caregiver can prioritize care tasks, simplify them, and pace their presentation to optimize participation by the care recipient. This process, known as task breakdown, is also available from occupational therapists (OTs) who are uniquely trained in these procedures.

Knowledge and Skill-based Characteristics

As with any clinical issue, the success of interactions with caregivers depends on a comprehensive assessment. However, it is difficult to know where to start the assessment process when confronted with an overwhelmed, stressed, and fatigued caregiver reciting a litany of complaints about the dependent family member. Experienced clinicians recognize the issues in such a litany and consider four overlapping areas to include in the assessment process. They are (1) the care context, (2) the caregiver's emotional and physical health, (3) the care recipient's level of *excess disability,* and (4) the caregiver's knowledge and skills. Each is discussed in more detail in the following paragraphs.

Context of Care. The context of care is described as consisting of three dimensions: objects, tasks, and supports. *Object* evaluation includes all physical items and structural attributes. The home should be observed to determine if necessary objects are present, easily accessible when needed, yet not so cluttered as to cause a home accident or confusion. In addition, the physical structure should support easy and safe access and ideally allow a balance of privacy, comfort, and utility. *Tasks* can be assessed through detailed interview, simulation, and observation. In particular, tasks should be evaluated for their complexity, efficiency, and timing. For instance, is the caregiver spreading care tasks over a period of time or rushing to fit them all in a few hours? *Support* evaluation primarily involves understanding the effectiveness of the caregiving network. Health care providers should evaluate the family in terms of who is available to help with caregiving, how care is coordinated, and how each family member interacts with the disabled older person.

The Caregiver's Emotional and Physical Health. In a comprehensive assessment of any person with a functional limitation, it is essential to include a caregiver assessment (Brown, Potter, and Foster, 1990). Caregiver assessments are used for two reasons: to assess the caregiver's capacity to provide care, and as outcome measure in effectiveness studies.

The Care Recipient's Level of Excess Disability. Although many behavioral and functional problems are a consequence of impairment, there may be aspects of the problem that represent *excess disability.* Excess disability refers to a level of dysfunction that is disproportionate to the degree of cognitive or physical impairment (Mace, 1990). This disparity between functional ability and level of physical and cognitive decline may be the consequence of factors external to the individual, such as environmental barriers or lack of stimulation (Lawton and Nahemow, 1973; Mace, 1990).

The Caregiver's Knowledge and Skills. As part of the comprehensive assessment, the health care providers should interview the caregiver to gain information about his or her knowledge and skills for managing the care recipient's condition. If needed, the caregiver can be asked directly to define the condition ("How would you explain this condition to a neighbor or friend?") and to describe his or her care techniques. As a result, the health care provider will gain important assessment information about the strengths and weaknesses of the caregiver that could be the basis for referral or intervention. See Table 30-2 for the key elements of a caregiver assessment.

TABLE 30-2 Assessment of Caregivers

Domain	Key Elements
Ethnic and cultural issues	Primary language Level of acculturation of caregiver versus majority culture Level of acculturation of caregiver versus other family members Values regarding elder care Values regarding help-seeking
Knowledge base	Expected signs, symptoms, and course Causal attributions for difficult behaviors Communication skills Behavioral management techniques Local services
Social support	Extent of social network Local presence of extended family Availability of support and instrumental aid Satisfaction with support
Psychiatric symptomatology and burden	Depression, including vegetative signs Anxiety and stress-related symptoms Caregiver's perception of adverse impact
Family conflict	Quality of past relationship Degree of unresolved family issues Hostility and criticism toward patient Elder abuse

From Dunkin J, Cay A: Dementia caregiver burden: a review of the literature and guidelines for assessment and intervention, *Neurology* 51(Suppl 1):S53-S60, 1998.

Caregiving Interventions

Typically the short-term services of a team of health care professionals are required for implementing the caregiver care plan. For instance, a physical therapist may use one session with the caregiver to teach proper body mechanics, in addition to any therapy or use of mobility equipment required for the care recipient. Occupational therapists help with task breakdown and use a range of methods to restore maximal functional independence (including adaptive equipment), make caregiving easier, and establish an energy-conserving routine. An OT may be indicated for the caregiver (to assist with dementia management strategies), the dependent family member (to improve function), or both. Social work is essential when financial or community resource needs are identified, especially a seasoned social worker who has an in-depth understanding of the local aging network.

A comprehensive intervention program dealing with the issue of caregiving can include treatments both for the person receiving the care and the family caregiver. One type of intervention is aimed at the behavior of the family member who is the being cared for. This type of intervention may serve to lessen the caregiver's problems indirectly.

Table 30-3 Interventions for Caregivers

Intervention	Appropriate for	Impact	Comment
Education	All caregivers	No known systematic studies	Should include access to local services
Support groups	Caregivers displaying minimal distress	Equivocal effect on burden and depression May delay long-term placement	Not appropriate as sole intervention for very distressed caregivers
Respite care	All caregivers	May delay long-term placement Equivocal effect on burden depression	Caregivers require education about respite before using it effectively
Family therapy	Families with unresolved issues affecting patient care	No known systematic studies	Can be reframed as education to engage more resistant families
Individual treatment	Caregivers with overt distress, psychopathology	Strongest effect on caregiver outcome	Little consensus as to essential components of treatment

From Dunkin J, Cay A: Dementia caregiver burden: a review of the literature and guidelines for assessment and intervention, *Neurology* 51(Suppl 1):S53-S60, 1998.

The caregiver may benefit from education concerning the particular illness that is afflicting his or her family member. Effective management techniques such as communication skills can be taught, which may prove to be a substantial benefit. Interventions aimed at reducing isolation and stress include support groups, respite care, and family therapy. See Table 30-3 for a list of interventions for caregivers.

Summary

The complexity of family caregiving requires a comprehensive approach to health care. As with any dynamic system that has multiple components, change in any one component will potentially resonate to the rest of the system. Therefore problems experienced by an elderly individual may have implications for the health and well-being of the rest of the family. In turn, an ineffective family care network is likely to promote further dependence and health issues for the elderly individual. The unique challenge in partnering with family caregivers to promote health is initially identifying who is experiencing negative consequences from caregiving. Because these negative consequences may not be the primary reason for contact with a health provider, their presence may go undetected. One solution to effectively identify family members who need additional knowledge and skills is for all health professionals to be vigilant about examining the status not only of a particular individual, but also the family system that supports that individual.

Resources

AGENET
http://www.caregivers.com

Caregiving Online Newsletter
http://www.caregiving.com

Administration on Aging
http://www.aoa.gov

Alzheimer's Caregiving Page
http://www.alzwell.com

Elderweb Online Eldercare Sourcebook
http://www.elderweb.com

References

Able E: *Who cares for the elderly? Public policy and the experiences of adult daughters,* Philadelphia, 1991, Temple University Press.

Brookmeyer R, Gray S, Kawas C: Projections of Alzheimer's disease in the United States and the public health impact of delaying disease onset, *Am J Public Health* 88(9):1337-1341, 1998.

Brown JJ, Potter JF, Foster GB: Caregiver burden should be evaluated during geriatric assessment, *J Am Geriatr Soc* 85:455-456, 1990.

Chang CF, White-Means SI: The men who care: An analysis of male primary caregivers who care for the frail elderly at home, *J Applied Gerontol* 10(3):343-358, 1991.

Colerick [Clipp] EJ, George LK: Predictors of institutionalization among caregivers of patients with Alzheimer's disease, *J Am Geriatr Soc* 34:493-498, 1986.

Corcoran MA: Gender differences in dementia management plans of spousal caregivers: implications for occupational therapy, *Am J Occup Ther* 46(11):1006-1011, 1992a.

Corcoran MA: *Spousal caregivers of elderly with dementia,* Ann Arbor, 1992b, University of Michigan.

Deimling GT: Caregiver functioning. In Lawton MP, Teresi JA, editors: *Annual review of gerontology and geriatrics,* vol 14, New York, 1994, Springer Publishing.

Dunkin J, Cay A: Dementia caregiver burden: a review of the literature and guidelines for assessment and intervention *Neurology* 51(suppl 1): S53-S60, 1998.

Fredman L, Daly MP, Lazur AM: Burden among white and black caregivers to elderly adults, *J Gerontol B Psychol Sci Soc Sci* 50(2):S110-S118, 1995.

Gwyther LP: *Clinician and family: a partnership for support.* In Mace NL, editor: Dementia care: patient, family, and community, Baltimore, 1990, Johns Hopkins University Press.

Haley WE et al: Psychological and health symptoms among black and white dementia caregivers, Paper presented at the American Psychological Association annual meeting, Washington, DC, 1992.

Jette AM, Tennstedt S, Crawford S: How does formal and informal community care affect nursing home use? *J Gerontol: Soc Sci* 50B(1):S4-S12, 1995.

Lawton MP, Nahemow L: *Ecology and the aging process.* In Eisedorfer C, Lawton MP, editors: *Psychology of Adult Development and Aging.* Washington, DC, 1973, American Psychological Association.

Le Navenec CL, Vonhof T: *One day at a time: how families manage the experience of dementia,* Westport, Conn, 1996, Auburn House.

Lyman K: *Day in, day out with Alzheimer's stress in caregiving relationships,* Philadelphia, 1993, Temple University Press.

Mace NL: *The management of problem behaviors.* In Mace NL, editor: *Dementia care: patient, family, and community,* Baltimore, 1990, Johns Hopkins University Press.

Miller B: Gender and control among spouses of the cognitively impaired: a research note, *Gerontologist* 27(4):447-453, 1987.

Miller B: Race, control, mastery and caregiver distress, *J Gerontol: Soc Sci* 50B(6):S374-S382, 1995.

National Institute on Aging: *Progress report on Alzheimer's disease,* NIA, NIH Publication No. 97-4014, 1997.

Petty D, Friss L: A balancing act of working and caregiving, *Business Health* October, 22-26, 1987.

Stone R, Cafferata GL, Sangl J: Caregivers of frail elderly: a national profile, *Gerontologist* 27:616-626, 1987.

Zarit SH: Dementia and the family: a stress management approach, *Clin Psychol* 39:103-105, 1996.

Unit V

31

Demographics: The Older Population in the United States

The growth in life expectancy is one of the great accomplishments of the twentieth century. In 1900, adults over age 65 accounted for 4% of the total population, and the life expectancy of a child born in that year was 46.4 years for boys and 49.0 years for girls. Advances in medical technology in combination with public health measures such as clean water, sanitation, work safety laws, and better nutrition have contributed to the increased life expectancy we are now experiencing. In the year 2000 older adults account for 12.7% of the total population, and life expectancy is 71.1 years for males and 79.5 years for females. The fastest growing segment of the older population is people over age 85. However, within the U.S. population there are significant differences in life expectancy at birth in relationship to race (Tables 31-1 and 31-2).

The proportion of elderly will remain constant until around 2010, when the baby boom cohort turns 65. This event will trigger large increases in the number and proportion of older people. In recent years the many articles discussing the impact of baby boomers on social services, pensions, the economy, the health care industry, and even national production have illustrated the concern and attention this population shift has been receiving. The growth rate in the older population has implications for the sheer number of people requiring elderly services (e.g., housing, health, nutrition, information, and entitlement programs).

The projections of a very high and increasing proportion of elderly from 2010 to 2030 are attributed to three factors: (1) declining and low fertility, (2) maturing of the baby boom cohort, and (3) sharp declines in mortality at older ages. Once the baby boom influx is over (i.e., has completely passed age 65) in 2030, the proportion of elderly in the total population will stabilize (Siegel, 1996).

TABLE 31-1 Projections of Percent of Individuals 65 Years and Older in Total Population by Race by Year

Year	White	Black	Hispanic	Other
1995	13.8	8.2	5.6	6.6
2000	13.7	8.1	6.0	7.2
2010	14.4	8.6	6.9	8.7

Source: US Department of Health and Human Services, Administration on Aging, 1996, based on US Bureau of the Census data.

TABLE 31-2 Life Expectancy at Birth, Age 65, and Age 85 by Sex and Race: 1995 and 2050

Sex	Race	Age	Life Expectancy: 1995	Life Expectancy: 2050
Male	White	Birth	73.6	82.0
		65	19.2	22.4
	Black	Birth	64.8	70.8
		65	13.6	16.5
	Hispanic	Birth	74.9	84.4
		65	18.5	25.6
Female	White	Birth	80.1	85.9
		65	19.4	23.6
		85	6.5	9.4
	Black	Birth	74.5	79.7
		65	17.6	20.3
	Hispanic	Birth	82.2	89.6
		65	21.8	27.9
All races	Male	85	5.2	6.8
	Female	85	6.5	9.4

Source: US Department of Health and Human Services, Administration on Aging, 1996, based on US Bureau of the Census data.

Socioeconomic Factors

The socioeconomic characteristics of the older population include elements such as income, gender, and race. An understanding of how various socioeconomic factors are interwoven and impact primary health care is more important than simply defining individual socioeconomic factors.

Income

In 1995 approximately 3.7 million people over age 65 lived below the poverty level ($9212 for older couples or $7309 for an older individual living alone) (U.S. Department of Health and Human Services, 1996). Thirty-nine percent have incomes below $10,000, and 6% have incomes under $5000. Eighteen percent of people age 65 or older were

TABLE 31-3 Percent Distribution of Income Source for Persons 65 Years and Older

Income Source	Percent
Social Security	42%
Public and Private Pensions	19%
Earnings	18%
Asset Income	18%
All Other Sources	3%

Source: US Department of Health and Human Services, Administration on Aging, 1996, based on US Bureau of the Census data.

classified as poor or near poor in 1995; that is, almost one fifth of older people had annual incomes under $11,515. More than half of older African-American women who live alone live in poverty. The poverty rate for older individuals is higher in the South, for those with less than 12 years of education, and for those who are ill or disabled. Only 16% have annual incomes of $25,000 or more. The median net worth (assets minus liabilities) of households headed by a person age 65 or older is $86,300. Table 31-3 illustrates the major sources of income for older people.

Employment. Although the elderly represent a growing proportion of the total population and although life expectancy has increased, the older population represents a much smaller share of the nation's labor force today than they did 50 years ago. The percentage of men over age 55 in the work force has decreased dramatically—from approximately 69% in 1950 to approximately 38% in 1993. The Bureau of Labor Statistics predicts that the percentage of men age 55 to 59 in the labor force will continue to decline through 2005, but at a slower rate. The change in labor force participation has not been as striking for older women, with participation actually increasing in the over-55 age-group—from 19% in 1950 to 23% in 1993. Thus women in their late fifties, unlike men, have been increasingly likely to be in the work force (Figure 31-1).

Assets. Because financial soundness include a person's lifetime accrual of assets in addition to net income, it is not surprising that the median net worth of the elderly is more than 15 times higher than that of households headed by the under-35 age-group (Hobbs and Damon, 1996). In fact, their median net worth is estimated to be approximately $88,000, compared with about $5500 for the under-35 age-group. More than 70% of elderly people's assets is made up of home equity, with interest-earning assets at financial institutions accounting for 21%, and stocks and mutual funds accounting for 9%. Despite the optimistic picture that their high median net worth presents, a large number of people reach retirement age with little or no savings. This may have considerable implications for their ability to finance potential long-term care services and to assume the burden of other health care expenditures, because the elderly face an increased risk for more serious and expensive health care problems.

Gender

Among the elderly, there are significantly more women than men (45% more women in the 1995 65+ age group). In the 55- to 64-year age-group, the number of men per 100

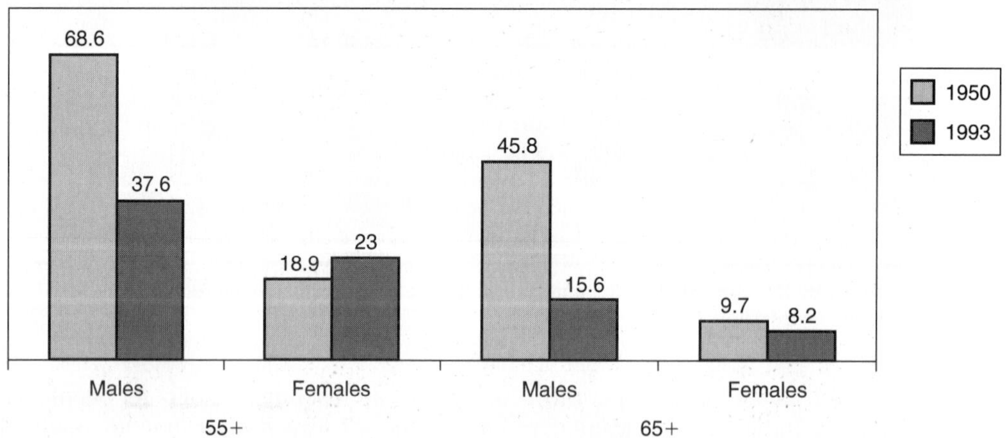

Figure 31-1 Percent of older population in the labor force by age group and sex: 1950 and 1993. (Source: US Bureau of Labor Statistics: 1950 from 1950 Current Population Survey, unpublished tabulations; 1993 from reprint of 1993 Annual Average Tables from the January 1994 issue, *Employment and Earning,* Table 3.)

women is 90.6. For 65- to 74-year-olds the number is 80, and for 75- to 84-year-olds the number is 63.4. The imbalance between genders in the elderly has implications for the types of integrated primary health care delivery systems that will be developed over the next decades. Planning and policy efforts regarding primary health care should reflect gender proportions within the population cohort. Although the projected gender imbalance in the 65+ age-group will decrease because of converging mortality rates, women are projected to continue to outnumber men, especially in the over-85 age-group (Figure 31-2).

Race

Projections for the racial composition of the U.S. population call for important changes. The Hispanic proportion of the over-65 age-group is projected to increase from 4.5% in 1995 to more than 17% in 2050. The proportion of African-Americans in the 65+ age-group is also projected to increase, but not so dramatically—from 8% in 1995 to almost 11% in 2050. The proportion of other races (mainly Asian and Pacific Islanders) is projected to increase significantly during this same time period—from 2.3% to 7.4%. The proportion of Caucasians in the 65+ age-group is projected to decrease from around 90% in 1995 to approximately 82% in 2050 (U.S. Bureau of the Census, 1990). These projections are estimates of future changes, and the proportion may vary; however, the undeniable fact is that the composition of the population in 2050 will be different than that of 2000.

Racial differences are important factors for primary care health policy. For example, African-Americans report higher rates of hypertension, diabetes, and arthritis than other races. People of Hispanic descent report higher rates of hypertension and diabetes and lower rates of heart conditions than other races. Although socioeconomic status accounts

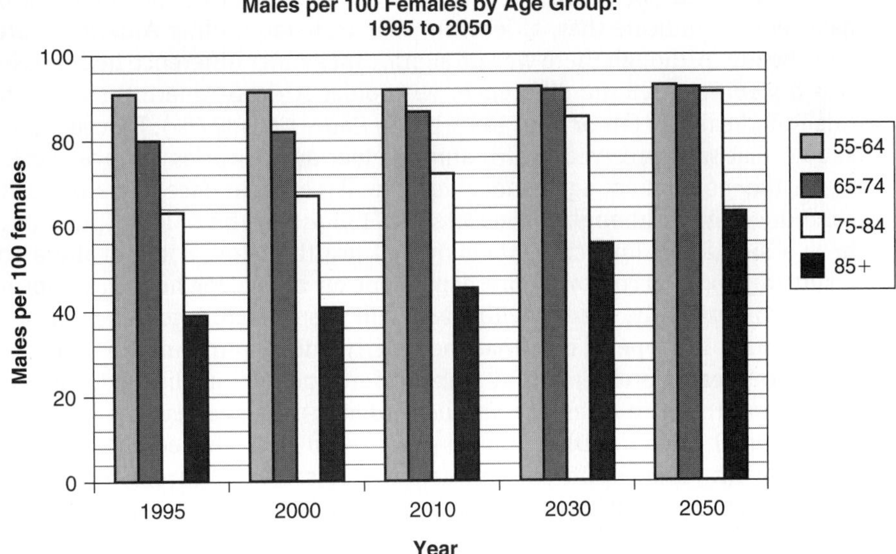

Figure 31-2 Males per 100 females by age group: 1995 to 2050. (Source: US Department of Health and Human Services, Administration on Aging, 1996, based on data from the US Bureau of the Census.)

for much of the difference in functional status associated with these chronic diseases, it does not explain the differences in the prevalence of these diseases among the different groups. These differences suggest varying causal pathways among racial and ethnic groups (Kington and Smith, 1997).

However, race alone is not necessarily the causative biologic factor determining health status and health services utilization. Martin and Soldo (1997) argue that race and ethnicity are fluid categories defined as much by social and historical context as by how a person responds to race questions on a survey. Intermarriage, socioeconomic integration, and cultural exchange will continue to contribute to significant changes in "standard" race definitions and the association between race and health or race and primary health care utilization.

Health Status

It has been shown in various life expectancy projections that elderly people can expect a longer average life by the year 2050. In fact, by the year 2050 the average 65-year-old Caucasian woman can expect to live to almost age 90. These projections are based partly on the estimates of decreasing mortality rates, particularly among the older age-groups. Although this indicates that the elderly are living longer, the question of quality of life is not addressed solely by number of years. The issue of a healthy life during the last years is an important consideration for all primary care providers.

When elderly people were asked to assess their own health, almost three out of four noninstitutionalized persons age 65 to 74 indicated that they thought their health was good, very good, or excellent (U.S. Department of Health and Human Services, 1996).

Thus only about one quarter of older people evaluated their health as fair or poor. These data seem to indicate that, at least in their viewpoint, older Americans are generally in good health. Although there was no significant gender difference in this assessment, there was a significant ethnic difference, with older African-Americans much more likely to rate their health as fair or poor (43%) than Caucasians (27%). Indeed, other studies have shown that self-perceived health among older adults varies by race (Peek et al., 1997).

As the population ages the elderly will come to face certain health states and conditions that, although not necessarily unique to the older population, nevertheless have a significant impact on their overall health status. Some of these conditions will result in people becoming more dependent on others for help in performing everyday tasks. Consequently, these health states will pose a challenge to health care providers in determining the type of care that the elderly will require and how best to provide that care. The health problems that many elderly people are likely to face are chronic in nature and result in disability and dependency on activities of daily living (ADLs) and instrumental ADLs (IADLs). Given any particular health condition, the proportion of actual healthy years of life vs. the years characterized by chronic illness and disability is an important factor in assessing the health status of the elderly.

Chronic Conditions

Chronic conditions such as arthritis and heart disease have become an increasingly important public health concern. This is especially true among the older population, who are most prone to chronic conditions. These types of health conditions have a significant impact on both health care utilization and expenditures in that people with chronic conditions usually require ongoing care, and thus their costs are proportionately high. For example, one study showed that although persons with activity limitations due to chronic conditions represented only about 17% of the general population in 1987, they accounted for about 47% of medical expenditures (Trupin et al., 1995). Thus with declining mortality rates, an aging population, and improved medical technology, the number of people with chronic conditions will continue to grow. These people will need medical and long-term care, which has an impact on the provision of appropriate health care services to meet their needs.

The majority of older people have at least one chronic condition, and many have multiple chronic conditions. According to a study conducted by Hoffman et al. (1996), rates of chronic conditions were highest among the elderly, with 88% of them having at least one chronic condition. The presence of more than one chronic condition (i.e., comorbidity) added significantly to the burden faced by those with chronic conditions, with the risk of comorbidities being the greatest among the elderly. In many cases having chronic health conditions leads to the development of limitations on an individual's daily tasks. In noninstitutionalized people age 65 and over, 38% report having some limitation of activity brought about by the existence of chronic health problems (National Center for Health Statistics, 1996). Within the same age-group, the proportion of elderly persons with a limitation in activity was 21% higher for African-Americans than for Caucasians, and the severity of the limitation was greater for African-Americans than for their Caucasian counterparts. Of importance to note is that although the Hoffman et al. study found the elderly far more likely to have a chronic condition than all other age-groups, the elderly accounted for only one quarter of all those living in the community with chronic conditions.

The most common chronic conditions in the noninstitutionalized elderly are arthritis, hypertension, heart disease, hearing impairments, cataracts, orthopedic impairments, sinusitis, and diabetes (U.S. Department of Health and Human Services, 1996). Figure 31-3 shows the most common chronic conditions affecting the elderly. For men, the three most prevalent chronic conditions are arthritis, heart disease, and hearing impairments. With increasing age (i.e., 75+ age group), heart disease and hearing impairments surpass arthritis as the leading chronic condition among older men. Among older women, arthritis, heart disease, and hypertension are consistently the top three chronic conditions and are irrespective of age-group. In general, arthritis and hypertension were more prevalent among women than among their male counterparts, but men had higher levels of heart disease and hearing impairments than women in every age-group. Thus despite the fact that men in general have a higher risk for fatal diseases than women, women are at greater risk for incurring nonfatal chronic conditions, such as arthritis.

Activities of Daily Living and Disability

Not surprisingly, the likelihood of having a disability increases with age. People age 65 and over account for a far larger share of all those with disabilities (34%) than does the total population (12%). They make up an even larger percentage (43%) of those with severe disabilities (U.S. Bureau of the Census, 1996). The Bureau of the Census defines having a severe disability as using a wheelchair or other special aid for 6 months or longer, being unable to perform one or more functional activities or needing assistance with an ADL or IADL, being prevented from working at a job or doing housework, or having a selected condition that includes autism, cerebral palsy, Alzheimer's disease, senility or dementia, or mental retardation. One study proposes that a small number of diseases and

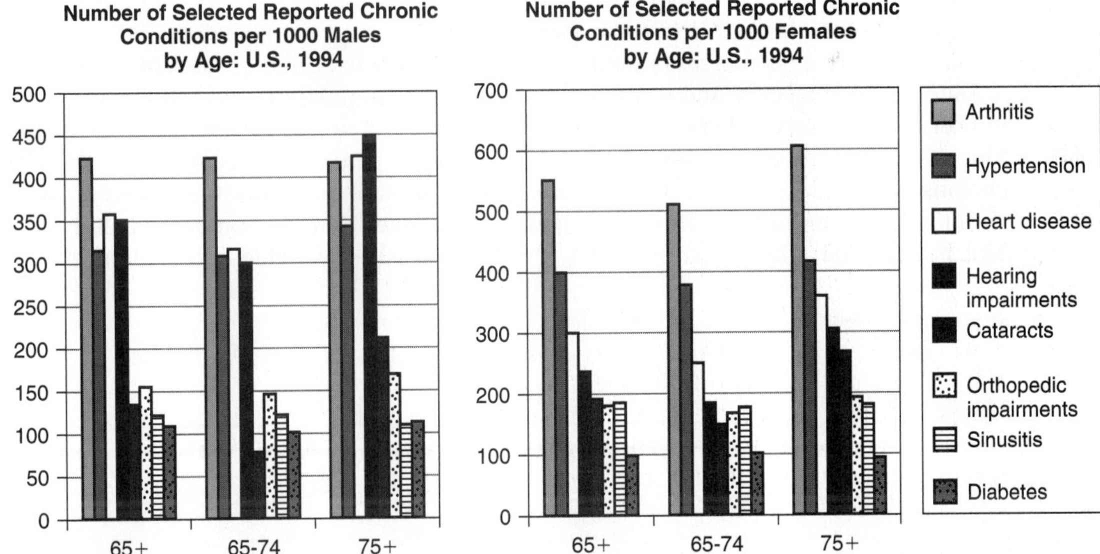

Figure 31-3 Number of selected reported chronic conditions per 1000 males by age: U.S. 1994; number of selected reported chronic conditions per 1000 females by age: U.S. 1994. (Source: Adams PF, Marano MA: Current estimates from the National Health Interview Survey 1994, National Center for Health Statistics, *Vital Health Stat* 10[193]:83-84, 1995.)

conditions are responsible for a large share of severe disability in older persons: stroke, hip fracture, congestive heart failure, pneumonia, coronary heart disease, diabetes, and dehydration. Targeting these conditions could help to decrease severe disability among the elderly and improve their independent functioning (Ferrucci et al., 1997).

Disability in the older population often is measured in terms of a person's ability to perform ADLs and IADLs. ADLs include bathing, dressing, toileting, walking, eating, and getting in and out of a bed or chair. IADLs include housekeeping tasks such as preparing meals, shopping, managing money, using the telephone, doing light housework, and doing heavy housework. Table 31-4 shows that the percentage of elderly requiring assistance with ADLs increases with age from 2.3% in the 65 to 69 age-group to 20% in the 85+ age-group. The percentage of those needing help with IADLs was higher, with 5% in the 65 to 69 age-group needing assistance and 22.3% of those in the 85+ age-group requiring help. In addition, in the age-groups of 65 to 74 and 75+, disability was more prevalent among elderly women than among elderly men (e.g., 32.9% vs. 22.8% in the 75+ age group). Indeed, given the longer life expectancy of women, women account for a larger share of older persons with a disability.

It is important to realize that if 22.3% of people over age 85 need formal assistance in IADLs, then 77.7% of people who are over age 85 and living in the community are managing to prepare their meals, shop for groceries, do housework, manage their finances, and use the telephone without any formal assistance. There are many projections concerning this group of older independent people, but it behooves all health professionals to recognize and affirm the strengths of older people and support them and their network of informal support.

Another way to look at the extent and impact of disability in the elderly is to consider the number of bed-disability days—the number of days when normal activities are restricted because of illness or injury to the extent that the day is spent in bed. Table 31-5 shows that the elderly average approximately 14.8 of these days annually (U.S. Department of Health and Human Services, 1996). These data also show that the number of bed-disability days increases with age and has remained quite consistent since 1982.

Data on the disability and limitations status of the noninstitutionalized elderly are of importance to policymakers, researchers, and service planners to assess service needs. Thus it is important to have an accurate estimate of the actual number of disabled elderly persons. Although the range of estimates of the future number of disabled elderly is wide (from 2.8 million to 22.6 million), it is generally believed that the number of elderly who will be disabled will increase (Siegel, 1996). Table 31-6 provides projections on the

TABLE 31-4 Percent of Elderly Needing Assistance with Activities of Daily Living, by Age

	Assistance Needs with ADL Only	Assistance Needs with IADL Only
65-69	2.3	5.0
70-74	4.4	7.5
75-84	8.6	13.9
85+	20.0	22.3

Based on data from the National Health Interview Survey, 1992.

number of older people who will become disabled through the year 2040. These figures estimate that in general there will be an increase in the percentage of the elderly population who will be disabled—from approximately 19% in 1990 to approximately 21% by the year 2040. The percentage of the elderly who will be severely disabled will also increase accordingly (Manton et al., 1993).

The statistics and information presented in this discussion of disability strongly indicate that the elderly are vulnerable to the onset of disability and ADL dependencies and that the number of disabled elderly will increase dramatically in the future. However, recent research conducted at Duke University brings forth another viewpoint. The findings suggest that disability rates among the elderly in the United States are actually declining dramatically and that this rate of reduction is increasing. Researchers found that the actual number of older people with disability in 1994 was 7.1 million and not the expected 8.3 million—an estimate based on the assumption that the 1982 disability rates would remain unchanged (Manton et al., 1993). This overestimation of the number of disabled elderly

TABLE 31-5 Number of Bed-Disability Days per Person per Year as a Result of Acute and Chronic Conditions for All Races and Sex, by Age: United States, 1982-1992

	1982	1983	1984	1985	1986	1987	1988	1989	1990	1991	1992
All ages	6.4	6.7	6.5	6.1	6.5	6.2	6.3	6.5	6.2	6.5	6.3
55-64 years	10.1	10.1	10.1	9.1	9.8	9.6	9.9	8.5	8.9	9.4	8.7
65-74 years	13.1	14.2	12.4	11.2	13.0	12.3	12.5	11.4	10.8	12.1	11.8
75-84 years	15.6	17.9	18.3	15.6	15.6	14.8	15.0	16.8	16.0	16.1	17.5
65+ years	14.7	16.7	15.1	13.7	14.9	14.0	14.4	14.2	13.6	14.7	14.8

Source: Cohen RA, Van Nostrand JF: Trends in the health of older Americans: United States, 1994, National Center for Health Statistics, *Vital and Health Statistics* 3(30), 1995, US Department of Health and Human Services, Public Health Service, Centers for Disease Control and Prevention, National Center for Health Statistics. Data based on interviews with civilian noninstitutionalized population.

TABLE 31-6 Projections of the Noninstitutionalized Population 65+ Years with ADL Limitations: 1990-2040

	Number (in Thousands)		Percent of Population*	
	With ADL Limitations	Severely Disabled	With ADL Limitations	Severely Disabled
1990	6,029	1,123	18.8	3.5
1995	6,712	1,265	19.3	3.6
2000	7,262	1,384	20.0	3.8
2020	10,118	1,927	19.2	3.7
2040	14,416	2,806	21.4	4.2

Calculated on the basis of projections of the US population prepared by the US Social Security Administration and preliminary data from the 1982 National Long-Term Care Survey.

*Base includes the institutional population.

may be attributed in part to improved public health measures and nutrition, higher levels of education, improved economic status, and technologic advances in medicine, all of which have helped to improve the health of the elderly. If this trend of declining disability among the elderly is indeed occurring, then it will change in part the way aging is viewed in this country. It would be important to maintain this decline by investigating further the factors involved in decreasing disability in the older population.

Other Illnesses and Disease Rates

The elderly account for approximately 1.6 million (or approximately 73%) of the 2.2 million total annual deaths in the United States. Heart disease, cancer, and stroke continue to be the leading causes of death among the elderly. In 1980 these three diseases accounted for 75% of deaths in the elderly and in 1993 were still responsible for approximately 70% of all elderly deaths. Respiratory conditions such as pneumonia and influenza, as well as chronic obstructive pulmonary diseases, were also significant causes of death in the elderly population.

A New Trend

Data show that deaths related to human immunodeficiency virus (HIV) are higher in the elderly than in the 20-year-old age-group (Table 31-7). In fact, the number of deaths related to acquired immunodeficiency syndrome (AIDS) in the elderly population more than doubled between 1987 and 1993, whereas this figure was quite stable for children during the same period. This is an important consideration for primary care providers, not only in terms of diagnosing but also in terms of preventing HIV in the older population.

Overview of Primary Health Care Service Utilization

As a person ages, the use of health services typically increases. Physician office visits and drug expenditures increase; among the older-old, nursing home services, home health, and durable medical equipment expenses may be incurred for the first time. Physician

TABLE 31-7 Death Rates for HIV Infection (per 100,000 population), All Races

Age Group	1987	1988	1989	1990	1991	1992	1993
<1	2.3	2.2	3.1	2.7	2.3	2.5	2.2
1-4	0.7	0.8	0.8	0.8	1.0	1.0	1.3
5-14	0.1	0.2	0.2	0.2	0.3	0.3	0.4
15-24	1.3	1.4	1.6	1.5	1.7	1.6	1.7
55-64	3.5	4.0	5.4	6.2	7.4	8.5	8.8
65-74	1.3	1.6	1.8	2.0	2.4	2.8	2.9
75-84	0.8	0.8	0.7	0.7	0.9	0.8	0.8

Source: National Center for Health Statistics (1996): *Health, United States,* Hyattsville, Md, 1995, Public Health Service, Table 43.

contact sites for those over age 65 vary, with the most common site being the physician's office (53%), followed by the hospital outpatient department (10%), telephone (9%), and home health (19%).

The site of physician contact is strongly associated with income. Age-adjusted contacts in a physician's office were 31% lower for people with incomes below $14,000 than for people whose income was over $50,000 (U.S. Department of Health and Human Services, 1995b). People with lower incomes are less likely to use the telephone and more likely to contact a physician in a hospital outpatient department or emergency department. The number and site of physician contacts also vary by race. The number of age-adjusted ambulatory visits was 15% lower for African-Americans than for Caucasians; physician office visits were 34% lower, and the use of hospital outpatient departments was double. It is quite possible that these observed differences between races actually reflect differences in income-related visits.

Women typically have more physician contacts than men. For example, women age 45 to 64 see physicians approximately 35% more often than men (National Center for Health Statistics, 1996). The gender difference dissipates somewhat with age. Both women and men age 64 to 74 make, on average, 10 physician visits per year. Men age 75 years and older make approximately 11.6 physician visits per year, compared with 12.4 for women in the same age-group.

The primary health care delivery system is often closely linked to Medicare or Medicaid eligibility because many services are reimbursed through these programs. Health maintenance organizations, health care prepayment plans, social HMOs, home health agencies, and hospital geriatric care networks with services emphasizing ambulatory care and prevention are some examples of delivery systems for the elderly that are usually funded through government programs.

Medicare managed care plans have the option of contracting with the Health and Human Services Department's Health Care Financing Administration to provide services to Medicare enrollees and to receive monthly payments based either on risk or on a set rate per capita. In 1996 approximately 4.4 million Medicare beneficiaries (11.2% of the Medicare population) were enrolled in managed care plans (Health Care Financing Administration, 1997). This number, as well as the percentage of total Medicare enrollees, is expected to increase as baby boomers become eligible for Medicare eligible. Based on past enrollment trends for managed care, Medicare managed care enrollment may level off around 15% of Medicare enrollees. However, based on population projections for those in the 65+ age-group, the total number of those eligible for Medicare who are enrolled in managed care plans in the future could be significantly greater than the 4.4 million Medicare beneficiaries currently enrolled.

The use of home health care has increased because changes and advances in medical technology have made it possible to deliver some primary care services at home. Corresponding changes in health insurance coverage, which is beginning to cover home health services, have contributed to the increasing use of home health services. In 1993 about 1.5 million people (20% in the 85+ age-group) used home health agencies, with the most common diagnoses being heart disease (13%), diseases of the musculoskeletal system (9%), and cerebrovascular disease (7%). Not surprisingly, the use of home health care increases with age, and women tend to use home health care more than men, with the differential increasing with age. Approximately three quarters of home health users are at least 65 years of age, and two thirds are women. Men and women 45 to 64 years old tend to have the same rate of use—about 0.3% of the population. However, among the older cohorts (85+ age-group), women's home health use tends to be higher than men's—more than 13% compared with 8% (National Center for Health Services, 1996).

The integration of primary health care services among and between delivery structures is imperative. Formal primary care providers do recognize the importance of incorporating existing organizational structures such as churches, informal support structures, and their formal delivery structure into effective primary health care delivery (Hatch, 1991). The Program for All-Inclusive Care for the Elderly (PACE) is an example of such an integrated care model. Jointly funded by Medicare and Medicaid, PACE focuses on delivering a continuum of care for frail elderly (who are state certified as needing nursing home care but are living in the community) by integrating providers and community-based long-term care programs. Primary care delivery is centered around adult day care centers and arranging for hospital or nursing home placement as necessary. The PACE program ensures that primary care needs are met through a single service delivery and financing system. Currently there are 15 PACE programs authorized nationwide (Prospective Payment Assessment Commission, 1997).

Factors Influencing Primary Care for the Older Population

Geographic Distribution

State Estimates. It is well known that the older population represents a fast-growing proportion of the total U.S. population. Hence it follows that most, if not all, states will experience an increase in their proportion of elderly residents. The largest increases during the 1980s were seen predominantly in the West (e.g., Nevada and Utah) and in the South (e.g., Florida and South Carolina). In 1993 nine states had more than 1 million elderly residents (California, Florida, New York, Pennsylvania, Texas, Illinois, Ohio, Michigan, and New Jersey). Although California had the most elderly residents, Florida had the highest proportion of elderly (19%). The migration of the elderly into Florida contributed to the state's high rankings, and Florida is expected to continue to have the country's highest proportion of elderly residents, at approximately 25% (Hobbs and Damon, 1996). The U.S. Census Bureau projects that by 2020 approximately half of all elderly people will be domiciled in the same nine states that had the most elderly residents in 1993, plus North Carolina. California and Florida will still be the top states with the largest number of elderly residents (Figure 31-4).

Older adults living in rural areas seem to have poorer health status than their urban counterparts. These differences in health status may be partly due to differences in access to care, adequacy of care, and income levels (Angel, 1995).

Migration

In general, the older population remains geographically quite stationary. The elderly represented only 4% of all individuals who moved in the United States; only 3% of all elderly who moved actually changed their county of residence, only 1% moved as far as another state, and 8% moved from a metropolitan area to a nonmetropolitan area. In addition, of all people age 65 and older, about 6% moved within the country as compared with approximately 18% of all younger people.

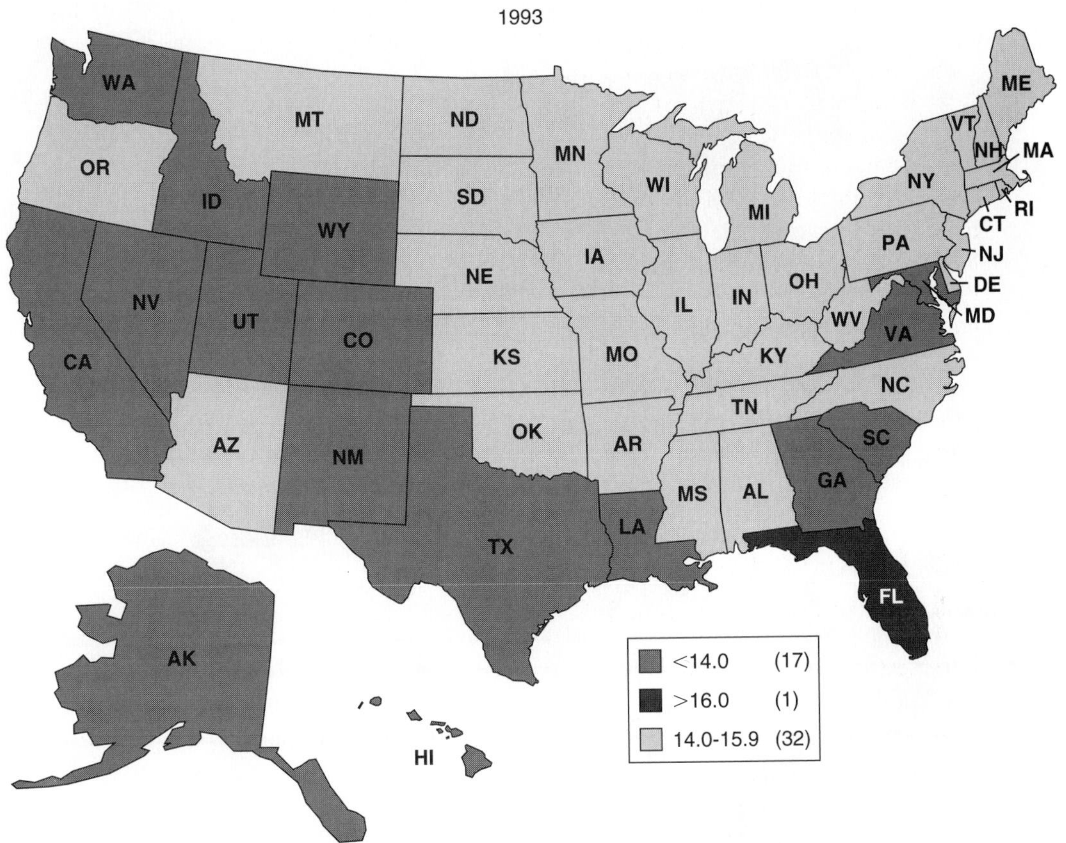

Figure 31-4 Percentage of total state population 65 years and over: 1993 and 2020. (Source: US Bureau of the Census 1993, from State age-sex population estimates consistent with census advisory CB94-43; 2020, *Population projections for states by age, sex, race, and Hispanic origin: 1993 to 2020,* Current Population Reports p 25-1111, Washington, DC, 1994, US Government Printing Office.) *Continued*

Research conducted on elderly migration has shown that households headed by men older than age 55 were inclined to move toward lower-crime and lower-cost areas, toward nonmetropolitan areas, and closer to the residences of families and friends (Kallan, 1993). However, the most salient fact to be drawn from these data is that most older people remain either in their primary residence or in the same geographic location where they have spent their adult lives, and this fact remains constant over time (Table 31-8).

Silverstein (1995) found that older people moving from warmer to colder states tend to be disproportionately disabled and widowed as compared with those moving from colder to warmer states. This phenomenon probably occurs after the death of a spouse in combination with other illness, which causes an older person to move closer to children or other family members in their original home communities, presumably to receive support.

Economic Factors

Twenty percent of personal health expenditures are paid for out of pocket; federal government and private health insurance each cover one third, and state and local

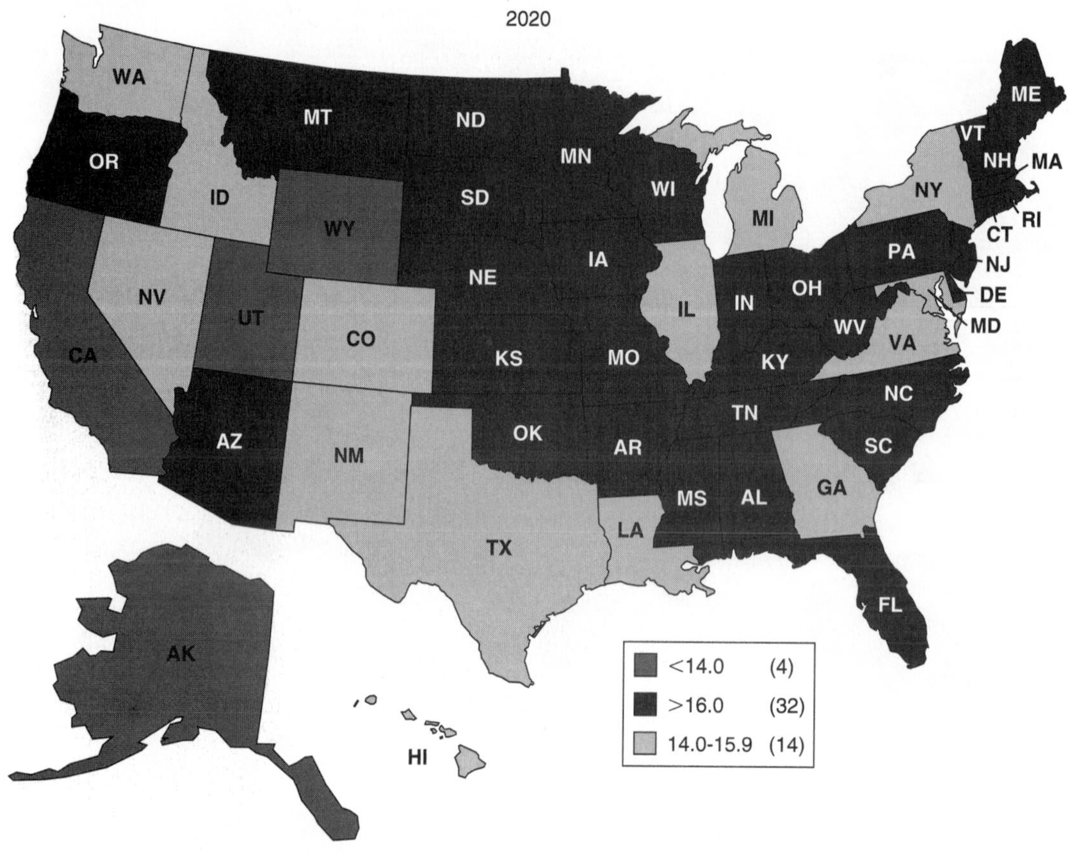

Figure 31-4, cont'd For legend see p. 601.

government pay one tenth. The average national health care expenditure per person was $3510 (National Center for Health Statistics, 1996). For those over age 65, the average national expenditure per capita increased to about $5500. The payment source across all sites of care for patients over age 65 was approximately 40% private, about 45% Medicare, about 11% Medicaid, and 6% other.

Based on a survey of office-based physicians, self-pay was the expected source of payment for the physician office visit almost half the time for 55- to 64-year-olds (U.S. Department of Health and Human Services, 1993b). For those age 65 and over, the expected source of payment for the physician office visit was Medicare (71% of time). Figure 31-5 illustrates source of payment by age-group.

Table 31-9 depicts the percent distribution of the interval since the last physician contact. Because this figure is closely linked with the number of physician contacts per year, it is not unexpected that the interval between physician contacts tends to be higher for men than for women. For example, almost 9% of men over age 65 had not had a physician contact for 2 or more years, compared with about 6% of women in the same age category. The frequency of physician contact is also closely linked to income. Individuals with higher income tend to have more frequent physician contact than those with lower incomes. The interval between physician contacts is highest in the West and

TABLE 31-8 Percent Distribution of Geographical Mobility for Elderly Population by Age: 1975-80, 1985-90

	65+ Years		65-74 Years		75-84 Years		85+ Years	
Mobility Type	**1975-80**	**1985-90**	**1975-80**	**1985-90**	**1975-80**	**1985-90**	**1975-80**	**1985-90**
Same house	77.0	77.4	77.8	80.8	77.5	77.9	70.3	68.3
Different house, U.S.	22.5	22.1	21.8	18.6	22.2	21.8	29.5	31.4
Same county	13.5	13.1	12.5	16.2	13.9	15.4	18.9	19.6
Different county	9.0	9.0	9.2	12.5	8.2	0.5	10.6	11.8
Same state	4.6	4.7	4.5	3.7	4.5	4.6	6.3	7.3
Different state	4.4	4.3	4.8	4.6	3.7	3.7	4.3	4.5
Abroad	0.4	0.5	0.5	0.6	0.3	0.4	0.3	0.2

Source: US Bureau of the Census, 1980 Census of Population, Summary Tape File 5, National Institute on Aging Special Tabulations, Table 5 and 1990 Census of Population, Special Tabulations for Administration of Aging, Table 5.

South, where more than 12% of the population has not had a physician contact for 2 or more years, compared with a little over 11% in the Midwest and about 8.5% in the Northeast. These are important facts when considering alternative primary health care delivery for the older population. Health policy considerations must take into account geographic location as well as income and gender.

The association between physician contacts and income has been demonstrated. Lower income categories have fewer physician contacts. However, health insurance

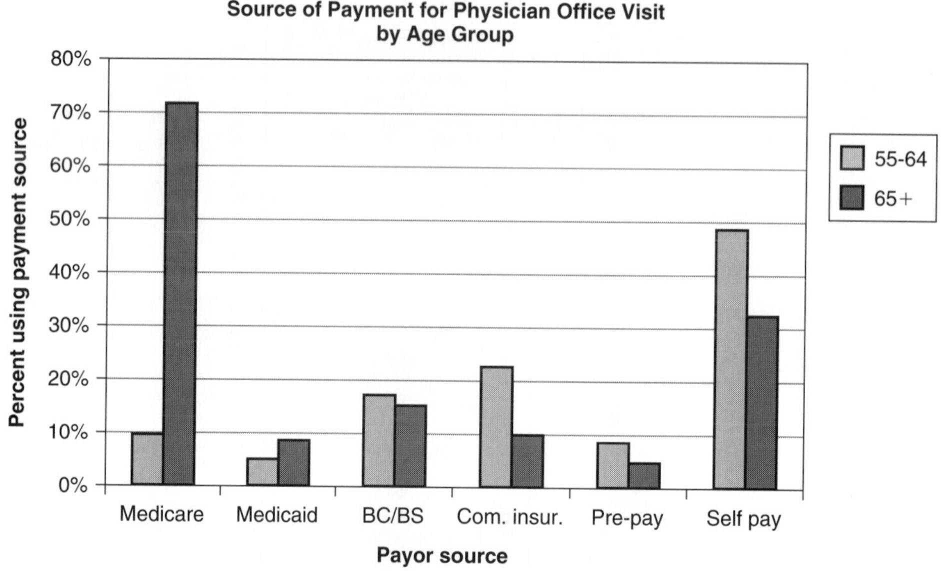

Figure 31-5 Source of payment for physician office visit by age group. (Source: National Center for Health Statistics, Centers for Disease Control and Prevention, Public Health Service, US Department of Health and Human Services, 1993.)

TABLE 31-9 Percent Distribution of Interval since Last Physician Contact by Selected Characteristics: 1994

	Less Than 1 Year	1 Year to <2 Years	2 Years or More
All 65+ Years	89.3	4.2	6.5
Males 65+ Years	85.9	5.2	8.9
Females 65+ Years	89.5	4.3	6.2
Income <$14,000 (all ages)	78.0	9.2	12.7
Income >$50,000 (all ages)	83.7	8.3	8.0
Northeast US (all ages)	83.4	8.1	8.6
Midwest US (all ages)	79.5	9.4	11.1
South US (all ages)	77.3	10.5	12.2
West US (all ages)	78.4	9.2	12.4

Source: Centers for Disease Control and Prevention, National Center for Health Statistics, Health Interview Statistics, National Health Interview Survey, 1994.

coverage is also directly linked to access to and utilization of primary care services. Grana and Stuart (1997) found insurance status to be statistically significant and positively associated with initial access to care and the amount of arthritis care for elderly patients. Medicare and supplemental insurance coverage are closely associated with women over age 65 and their use of mammography screening (Blustein, 1995).

During people's working years, income and employment are closely associated with health insurance availability through the employer. Approximately 66% of people over age 85 are covered by private health insurance as well as Medicare. The National Center for Health Statistics reports that both Medicare and private insurance are held by almost 80% of elderly Caucasians, almost 40% of elderly African-Americans, and 36% of elderly Hispanics. Medicare was more likely to be the sole source of health insurance for African-American (37%) and Hispanic (30%) elderly than for Caucasian (13%) elderly. Health status and functional limitations are important determinants in an elderly patient's decision to purchase private health insurance (Wilcox-Gov and Rubin, 1994).

Education

An individual's educational level is often used as a gauge for both economic well-being and health status. Indeed, research has shown that mortality more than doubles for those who did not finish high school compared with those who did graduate from high school. The death rate among high school graduates is 79% higher than for those whose education continued beyond high school. In addition, those without a high school education were more likely to have a disability than better-educated people (U.S. Bureau of the Census, 1996).

People over age 65 are less likely than those in the 25 to 64 age-group to have completed a high school education. In 1993, about 60% of people 65 or older had obtained at least a high school education; the high school completion rate is about 85% for those 25 to 64 years old (Figure 31-6). Among elderly African-Americans and Hispanics, only 33% and 26%, respectively, are high school graduates or higher. In addition, approximately one fourth of all those age 65 and over had less than a ninth-grade education level, compared with 6% in the 25 to 64 age-group. This proportion was even lower for African-Americans (46%) and Hispanics (62%) (US Bureau of the Census, 1993).

The educational level of the elderly population is rising, and the proportion of the older population with at least a high school education will notably increase. Therefore the elderly of the future will be better educated. This significant progression in educational attainments by the elderly will presumably have a positive impact on their overall well-being.

Living Arrangements

Lifestyle components significantly affect both the access to and the use of primary health care. Factors such as marital status, housing arrangements, and availability of community or home services are closely associated with an older person's ability to perform ADLs. Close family connections, such as living in the same household with one's spouse or child, may encourage the use of primary health care and result in increased access to care (e.g., better transportation opportunities).

Because women live longer than men, it is not surprising that more women than men

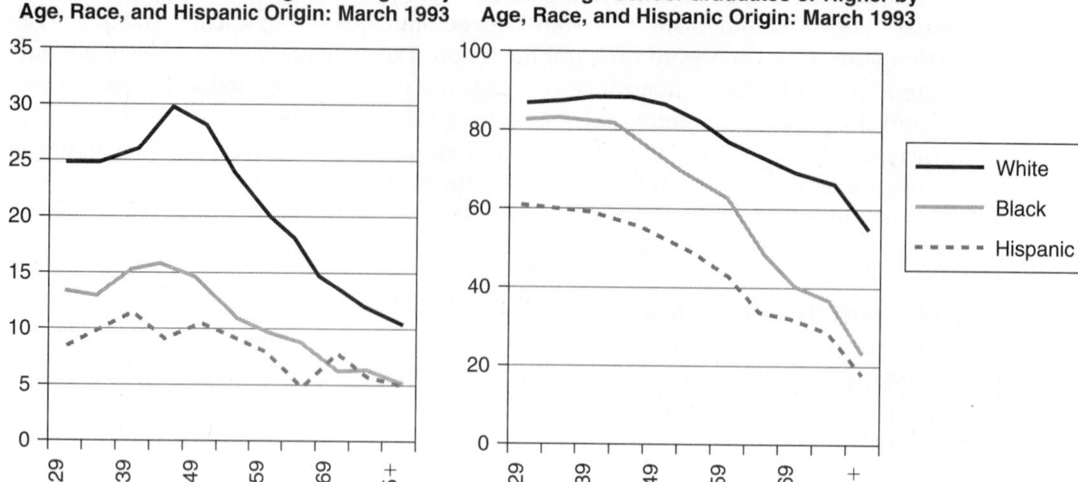

Figure 31-6 Percent with bachelor's degree or higher by age, race, and Hispanic origin: March 1993; percent of high school graduates or higher by age, race, and Hispanic origin: March 1993. (Source: US Bureau of the Census: *Educational attainment in the United States: March 1993 and 1992,* Current Population Reports p20-476, Washington, DC, 1993, US Government Printing Office.)

live alone or with nonrelatives and that 75% of men age 65 and over live with their spouses as compared with 41% of women (Table 31-10).

One study suggests that national origin or heritage is associated with living arrangement preference (Zsembik, 1996). The majority of older Latinos who live alone prefer it to coresidence. Central and South American men living in the United States and Puerto Rican women are most likely to live alone (Zsembik, 1993). Kin availability is highly associated with living arrangements.

Not surprisingly, older adults with declining health and economic resources are more likely to form a household with one of their children (Burr and Mutchler, 1995). On the other extreme, one in 10 grandparents raises a grandchild for at least 6 months, and often for longer (Gerontological Society of America, 1997).

The ability to stay in one's own home depends on securing the necessary primary health care support. In response to this growing need, assisted living arrangements have

TABLE 31-10 Living Arrangement of Persons 65 Years and Older by Gender

Living Arrangement	Percent of Men	Percent of Women
With spouse	75%	41%
With other relative	6%	17%
Alone or with nonrelative	19%	42%

Source: US Department of Health and Human Services, Administration on Aging, 1996, based on US Bureau of the Census data.

increased greatly in the past 10 years. The demand for assisted living or support services (nursing or other) delivered in a residential environment grows with the increase in the elderly population. With the addition of services or modifications to the environment, frail elderly are able to live in a variety of settings. Terms such as "aging in place" and "noninstitutional alternative living arrangements" become a reality. By 1996, 30 states had an assisted living licensure category and had passed legislation authorizing the category (Mollica and Snow, 1996).

Community-based elderly primary health care follows growth patterns similar to assisted living. In the more successful systems, community-based care is an integrated care delivery system that coordinates all primary, acute, and long-term care services for the older population (Henderson and Lipson, 1997). The success of community-based care depends on closely monitored service integration and a willingness to invest in clinical caregivers, appropriate equipment, and clinical care planning. Federal and state regulations are only beginning to emerge in this area and, at present, provide little guidance in defining an integrated community-based delivery system. As such, the most successful community-based systems plan and provide care beyond the current minimum legal requirements. Growth in community-based primary health care is due to an increase in the percentage and number of the older population who have the economic resources to purchase community-based health services or alternative community housing arrangements. The growth of these services is accentuated by the combination of need for health care and supportive services and the demand or ability to pay for services that allow the elderly to remain in the community (National Academy on Aging, 1997).

Summary

This chapter has provided an overview of the nation's older population, with an emphasis on the importance of the relationship between demographic data and the development and provision of primary care to the older population. Primary care providers need to be able to access this information for their community in order to advocate health policy developments that will meet the needs of the older population they serve.

Resources

Administration on Aging
http://www.aoa.dhhs.gov

American Association of Retired Persons
http://www.aarp.org

American Public Health Association (APHA)
http://www.apha.org

Bureau of Labor Statistics
http://stats.bls.gov

Health Care Financing Administration (HCFA)
http://www.hcfa.gov

National Center for Health Statistics
http://www.cdc.gov/nchs

National Institute on Aging
http://www.nih.gov/nia

National Library of Medicine (includes free MEDLINE service)
http://www.nlm.nih.gov

References

Angel J et al: Diminished health and living arrangement of rural elderly Americans, *Nat J Soc* 9(1):31-57, 1995.

Blustein J: Medicare coverage, supplemental insurance, and the use of mammography by older women, *N Engl J Med* 332:1138-1143, 1995.

Burr J, Mutchler J: *Intergenerational living arrangements: new evidence from the national survey of families and households,* paper presented at the American Sociological Association, Amherst, NY, 1995.

Ferrucci L et al: Hospital diagnoses, Medicare charges, and nursing home admissions in the year when older persons become severely disabled, *JAMA* 277:728-734, 1997.

Gerontological Society of America: *One in ten grandparents raises a grandchild,* news release, May 29, 1997, http://gsa.iog.wayne.edu/press.html.

Graña J, Stuart B: The impact of insurance on access to physician services for elderly people with arthritis, *Inquiry* 33(4):326-338, 1997.

Hatch L: Informal support patterns of older African-American and white women: examining effects of family, paid work, and religious participation, *Res Aging* 13(2):144-170, 1991.

Health Care Financing Administration: *Health care financing review: Medicare and Medicaid statistical supplement,* Baltimore, 1997, US Department of Health and Human Services.

Henderson T, Lipson L: *Primary care for older Americans: a primer,* Washington, DC, 1997, Primary Care Resource Center, Intergovernmental Health Policy Project.

Hobbs FB, Damon BL. *65+ in the United States* (Current Population Reports, Special Studies, P23-190), Washington, DC, 1996, US Department of Commerce, Economics and Statistics Administration, Bureau of the Census.

Hoffman C et al: Persons with chronic illness: their costs and prevalence, *JAMA* 276:1473-1479, 1996.

Kallan JE: A multilevel analysis of elderly migration, *Soc Sci Quart* 74(2):405-416, 1993.

Kington R, Smith J: Socioeconomic status and racial and ethnic differences in functional status associated with chronic diseases, *Am J Public Health* 87(5):805-810, 1997.

Manton KG et al: Estimates of change in chronic disability and institutional incidence and prevalence rates in the U.S. elderly population from the 1982, 1984, and 1989 National Long Term Care Survey, *J Gerontol* 48(4):S153-S166, 1993.

Martin L, Soldo B, editors: *Racial and ethnic differences in the health of older Americans,* Washington, DC, 1997, National Academy of Science, National Academy Press.

Mollica R, Snow K: *Assisted living and state policy: 1996,* Portland, ME, 1996, National Academy for State Health Policy.

National Academy on Aging: *Public Policy and Aging Report* 8(2), 1997.

National Center for Health Statistics: *Health, United States, 1995,* Hyattsville, Md, 1996, Public Health Service.

Peek C et al: Race differences in the health of elders who live alone, *J Aging Health* 9(2):147-170, 1997.

Prospective Payment Assessment Commission: *Medicare and the American health care system: report to the Congress,* Washington, DC, 1997, The Commission.

Siegel J: *Aging into the 21st century* (National Aging Information Center report prepared under contract number HHS-100-95-0017 with the Administration on Aging), Washington, DC, 1996, US Department of Health and Human Services.

Silverstein M: Stability and change in temporal distance between the elderly and their children, *Demography* 32(1):29-45, 1995.

Trupin L et al: *Medical expenditures for people with disabilities in the United States, 1987,* Washington, DC, 1995, US Department of Education, National Institute on Disability and Rehabilitation Research.

US Bureau of the Census: *Population projection of the United States by age, sex, race, and Hispanic origin: 1992-2050* (Current Population Report, p25-1092), Washington, DC, 1990, US Government Printing Office.

US Bureau of the Census: *Educational attainment in the United States: March 1992 and 1993* (Current Population Report, p20-476), Washington, DC, 1993, US Government Printing Office.

US Bureau of the Census: *Americans with disabilities: statistical brief,* Washington, DC, 1996, US Department of Commerce, Economics and Statistics Administration.

US Department of Health and Human Services: *A profile of older Americans,* Washington, DC, 1996, Administration on Aging.

US Department of Health and Human Services: *With the passage of time: the Baltimore longitudinal study of aging* (NIH pub [PHS]93-3685), Washington, DC, 1993a, Public Health Service, National Institutes of Health, National Institute on Aging.

US Department of Health and Human Services: *Vital and health statistics: health data on older Americans—United States, 1992* (DHHS pub [PHS]93-1411), Washington, DC, 1993b, Public Health Service, Centers for Disease Control and Prevention, National Center for Health Statistics.

US Department of Health and Human Services: *Monthly report, Medicare prepaid health plans,* Washington, DC, 1995a, Health Care Financing Administration Office of Prepaid Health Care Operations and Oversight.

US Department of Health and Human Services: *Health: United States,* Washington, DC, 1995b, Health Care Financing Administration.

Wilcox-Gov V, Rubin J: Health insurance coverage among the elderly, *Soc Sci Med* 38(11):1521-1529, 1994.

Zsembik B: Determinants of living alone among older Hispanics, *Res Aging* 15(4):449-464, 1993.

Zsembik B: Preference for coresidence among older Latinos, *J Aging Stud* 10(1):69-81, 1996.

32

Health Care Delivery System

The organizational, financial, and even legal framework of health care in the United States is an emerging system of integrated care that combines primary, specialty, and hospital services. The integrated delivery system manages care for a specific population, with the goals and objectives being cost containment, patient satisfaction, and improvement of health care outcomes. It is projected that within another decade between 80% and 90% of the insured U.S. population will receive its care through one of these management systems (Pew Health Professions Commission, 1998).

Gerontologic Primary Health Care System

The structure of the gerontologic primary health care system must account for the integration of individual, socioeconomic, and cultural factors within the existing health care system in order to obtain comprehensive, continuous, accountable, accessible, and coordinated health care for the elderly (Eisenberg, 1997). Primary care for the elderly includes health promotion and preventive medicine, treatment of acute episodes of disease, cure of disease when possible, and stabilization of chronic diseases. An integrated primary health care delivery system reflects the dynamic life transitions of the older adult population and accounts for the changing social and physical conditions of the elderly (U.S. Department of Health and Human Services, 1995). It also results in an educated, healthy lifestyle for the individual, with the health care institutions focused on prevention of disease and promotion of health and well-being of patients.

The health care delivery system continues to evolve. The delivery system changes with respect to health care knowledge and technologies, social commitment of scarce resources, and identification of the costs to meet social needs. It is quite clear that the health care demands of an aging U.S. population (which constitutes an ever-increasing proportion of the population) will drive changes in the health care delivery system.

The structure of health care delivery has developed from a system based mainly on acute care to one directed toward the needs of people with chronic illness, which is especially important among the elderly. The U.S. Department of Health and Human Services, Administration on Aging, projects that by the year 2050 more than 30% of the population will be over 65 years old, compared with around 14% today. Furthermore, in the year 2050 more than 20% of these older adults will have some type of limitation in terms of activities of daily living. This is well over 14 million people in the United States (Health Care Financing Administration, 1998). Any primary care delivery system for the elderly must be structured to accommodate these needs. An integrated gerontologic primary health care system reflects the dynamic life transitions of the older population, accounts for the changing social and physical conditions of the elderly, and results in individual patients and primary care providers being focused on prevention and early recognition of disease and promotion of health and well-being.

In the recent past, the fragmented system of acute care focus, hospital-based practice, lack of utilization of geriatric medicine, and physician specialization led to the overuse of certain procedures and inappropriate care for elderly patients. For this and other reasons, it is best to include the following elements when considering a definition of primary care for older adults:

- Provision of initial point of entry into the health care system
- Management of the majority of health problems for individual patients
- Responsibility for patients' overall health care to include comprehensive, preventive, emergency, coordination, and continuity of care through end of life
- A holistic approach that considers the biologic, psychologic, social, cultural, and environmental elements
- Community involvement to include surveillance of health problems and provision of health services (Sloane and Ham, 1997)
- Clinical teams made up of multiple disciplines as the most effective method to manage a patient's overall health care

As the primary health care system has changed to meet the present and future needs of the growing older population, the education of primary care providers has undergone significant change. Health care educators have defined education standards and have made recommendations for its practitioners (American Association of Colleges of Nursing, 1996).

There has been a recent expansion of nurse practitioner (NP) programs throughout the United States, with the number of programs rising from 100 in 1992 to 250 in 1997 (Cooper et al., 1998). During this same period the number of NP students rose from 4000 to 20,000. It is the hope of many NP and medical school faculty that NP and medical students will be trained and educated in cooperative programs that foster collegial attitudes (Catlin and McAuliffe, 1999). This type of education may alleviate the rancor in battles concerning the scope of practice, which the Pew Foundation reports as time-consuming and costly. Often decisions are based not on quality, cost containment, or access but rather on lobbying and power struggles (Catlin and McAuliffe, 1999; Pew Commission, 1998).

Americans age 65 and older make up approximately 12% of the total population but use 20% of all physician services, 40% of all hospital days, and more than 90% of all nursing home days, accounting for 36% of total health care expenditures, or $300 billion dollars (Pawlson, Infield, and Lastinger, 1997). National health spending as a share of the gross national product is projected to increase from 13.6% to 16.6% by the year 2007. However, the Balanced Budget Act of 1997 (BBA) is expected to slow growth in Medicare spending between 1998 and 2002 (Health Care Financing Administration, 1998). The introduction of prospective payment systems for different services (nursing home, home health) and cutbacks in payment formulas (managed care contracts) are the reasons for the government projection of slowed growth in Medicare costs for the near future. At this time it is too early to tell what actually will be the result of the cost-cutting measures, because many provider organizations are not in favor of the prospective payment system, and the government will need more data to accurately gauge the impact of the BBA on the access and quality of care received by Medicare beneficiaries. The 1999 budget act rescinded some of the 1997 cutbacks and restored $12 million of the cuts in the Medicare program (*Washington Post,* Nov. 19, 1999).

Federal Health Care Insurance Programs

Medicare and Medicaid

In 1965 Congress passed the Title 18 and 19 amendments to the Social Security Act, which enacted the Medicare and Medicaid programs. Medicare is a federal government entitlement program, and Medicaid is a joint federal and state need-based program.

Medicare covers 37 million Americans. People over age 65 who are eligible for Social Security, people who have been disabled for at least 2 years, people with end-stage renal disease, and all people over 80 years of age are eligible for Medicare. Medicare part A includes coverage of inpatient hospital services, skilled nursing facilities, home health, and hospice benefits. There are copayments and caps on most part A benefits. Optional Medicare part B covers partial physician services, outpatient hospital services, medical equipment and supplies, and other health services and supplies (Health Care Financing Administration, 1997). Beneficiaries must pay a monthly fee for part B coverage. A beneficiary who is enrolled in a managed care system must carry part B.

Medicaid, the federal-state matching entitlement program (administered by the state) provides health care services for the poor and near poor. Medicaid is the health care safety net for the elderly. Many of the expenditures are for nursing home care after older people have spent their life savings for nursing home care and have become destitute. The Health Care Financing Administration within the Health and Human Services Department regulates and provides national standards for both the Medicaid and Medicare programs. Medicare and/or Medicaid coverage usually determines where the elderly will seek primary care.

Medicare coverage includes primary health care services. Typical Medicare coverage allows the Medicare beneficiary to select a physician of choice, although there is an increased focus on persuading beneficiaries to enroll in managed care programs. In 1988 the Medicare managed care program reported an enrollment of more than 6 million older beneficiaries (Health Care Financing Administration, 1998).

Not all primary care costs and/or services are covered by Medicare. Medicare managed care plans currently offer prescription drug benefits and vision care that are not covered in the conventional Medicare program. The proportion of health maintenance organizations (HMOs) plans offering these services is predicted to decline in the coming years as Medicare reimbursement rates decline (Consumer Reports, 1998).

Sources of Primary Care for the Elderly

Primary care is delivered in a myriad of settings: physician offices, HMOs, other managed care systems, outpatient departments, emergency departments, community health centers, and nursing homes. The National Ambulatory Medical Care Survey reported 155,870,000 office visits by patients age 65 and over; 21% were to generalists and family practitioners, 25% to internists, and 14% to ophthalmologists. The remainder was spread over other specialists and subspecialists (U.S. Department of Health and Human Services, 1994).

Physician's Office

Of the 37 million Medicare enrollees, more than 28 million had a physician's office contact (Health Care Financing Administration, 1997). Fifty-three percent of people age 65 and over reported the physician's office as their point of contact. On average the elderly made between 5 visits (65 to 74 age-group) and 6.5 visits (75+ age-group) to a physician's office per year (National Center for Health Statistics, 1998). Of these, more than 70% were covered by Medicare, approximately 15% were self-pay, and approximately 5% were covered by Medicaid. The physician is reimbursed by Medicare up to a certain amount. Unless otherwise specified, the physician may "balance bill" the patient for the amount Medicare does not reimburse. Physicians may or may not choose to participate in the Medicare program. The usual incentive not to participate is remuneration—the physician is unable to recoup costs incurred for delivering primary care services to the elderly. To protect themselves from the circumstances of "balance billing," Medicare recipients may purchase supplemental health insurance. These supplemental insurance policies (Medi-gap policies) fill in the gaps in Medicare coverage for physicians and hospitals.

Great strides have been made regarding the physician's office as the initiator of integrated care for the elderly. Physicians are increasingly aware of the importance of educating the patient and accounting for the patient's other sources of primary care. A survey of primary care physicians in Massachusetts reported that health promotion is becoming more a part of usual primary health care delivery than in the past. However, a lack of valid and consistent data and patient education materials diminishes their abilities to focus on healthy aging education. Although the vast majority of respondents believe it is definitely their responsibility to educate patients about risk factors and help them adhere to their regimens, many feel inadequate and ill prepared to do so (Wechsler, 1996).

What is called primary care by many fee-for-service providers actually lacks the critical component of continuity of care by a physician or another health professional who is specifically trained and skilled in the comprehensive first contact with and ongoing care of a population (Henley, 1996). An integrated primary health care delivery system for the elderly is one way to ensure appropriate primary care.

Health Maintenance Organizations and Managed Geriatric Primary Care

The current Medicare managed care program has 6 million enrollees. After the 1997 BBA cost reduction in the payment formula for the Medicare managed care system, 33 managed care contractors (HMOs) opted not to renew their 1999 contracts, thereby disenrolling 400,000 Medicare beneficiaries. In other words the health care system terminated 400,000 people with no warning and for no health reasons. Luckily these people still have Medicare coverage, but for many there were significant problems that required them to make multiple, somewhat complex decisions in a short space of time and designate certain options to ensure health care coverage within the Medicare program. The process is complicated; in fact, the government established an Internet Web site with six information pages to assist older people in finding their way through the myriad of regulations so they can continue some form of appropriate coverage. This was not an easy task for many older people. It seems obvious in a free market system that capitation for older adults is a disincentive to providing optimum care in systems in which the primary mission is to achieve a profit margin that satisfies shareholders and other market demands.

In general, members of an HMO pay a set amount each month for complete health care services, regardless of utilization. Conventional HMOs participating in the Medicare program are required to provide a full range of benefits, including postacute benefits that are especially important for the elderly. The elderly themselves must be astute purchasers of health care, even in instances (such as an HMO) in which it appears that all their primary care needs and associated costs will be covered.

There are numerous versions of Medicare managed care plans that deliver health care services to the elderly. The typical Medicare managed care plan contracts with the Health Care Financing Administration to provide services to Medicare enrollees. These plans receive monthly payments based on risk or cost. Calculations regarding current health care expenditures are made by adding the annual premium and annual copayment amount. In addition, expenditures beyond the maximum annual benefit (sometimes called the *cap*) are estimated. Finally, an estimated health risk of using other services in the future that are outside the HMO-reimbursed services are made and added to current expenditures.

As part of the health care coverage, Medicare HMOs provide primary care services for the elderly. They may pay a specific provider group a set amount each month to provide health care services for a Medicare beneficiary. The beneficiary must use specific providers unless the HMO offers a point-of-service option by which the beneficiary is permitted to use other providers, usually at an increased cost.

Another Medicare arrangement is the provider-sponsored organization (PSO). With a PSO group of physicians and/or hospitals form a legal arrangement (usually under federal waiver) to contract, as a group, with Medicare to provide both part A and part B services. The organization bears all risk for the health care delivery costs of the Medicare beneficiary. The Medicare beneficiary pays a low premium and must secure all health care from the PSO.

Despite some demonstration failings, in general the HMO delivery system increases both access to and the quality of care for HMO enrollees, especially among the elderly with chronic conditions and diseases. Organizational structure changes positively affect both access to care and the quality of outcomes (Miller, 1998). For example, a shift from fragmented clinical management of specific services at one point in time toward a more integrated clinical management of chronic conditions would not only increase access to care but also attract and retain elderly enrollees.

Brummel-Smith (1998) states that managed care is much better than a fee-for-service system in caring for older people, frail people, and people with disabilities. Managed health care delivery focuses on a function-management health care delivery system rather than on the disease-based health care delivery system typical of a fee-for-service arrangement. Function management makes outcomes tracking possible and consequently allocates scarce resources to clearly effective types of care. Managed care incorporates accountability and quality into health care delivery with less emphasis on specialization.

Before one jumps too quickly on the managed care bandwagon, careful consideration should be given to the organizational incentives inherent within a managed care system. Mirvis, Chang, and Morreim (1997) point out the complex and often competing incentives in a managed care delivery system for the elderly. They begin by stating that, given multiple health problems, the elderly would benefit the most from high-quality managed care that coordinates primary care across chronic conditions. However, managed care generally limits elderly enrollment, inappropriately uses advance directives, and applies selective criteria to limit care. The limited enrollment techniques are often called "cherry picking." This term refers to the practice of enticing into the managed care programs younger beneficiaries who are less costly and avoiding the more costly oldest old. Under a poor-quality managed care system, the elderly are most vulnerable to financial manipulation in that they consume a disproportionate amount of resources—making them a target for cost containment measures (Lachs et al., 1997).

Social Health Maintenance Organizations

A Medicare demonstration project sponsored by the Health Care Financing Administration is the social health maintenance organization (SHMO). The SHMO is a Medicare HMO that includes long-term care benefits. The program seeks to enroll a broad cross-section of elderly in terms of disability and financial status. Another project is the Program for All-Inclusive Care for the Elderly (PACE). This program provides an extensive set of acute and long-term care services on a capitated basis to frail elderly who wish to continue to live at home (avoiding nursing home placement) (Irvin, Massey, and Dorsey, 1997). The program aims to integrate a wide range of primary care services the elderly typically need into one delivery program that coordinates these services. The success of programs that offer an extensive array of services varies. Much depends on the primary care delivery structure in relation to the preferences of the Medicare recipient. For example, the PACE program offers adult day care. This structure is designed to monitor and deliver primary care for a chronically ill elderly population. Although the structure is inherently designed for successful health care delivery, it cannot account for the fact that some elderly people prefer the costly route in order of remaining in their homes during the day or that any capitated payment structure creates an incentive for the program to avoid costly individuals.

Medicaid Programs

Quite often the entry of the Medicaid recipient into the primary care system is fraught with discontinuity and ill-coordinated care (Ormond and Bovbjerg, 1998). Although the state may structure primary health care services to encourage coordinated care, Medicaid recipients often move in and out of the health care delivery system depending on a number of factors, including the state benefits structure, health status, knowledge of program benefits, and personal preference. Reentry into the health care system may not be the same primary care contact used previously. In 1995 20% of the elderly Medicaid patients who received care received inpatient hospital services, 67% received physician visits, 38% received hospital outpatient department services, and approximately 12% received home health services (Health Care Financing Administration, 1997).

State community health centers (CHCs) were very popular in the 1960s and continue to provide primary care services for some elderly Medicaid recipients. The CHC was typically located in low-income areas and served by a blend of providers aimed to meet the multiple primary health care needs of the poor and near poor. However, office waiting time was usually long, and patient satisfaction and staff morale were low. The organization of the CHC as a stand-alone delivery site has evolved over time to become better integrated with other state health and social services.

A variation of the CHC is the establishment of women's health centers. Twelve National Centers of Excellence in Women's Health currently exist and are funded by the Public Health Service's Office on Women's Health (Nation's Health, 1998). The centers aim to meet the health needs of minority women (including the elderly) through a "one-stop-shopping" design that focuses on preventive and early detection health care. The centers coordinate services in academic centers and surrounding communities, provide education programs and materials, and network with local businesses, consumer groups, scientific organizations, and public health leaders.

Hospitals

For the majority of the elderly the hospital is not the source of primary care. However, about 10% of the elderly report the hospital outpatient department as their usual source of care, and under 1% report the hospital emergency department as their usual source of care (Agency for Health Care Policy and Research, 1998). On average, these elderly visit less often than once per year either the hospital outpatient department or the emergency department (National Center for Health Statistics, 1998).

The attitude of Medicare beneficiaries regarding the use of health care services determines the site of primary health care as well as the frequency of visits. Medicare beneficiaries who say they avoid going to the doctor are less likely to have a hospital outpatient visit or physician office visit but are just as likely to visit a hospital emergency department (Eppig et al., 1997). This suggests that, when reported as the usual source of care, the hospital emergency department may in fact be the health care site of last resort for the Medicare beneficiary population.

The hospital emergency department and even the outpatient department are not structured to deliver integrated primary care services for the elderly. Primary care services are typically delivered a la carte—on an as-needed, one-time-only basis. Given the structure of the hospital outpatient setting, there may be little attempt to monitor chronic conditions or incorporate (or even know about) confounding diseases. Among the elderly who use the hospital as a source of primary care, it is usually the lack of comprehensive health insurance that makes the hospital site an attractive alternative to a physician office setting.

Home Health

Primary health care delivery in the home setting has increased dramatically within the last 10 years. Changes in medical technology and information technology make it possible to deliver effective primary care services to the elderly within their own homes. Corresponding changes in health insurance coverage, now more recently covering home health services, have contributed to the increasing use of home health services. In 1993 more than 1.5 million people (20% of whom were age 85 and over) used home health care (National Center for Health Statistics, 1996). More than 19% of those age 65 and over use home health services. The number of home health users increases daily. An increasing number of elderly people, insurance changes that encourage home care, and effectively designed demonstrations (e.g., PACE) have contributed to the increasing use.

Although primary home health care appears to be on the rise, there are serious concerns regarding quality-monitoring systems. There have been recent advances to correct this problem (e.g., OASIS home health assessment form, see Appendix B) and integrate primary home health care delivery into the primary care delivery system.

Satisfaction with Usual Source of Primary Care

In general, the elderly are very satisfied with their usual source of care (National Center for Health Statistics, 1998). Between 95% and 97% of the elderly gave high marks for overall quality, professional staffing, a provider who listens, and confidence in the provider's ability to deliver effective health care. However, only 77% indicated that the provider asked about their prescription drugs. This latter finding is reflective of a primary health care system that has yet to focus on integrated health care delivery. Reasons for changing the usual source of care include dissatisfaction with quality (19%), insurance-related reasons (24%), and location—being too far away or moving (39%).

Impact of Information Technology on Primary Health Care Delivery for the Elderly

Health care delivery flows from a constantly changing organizational structure that is heavily influenced by communication and technology. For example, information technology can be aimed at improving consistency and efficiency in terms of strategies for health promotion and disease prevention in older adults (Grant, Niyonsenga, and Bernier, 1994). It can also provide information for the patient in terms of responsibility and for the provider in terms of accountability. Pollock and Rice (1997) write that patient care will become more fragmented unless patient data are standardized and disseminated uniformly across different settings. The Health Insurance Portability and Accountability Act of 1996 is a step toward standardizing health information.

Currently there are accreditation structures in place to measure quality of care provided by primary care sites in the health systems. These structures include the National Committee for Quality Assurance (NCQA) and the Joint Commission on Accreditation of Healthcare Organizations (JCAHO) (O'Malley, 1997). There are health systems report cards, including NCQA's Health Plan Employer Data and Information Set, which includes outcomes measures; JCAHO's requirements of performance data (Oryx); a consumer-oriented report on HMOs; and survey data on skilled nursing facilities available on the World Wide Web. Others measures depict quality outcomes as total quality management. This is a loosely defined health care delivery structure that focuses on the process of primary care delivery and is guided by data (e.g., patient records) (Chambers, 1998). Still other measures address data standardization, care planning, and cross-setting integration (e.g., the Minimum Data Set Resident Assessment Instrument for skilled nursing facilities). All of these quality measures are intended to standardize and enhance outcomes measurement and provider-patient accountability.

Summary

The development of an integrated health care system to provide appropriate services across settings for the elderly population is the challenge of the twenty-first century. Creative concepts regarding organization of primary care services, intradisciplinary practice, and education of primary care providers that support accountability for improving the elderly's health are the hope for the future (Welton, Kantner, and Katz 1997). Policymakers are challenged by the constraints of a society that is unable or unwilling to accept tax increases to pay for the service increases that appear necessary to protect the health of the aging population. The government is mounting a wide campaign to contain costs through the 1997 BBA and also by accosting the seemingly large amount of fraud and abuse in the Medicare system. If successful in changing practices, these programs may have results that have an impact on costs. How that movement or change will occur is not currently clear. However, all health care professionals have a responsibility to be part of the solution that protects and provides appropriate primary health care for older Americans.

Resources

Healthy People 2000
U.S. Department of Health and Human Services
Pub #PHS 93-1411
U.S. Department of Health and Human Services
http://www.os.dhhs.gov

Health Care Financing Administration
http://www.hcfa.gov

References

Agency for Health Care Policy and Research: *Medical expenditure panel survey, household component, 1996,* Rockville, Md, 1998, Center for Cost and Financing Studies.

American Association of Colleges of Nursing: *The essentials of master's education for advanced practice nursing,* Washington, DC, 1996, American Association of Colleges of Nursing.

Brummel-Smith K: *Managed geriatric primary care,* 1998, posted by the American Society on Aging Website at http://www.asaging.org/mcan.html.

Catlin A, McAuliffe M: Proliferation on non-physician providers as reported in the Journal of the American Medical Association (JAMA), 1998, *Image J Nurs Sch* 31(2):175-179, 1999.

Chambers D: TQM: the essential concepts, *J Am Coll Dent* 65(2):6-13, 1998.

Consumer Reports: *Medicare: new choices, new worries,* September 1998.

Cooper RA et al: Current and projected workforce of non-physician clinicians. *JAMA* 280(9):788-794, 1998.

Eisenberg J: Comment on *Primary care: America's health in a new era,* by Donaldson M et al, editors. Washington, DC, 1996, National Academy Press. *N Engl J Med* 336(22), 1997.

Eppig FJ et al: Medicare beneficiaries' attitudes about seeking healthcare: 1996. *Health Care Financ Rev* 19(2):155-157, 1997.

Grant A, Niyonsenga T, Bernier R: The role of medical informatics in health promotion and disease prevention, *Generations* 18:74-77, 1994.

Health Care Financing Administration: *Health care financing review: Medicare and Medicaid statistical supplement,* Baltimore, 1997, Health and Human Services.

Health Care Financing Administration: *Highlights of the national health expenditure projections 1997-2007,* updated September 14, 1998, http://www.hfca.gov/stats/NHE-Proj/hilites.htm.

Henley D: Comment from the American Academy of Family Physicians, *N Engl J Med* 335(12):897-898, 1996.

Irvin C, Massey S, Dorsey T: Determinants of enrollment among applicants to PACE, *Health Care Financ Rev* 19(2):135-151, 1997.

Lachs MS et al: Is managed care good or bad for geriatric medicine? *J Am Geriatr Soc* 45(9):1123-1127, 1997.

Miller R: Healthcare organizational change: implications for access to care and its measurement, *Health Serv Res* 33(3):653-680, 1998.

Mirvis D, Chang C, Morreim H: Protecting older people while managing their care, *J Am Geriatr Soc* 45:645-646, 1997.

National Center for Health Statistics: *Health, United States, 1995,* Hyattsville, Md, 1996, Public Health Service.

National Center for Health Statistics: *1996 National Ambulatory Medical Care Survey,* Hyattsville, Md, 1998, Public Health Service.

Nation's Health (official newspaper of the American Public Health Association; published monthly), Washington, DC, 1998, The Association.

O'Malley C: Quality measurement for health systems: accreditation and report cards, *Am J Health Syst Pharm* 54(13):1528-1535, 1997.

Ormond B, Bovbjerg R: *The changing hospital sector in Washington, DC: implications for the poor,* Washington, DC, 1998, Urban Institute.

Pawlson G, Infield D, Lastinger D: The health care system. In Ham RJ, Sloane PD, editors: *Primary care geriatrics,* ed 3, St Louis, 1997, Mosby.

Pew Commission: Recreating health professional practice for a new century: executive summary, 1998. Pew Website: www.futurehealth.ucsf.edu/pubs.html.

Pew Health Professions Commission in HCFA: *National health care expenditures projections,* Washington, DC, 1998, US Department of Health and Human Services.

Pollock A, Rice D: Monitoring health care in the United States: a challenging task, *Public Health Rep* 112:108-113, 1997.

Prospective Payment Assessment Commission: *Medicare and the American health care system: report to the Congress,* Washington, DC, 1997, The Commission.

Sloane PD, Ham RJ: Primary care. In Ham RJ, Sloane PD, editors: *Primary care geriatrics,* ed 3, St Louis, 1997, Mosby.

US Department of Health and Human Services: *Vital and health statistics: health data on older Americans—United States, 1992* (DHHS pub [PHS]93-1411), Washington, DC, 1993, Public Health Service, Centers for Disease Control and Prevention, National Center for Health Statistics.

US Department of Health and Human Services: *Public Health Service: national ambulatory medical survey: 1991 summary vital and health statistics* (series 13, 116), May 1994.

US Department of Health and Human Services: *Health: United States,* Washington, DC, 1995, Health Care Financing Administration.

Washington Post, November 19, 1999, p. A1.

Wechsler H et al: The physician's role in health promotion revisited: a survey of primary care practitioners, *N Engl J Med* 334(15):996-998, 1996.

Welton W, Kantner T, Katz S: Developing tomorrow's integrated community health systems: a leadership challenge for public health and primary care, *Milbank Q* 75(2):261-288, 1997.

33

Ethics

A headline in the *Washington Post* reads, "Medical Competency Tests Proposed: Panel Recommends Periodic Exams for Doctors and Nurses." The accompanying article described the conclusion by the Pew Health Professions Commission that the nation's method of policing health care workers provides patients far too little protection. This influential commission of health advisors recommended that all physicians, nurses, and other health workers be compelled to pass written examinations and allow state regulators to watch them work and inspect their patient records at least every 6 years. The article linked the idea of tighter government controls to growing fears about whether managed care has damaged the quality of the nation's health care system.

Sadly, no board examination can guarantee the public that health care professionals will be both clinically competent and, equally important, committed to using that competence to secure the public's health and well-being. For this reason the health professions must find a way to ensure that their members are ethically, intellectually, technically, and interpersonally competent (Taylor, 1997). Although this holds for health professionals in all practice areas, it is particularly compelling for primary care providers specializing in gerontologic care. The chronicity, frailty, and special needs that characterize many of the elderly expose them to particular risk in today's efficiency-driven health culture. It does not take long for an older patient's hearing problem, mobility problem, or dexterity problem to dangerously threaten a provider's prescribed clinician-patient ratio. And the hope of "making up time" with the next older person is usually not realized.

In 1998 the National Academies of Practice developed ethical guidelines to set forth their positions on issues related to the shifting of financial risk from payers to health professionals in today's managed care environment. The Academies stated that "this transfer of financial risk has the potential to invite ethical conflicts by way of creating a tension between economic availability and clinical care considerations bearing on patient care, patient rights and advancing the knowledge base of the health care professions" (National Academies of Practice, 1998). Citing the economic pressures to abbreviate the utilization and scope of professional service, the National Academies of Practice set as its first guideline: *Professional Commitment to Patient Needs Must Remain the Primary Concern.*

The benefits offered by all health care providers should:

- Provide access by patients to appropriate professional services
- Meet with patient satisfaction
- Avoid contamination by an overly rigid adherence to clinical guidelines such that the practitioner's decision making is hampered
- Provide delivery by uniquely trained personnel, such as medical specialists and other professionals trained in delivering psychosocial services, when the complexity of the patient's condition requires a knowledge base and expertise beyond those of the primary care provider

Other guidelines address information disclosure, teaching and research in patient care, confidentiality, and prevention. The guideline on prevention charges each health care enterprise to acknowledge the critical importance of the teaching and inculcation of prevention as well as the need for competently delivered patient care services.

Ethical Standards

Those responsible for educating today's health care professionals have also taken measures to ensure that graduates possess the ethical competence necessary to faithfully execute their public charge. In 1995 the American Association of Colleges of Nursing (AACN) charged a task force to define the essential elements of baccalaureate education for professional nursing practice. Their report, published in 1998, identifies the following core values for caring professional nurses: altruism, autonomy, human dignity, integrity, and social justice (American Association of Colleges of Nursing, 1998). The AACN report on the essentials of master's education for advanced practice nursing (1996) charged master's nursing education to develop an understanding of the principles, personal values, and beliefs that provide a framework for nursing practice.

The graduate educational experience should provide students the opportunity to explore their values, analyze how these values shape their professional practice and influence their decisions, and analyze systems of health care and determine how the values underpinning them influence the interventions and care delivered. Course work should provide graduates with the knowledge and skills to do the following:

1. Identify and analyze common ethical dilemmas and the ways in which these dilemmas impact patient care
2. Evaluate ethical methods of decision making and engage in an ethical decision-making process
3. Evaluate ethical decision making from both personal and organizational perspectives and develop an understanding of how these two perspectives may create conflicts of interest
4. Identify areas in which a personal conflict of interest may arise; propose resolutions or actions to resolve the conflict
5. Understand the role of an ethics committee in health delivery systems; serve on ethics committees
6. Assume accountability for the quality of one's own practice

Similarly, in January 1996 the Association of American Medical Colleges (AAMC) embarked on a major new initiative—the Medical School Objectives Project—to assist medical schools in responding to concerns that new doctors are not as well prepared as they should be to meet society's expectations of them. In 1998 AAMC published a broad set of objectives designed to ensure that physicians possess the attributes necessary in meeting their individual and collective responsibilities to society (Association of American Medical Colleges, 1998):

- Physicians must be altruistic.
- Physicians must be knowledgeable.
- Physicians must be skillful.
- Physicians must be dutiful.

Because many primary care providers are precepting advanced practice nurses and medical students and residents, it is helpful to seize the "teachable moments" that occur in daily practice to explore the ethical dimensions of gerontologic care. This chapter uses practice vignettes to highlight challenges to ethical competence and concludes with a description of strategies to develop ethical competence.

Challenges to Ethical Competence

A primary care provider's ethical competence is the patient's (and the public's) best security that health care needs will be adequately met. Ethically competent primary care providers have the following characteristics (Taylor, 1997):

1. Are clinically competent
2. Can be trusted to act in ways that advance the best interests of the patients entrusted to their care
3. Hold themselves and their colleagues accountable for their practice
4. Work collaboratively to advocate for patients, families, and communities
5. Mediate ethical conflicts among the patient, significant others, the health care team, and other interested parties
6. Critique new health care technologies and changes in the way health care is defined, administered, delivered, and financed in light of their potential to influence human well-being

Clinical Competence

Clinical competence is obviously a prerequisite of ethical competence. Effective practitioners today value evidence-based practice and work hard to develop the interpersonal and therapeutic skills that equate with high-quality care. The Institute of Medicine defines *quality of care* as the degree to which health services for individuals and populations increase the likelihood of desired health outcomes and are consistent with current professional knowledge. It has also identified three fundamental quality-of-care issues: (1) use of unnecessary or inappropriate care; (2) underuse of needed, effective, and appropriate care; and (3) shortcomings in technical and interpersonal aspects of care (Institute of Medicine, 1994).

Deficient Clinical Competence: Case Studies

The following scenarios illustrate one or more types of deficiency in clinical competence. In the first case study, a family nurse practitioner notices that an elderly oncology patient is becoming more and more depressed, but the practitioner fails to explore or treat the patient's depression. The patient moved in with her daughter 14 months earlier after learning that she most likely had fewer than 6 months to live. When the patient's daughter asks about her mother's growing depression, the nurse practitioner responds, "Well, she certainly has lots to be depressed about" and changes the subject. In the second scenario, a surgical resident explains his practice of undermedicating older patients postoperatively by telling a medical student that older patients do not experience pain to the same degree as younger patients, as evidenced by their lack of complaints. In the third example, the neurology practice responsible for a large population of patients with Alzheimer's disease, Parkinson's disease, and other predictably debilitating neurologic disorders makes no effort to encourage its members to talk with patients about their end-of-life treatment preferences and advance directives and to document these discussions. When questioned, they reply that they have no time for these conversations.

These scenarios illustrate why it is important to assess whether or not the goals being sought for a particular patient or population aggregate are adequate and whether or not the provider or caregiving team's competence, motivation, and resources are adequate. An oncologist recently confided how "beaten and defeated" he felt after the death of a woman he had cared for over several years. He shared his puzzlement on learning that the chaplain who had cared for this woman in her last days found the experience "transcendent and transforming." A physician unable to accept "helping people die well" as a legitimate goal of medicine may never be able to feel a sense of accomplishment or peace when one of his patients dies. More important, he will be deficient clinically if he cannot bring his otherwise powerful clinical skills to bear in helping his patients experience a comfortable and dignified death.

Trustworthiness

Clinical competence in and of itself cannot guarantee that patients and the public will be well served. Most of us can remember hiring a practitioner who "looked good on paper" but whose presence in the clinic was frustrating because the promised skills were rarely or erratically displayed. Trustworthiness is the character criterion. Can patients and their families, the public, count on the clinician to secure their interests? In today's culture, where the overwhelming majority of Americans surveyed believe that the rush to manage costs has sacrificed safety and quality, trustworthiness is paramount. Clinicians are trustworthy to the extent that they habitually display those human qualities or virtues that equate with excellent care. Fletcher, Miller, and Spencer (1995) define *virtues* as "those dispositions of character and conduct which motivate and enable clinicians to provide good care to patients. The clinical virtues function as habits conducive to good practice as well as guides to healing and caring interactions with patients." Their list of clinical virtues includes technical competence, objectivity and detachment, caring, clinical benevolence, subordination of self-interest to patient care, reflective intelligence, humility, practical wisdom, and courage. Imagine that you learned at the end of a clinical day that someone had secretly videotaped each interaction you had with patients, families, and colleagues. Would you greet with pride or horror the announcement that your videotape was to be shown to colleagues as an example of "excellence in practice"? Which of the preceding clinical virtues would be glaring by their preponderance or absence?

The trustworthiness criterion is displayed in the following scenarios. In the first example a new gerontologic case manager in a Medicare managed care program becomes convinced that deficient screening and follow-up services for a large cohort of enrolled elderly patients with diabetes are resulting in unnecessary complications and repeat hospitalizations. When she reports this to the medical director, she is thanked for her observation but is told that the health plan simply cannot afford to routinize the benefits she is recommending. Undaunted, she begins to gather data about the costs associated with the repeat hospitalizations in order to convince senior management by talking in terms they understand. Choosing to remain an advocate for this population illustrates her ability to be trusted. A more mundane example is that of a clinician who is tempted to abbreviate an intake examination on an "ornery" patient because of extreme fatigue, feelings of impatience or natural aversion, or simply time constraints. The clinician's decision to be faithful to the time needed to conduct a thorough examination in the face of personal constraints to do less is a decision to be trustworthy.

Accountability

As the preceding illustrations make clear, it is often difficult to hold *ourselves* accountable for high-quality practice, let alone our colleagues. Self-regulation is one of the hallmarks of a moral profession. We earn the right to practice by professing to the public that we can be accountable. Because trustworthiness in individuals and health care institutions and systems is not a given, accountability is another criterion of ethical competence. What does it mean to hold health care professionals accountable for safe and good-quality practice? At the very least this entails periodically stepping back from practice to gain enough distance to be critically reflective about what is being done. A helpful practice is to perform a chart review on an individual patient for whom you established a treatment plan to determine the weight each of the following has in determining the interventions selected:

- Maintenance of status quo
- Clear demonstration by research that this is the best option for the condition(s) being treated
- Availability of resources to execute this plan of care
- Willingness of payers to reimburse for all aspects of the proposed treatment plan
- Patient preferences for the plan of care
- Convenience for providers with the plan of care
- Past experience that demonstrates a high level of patient and/or family satisfaction with this approach

Obviously the ideal is to give greatest weight to the variables that best serve patients and the public.

Another helpful exercise is to think back to the quality-of-care issues identified previously: (1) use of unnecessary or inappropriate care; (2) underuse of needed, effective, and appropriate care; and (3) shortcomings in technical and interpersonal aspects of care. Then identify a recent practice situation where you noted one or more of these problems, and think carefully about how you responded to your initial sense that something was wrong. Which of the following characterizes your typical response to problems of quality (Exercises adapted from Taylor and Barnet, 1999)?

- Try to ignore discomfort and pretend there is no problem
- Experience the frustration of knowing that conditions are less than optimal but accept that you are powerless to effect a solution
- Commit your best energies to attempting to resolve the problem

Reflection on this sort of challenge and your characteristic responses will yield valuable information about your competence, willingness, and confidence to address challenges to quality. Deficient accountability occurs in many forms:

- Unwillingness to challenge a colleague who often prejudices caregivers negatively toward patients and families by the tone and content of his report
- Doing nothing to address staff concerns about certain practitioners or departments who routinely do poorly on measures of performance and patient outcome
- Accepting the new "playing rules" when changes in the reimbursement levels result in a dangerous reduction of services to older adults

Advocacy

The ability to collaborate with others to secure the health care resources and services needed by older adults is essential to ethical competence. Because few providers work independently, advocacy strengths must include strong interpersonal skills to facilitate the coordination of resources needed in any clinical situation. Any attempt to rely solely on oneself to "make up" for deficient resources in the system or the team is bound to result in failure and burnout. Increasingly today this includes being able to work with payers and community-based support groups. Professional barriers to effective advocacy include the following:

- Low value attached to advocacy ("It's not my job!")—the *character* issue
- Inadequate knowledge or interpersonal skills—the *competence* issue
- Low morale and the mediocrity-sustaining cycle; initial enthusiasm, frustration when things do not change, and cynicism (e.g., "nothing ever changes around here for the better" syndrome)—the *motivation* issue
- Fear of reprisal: how much are we willing to risk to secure valued health outcomes for the patients and/or communities entrusted to our care?—the *balancing* issue

Chief among the professional barriers to effective advocacy is the degree to which external forces are redefining the nature of professional health care practice (threats to health care professional-patient relationships, policies that compromise clinical judgments, increasing demand to resolve conflicting obligations). System barriers to effective advocacy are unresponsive or ineffective systems and unsafe systems resulting from the increasing tendency to prioritize cost containment over quality, a preference toward underutilization of services, the gradual de-skilling of the work force, and financial incentives that reward denying or reducing indicated treatment and care. The many examples of excellence in advocacy that can be found in practice range from the simple confrontation of a colleague whose commitment to excellence seems to be slipping to testifying before Congress on the health needs of older Americans. The major changes needed to ensure a "basic decent minimum of care" for all older Americans mandate that we work collectively to advocate for older adults. No one is capable of orchestrating the needed change alone; participation in professional societies and organizations that can lobby for better gerontologic care is needed more now than ever before.

Conflict Mediation

Ethically competent primary care providers mediate ethical conflict among patients, families, health care professionals, payers, and other interested parties. The first trick in mediating ethical conflict is to identify it early and begin to intervene. Although it is easy to identify older adults at risk for skin impairment or falls, the families and caregiving teams at high risk for decisional conflict are often ignored, and intervention does not occur until adversarial camps have developed. At this point resort to a legal court often seems to be the only option.

Successful conflict mediation entails recognizing conflict early, developing the trusting relationships and communication skills that facilitate the identification of variables causing or contributing to the conflict, becoming skilled in facilitating the type of dialogue that results in consensus about prudential judgments that best serve the interested parties, and knowing and assessing the resources available to facilitate conflict resolution. Central to its process is the identification of key stakeholders and their interests, values, and beliefs. We often presume to know what other stakeholders value and believe when nothing is further from the truth.

When conflicts develop between patients and providers about treatment decisions, a patient advocate stands in the middle and does the hard work of uncovering exactly what underlies the patient's and surrogate's demands, as well as what makes providers uncomfortable with these demands. Providers often dismiss patients and family members as being "unreasonable" or "sick in the head" because what they want is something other than what the provider has decided ought to be done. The objective is to facilitate patient autonomy without compromising the autonomy of individual health care providers or the internal morality of the health professions. At issue is the patient's right to be self-determining, to demand treatment believed to be in his or her best interests, and to refuse treatment not believed to be in his or her best interests, as well as the health care professional's right to control practice and to use only those diagnostic and therapeutic measures consistent with the internal morality of the profession.

In the case that follows it is easy to predict two very different outcomes on the basis of the ability of the professional caregivers to be a patient advocate and their willingness to get involved.

Case Study

A 74-year-old man develops a mesenteric infarct after a resection for a meningioma that impaired his vision. His wife withholds consent for surgical repair of the bowel, to the consternation of the neurosurgeon and consulting gastroenterologist. They explain to her that this is a reversible problem that must be treated. The wife explains that the patient, who "crashed" after surgery and is now incapacitated, on a ventilator, and receiving vasopressors, would never want anything done to prolong his life in this condition. The patient is a lawyer who has been married for 49 years, has five children and, according to his wife, did not want surgery the second time around for the meningioma but allowed himself to be "talked into it" by his children. He places a very high value on being active and independent. The wife consults you, the primary care provider who initially referred her husband to a specialist for the meningioma, and asks you to plead their case.

Commitment to Human Well-Being

The ability to critique new health care technologies and changes in the way health care is defined, administered, delivered, and financed *in light of their potential to influence human well-being* is critical for gerontologic providers. Upon entry to the health professions, each of us adopts, along with our white coats or uniforms, a particular lens for viewing the world. This lens focuses our attention on certain phenomena and screens out others. We would go crazy if we ever attempted to pay attention to everything that is going on around us at any point in time. The phenomena of concern to health professionals must be health and human well-being. As we sit at decision-making tables, our voices should be raised on behalf of the people we serve and should ask, "What are the human consequences of what we are proposing?" "How will the people we serve be affected by our decisions?" Although this point might seem self-evident, the fact is that often we are not present when decisions that affect health care for older adults are made and that, when present, we fail to articulate concerns about the human consequences of what is being decided. In today's health culture we can be sure that someone is examining the economic and legal implications of our decisions, which affect health care for older adults in both small and major ways. If we think carefully about how our death-denying culture affects end-of-life care for the elderly or how our car-repair-shop model of health care, with its focus of wholeness of body vs. wholeness of being influences reimbursable health care priorities, we begin to see problems. When the old family car is no longer deemed "worthy" of an expensive repair, it is likely to be driven or towed to a junkyard. Some find striking parallels with the nursing home industry. We need to be able to think critically about how the explosion of genetic information, Medicare managed care alternatives, and research to prevent aging will affect the daily lives of older adults and their families. Never has so much change occurred in so little time. Ethically competent providers are committed to shaping change to ensure that the elderly are well served. This stance is very different from an after-the-fact accommodation to change dictated by a lust for profit, misguided altruism, or faulty reasoning.

Developing Ethical Competence

A commitment to develop ethical competence requires taking a careful inventory of our knowledge and skills. Once we know our personal strengths and limitations, we can strategize to address the deficits. This chapter concludes with a discussion of practical strategies to develop ethical competence.

Knowledge

As with clinical reasoning, ethical reasoning and analysis requires a knowledge base. Familiarity with major theoretical and practical ways of "doing" clinical ethics may be obtained by reading, taking a formal course in bioethics at a neighboring university, or attending a continuing education workshop or seminar. Although many specialty practice journals routinely address ethical issues, the most accessible journals devoted exclusively to bioethics and/or health care ethics are the *Hastings Center Report* and the *Journal of Clinical Ethics.* One of the chief objectives in acquiring some formal knowledge of ethical theory and systems of justification is to provide a language by which to facilitate conversation and dialogue about ethical matters. The ideal would be for us to consult both formally and informally with our colleagues about perplexing ethical matters in the same way that we consult on interesting clinical questions. Just as we confer with a colleague about a drug regimen—"I'm not sure why she isn't responding to this drug, given its pharmacokinetics"—we should be able to confer about our role in working with proxy decision makers to get the best decision for a patient—"I'm not sure why this family is so reluctant to do any sort of advance planning. Clearly the patient is not responding to treatment, and we are very close to that time when aggressive interventions will be futile." Initiating some regular forum for the discussion of ethical concerns is an important way to "own the language" of ethics and to develop facility in ethical discourse. Structured ways to do this include having ethics as a topic for a regular team meeting, discussing ethical issues in regularly scheduled team meetings as appropriate, having brown bag lunch conferences on interesting "cases" or issues, or dedicating one grand round a semester to an ethics case or topic.

Skills

Ethically competent providers possess a variety of ethical skills that range from the ability to establish trusting professional relationships to sophisticated conflict-mediation skills. Providers working with older patients and their families should be skilled in most of the following:

- Establishing trusting professional relationships with patients, family members, colleagues, payers, and other interested parties

- Communicating respect and promoting dignity
- Identifying and supporting appropriate decision makers
- Using the shared decision-making model to facilitate health care decision making that best advances patient interests
- Patient advocacy
- Advance care planning (advance directives, special orders: do-not-resuscitate, comfort measures only, do-not-hospitalize)
- Preventing and resolving conflicts
- Initiating and facilitating an ethics consult
- Distributing scarce resources
- Preparing for comfortable, dignified deaths
- Reporting unethical, illegal, and incompetent practice

Because most educational programs do not guarantee mastery of these skills, it is helpful for providers to determine their competence and confidence level in the skills that equate with excellent care in their practice setting and then strategize to remedy any deficiencies. For example, a provider who has never initiated an ethics consult and who routinely "muddles through" dilemmas that divide patients, families, and caregiving teams would be well advised to explore the ethics resources available within his or her setting and to practice the skill of facilitating an ethics consult or committee meeting. A provider who works in a culture that routinely dehumanizes older adults and their spouses and families may call a group meeting to explore how staff can change the culture of care and can practice developing and monitoring outcomes that reverse the forces of objectification and dehumanization.

Methodology for Values-Conflict Resolution: Georgetown University Center for Clinical Bioethics*

Recognizing and Acknowledging the Conflict or Uncertainty

Although recognizing the conflict seems to be a self-evident step of the process, it is often the source of unresolved conflicts. Participants may deny the actual conflict or uncertainty and reject the idea that there are *legitimate* competing ethical principles and values. Resolutions begin by recognizing that others hold legitimate values and have ethical traditions that must be respected and taken into account. Once this step is taken, the conflicts become evident and can be acknowledged publicly—regardless of the specific resolution each stakeholder initially made.
PREREQUISITE: Moral sensitivity and responsibility

---

*Used with permission. This methodology is modified from materials from the Woodstock Theological Center, Washington, DC, and the Health Policy and Bioethics Consultation Group, Berkeley, California.

Gathering Information

In gathering information, participants attempt to learn all they can about the conflict itself. What is the source of the conflict and related uncertainties? What is at stake? What information is needed to facilitate resolution of the conflict? Who are the stakeholders, and what are their values and interests? During the data-gathering phase it is essential to distinguish *factual judgments* from *individual or collective perceptions,* which may or may not be true.
PREREQUISITE: Intellectual humility, openness, respect, empathy

Identifying the Stakeholders

Who are the stakeholders in the decision? That is, who will be affected by it, either through responsibility for making decisions or implementing the decision, or through experiencing the outcomes of its implementation?

Identifying the Stakeholders' Interests

Each stakeholder should talk freely about his or her perspective on the issue in question. (Note: It is important for all stakeholders to be present at the table and to have a voice. Examples abound of discrepancies between perceived and actual values/interests of particular individuals and groups.) The aim of this phase is to have people talk freely and fully, without contradiction or analysis, so that all the relevant perspectives and data get put on the table.

Articulating and Ranking Values

Begin by articulating, and listing, the cherished values of each stakeholder group. Rank these so that the most important values of each stakeholder are known to the group at large. Use some process to reach consensus about the core values, which then ought to direct the resolution of the problem at hand.
PREREQUISITE: Respect and trust

Achieving agreement on a decision will depend in large part on the extent to which the participants in the discussion have gained an appreciation of and respect for the concerns and values of the varying perspectives they represent. Ideally, they come to respect and trust one another as honest, decent, well-motivated people—not as members of hostile "interest groups."

Identifying the Issue

After hearing the different perspectives, the group tries to define the disputed issue or issues as precisely as possible and identify the reasons for or root causes of the problem. The aim here is for the group to understand the problem as accurately as possible. The group then reflects on the various explanations for the problem, tests them for their

relative adequacy, and sees which best "fits" the data gathered in the first phase of the discussion. The aim of this phase is for all stakeholders to reach a common judgment on the best explanation of the issue, which will also involve overcoming partial ignorance or personal bias.
PREREQUISITE: Intellectual clarity

Generating Possible Courses of Action

Crafting a response to the issue involves identifying various plans of actions, which are then critiqued in light of the most cherished values of the full group.
PREREQUISITE: Critical thinking and creativity

Making the Decision

Ideally a consensus is reached and a decision is made on the basis of a relatively adequate understanding of all the dimensions of the problem and a generous concern for the most cherished among the values of each of the stakeholder representatives.
PREREQUISITE: Responsibility and accountability

If Deadlock Results

If a group of representatives cannot reach consensus and is deadlocked in opposing positions, redo the preceding steps to make sure participants genuinely understand and empathize with the cherished values of each. In this way they can rank by priority the most compelling concerns in order to reach consensus:

- Strive anew to design a new, creative, and imaginative course of action in which all the required values are promoted.
- Ask the opposing parties if their disagreement is nonnegotiable (i.e., is a matter of serious violation of conscience) or whether they could move ahead with the majority's plan of action, even if it is not their preference.
- Check the past history to see if there is precedent for one or another of the opposed positions and how, and how satisfactorily, the issue was resolved at that time.
- If possible, the group might be asked to agree on one of the opposed views on the condition that those who disagree with the view are not obliged to implement it themselves.
- If time is not of the essence, the decision can be deferred to give everyone opportunity for further thought and reflection.

Implementing and Evaluating the Decision

Once the decision is made about a possible course of action, it is important to discern how best to implement the decision given the interests and values at stake. Likewise, there

should be some advance discussion regarding the best way to evaluate the consequences of the selected course of action. The aim of this evaluation is to critique the adequacy of the process used in order to facilitate future decision making.
PREREQUISITE: Responsibility and accountability

Summary

Older adults have much to lose if a practitioner's ethical competence is undeveloped or undervalued. Long presumed to be somehow inherently present in health care professionals ("only good people are attracted to the health professions for all the right reasons, so it is safe to presume that ethical competence is a given"), ethical competence is beginning to get the attention it deserves. Until all health professionals hold themselves and one another accountable for ethical competence, high-quality health care will continue to be at best a fond hope and a sometimes reality.

Resources

Ethics in Aging
http://www.grants.cohpa.ucf.ed/age-ethics

The Ability Project
http://www.ability.org.uk/bioethics.html

References

American Association of Colleges of Nursing: *The essentials of master's education for advanced practice nursing,* Washington, DC, 1996, The Association.

American Association of Colleges of Nursing: *The essentials of baccalaureate education for professional nursing practice,* Washington, DC, 1998, The Association.

Association of American Medical Colleges: *Report 1: learning objectives for medical student education—guidelines for medical schools,* Washington, DC, 1998, The Association.

Fletcher JC, Miller FG, Spencer EM: Clinical ethics: history, content and resources. In Fletcher JC et al: *Introduction to clinical ethics,* Frederick, Md, 1995, University Publishing Group.

Goldstein A: Medical competency tests proposed, *Washington Post,* p A2, October 24, 1998.

Institute of Medicine: *America's health in transition: protecting and improving quality,* Washington, DC, 1994, National Academy Press.

National Academies of Practice: *Ethical guidelines for professional care and services in a managed health care environment,* Washington, DC, 1998.

Taylor C: Ethical issues in case management. In Cohen E, Cesta T, editors: *Nursing case management: from concept to evaluation,* ed 2, St Louis, 1997, Mosby.

Taylor C, Barnet R: The ethics of case management: the quality/cost conundrum. In Cohen E, DeBack V, editors: *The outcomes mandate: case management in health care today,* St Louis, 1999, Mosby.

Appendix

A

Minimum Data Set for Nursing Home Resident Assessment and Care Screening (v2)

Basic Assessment Tracking Form

General Instructions

Complete this information for submission with all full and quarterly assessments (admission, annual, significant change, quarterly review, discharge, reentry).

SECTION AA: IDENTIFICATION INFORMATION

1	RESIDENT NAME	a. First b. Middle Initial c. Last d. Jr/Sr
2	GENDER	1. Male 2. Female
3	BIRTHDATE	Month - Day - Year
4	RACE/ ETHNICITY	1. American Indian or Alaska Native 2. Asian or Pacific Islander 3. Black, not of Hispanic origin 4. Hispanic 5. White, not of Hispanic origin
5	SOCIAL SECURITY and MEDICARE NUMBERS	a. Social Security number b. Medicare number (or comparable railroad insurance number) ("C" in 1st box if non-Medicare number)
6	FACILITY PROVIDER No.	a. State number b. Federal number
7	MEDICAID No.	("+" if pending, "N" if not a Medicaid recipient)
8	REASONS FOR ASSESSMENT	a. Primary reason for assessment 1. Admission assessment (required by day 14) 2. Annual assessment 3. Significant change in status assessment 4. Significant correction of prior full assessment 5. Quarterly review assessment 10. Significant correction of prior quarterly assessment 6. Discharged – Return not anticipated 7. Discharged – Return anticipated 8. Discharged prior to completing initial assessment 9. Reentry 0. NONE OF ABOVE b. Codes for assessments required for Medicare PPS or the state 1. Medicare 5-day assessment 2. Medicare 30-day assessment 3. Medicare 60-day assessment 4. Medicare 90-day assessment 5. Medicare readmission or return assessment 6. Other state-required assessment 7. Medicare 14-day assessment 8. Other Medicare required assessment

9 SIGNATURES OF PERSONS COMPLETING THESE ITEMS:

	Signature	Title	Date
a.			
b.			
c.			

Reentry Tracking Form

On reentry, complete the Reentry Tracking Form and also the Basic Assessment Tracking Form, at left. In item AA8 *Reason for Assessment* enter a code of "9".

SECT A: IDENTIFICATION AND BACKGROUND INFORMATION

4a	DATE OF REENTRY	Month - Day - Year
4b	ADMITTED FROM (at reentry)	1. Private home / apartment with no home health services 2. Private home / apartment with home health services 3. Board and care / assisted living 4. Another nursing facility 5. Acute care hospital 6. Psychiatric hospital, MR/DD facility 7. Rehabilitation hospital 8. Other
6	MEDICAL RECORD NO.	

Discharge Tracking Form

(Do not use for temporary visits home.)

On discharge, complete the Discharge Tracking Form and also the Basic Assessment Tracking Form, at left. In item AA8a *Reason for Assessment* enter a code of "6" or "7" or "8". Leave item AA8b blank.

AB. DEMOGRAPHIC INFORMATION

1	DATE OF ENTRY	Month - Day - Year
2	ADMITTED FROM (at entry)	1. Private home or apt with no home health services 2. Private home or apt with home health services 3. Board and care or assisted living or group home 4. Nursing home 5. Acute care hospital 6. Psychiatric hospital or MR/DD facility 7. Rehabilitation hospital 8. Other

SECT A: IDENTIFICATION AND BACKGROUND INFORMATION

6	MEDICAL RECORD NO.	

SECTION R: DISCHARGE STATUS

3	DISCHARGE STATUS	*(Skip if not discharged.)* a. Code for resident disposition upon discharge. 1. Private home / apartment with no home health services 2. Private home / apartment with home health services 3. Board and care / assisted living 4. Another nursing facility 5. Acute care hospital 6. Psychiatric hospital, MR/DD facility 7. Rehabilitation hospital 8. Deceased 9. Other b. Optional state code
4	DISCHARGE DATE	Month - Day - Year

SECT A: IDENTIFICATION AND BACKGROUND INFORMATION

1	RESIDENT NAME	a. First b. Middle Initial c. Last d. Jr/Sr
2	ROOM No.	
3	ASSESSMENT REFERENCE DATE	a. Last day of MDS observation period Month - Day - Year a. Original (0) or corrected copy of form (enter number of correction)
4	DATE OF REENTRY	*Date of reentry from most recent temporary discharge to a hospital in last 90 days (or since last assessment or admission if less than 90 days).* Month - Day - Year
5	MARITAL STATUS	1. Never married 3. Widowed 5. Divorced 2. Married 4. Separated
6	MEDICAL RECORD NO.	
7	CURRENT PAYMENT SOURCES FOR NURSING HOME STAY	(*Billing office to indicate; check all that apply in LAST 30 DAYS.*) a. Medicaid *per diem* [a] b. Medicare *per diem* [b] c. Medicare ancillary Part A [c] d. Medicare ancillary Part B [d] e. CHAMPUS *per diem* [e] f. VA *per diem* [f] g. Self or family pays for full *per diem* [g] h. Medicaid resident liability or Medicare co-payment [h] i. Private insurance *per diem* (including co-payment) [i] j. Other *per diem* [j]
8	REASONS FOR ASSESSMENT Note: If this is a discharge or reentry assessment, only a limited subset of MDS items needs to be completed	a. Primary reason for assessment 1. Admission assessment (required by day 14) 2. Annual assessment 3. Significant change in status assessment 4. Significant correction of prior full assessment 5. Quarterly review assessment 10. Significant correction of prior quarterly assessment 6. Discharged – Return not anticipated 7. Discharged – Return anticipated 8. Discharged prior to completing initial assessment 9. Reentry 0. NONE OF ABOVE b. Codes for assessments required for Medicare PPS or the state 1. Medicare 5-day assessment 2. Medicare 30-day assessment 3. Medicare 60-day assessment 4. Medicare 90-day assessment 5. Medicare readmission or return assessment 6. Other state-required assessment 7. Medicare 14-day assessment 8. Other Medicare required assessment
9	RESPONSIBILITY/ LEGAL GUARDIAN	(*Check all that apply.*) a. Legal guardian [a] b. Other legal oversight [b] c. Durable power of attorney/health care [c] d. Durable power of attorney/financial [d] e. Family member responsible [e] f. Resident responsible for self [f] g. *NONE OF ABOVE* [g]
10	ADVANCED DIRECTIVES	(*For those items with supporting documentation in the medical record, check all that apply.*) a. Living will [a] b. Do not resuscitate [b] c. Do not hospitalize [c] d. Organ donation [d] e. Autopsy request [e] f. Feeding restrictions [f] g. Medication restrictions [g] h. Other treatment restrictions [h] i. *NONE OF ABOVE* [i]

SECTION B: COGNITIVE PATTERNS

1	COMATOSE	(*Persistent vegetative state or no discernible consciousness.*) 0. No 1. Yes (Skip to item G1) ◇0
2	MEMORY	Recall of what was learned or known. a. Short-term memory OK – seems or appears to recall after 5 minutes 0. Memory OK 1. Memory problem ❷ ◇0 b. Long-term memory OK – seems or appears to recall long past 0. Memory OK 1. Memory problem ❷
3	MEMORY/ RECALL ABILITY	(*Check all that resident was normally able to recall during the last 7 days.*) a. Current season [a] b. Location of own room [b] c. Staff names or faces [c] d. That he / she is in a nursing home [d] e. *NONE OF ABOVE* are recalled [e]
4	COGNITIVE SKILLS FOR DAILY DECISION-MAKING ◇0	(*Made decisions regarding tasks of daily life.*) 0. INDEPENDENT – decisions consistent and reasonable 1. MODIFIED INDEPENDENCE – some difficulty in new situations only ❷ 2. MODERATELY IMPAIRED – decisions poor; cues or supervision required 3. SEVERELY IMPAIRED – never / rarely made decisions ❺
5	INDICATORS OF DELIRIUM– PERIODIC DISORDERED THINKING/ AWARENESS	(*Code for behavior in last 7 days.*) *Accurate assessment requires conversations with staff and family who have direct knowledge of resident's behavior over this time.* 0. Behavior not present 1. Behavior present, not of recent onset — Any 2 below = ❶ ⓱ 2. Behavior present, over last 7 days appears different from resident's usual functioning (*e.g.*, new onset or worsening) a. EASILY DISTRACTED (*e.g.*, difficulty paying attention, gets sidetracked). b. PERIODS OF ALTERED PERCEPTION OR AWARENESS OF SURROUNDINGS (*e.g.*, moves lips or talks to someone not present; believes he or she is somewhere else, confuses night and day). c. EPISODES OF DISORGANIZED SPEECH (*e.g.*, speech is incoherent, nonsensical, irrelevant, or rambling from subject to subject; loses train of thought). d. PERIODS OF RESTLESSNESS (*e.g.*, fidgeting or picking at skin, clothing, napkins, etc.; frequent position changes; repetitive physical movements or calling out). e. PERIODS OF LETHARGY (*e.g.*, sluggishness, staring into space, difficult to arouse, little bodily movement). f. MENTAL FUNCTION VARIES OVER THE COURSE OF THE DAY (*e.g.*, sometimes better, sometimes worse; behaviors sometimes present, sometimes not).
6	CHANGE IN COGNITIVE STATUS	*Resident's cognitive status, skills, or abilities have changed as compared to status of 90 DAYS AGO (or since last assessment if less than 90 days).* 0. No change 1. Improved 2. Deteriorated ❶ ⓱

[ ] When box is empty, enter a letter or number.
[a] When box holds a letter, check if condition applies.

Resident Assessment Protocols (RAPs)

1. Delirium
2. Cognitive Loss / Dementia
3. Visual Function
4. Communication
5. ADL Functional / Rehabilitation Potential
6. Urinary Incontinence and Indwelling Catheter
7. Psychosocial Well-Being
8. Mood State
9. Behavior Problems
10. Activities
11. Falls
12. Nutritional Status
13. Feeding Tubes
14. Dehydration / Fluid Maintenance
15. Dental Care
16. Pressure Ulcers
17. Psychotropic Drug Use
18. Physical Restraints

SECTION C: COMMUNICATION / HEARING PATTERNS

1	HEARING	(*With hearing appliance, if used.*) 0. HEARS ADEQUATELY – normal talk, TV, phone 1. MINIMAL DIFFICULTY when not in quiet setting ❹ 2. HEARS IN SPECIAL SITUATION ONLY – speaker has to adjust tonal quality and speak distinctly ◇Q 3. HIGHLY IMPAIRED or absence of useful hearing ◇Q	
2	COMMUNI-CATION DEVICES / TECHNIQUES	(*Check all that apply during last 7 days.*) a. Hearing aid, present and used b. Hearing aid, present and not used regularly c. Other receptive communication techniques used (*e.g.*, lip reading) d. *NONE OF ABOVE* ◇Q	a b c d
3	MODES OF EXPRESSION	(*Check all used by resident to make needs known.*) a. Speech [a] b. Writing messages to express or clarify needs [b] c. American sign language or Braille [c] d. Signs or gestures or sounds e. Communication board f. Other g. *NONE OF ABOVE*	d e f g
4	MAKING SELF UNDERSTOOD	(*Expressing information content – however able.*) 0. UNDERSTOOD 1. USUALLY UNDERSTOOD – difficulty finding words or finishing thoughts ❹ 2. SOMETIMES UNDERSTOOD – ability is limited to making concrete requests ◇Q 3. RARELY OR NEVER UNDERSTOOD ◇Q	
5	SPEECH CLARITY	(*Code for speech in last 7 days.*) 0. CLEAR SPEECH – distinct, intelligible words 1. UNCLEAR SPEECH – slurred, mumbled words ◇Q 2. NO SPEECH – absence of spoken words	
6	ABILITY TO UNDERSTAND OTHERS	(*Understanding verbal information content – however able.*) 0. UNDERSTANDS 1. USUALLY UNDERSTANDS – may miss some part or intent of message 2. SOMETIMES UNDERSTANDS – responds adequately to simple, direct communication ◇Q ❷ 3. RARELY OR NEVER UNDERSTANDS ◇Q ❹	
7	CHANGE IN COMMUNICATION / HEARING	*Resident's ability to express, understand, or hear information has changed as compared to status of 90 DAYS AGO (or since last assessment if less than 90 days)* 0. No Change 1. Improved 2. Deteriorated ⓱	

SECTION D: VISION PATTERNS

1	VISION ◇Q	(*Able to see in adequate light and with glasses, if used.*) 0. ADEQUATE – sees fine detail, including regular print in newspapers or books 1. IMPAIRED – sees large print, but not regular print in newspapers or books ❸ 2. MODERATELY IMPAIRED – limited vision; not able to see newspaper headlines, but can identify objects ❸ 3. HIGHLY IMPAIRED – object identification in question, but eyes appear to follow objects ❸ 4. SEVERELY IMPAIRED – no vision or sees only light, color or shapes; eyes do not appear to follow objects	
2	VISUAL LIMITATIONS / DIFFICULTIES ◇Q	a. Side vision problems – decreased peripheral vision (*e.g.*, leaves food on one side of tray, difficulty traveling, bumps into people and objects, misjudges placement of chair when seating self) ❸ b. Experiences any of the following: sees halos or rings around lights, sees flashes of light, sees "curtains" over eyes c. *NONE OF ABOVE*	a b c
3	VISUAL APPLIANCES	Glasses; contact lenses; magnifying glass 0. No ◇Q 1. Yes	

SECTION E: MOOD AND BEHAVIOR PATTERNS

1	INDICATORS OF DEPRESSION, ANXIETY, SAD MOOD Any 1, 2 = ❽	(*Code for indicators observed in LAST 30 DAYS, irrespective of the assumed cause.*) 0. Indicator not exhibited in last 30 days 1. Indicator of this type exhibited up to 5 days a week 2. Indicator of this type exhibited daily or almost daily (6, 7 days) **VERBAL EXPRESSIONS OF DISTRESS** ◇Q a. Resident made negative statements – *e.g.*, "Nothing matters; Would rather be dead; What's the use; Regrets having lived so long; Let me die." ◇Q b. Repetitive questions: "Where do I go? What do I do?" ◇Q c. Repetitive verbalizations – *e.g.*, Calling out for help ("God help me") ◇Q d. Persistent anger with self or others (*e.g.*, easily annoyed, anger at placement in nursing home; anger at care received) e. Self deprecation (*e.g.*, "I am nothing, of no use to anyone") f. Expressions of what appear to be unrealistic fears (*e.g.*, fear of being abandoned, left alone, being with others) ◇Q g. Recurrent statements that something terrible is about to happen (*e.g.*, believes is about to die, have a heart attack) h. Repetitive health complaints (*e.g.*, persistently seeks medical attention, obsessive concern with body functions) i. Repetitive anxious complaints or concerns – non-health (*e.g.*, persistently seeks attention or reassurance regarding schedules, meals, laundry or clothing, relationship issues) **SLEEP-CYCLE ISSUES** ◇Q j. Unpleasant mood in morning k. Insomnia or change in usual sleep pattern **SAD, APATHETIC, ANXIOUS APPEARANCE** l. Sad, pained, worried facial expressions (*e.g.*, furrowed brow) m. Crying, tearfulness ◇Q n. Repetitive physical movements (*e.g.*, pacing, hand wringing, restlessness, fidgeting, picking) ⓱ **LOSS OF INTEREST** ◇Q o. Withdrawal from activities of interest (*e.g.*, no interest in longstanding activities or being with family, friends) ❼ ◇Q p. Reduced social interaction	
2	MOOD PERSISTENCE	One or more indicators of depressed, sad or anxious mood were not easily altered by attempts to "cheer up," console, or reassure the resident in last 7 days. 0. No mood indicators 1. Indicators present, easily altered ◇Q ❽ 2. Indicators present, not easily altered	
3	CHANGE IN MOOD	Resident's mood status has changed as compared to status of 90 DAYS AGO (or since last assessment if less than 90 days ago) 0. No change 1. Improved 2. Deteriorated ❶⓱	
4	BEHAVIORAL SYMPTOMS	(*Code for behavior in last 7 days.*) A. Behavioral symptom frequency in last 7 days 0. Behavior not exhibited in last 7 days 1. Behavior of this type occurred on 1 to 3 days in last 7 days 2. Behavior of this type occurred 4 to 6 days, but less than daily 3. Behavior of this type occurred daily B. Behavioral symptom alterability in last 7 days 0. Behavior not present -OR- behavior was easily altered 1. Behavior was not easily altered ❾ a. **WANDERING** (moved with no rational purpose, seemingly oblivious to needs or safety) ⓫ ◆Q❾ b. **VERBALLY ABUSIVE** behavioral symptoms (others were threatened, screamed at, cursed at) ◆Q❾ c. **PHYSICALLY ABUSIVE** behavioral symptoms (others were hit, shoved, scratched, sexually abused) ◆Q❾ d. **SOCIALLY INAPPROPRIATE or DISRUPTIVE** behavioral symptoms (made disruptive sounds, noisiness, screaming, self-abusive acts, sexual behavior or disrobing in public, smeared or threw food or feces, hoarding, rummaged in others' belongings) ❾ e. **RESISTS CARE** (resisted taking meds or injections, ADL assistance, or eating) ◇Q	A B
5	CHANGE IN BEHAVIORAL SYMPTOMS	Resident's behavioral status has changed as compared to status of 90 DAYS AGO (or since last assessment if less than 90 days ago) 0. No change 1. Improved ❾ 2. Deteriorated ❶⓱	

SECTION F. PSYCHOSOCIAL WELL-BEING

1	SENSE OF INITIATIVE / INVOLVEMENT	a. At ease interacting with others	a
		b. At ease doing planned or structured activities	b
		c. At ease doing self-initiated activities	c
		d. Establishes own goals ❼	d
		e. Pursues involvement in life of facility (*e.g.*, makes and keeps friends; involved in group activities; responds positively to new activities; assists at religious services)	e
		f. Accepts invitations into most group activities	f
		g. *NONE OF ABOVE*	g
2	UNSETTLED RELATIONSHIPS	a. Covert/open conflict with or repeated criticism of staff ❼	a
		b. Unhappy with roommate ❼	b
		c. Unhappy with residents other than roommate ❼	c
		d. Openly expresses conflict / anger with family / friends ❼	d
		e. Absence of personal contact with family or friends	e
		f. Recent loss of close family member or friend	f
		g. Does not adjust easily to change in routines	g
		h. *NONE OF ABOVE*	h
3	PAST ROLES	a. Strong identification with past roles and life status ❼	a
		b. Expresses sadness, anger or empty feeling over lost roles or status ❼	b
		c. Resident perceives that daily life (customary routine, activities) is very different from prior pattern in the community ❼	c
		d. *NONE OF ABOVE*	d

G. PHYSICAL FUNCTIONING AND STRUCTURAL PROBLEMS

1 **A. ADL SELF-PERFORMANCE** (Code for resident's ***PERFORMANCE OVER ALL SHIFTS*** *during last 7 days*, not including setup.)

0. INDEPENDENT. No help or oversight –OR– Help / oversight provided only 1 or 2 times during last 7 days.

1. SUPERVISION. Oversight, encouragement or cueing provided 3 or more times during last 7 days –OR– Supervision plus physical assistance provided only 1 or 2 times during last 7 days.

2. LIMITED ASSISTANCE. Resident highly involved in activity; received physical help in guided maneuvering of limbs, or other nonweight-bearing assistance 3 or more times –OR– More help provided only 1 to 2 times during last 7 days.

3. EXTENSIVE ASSISTANCE. Although resident performed part of activity, over last 7-day period, help of the following type(s) was provided 3 or more times:
- Weight-bearing support
- Full staff performance during part (but not all) of last 7 days

4. TOTAL DEPENDENCE. Full staff performance of activity during entire 7 days.

8. ACTIVITY DID NOT OCCUR during entire 7 days. **Any 1, 2, 3, 4 in col. A = ❺**

B. ADL SUPPORT PROVIDED (Code for ***MOST SUPPORT PROVIDED OVER ALL SHIFTS during last 7 days;*** code regardless of resident's self-performance classification.)

0. No setup or physical help from staff
1. Setup help only
2. One-person physical assist
3. Two + persons physical assist
8. ADL activity did not occur during entire 7 days

			A SELF-PERFORMANCE	B SUPPORT
a	BED MOBILITY	How resident moves to and from lying position, turns from side to side, and positions body while in bed ⓰		
b	TRANSFER	How resident moves between surfaces – to and from: bed, chair, wheelchair, standing position (EXCLUDE to and from bath and toilet)		
c	WALK IN ROOM	How resident walks between locations in own room.		
d	WALK IN CORRIDOR	How resident walks in corridor on unit.		
e	LOCOMOTION ON UNIT	How resident moves between locations in own room and adjacent corridor on same floor. If in wheelchair, self-sufficiency once in chair.		
f	LOCOMOTION OFF UNIT	How resident moves to and returns from off-unit locations (*e.g.*, areas set aside for dining, activities, or treatments). If facility has only one floor, how resident moves to and from distant areas on the floor. If in wheelchair, self-sufficiency once in chair.		
g	DRESSING	How resident puts on, fastens, and takes off all items of street clothing, including donning and removing prosthesis		

G. Physical Functioning and Structural Problems (continued)

Any 1, 2, 3, 4 in column A = ❺

			A	B
h	EATING	How resident eats and drinks (regardless of skill). Includes intake of nourishment by other means (*e.g.*, tube feeding, total parental nutrition)		
i	TOILET USE	How resident uses the toilet room (or commode, bed-pan, urinal); transfers on / off toilet, cleanses, changes pad, manages ostomy or catheter, adjusts clothes		
j	PERSONAL HYGIENE	How resident maintains personal hygiene, including combing hair; brushing teeth; shaving; applying makeup; washing and drying face, hands, and perineum (EXCLUDE baths and showers)		

2	BATHING	How resident takes full-body bath or shower, sponge bath, and transfers in and out of tub or shower (EXCLUDE washing of back and hair). Code for most dependent in self-performance and support. Bathing self-performance codes are: 0. Independent – No help provided 1. Supervision – Oversight help only ❺ 2. Physical help limited to transfer only ❺ 3. Physical help in part of bathing activity ❺ 4. Total dependence ❺ 8. Bathing did not occur during the entire 7 days (Bathing support codes are as defined in item 1B above)	A SELF-PERFORMANCE / B SUPPORT
3	TEST FOR BALANCE	(*Code for ability during test in the last 7 days.*) 0. Maintained position as required in test 1. Unsteady, but able to rebalance self without physical support 2. Partial physical support during test or doesn't follow directions 3. Not able to attempt test without physical help	
		a. Balance while standing	
		b. Balance while sitting – position, trunk control ⓱	
4	FUNCTIONAL LIMITATION IN RANGE OF MOTION ◈	(*Code for limitations during last 7 days that interfered with daily functions or put resident at risk of injury.*) **A.** RANGE OF MOTION: 0. No limitation; 1. Limitation on 1 side; 2. Limitation on both sides **B.** VOLUNTARY MOVEMENT: 0. No loss; 1. Partial loss; 2. Full loss	A / B
		a. Neck	
		b. Arm – including shoulder or elbow	
		c. Hand – including wrist or finger	
		d. Leg – including hip or knee	
		e. Foot – including ankle or toes	
		f. Other limitation or loss	
5	MODES OF LOCOMOTION	(*Check all that apply during last 7 days.*)	
		a. Cane, walker, or crutch	a
		b. Wheeled self	b
		c. Other person wheeled	c
		d. Wheelchair primary mode of locomotion	d
		e. *NONE OF ABOVE*	e
6	MODES OF TRANSFER	(*Check all that apply during last 7 days.*)	
		a. Bedfast all or most of the time ◈ ⓰	a
		b. Bed rails used for bed mobility or transfer	b
		c. Lifted manually	c
		d. Lifted mechanically	d
		e. Transfer aid (*e.g.*, slide board, trapeze, cane, walker, brace)	e
		f. *NONE OF ABOVE*	f
7	TASK SEGMENTATION	Some or all of ADL activities were broken into sub-tasks during last 7 days so that resident could perform them. 0. No 1. Yes	
8	ADL FUNCTIONAL REHAB. POTENTIAL	a. Resident believes self to be capable of increased independence in at least some ADLs ❺	a
		b. Direct care staff believe resident is capable of increased independence in at least some ADLs ❺	b
		c. Resident able to perform tasks / activity but is very slow	c
		d. Difference in ADL self-performance or ADL support, comparing mornings to evenings	d
		e. *NONE OF ABOVE*	e
9	CHANGE IN ADL FUNCTION	Resident's ADL Self-Performance status has changed as compared to status of 90 DAYS AGO (or since last assessed). 0. No change 1. Improved 2. Deteriorated ◈	

SECTION H. CONTINENCE IN LAST 14 DAYS

1	CONTINENCE SELF-CONTROL CATEGORIES (Code for performance over all shifts.) 0. CONTINENT – Complete control 1. USUALLY CONTINENT – BLADDER, incontinent episodes once a week or less; BOWEL, less than weekly 2. OCCASIONALLY INCONTINENT – ◇0 BLADDER, 2 + times a week but not daily; BOWEL, once a week ◇0 3. FREQUENTLY INCONTINENT – BLADDER, tended to be incontinent daily, but some control present (*e.g.*, on day shift); BOWEL, 2 or 3 times a week ◇0 4. INCONTINENT – Had inadequate control. BLADDER, multiple daily episodes; BOWEL, all (or almost all) of the time	
a	**BOWEL CONTINENCE**	Control of bowel movement, with appliance or bowel continence programs, if used (16)
b	**BLADDER CONTINENCE**	Control of urinary bladder function (if dribbles, volume insufficient to soak through underpants), with appliances (*e.g.*, foley) or continence programs, if used 2, 3, 4 = (6)
2	**BOWEL ELIMINATION PATTERN**	a. Bowel elimination pattern regular – at least 1 movement every 3 days [a] b. Constipation (17) [b] c. Diarrhea [c] d. Fecal impaction [d] ◇0 (17) e. *NONE OF ABOVE* [e]
3	**APPLIANCES AND PROGRAMS**	a. Any scheduled toileting plan ◇0 [a] b. Bladder retraining program ◇0 [b] c. External (condom) catheter (6) [c] ◇0 d. Indwelling catheter (6) [d] e. Intermittent catheter (6) [e] f. Did not use toilet room, commode, urinal [f] g. Pads or briefs used (6) [g] h. Enemas, irrigation [h] i. Ostomy present ◇0 [i] j. *NONE OF ABOVE* [j]
4	**CHANGE IN URINARY CONTINENCE**	Resident's urinary continence has changed as compared to status of 90 DAYS AGO (or since last assessment if less than 90 days) 0. No change 1. Improved 2. Deteriorated

SECTION I. DISEASE DIAGNOSES

Check only those diseases that have a relationship to current ADL status, cognitive status, mood and behavior status, medical treatments, nurse monitoring, or risk of death. (Do not list inactive diagnoses.)

1	**DISEASES**	(*If none apply, CHECK item I1rr, NONE OF ABOVE*)

ENDOCRINE / METABOLIC / NUTRITIONAL
- a. Diabetes mellitus ◇0 [a]
- b. Hyperthyroidism [b]
- c. Hypothyroidism [c]

HEART / CIRCULATION
- d. Arteriosclerotic heart disease (ASHD) [d]
- e. Cardiac dysrhythmia [e]
- f. Congestive heart failure [f]
- g. Deep vein thrombosis [g]
- h. Hypertension [h]
- i. Hypotension (17) [i]
- j. Peripheral vascular disease (16) [j]
- k. Other cardiovascular disease [k]

MUSCULOSKELETAL
- l. Arthritis [l]
- m. Hip fracture [m]
- n. Missing limb (*e.g.*, amputation) [n]
- o. Osteoporosis [o]
- p. Pathological bone fracture [p]

NEUROLOGICAL
- q. Alzheimer's disease [q]
- r. Aphasia [r]
- s. Cerebral palsy [s]
- t. Cerebrovascular accident (stroke) [t]
- u. Dementia other than Alzheimer's disease [u]
- v. Hemiplegia / hemiparesis [v]
- w. Multiple sclerosis [w]
- x. Paraplegia [x]
- y. Parkinson's disease [y]
- z. Quadriplegia [z]
- aa. Seizure disorder [aa]
- bb. Transient ischemic attack (TIA) [bb]
- cc. Traumatic brain injury [cc]

PSYCHIATRIC / MOOD
- dd. Anxiety disorder [dd]
- ee. Depression ◇0 (17) [ee]
- ff. Manic depressive (bipolar disease) ◇0 [ff]
- gg. Schizophrenia [gg]

PULMONARY
- hh. Asthma [hh]
- ii. Emphysema / COPD [ii]

SENSORY
- jj. Cataracts (3) [jj]
- kk. Diabetic retinopathy [kk]
- ll. Glaucoma (3) [ll]
- mm. Macular degeneration [mm]

OTHER
- nn. Allergies [nn]
- oo. Anemia [oo]
- pp. Cancer [pp]
- qq. Renal failure [qq]
- rr. *NONE OF ABOVE* [rr]

Section I. Disease Diagnoses (continued)

2	**INFECTIONS**	(*If none apply, CHECK the NONE OF ABOVE box*) a. Antibiotic resistant infection (*e.g.*, methicillin resistant staph) [a] b. Clostridium difficile [b] c. Conjunctivitis [c] d. HIV infection [d] e. Pneumonia [e] f. Respiratory infection [f] g. Septicemia [g] h. Sexually transmitted diseases [h] i. Tuberculosis (active) [i] j. Urinary tract infection in last 30 days ◇0 (14) [j] k. Viral hepatitis [k] l. Wound infection [l] m. *NONE OF ABOVE* [m]
3	**OTHER CURRENT OR MORE DETAILED DIAGNOSES AND ICD-9-CM CODES**	276.5 = (14) a. ____ ☐☐☐☐.☐☐ b. ____ ☐☐☐☐.☐☐ c. ____ ☐☐☐☐.☐☐ d. ____ ☐☐☐☐.☐☐ e. ____ ☐☐☐☐.☐☐

SECTION J: HEALTH CONDITIONS

1	**PROBLEM CONDITIONS**	(*Check all problems present in last 7 days UNLESS OTHER TIME FRAME IS INDICATED*) **INDICATORS OF FLUID STATUS** a. Weight gain or loss of 3 or more lbs in last 7 days (14) [a] b. Inability to lie flat due to shortness of breath [b] c. Dehydrated; output exceeds intake ◇0 (14) [c] d. Insufficient fluid; did NOT consume all or almost all liquids provided during LAST 3 DAYS (14) [d] **OTHER** e. Delusions [e] f. Dizziness/vertigo (11) (17) [f] g. Edema [g] h. Fever (14) [h] i. Hallucination (17) [i] j. Internal bleeding (14) [j] k. Recurrent lung aspirations in LAST 90 DAYS (17) [k] l. Shortness of breath [l] m. Syncope (fainting) (17) [m] n. Unsteady gait (17) [n] o. Vomiting [o] p. *NONE OF ABOVE* [p]
2	**PAIN SYMPTOMS**	(*Code for the highest level of pain present in last 7 days*) **a. FREQUENCY** with which resident complains or shows evidence of pain: 0. No pain (*Skip to J4*) 1. Pain less than daily 2. Pain daily **b. INTENSITY** of pain: 1. Mild pain 2. Moderate pain 3. Times when pain is horrible or excruciating
3	**PAIN SITE**	(*Check all sites where pain was present in last 7 days*) a. Back pain [a] b. Bone pain [b] c. Chest pain during usual activities [c] d. Headache [d] e. Hip pain [e] f. Incisional pain [f] g. Joint pain (other than hip) [g] h. Soft tissue pain (*e.g.*, lesion, muscle) [h] i. Stomach pain [i] j. Other [j]
4	**ACCIDENTS**	a. Fell in LAST 30 DAYS ◇0 (11) (17) [a] b. Fell in LAST 31 to 180 DAYS (11) (17) [b] c. Hip fracture in LAST 180 DAYS ◇0 (17) [c] d. Other fracture in LAST 180 DAYS ◇0 [d] e. *NONE OF ABOVE* [e]
5	**STABILITY OF CONDITIONS**	a. Conditions or diseases make resident's cognitive, ADL, mood, or behavior patterns unstable (fluctuating, precarious, or deteriorating) [a] b. Resident experiencing an acute episode or a flare-up of a recurrent or chronic problem [b] c. End-stage disease; 6 months or less to live [c] d. *NONE OF ABOVE* [d]

SECTION K. ORAL / NUTRITIONAL STATUS

1	ORAL PROBLEMS	a. Chewing problem a b. Swallowing problem ⓱ b c. Mouth pain ⓯ c d. *NONE OF ABOVE* d	
2	HEIGHT AND WEIGHT	a. **Record height** in inches b. **Record weight** in pounds Base weight on most recent measure in LAST 30 DAYS; measure weight consistently in accord with standard facility practice (*e.g.*, in AM after voiding, before meal, with shoes off, and in nightclothes).	a. HEIGHT (in.) b. WEIGHT (lb.)
3	WEIGHT CHANGE	**a. Weight loss** – 5 % or more in LAST 30 DAYS or 10% or more in LAST 180 DAYS. 0. No 1. Yes ⓬ **b. Weight gain** – 5 % or more in LAST 30 DAYS or 10% or more in LAST 180 DAYS. 0. No 1. Yes	
4	NUTRITIONAL PROBLEMS	a. Complains about the taste of many foods ⓬ a b. Regular or repetitive complaints of hunger b c. Leaves 25% or more of food uneaten at most meals ⓬ c d. *NONE OF ABOVE* d	
5	NUTRITIONAL APPROACHES	(*Check all that apply in last 7 days.*) a. Parenteral / IV ⓬⓮ a b. Feeding tube ⓭⓮ b c. Mechanically altered diet ⓬ c d. Syringe (oral feeding) ⓬ d e. Therapeutic diet ⓬ e f. Dietary supplement between meals f g. Plate guard, stabilized built-up utensil, etc. g h. On a planned weight change program h i. *NONE OF ABOVE* i	
6	PARENTERAL OR ENTERAL INTAKE	(*Skip to Section L if neither 5a nor 5b is checked.*) a. Code the proportion of total calories the resident received through parenteral or tube feedings in the last 7 days 0. None 1. 1% to 25% 2. 26% to 50% 3. 51% to 75% 4. 76% to 100% b. Code the average fluid intake per day by IV or tube in the last 7 days 0. None 1. 1 to 500 cc/day 2. 501 to 1000 cc/day 3. 1001 to 1500 cc/day 4. 1501 to 2000 cc/day 5. 2001 or more cc/day	

SECTION L. ORAL / DENTAL STATUS

1	ORAL STATUS AND DISEASE PREVENTION	a. Debris (soft, easily movable substances) present in mouth prior to going to bed at night ⓯	a
		b. Has dentures and/or removable bridge	b
		c. Some or all natural teeth lost – does not have or does not use dentures (or partial plates) ⓯	c
		d. Broken, loose, or carious teeth ⓯	d
		e. Inflamed gums (gingiva); swollen or bleeding gums; oral abscesses, ulcers, or rashes ⓯	e
		f. Daily cleaning of teeth or dentures, or daily mouth care – by resident or staff Not ✓ed = ⓯	f
		g. *NONE OF ABOVE*	g

SECTION M. SKIN CONDITION

1	ULCERS (due to any cause)	(*Record the number of ulcers at each ulcer stage – regardless of cause. If none present at a stage, record "0" (zero). Code all that apply in last 7 days. Code 9 = 9 or more.*) **Requires a full body exam.** a. **Stage 1** A persistent area of skin redness (without a break in the skin) that does not disappear when pressure is relieved. b. **Stage 2** A partial thickness loss of skin layers that presents clinically as an abrasion, blister or shallow crater. c. **Stage 3** A full thickness of skin is lost, exposing the subcutaneous tissues – presents as a deep crater with or without undermining adjacent tissue. d. **Stage 4** A full thickness of skin and subcutaneous tissue is lost, exposing muscle or bone.
2	TYPE OF ULCER	(*For each type of ulcer, code for the highest stage in last 7 days using scale in item M1 – i.e., 0 = none; stages 1, 2, 3, 4*) a. Pressure ulcer – any lesion caused by pressure resulting in damage of underlying tissue ⓬⓰ b. Stasis ulcer – open lesion caused by poor circulation in the lower extremities
3	HISTORY OF RESOLVED ULCERS	Resident had an ulcer that resolved or was cured in LAST 90 DAYS. 0. No 1. Yes ⓰
4	OTHER SKIN PROBLEMS OR LESIONS PRESENT	(*Check all that apply during last 7 days.*) a. Abrasions, bruises a b. Burns (second or third degree) b c. Open lesions other than ulcers, rashes or cuts (*e.g.*, cancer lesions) c d. Rashes (*e.g.*, impetigo, eczema, drug/heat rash, herpes) d e. Skin desensitized to pain or pressure ⓰ e f. Skin tears or cuts (other than surgery) f g. Surgical wounds g h. *NONE OF ABOVE* h
5	SKIN TREATMENTS	(*Check all that apply during last 7 days.*) a. Pressure relieving device(s) for chair a b. Pressure relieving device(s) for bed b c. Turning or repositioning program c d. Nutrition or hydration intervention to manage skin problems d e. Ulcer care e f. Surgical wound care f g. Application of dressings (with or without topical medications) other than to feet g h. Application of ointments or medications (except to feet) h i. Other preventive or protective skin care (except to feet) i j. *NONE OF ABOVE* j
6	FOOT PROBLEMS AND CARE	(*Check all that apply during last 7 days.*) a. Resident has one or more foot problems (*e.g.*, corns, callouses, bunions, hammer toes, overlapping toes, pain, structural problems) a b. Infection of the foot (*e.g.*, cellulitis, purulent drainage) b c. Open lesions on the foot c d. Nails or callouses trimmed during last 90 days d e. Received preventative or protective foot care (*e.g.*, used special shoes, inserts, pads, toe separators) e f. Application of dressings (with or w/o topical meds.) f g. *NONE OF ABOVE* g

SECTION N. ACTIVITY PURSUIT PATTERNS

1	TIME AWAKE	(*Check appropriate time periods over last 7 days.*) Resident awake all or most of the time (*i.e.*, naps no more than 1 hour per time period) in the: a. Morning ⑩ a b. Afternoon b c. Evening c d. *NONE OF ABOVE* d
		(*If resident is comatose, skip to Section O.*)
2	AVERAGE TIME INVOLVED IN ACTIVITIES	(*When awake and not getting treatment or ADL care*) 0. Most – more than $^2/_3$ of time ⑩ 1. Some – from $^1/_3$ to $^2/_3$ of time 2. Little – less than $^1/_3$ of time ⓾ 3. None ⓾
3	PREFERRED ACTIVITY SETTINGS	(*Check all settings in which activities are preferred.*) a. Own room a b. Day or activity room b c. Inside NH / off unit c d. Outside facility d e. *NONE OF ABOVE* e
4	GENERAL ACTIVITY PREFERENCES (adapted to resident's current abilities)	(*Check all PREFERENCES whether or not activity is currently available to resident.*) a. Cards, other games a b. Crafts or arts b c. Exercise or sports c d. Music d e. Reading, writing e f. Spiritual or religious activities f g. Trips or shopping g h. Walk / wheeling outdoors h i. Watching TV i j. Gardening or plants j k. Talking or conversing k l. Helping others l m. *NONE OF ABOVE* m
5	PREFERS CHANGE IN DAILY ROUTINE	Code for resident preferences in daily routine. 0. No change 1. Slight change ⓾ 2. Major change ⓾ a. Type of activities in which resident is currently involved b. Extent of resident involvement in activities

SECTION O. MEDICATIONS

1	NUMBER OF MEDICATIONS	(Record the number of different medications used in the last 7 days. *Enter 0 if none used.*) > 8 = ◈
2	NEW MEDICATIONS	Resident currently receiving medications that were initiated during the LAST 90 DAYS. 0. No 1. Yes
3	INJECTIONS	(Record the number of DAYS injections of any type were received during the last 7 days. *Enter 0 if none used.*)
4	DAYS RECEIVED THE FOLLOWING MEDICATION	(Record the number of DAYS during last 7 days; enter 0 if not used. *n.b., Enter 1 for long-acting meds used less than weekly.*) ◈ a. Antipsychotic ◈ b. Antianxiety drug ◈ 11 c. Antidepressant 11 d. Hypnotic ◈ 11 e. Diuretic 14

SECTION P. SPECIAL TREATMENTS AND PROCEDURES

1	SPECIAL TREATMENTS, PROCEDURES, AND PROGRAMS	*SPECIAL CARE – (Check treatments or programs received in LAST 14 DAYS.)* **TREATMENTS** a. Chemotherapy b. Dialysis c. IV medication d. Intake / output e. Monitoring acute medical condition f. Ostomy care g. Oxygen therapy h. Radiation i. Suctioning j. Trach. care k. Transfusion l. Ventilator or respirator **PROGRAMS** m. Alcohol or drug treatment program n. Alzheimer's or dementia special care unit o. Hospice care p. Pediatric care q. Respite care r. Training in skills required to return to the community (*e.g.*, taking medications, housework, shopping, transportation, ADLs) s. *NONE OF ABOVE*
		THERAPIES – *Record the number of days and total minutes each of the following therapies was administered (for at least 15 minutes a day) in the last 7 days. (Enter 0 if none or less than 15 minutes daily.) Note: Count only post-admission therapies.* Box **A = # of days** administered for 15 minutes or more Box **B = total # of minutes** provided in last 7 days (A, B) a. Speech – language pathology, audiology service ◈ b. Occupational therapy c. Physical therapy d. Respiratory therapy e. Psychological therapy (by any licensed mental health professional) ◈
2	INTERVENTION PROGRAMS FOR MODD, BEHAVIOR, COGNITIVE LOSS	*(Check all interventions or strategies used in the last 7 days, no matter where received.)* a. Special behavior symptom evaluation program b. Evaluation by a licensed mental health specialist in LAST 90 DAYS c. Group therapy d. Resident-specific deliberate changes in the environment to address mood or behavior patterns (*e.g.*, providing bureau in which to rummage) e. Reorientation (*e.g.*, cueing) f. *NONE OF ABOVE*
3	NURSING REHABILITATION / RESTORATIVE CARE ◈	Record the NUMBER OF DAYS each of the following rehabilitation or restorative techniques or practices was provided to the resident for more than or equal to 15 minutes per day in the last 7 days. (*Enter 0 if none or less than 15 minutes daily.*) a. Range of motion (passive) b. Range of motion (active) c. Splint or brace assistance **Training and skill practice in:** d. Bed mobility e. Transfer f. Walking g. Dressing or grooming h. Eating or swallowing i. Amputation or prosthesis care j. Communication k. Other

Section P. Special Treatments and Procedures (continued)

4	DEVICES AND RESTRAINTS	(*Use the following codes for the last 7 days:*) 0. Not used 1. Used less than daily 2. Used daily ◈ **Bed Rails** 0. No 1. Yes 11 a. Full bed rails on all open sides of bed b. Other types of side rails used (*e.g.*, half rail, 1 side) c. Trunk restraint 16 18 d. Limb restraint 18 18 e. Chair prevents rising
5	HOSPITAL STAY(s)	Record number of times resident was admitted to hospital with an overnight stay in the LAST 90 DAYS (or since last assessment if less than 90 days). (*Enter 0 if no admission.*)
6	EMERGENCY ROOM (ER) VISIT(s)	Record number of times resident visited ER without an overnight stay in the LAST 90 DAYS (or since last assessment if less than 90 days). (*Enter 0 if no ER visits.*)
7	PHYSICIAN VISITS	In the LAST 14 DAYS (or since admission, if less than 14 days in facility), on how many days has the physician (or authorized assistant or practitioner) examined the resident? (*Enter 0 if none.*)
8	PHYSICIAN ORDERS	In the LAST 14 DAYS (or since admission, if less than 14 days in facility), on how many days has the physician (or authorized assistant or practitioner) changed the resident's orders? *Do not include order renewals without change.* (*Enter 0 if none.*)
9	ABNORMAL LAB VALUES	Has the resident had any abnormal lab values during the LAST 90 DAYS (or since admission)? 0. No 1. Yes

SECTION Q. DISCHARGE POTENTIAL AND OVERALL STATUS

1	DISCHARGE POTENTIAL	a. Resident expresses or indicates preference to return to the community. 0. No 1. Yes b. Resident has a support person who is positive towards discharge. 0. No 1. Yes c. Stay projected to be of a short duration – Discharge projected WITHIN 90 DAYS (do not include expected discharge due to death) 0. No 1. Within 30 days 2. Within 31 – 90 days 3. Discharge status uncertain
2	OVERALL CHANGE IN CARE NEEDS	Resident's overall level of self-sufficiency has changed significantly as compared to status of 90 DAYS AGO (or since last assessment if less than 90 days ago) 0. No change 1. Improved – receives fewer supports, needs less restrictive level of care 2. Deteriorated – receives more support

SECTION R. ASSESSMENT INFORMATION

1	PARTICIPATION IN ASSESSMENT	a. Resident: 0. No 1. Yes b. Family: 0. No 1. Yes 2. No family c. Significant Other: 0. No 1. Yes 2. None

2 SIGNATURES OF THOSE COMPLETING THE ASSESSMENT:

a. Signature of RN Assessment Coordinator (sign on above line)

b. Date RN Assessment Coordinator signed as complete — Month - Day - Year

Other Signatures — Title — Sections — Date

c.

d.

e.

f.

g.

h.

	SECTION S. NEW YORK SPECIFIC ITEMS	
1	UNIT NUMBER	(*Enter current number. Follow instructions in manual.*)
2	PRESSURE ULCERS	Stage 3 or 4 pressure ulcer sites present upon admission or readmission. (*Code the appropriate response.*) 1. All currently reported sites were present on admission or readmission. 2. Some of the currently reported sites were present on admission or readmission. 3. None of the currently reported sites were present on admission or readmission. 4. No stage 3 or 4 sites currently reported.
3	SUBSTANCE ABUSE	SUBSTANCE ABUSE HISTORY. Has the resident with HIV engaged in substance abuse behaviors more than one month ago, which continue to influence care currently given to the resident? *Code the appropriate response.* 0. No 1. Yes 2. Resident does not have HIV.
4	DISEASE DIAGNOSES	(*Record ONLY those disease diagnoses that have a relationship to current ADL status, cognitive status, mood and behavior status, medical treatments, nursing monitoring, or risk of death during the last 30 days. Do not list inactive diagnoses. Check all that apply.*) a. HIV dementia (a) b. HIV wasting syndrome (b) c. Non-psychotic disorder following organic brain damage (c) d. Psychotic disorder following organic brain damage (d) e. Spinal cord injury (e) f. Hemiplegia (f) g. Hemiparesis (g) h. Huntington's Disease (h) i. Dementia Registry Reporting (i) 1. County (FIPS) code of prior residence ____ 2. Physician license number ____ j. *NONE OF ABOVE* (j)
5	MEDICARE and MEDICAID	a. PARTICIPATION IN MEDICARE PROSPECTIVE PAYMENT SYSTEM (PPS). Is this assessment for a Medicare Prospective Payment System (PPS) covered resident? (*Code the appropriate response.*) 0. No. (*Complete item S5b, then skip to Section V if required.*) 1. Yes. This assessment is for a Medicare PPS covered resident. (*Complete Sections T and V if required.*) b. CASE MIX GROUP – State. (*Enter the current Medicaid Resource Utilization Group (RUG) score.*)

	SECTION S. CONNECTICUT SPECIFIC ITEMS	
1	LEVEL OF CARE	1. Chronic and Convalescent Nursing Home (CCNH) 2. Rest Home with Nursing Supervision (RHNS)
2	ADMITTED FROM (at entry)	(*Skip unless AB2 = 4 or A4b = 4 Nursing Home.*) 1. Chronic and Convalescent Nursing Home (CCNH) 2. Rest Home with Nursing Supervision (RHNS)
3	CURRENT PAYMENT SOURCES FOR NURSING HOME STAY	a. TYPE OF MEDICAID (If A7a Medicaid per diem is checked) 1. Medicaid managed care per diem 2. Medicaid per diem (not managed care) b. MEDICAID SOURCE (If A7a Medicaid per diem is checked) 1. Connecticut Medicaid 2. Out-of-state Medicaid c. TYPE OF MEDICARE (If A7b Medicare per diem is checked) 1. Medicare managed care per diem 2. Medicare per diem (not managed care) d. TYPE OF INSURANCE (If A7i Private insurance per diem is checked). Does the resident have a private long term care insurance policy? 1. No 2. Yes d. TYPE OF LONG TERM CARE INSURACE (If Yes, is it a Connecticut Partnership for Long-Term Care approved policy? 1. No 2. Yes

	SECTION T. THERAPY SUPPLEMENT FOR MEDICARE PPS	
1	SPECIAL TREATMENTS AND PROCEDURES	**a. RECREATION THERAPY** – *Enter number of days and total minutes of recreation therapy administered (for at least 15 minutes a day) in the last 7 days. (Enter "0" if none.)* **A = # of days** administered for 15 minutes or more (A) **B = total # of minutes** provided in last 7 days (B) Skip unless this is a Medicare 5-day or Medicare readmission / return assessment. b. ORDERED THERAPIES – Has physician ordered any of following therapies to begin in FIRST 14 days of stay: physical therapy, occupational therapy, or speech pathology service? 0. No 1. Yes If not ordered, skip to item 2 c. Through day 15, provide an estimate of the number of days when at least one therapy service can be expected to have been delivered. d. Through day 15, provide an estimate of the number of therapy minutes (across the therapies) that can be expected to be delivered?
2	WALKING WHEN MOST SELF-SUFFICIENT	Complete item 2 if ADL self-performance score for TRANSFER (G1bA) is 0, 1, 2, or 3 -AND- at least one of the following is present: • Resident received physical therapy involving gait training (P1bc) • Physical therapy was ordered for the resident involving gait training (T1b) • Resident received nursing rehabilitation for walking (P3f) • Physical therapy involving walking has been discontinued within the past 180 days Skip to item 3 if resident did not walk in last 7 days. (For the following five items, base coding on the episode when the resident walked the farthest without sitting down. Include walking during rehabilitation sessions.) **a. Farthest distance** walked without sitting down during this episode. 0. 150+ feet 3. 10 - 25 feet 1. 51 - 149 feet 4. Less than 10 feet 2. 26 - 50 feet **b. Time walked** without sitting down during this episode. 0. 1 - 2 minutes 3. 11 - 15 minutes 1. 3 - 4 minutes 4. 16 - 30 minutes 2. 5 - 10 minutes 5. 31+ minutes **c. Self-Performance in walking** during this episode. 0. INDEPENDENT – No help or oversight 1. SUPERVISION – Oversight, encouragement or cueing provided 2. LIMITED ASSISTANCE – Resident highly involved in walking; received physical help in guided maneuvering of limbs or other non-weightbearing assistance 3. EXTENSIVE ASSISTANCE – Resident received weight bearing assistance while walking **d. Walking support** provided associated with this episode (code regardless of resident's self-performance classification). 0. No setup or physical help from staff 1. Setup help only 2. One person physical assist 3. Two+ persons physical assist **e. Parallel bars** used by resident in association with this episode. 0. No 1. Yes
3	CASE MIX GROUP	Medicare State

Appendix

B

Medicare Home Health Care Quality Assurance and Improvement Demonstration Outcome and Assessment Information Set (OASIS-B)

This data set should not be reviewed or used without first reading the accompanying narrative prologue that explains the purpose of the OASIS and its past and planned evolution.

OASIS Items to be Used at Specific Time Points

Start of Care (or Resumption of Care Following Inpatient Facility Stay): 1-69

Follow-Up: 1, 4, 9-11, 13, 16-26, 29-71

Discharge (not to inpatient facility): 1, 4, 9-11, 13, 16-26, 29-74, 78-79

Transfer to Inpatient Facility (with or without agency discharge): 1, 70-72, 75-79

Death at Home: 1, 79

Note: For items 51-67, please note special instructions at the beginning of the section.

CLINICAL RECORD ITEMS

a. (M0010) Agency ID: ___ ___ ___ ___ ___ ___ ___ ___

b. (M0020) Patient ID Number: ______________________

c. (M0030) Start of Care Date: __ __/__ __/__ __ __ __
month day year

d. (M0040) Patient's Last Name:
___ ___ ___ ___ ___ ___ ___ ___ ___ ___ ___ ___

e. (M0050) Patient State of Residence: ___ ___

f. (M0060) Patient Zip Code: __ __ __ __ __

g. (M0063) Medicare Number: (including suffix if any)
__ __ __ __ __ __ __ __ __ __ __ __

☐ NA - No Medicare

h. (M0066) Birth Date: __ __/__ __/__ __ __ __
month day year

i. (M0080) Discipline of Person Completing Assessment:
☐ 1 -RN ☐ 2-LPN ☐ 3-PT
☐ 4-SLP/ST ☐ 5-OT ☐ 6-MSW

j. (M0090) Date Assessment Information Recorded:
__ __/__ __/__ __ __ __
month day year

DEMOGRAPHICS AND PATIENT HISTORY

1. (M0100) This Assessment is Currently Being Completed for the Following Reason:

☐ 1 - Start of care
☐ 2 - Resumption of care (after inpatient stay)
☐ 3 - Discharge from agency - not to an inpatient facility **[Go to *M0150*]**
☐ 4 - Transferred to an inpatient facility - discharged from agency **[Go to *M0830*]**
☐ 5 - Transferred to an inpatient facility - not discharged from agency **[Go to *M0830*]**
☐ 6 - Died at home **[Go to *M0906*]**
☐ 7 - Recertification reassessment (follow-up) **[Go to *M0150*]**
☐ 8 - Other follow-up **[Go to *M0150*]**

2. (M0130) Gender:

☐ 1 - Male
☐ 2 - Female

3. (M0140) Race/Ethnicity (as identified by patient):

☐ 1 - White, non-Hispanic
☐ 2 - Black, African-American
☐ 3 - Hispanic
☐ 4 - Asian, Pacific Islander
☐ 5 - American Indian, Eskimo, Aleut
☐ 6 - Other
☐ UK - Unknown

4. (M0150) Current Payment Sources for Home Care: (Mark all that apply.)

- ☐ 0 - None; no charge for current services
- ☐ 1 - Medicare (traditional fee-for-service)
- ☐ 2 - Medicare (HMO/managed care)
- ☐ 3 - Medicaid (traditional fee-for-service)
- ☐ 4 - Medicaid (HMO/managed care)
- ☐ 5 - Workers' compensation
- ☐ 6 - Title programs (e.g., Title III, V, or XX)
- ☐ 7 - Other government (e.g., CHAMPUS, VA, etc.)
- ☐ 8 - Private insurance
- ☐ 9 - Private HMO/managed care
- ☐ 10 - Self-pay.
- ☐ 11 - Other (specify) ______________
- ☐ UK - Unknown

5. (M0160) Financial Factors limiting the ability of the patient/family to meet basic health needs: (Mark all that apply.)

- ☐ 0 - None
- ☐ 1 - Unable to afford medicine or medical supplies
- ☐ 2 - Unable to afford medical expenses that are not covered by insurance/Medicare (e.g., copayments)
- ☐ 3 - Unable to afford rent/utility bills
- ☐ 4 - Unable to afford food
- ☐ 5 - Other (specify) ______________

6. (M0170) From which of the following Inpatient Facilities was the patient discharged *during the past 14 days*? (Mark all that apply.)

- ☐ 1 - Hospital
- ☐ 2 - Rehabilitation facility
- ☐ 3 - Nursing home
- ☐ 4 - Other (specify) ______________
- ☐ NA - Patient was not discharged from an inpatient facility **[If NA, go to *M0200*]**

7. (M0180) Inpatient Discharge Date (most recent):

__ __/__ __/__ __ __ __
month day year

- ☐ UK - Unknown

8. (M0190) Inpatient Diagnosis and three digit ICD code categories *for only those conditions treated during an inpatient facility stay within the last 14 days* (no surgical or V-codes):

Inpatient Facility Diagnosis	ICD
a. ______________	(__ __ __)
b. ______________	(__ __ __)

9. (M0200) Medical or Treatment Regimen Change Within Past 14 Days: Has this patient experienced a change in medical or treatment regimen (e.g., medication, treatment, or service change due to new or additional diagnosis, etc.) within the last 14 days?

- ☐ 0 - No **[If No, go to *M0220*]**
- ☐ 1 - Yes

10. (M0210) List the patient's Medical Diagnoses and three-digit ICD code categories *for those conditions requiring changed medical or treatment regimen* (no surgical or V-codes):

Changed Medical Regimen Diagnosis	ICD
a. ______________	(__ __ __)
b. ______________	(__ __ __)
c. ______________	(__ __ __)
d. ______________	(__ __ __)

11. (M0220) Conditions Prior to Medical or Treatment Regimen Change or Inpatient Stay Within Past 14 Days: If this patient experienced an inpatient facility discharge or change in medical or treatment regimen within the past 14 days, indicate any conditions which existed *prior to* the inpatient stay or change in medical or treatment regimen. (Mark all that apply.)

- ☐ 1 - Urinary incontinence
- ☐ 2 - Indwelling/suprapubic catheter
- ☐ 3 - Intractable pain
- ☐ 4 - Impaired decision-making
- ☐ 5 - Disruptive or socially inappropriate behavior
- ☐ 6 - Memory loss to the extent that supervision required
- ☐ 7 - None of the above
- ☐ NA - No inpatient facility discharge *and* no change in medical or treatment regimen in past 14 days
- ☐ UK - Unknown

12. (M0230/M0240) Diagnoses and Severity Index: List each medical diagnosis or problem for which the patient is receiving home care and ICD code category (no surgical or V-codes) and rate them using the following severity index. (Choose one value that represents the most severe rating appropriate for each diagnosis.)

- 0 - Asymptomatic, no treatment needed at this time
- 1 - Symptoms well controlled with current therapy
- 2 - Symptoms controlled with difficulty, affecting daily functioning; patient needs ongoing monitoring
- 3 - Symptoms poorly controlled, patient needs frequent adjustment in treatment and dose monitoring
- 4 - Symptoms poorly controlled, history of rehospitalizations

	Primary Diagnosis	ICD	Severity Rating
a.	______________	(__ __ __)	☐ 0 ☐ 1 ☐ 2 ☐ 3 ☐ 4
	Other Diagnoses	**ICD**	**Severity Rating**
b.	______________	(__ __ __)	☐ 0 ☐ 1 ☐ 2 ☐ 3 ☐ 4
c.	______________	(__ __ __)	☐ 0 ☐ 1 ☐ 2 ☐ 3 ☐ 4
d.	______________	(__ __ __)	☐ 0 ☐ 1 ☐ 2 ☐ 3 ☐ 4
e.	______________	(__ __ __)	☐ 0 ☐ 1 ☐ 2 ☐ 3 ☐ 4
f.	______________	(__ __ __)	☐ 0 ☐ 1 ☐ 2 ☐ 3 ☐ 4

13. (M0250) Therapies the patient receives *at home*: (Mark all that apply.)

- ☐ 1 - Intravenous or infusion therapy (excludes TPN)
- ☐ 2 - Parenteral nutrition (TPN or lipids)
- ☐ 3 - Enteral nutrition (nasogastric, gastrostomy, jejunostomy, or any other artificial entry into the alimentary canal)
- ☐ 4 - None of the above

14. (M0260) Overall Prognosis: BEST description of patient's overall prognosis for *recovery from this episode of illness.*

- ☐ 0 - Poor: little or no recovery is expected and/or further decline is imminent
- ☐ 1 - Good/Fair: partial to full recovery is expected
- ☐ UK - Unknown

15. (M0270) Rehabilitative Prognosis: BEST description of patient's prognosis for *functional status.*

- ☐ 0 - Guarded: minimal improvement in functional status is expected; decline is possible
- ☐ 1 - Good: marked improvement in functional status is expected
- ☐ UK - Unknown

16. (M0280) Life Expectancy: (Physician documentation is not required.)

- ☐ 0 - Life expectancy is greater than 6 months
- ☐ 1 - Life expectancy is 6 months or fewer

17. (M0290) High Risk Factors characterizing this patient: (Mark all that apply.)

- ☐ 1 - Heavy smoking
- ☐ 2 - Obesity
- ☐ 3 - Alcohol dependency
- ☐ 4 - Drug dependency
- ☐ 5 - None of the above
- ☐ UK - Unknown

LIVING ARRANGEMENTS

18. (M0300) Current Residence:

- ☐ 1 - Patient's owned or rented residence (house, apartment, or mobile home owned or rented by patient/couple/significant other)
- ☐ 2 - Family member's residence
- ☐ 3 - Boarding home or rented room
- ☐ 4 - Board and care or assisted living facility
- ☐ 5 - Other (specify) ______________

19. (M0310) Structural Barriers in the patient's environment limiting independent mobility: (Mark all that apply.)

- ☐ 0 - None
- ☐ 1 - Stairs inside home which *must* be used by the patient (e.g., to get to toileting, sleeping, eating areas)
- ☐ 2 - Stairs inside home which are used optionally (e.g., to get to laundry facilities)
- ☐ 3 - Stairs leading from inside house to outside
- ☐ 4 - Narrow or obstructed doorways

20. (M0320) Safety Hazards found in the patient's current place of residence: (Mark all that apply.)

- ☐ 0 - None
- ☐ 1 - Inadequate floor, roof, or windows
- ☐ 2 - Inadequate lighting
- ☐ 3 - Unsafe gas/electric appliance
- ☐ 4 - Inadequate heating
- ☐ 5 - Inadequate cooling
- ☐ 6 - Lack of fire safety devices
- ☐ 7 - Unsafe floor coverings
- ☐ 8 - Inadequate stair railings
- ☐ 9 - improperly stored hazardous materials
- ☐ 10 - Lead-based paint
- ☐ 11 - Other (specify) ______________

21. (M0330) Sanitation Hazards found in the patient's current place of residence: (Mark all that apply.)

- ☐ 0 - None
- ☐ 1 - No running water
- ☐ 2 - Contaminated water
- ☐ 3 - No toileting facilities
- ☐ 4 - Outdoor toileting facilities only
- ☐ 5 - Inadequate sewage disposal
- ☐ 6 - Inadequate/improper food storage
- ☐ 7 - No food refrigeration
- ☐ 8 - No cooking facilities
- ☐ 9 - Insects/rodents present
- ☐ 10 - No scheduled trash pickup
- ☐ 11 - Cluttered/soiled living area
- ☐ 12 - Other (specify) ______________

22. (M0340) Patient Lives With: (Mark all that apply.)

- ☐ 1 - Lives alone
- ☐ 2 - With spouse or significant other
- ☐ 3 - With other family member
- ☐ 4 - With a friend
- ☐ 5 - With paid help (other than home care agency staff)
- ☐ 6 - With other than above

SUPPORTIVE ASSISTANCE

23. (M0350) Assisting Person(s) Other than Home Care Agency Staff: (Mark all that apply.)

- ☐ 1 - Relatives, friends, or neighbors living outside the home
- ☐ 2 - Person residing in the home (EXCLUDING paid help)
- ☐ 3 - Paid help
- ☐ 4 - None of the above **[If None of the above, go to *M0390*]**
- ☐ UK - Unknown **[If Unknown, go to *M0390*]**

24. (M0360) Primary Caregiver taking *lead* responsibility for providing or managing the patient's care, providing the most frequent assistance, etc. (other than home care agency staff):

- ☐ 0 - No one person **[If No one person, go to *M0390*]**
- ☐ 1 - Spouse or significant other
- ☐ 2 - Daughter or son
- ☐ 3 - Other family member
- ☐ 4 - Friend or neighbor or community or church member
- ☐ 5 - Paid help
- ☐ UK - Unknown **[If Unknown, go to *M0390*]**

25. (M0370) How Often does the patient receive assistance from the primary caregiver?

- ☐ 1 - Several times during day and night
- ☐ 2 - Several times during day
- ☐ 3 - Once daily
- ☐ 4 - Three or more times per week
- ☐ 5 - One to two times per week
- ☐ 6 - Less often than weekly
- ☐ UK - Unknown

26. (M0380) Type of Primary Caregiver Assistance: (Mark all that apply.)

- ☐ 1 - ADL assistance (e.g., bathing, dressing, toileting, bowel/bladder, eating/feeding)
- ☐ 2 - IADL assistance (e.g., meds, meals, housekeeping, laundry, telephone, shopping, finances)
- ☐ 3 - Environmental support (housing, home maintenance)
- ☐ 4 - Psychosocial support (socialization, companionship, recreation)
- ☐ 5 - Advocates or facilitates patient's participation in appropriate medical care
- ☐ 6 - Financial agent, power of attorney, or conservator of finance
- ☐ 7 - Health care agent, conservator of person, or medical power of attorney
- ☐ UK - Unknown

SENSORY STATUS

27. (M0390) Vision with corrective lenses if the patient usually wears them:

- ☐ 0 - Normal vision: sees adequately in most situations; can see medication labels, newsprint.
- ☐ 1 - Partially impaired; cannot see medication labels or newsprint, but *can* see obstacles in path, and the surrounding layout; can count fingers at arm's length.
- ☐ 2 - Severely impaired: cannot locate objects without hearing or touching them *or* patient nonresponsive.

28. (M0400) Hearing and Ability to Understand Spoken Language in patient's own language (with hearing aids if the patient usually uses them):

- ☐ 0 - No observable impairment. Able to hear and understand complex or detailed instructions and extended or abstract conversation.
- ☐ 1 - With minimal difficulty, able to hear and understand most multi-step instructions and ordinary conversation. May need occasional repetition, extra time, or louder voice.
- ☐ 2 - Has moderate difficulty hearing and understanding simple, one-step instructions and brief conversation; needs frequent prompting or assistance.
- ☐ 3 - Has severe difficulty hearing and understanding simple greetings and short comments. Requires multiple repetitions, restatements, demonstrations, additional time.
- ☐ 4 - *Unable* to hear and understand familiar words or common expressions consistently, *or* patient nonresponsive.

29. (M0410) Speech and Oral (Verbal) Expression of Language (in patient's own language):

- ☐ 0 - Expresses complex ideas, feelings, and needs clearly, completely, and easily in all situations with no observable impairment.
- ☐ 1 - Minimal difficulty expressing ideas and needs (may take extra time; makes occasional errors in word choice, grammar or speech intelligibility; needs minimal prompting or assistance).
- ☐ 2 - Expresses simple ideas or needs with moderate difficulty (needs prompting or assistance, errors in word choice, organization or speech intelligibility). Speaks in phrases or short sentences.
- ☐ 3 - Has severe difficulty expressing basic ideas or needs and requires maximal assistance or guessing by listener. Speech limited to single words or short phrases.
- ☐ 4 - *Unable* to express basic needs even with maximal prompting or assistance but is not comatose or unresponsive (e.g., speech is nonsensical or unintelligible).
- ☐ 5 - Patient nonresponsive or unable to speak.

30. (M0420) Frequency of Pain interfering with patient's activity or movement.

- ☐ 0 - Patient has no pain or pain does not interfere with activity or movement
- ☐ 1 - Less often than daily
- ☐ 2 - Daily, but not constantly
- ☐ 3 - All of the time

31. (M0430) Intractable Pain: Is the patient experiencing pain that is *not easily relieved*, occurs at least daily, and affects the patient's sleep, appetite, physical or emotional energy, concentration, personal relationships, emotions, or ability or desire to perform physical activity?

- ☐ 0 - No
- ☐ 1 - Yes

INTEGUMENTARY STATUS

32. (M0440) Does this patient have a Skin Lesion or an Open Wound? This excludes "OSTOMIES."

☐ 0 - No **[If No, go to *M0490*]**
☐ 1 - Yes

33. (M0445) Does this patient have a Pressure Ulcer?

☐ 0 - No **[If No, go to *M0468*]**
☐ 1 - Yes

33a. (M0450) Current Number of Pressure Ulcers at Each Stage: (Circle one response for each stage.)

Pressure Ulcer Stages	Number of Pressure Ulcers				
a) Stage 1: Nonblanchable erythema of intact skin; the heralding of skin ulceration. In darker-pigmented skin, warmth, edema, hardness, or discolored skin may be indicators.	0	1	2	3	4 or more
b) Stage 2: Partial thickness skin loss involving epidermis and/or dermis. The ulcer is superficial and presents clinically as an abrasion, blister, or shallow crater.	0	1	2	3	4 or more
c) Stage 3: Full thickness skin loss involving damage or necrosis of subcutaneous tissue which may extend down to, but not through, underlying fascia. The ulcer presents clinically as a deep crater with or without undermining of adjacent tissue.	0	1	2	3	4 or more
d) Stage 4: Full thickness skin loss with extensive destruction, tissue necrosis, or damage to muscle, bone, or supporting structures (e.g., tendon, joint capsule, etc.)	0	1	2	3	4 or more
e) In addition to the above, is there at least one pressure ulcer that cannot be observed due to the presence of eschar or a nonremovable dressing, including casts? ☐ 0 - No ☐ 1 - Yes					

33b. (M0460) Stage of Most Problematic (Observable) Pressure Ulcer:

☐ 1 - Stage 1
☐ 2 - Stage 2
☐ 3 - Stage 3
☐ 4 - Stage 4
☐ NA - No observable pressure ulcer

33c. (M0464) Status of Most Problematic (Observable) Pressure Ulcer:

☐ 1 - Fully granulating
☐ 2 - Early/partial granulation
☐ 3 - Not healing
☐ NA - No observable pressure ulcer

34. (M0468) Does this patient have a Stasis Ulcer?

☐ 0 - No **[If No, go to *M0482*]**
☐ 1 - Yes

34a. (M0470) Current Number of Observable Stasis Ulcer(s):

☐ 0 - Zero
☐ 1 - One
☐ 2 - Two
☐ 3 - Three
☐ 4 - Four or more

34b. (M0474) Does this patient have at least one Stasis Ulcer that Cannot be Observed due to the presence of a nonremovable dressing?

☐ 0 - No
☐ 1 - Yes

34c. (M0476) Status of Most Problematic (Observable) Stasis Ulcer:

☐ 1 - Fully granulating
☐ 2 - Early/partial granulation
☐ 3 - Not healing
☐ NA - No observable stasis ulcer

34. (M0482) Does this patient have a Surgical Wound?

☐ 0 - No **[If No, go to *M0490*]**
☐ 1 - Yes

35a. (M0484) Current Number of (Observable) Surgical Wounds: (If a wound is partially closed but has *more* than one opening, consider each opening as a separate wound.)

☐ 0 - Zero
☐ 1 - One
☐ 2 - Two
☐ 3 - Three
☐ 4 - Four or more

35b. (M0486) Does this patient have at least one Surgical Wound that Cannot be Observed due to the presence of a nonremovable dressing?

☐ 0 - No
☐ 1 - Yes

35c. (M0488) Status of Most Problematic (Observable) Surgical Wound:

☐ 1 - Fully granulating
☐ 2 - Early/partial granulation
☐ 3 - Not healing
☐ NA - No observable surgical wound

RESPIRATORY STATUS

36. (M0490) When is the patient dyspneic or noticeably Short of Breath?

- ☐ 0 - Never, patient is not short of breath
- ☐ 1 - When walking more than 20 feet, climbing stairs
- ☐ 2 - With moderate exertion (e.g., while dressing, using commode or bedpan, walking distances less than 20 feet)
- ☐ 3 - With minimal exertion (e.g., while eating, talking, or performing other ADLs) or with agitation
- ☐ 4 - At rest (during day or night)

37. (M0500) Respiratory Treatments utilized at home: (Mark all that apply.)

- ☐ 1 - Oxygen (intermittent or continous)
- ☐ 2 - Ventilator (continually or at night)
- ☐ 3 - Continous positive airway pressure
- ☐ 4 - None of the above

ELIMINATION STATUS

38. (M0510) Has this patient been treated for Urinary Tract Infection in the past 14 days?

- ☐ 0 - No
- ☐ 1 - Yes
- ☐ NA - Patient on prophylactic treatment
- ☐ UK - Unknown

39. (M0520) Urinary Incontinence or Urinary Catheter Presence:

- ☐ 0 - No incontinence or catheter (includes anuria or ostomy for urinary drainage) **[If No, go to *M0540*]**
- ☐ 1 - Patient is incontinent
- ☐ 2 - Patient requires a urinary catheter (i.e., external, indwelling, intermittent, suprapubic) **[Go to *M0540*]**

40. (M0530) When does Urinary Incontinence occur?

- ☐ 0 - Timed-voiding defers incontinence
- ☐ 1 - During the night only
- ☐ 2 - During the day and night

41. (M0540) Bowel Incontinence Frequency:

- ☐ 0 - Very rarely or never has bowel incontinence
- ☐ 1 - Less than once weekly
- ☐ 2 - One to three times weekly
- ☐ 3 - Four to six times weekly
- ☐ 4 - On a daily basis
- ☐ 5 - More often than once daily
- ☐ NA - Patient has ostomy for bowel elimination
- ☐ UK - Unknown

42. (M0550) Ostomy for Bowel Elimination: Does this patient have an ostomy for bowel elimination that (within the last 14 days): a) was related to an inpatient facility stay, *or* b) necessitated a change in medical or treatment regimen?

- ☐ 0 - Patient does *not* have an ostomy for bowel elimination.
- ☐ 1 - Patient's ostomy was *not* related to an inpatient stay and did *not* necessitate change in medical or treatment regimen.
- ☐ 2 - The ostomy *was* related to an inpatient stay or *did* necessitate change in medical or treatment regimen.

NEURO/EMOTIONAL/BEHAVIORAL STATUS

43. (M0560) Cognitive Functioning: (Patient's current level of alertness, orientation, comprehension, concentration, and immediate memory for simple commands.)

- ☐ 0 - Alert/oriented, able to focus and shift attention, comprehends and recalls task directions independently.
- ☐ 1 - Requires prompting (cuing, repetition, reminders) only under stressful or unfamiliar conditions.
- ☐ 2 - Requires assistance and some direction in specific situations (e.g., on all tasks involving shifting of attention), or consistently requires low stimulus environment due to distractibility.
- ☐ 3 - Requires considerable assistance in routine situations. Is not alert and oriented or is unable to shift attention and recall directions more than half the time.
- ☐ 4 - Totally dependent due to disturbances such as constant disorientation, coma, persistant vegetative state, or delirium.

44. (M0570) When Confused (Reported or Observed):

- ☐ 0 - Never
- ☐ 1 - In new or complex situations only
- ☐ 2 - On awakening or at night only
- ☐ 3 - During the day and evening, but not constantly
- ☐ 4 - Constantly
- ☐ NA - Patient nonresponsive

45. (M0580) When Anxious (Reported or Observed):

- ☐ 0 - None of the time
- ☐ 1 - Less often than daily
- ☐ 2 - Daily, but not constantly
- ☐ 3 - All of the time
- ☐ NA - Patient nonresponsive

46. (M0590) Depressive Feelings Reported or Observed in Patient: (Mark all that apply.)

- ☐ 1 - Depressed mood (e.g., feeling sad, tearful)
- ☐ 2 - Sense of failure or self reproach
- ☐ 3 - Hopelessness
- ☐ 4 - Recurrent thoughts of death
- ☐ 5 - Thoughts of suicide
- ☐ 6 - None of the above feelings observed or reported

47. (M0600) Patient Behaviors (Reported or Observed): (Mark all that apply.)

- ☐ 1 - Indecisiveness, lack of concentration
- ☐ 2 - Diminished interest in most activities
- ☐ 3 - Sleep disturbances
- ☐ 4 - Recent change in appetite or weight
- ☐ 5 - Agitation
- ☐ 6 - A suicide attempt
- ☐ 7 - None of the above behaviors observed or reported

48. (M0610) Behaviors Demonstrated *at Least Once a Week* (Reported or Observed): (Mark all that apply.)

- ☐ 1 - Memory deficit: failure to recognize familiar persons/places, inability to recall events of past 24 hours, significant memory loss so that supervision is required
- ☐ 2 - Impaired decision-making: failure to perform usual ADLs or IADLs, inability to appropriately stop activities, jeopardizes safety through actions
- ☐ 3 - Verbal disruption: yelling, threatening, excessive profanity, sexual references, etc.
- ☐ 4 - Physical aggression; aggressive or combative to self and others (e.g., hits self, throws objects, punches, dangerous maneuvers with wheelchair or other objects)
- ☐ 5 - Disruptive, infantile, or socially inappropriate behavior (excludes verbal actions)
- ☐ 6 - Delusional, hallucinatory, or paranoid behavior
- ☐ 7 - None of the above behaviors demonstrated

49. (M0620) Frequency of Behavior Problems (Reported or Observed) (e.g., wandering episodes, self abuse, verbal disruption, physical aggression, etc.):

- ☐ 0 - Never
- ☐ 1 - Less than once a month
- ☐ 2 - Once a month
- ☐ 3 - Several times each month
- ☐ 4 - Several times a week
- ☐ 5 - At least daily

50. (M0630) Is the patient receiving Psychiatric Nursing Services at home provided by qualified psychiatric nurse?

- ☐ 0 - No
- ☐ 1 - Yes

ADL/IADLs

For Questions 51-67, complete the "current" column for all patients. For these same items, complete the "prior" column at start of care or resumption of care; mark the level that corresponds to the patient's condition 14 days prior to start of care. In all cases, record what the patient is *able to do*.

51. (M0640) Grooming: Ability to tend to personal hygiene needs (i.e., washing face and hands, hair care, shaving or make up, teeth or denture care, fingernails care).

Prior	Current	
☐	☐	0 - Able to groom self unaided, with or without the use of assistive devices or adapted methods.
☐	☐	1 - Grooming utensils must be placed within reach before able to complete grooming activities.
☐	☐	2 - Someone must assist the patient to groom self.
☐	☐	3 - Patient depends entirely upon someone else for grooming needs.
☐		UK - Unknown

52. (M0650) Ability to Dress *Upper* Body (with or without dressing aids) including undergarments, pullovers, front-opening shirts and blouses, managing zippers, buttons, and snaps:

Prior	Current	
☐	☐	0 - Able to get clothes out of closets and drawers, put them on and remove them from the upper body without assistance.
☐	☐	1 - Able to dress upper body without assistance if clothing is laid out or handed to patient.
☐	☐	2 - Someone must help the patient put on upper body clothing.
☐	☐	3 - Patient depends entirely upon another person to dress the upper body.
☐		UK - Unknown

53. (M0660) Ability to Dress *Lower* Body (with or without dressing aids) including undergarments, slacks, socks or nylons, shoes:

Prior	Current	
☐	☐	0 - Able to obtain, put on, and remove clothing and shoes without assistance.
☐	☐	1 - Able to dress lower body without assistance if clothing and shoes are laid out or handed to patient.
☐	☐	2 - Someone must help the patient put on undergarments, slacks, socks or nylons, and shoes.
☐	☐	3 - Patient depends entirely upon another person to dress lower body.
☐		UK - Unknown

54. (M0670) Bathing: Ability to wash entire body. *Excludes* grooming (washing face and hands only).

Prior	Current	
☐	☐	0 - Able to bathe self in *shower or tub* independently.
☐	☐	1 - With the use of devices, is able to bathe self in shower or tub independently.
☐	☐	2 - Able to bathe in shower or tub with the assistance of another person: (a) for intermittent supervision or encouragement or reminders, *OR* (b) to get in and out of the shower or tub, *OR* (c) for washing difficult to reach areas.
☐	☐	3 - Participates in bathing self in shower or tub, *but* requires presence of another person throughout the bath for assistance or supervision.
☐	☐	4 - *Unable* to use shower or tub and is bathed in *bed or bedside chair.*
☐	☐	5 - Unable to effectively participate in bathing and is totally bathed by another person.
☐		UK - Unknown

55. (M0680) Toileting: Ability to get to and from the toilet or bedside commode.

Prior	Current	
☐	☐	0 - Able to get to and from the toilet independently with or without a device.
☐	☐	1 - When reminded, assisted, or supervised by another person, able to get to and from toilet.
☐	☐	2 - *Unable* to get to and from the toilet but is able to use a bedside commode (with or without assistance)
☐	☐	3 - *Unable* to get to and from the toilet or bedside commode but is able to use bedpan/urinal independently.
☐	☐	4 - Is totally dependent in toileting.
☐		UK - Unknown

56. (M0690) Transferring: Ability to move from bed to chair, on and off toilet or commode, into and out of tub or shower, and ability to turn and position self in bed if patient is bedfast.

Prior *Current*

- ☐ ☐ 0 - Able to independently transfer.
- ☐ ☐ 1 - Transfers with minimal human assistance or with use of an assistive device.
- ☐ ☐ 2 - *Unable* to transfer self but is able to bear weight and pivot during the transfer process.
- ☐ ☐ 3 - Unable to transfer self and is *unable* to bear weight or pivot when transferred by another person.
- ☐ ☐ 4 - Bedfast, unable to transfer but is able to turn and position self in bed.
- ☐ ☐ 5 - Bedfast, unable to transfer and is *unable* to turn and position self.
- ☐ UK - Unknown

57. (M0700) Ambulation/Locomotion: Ability to *SAFELY* walk, once in a standing position, or use a wheelchair, once in a seated position, on a variety of surfaces.

Prior *Current*

- ☐ ☐ 0 - Able to independently walk on even and uneven surfaces and climb stairs with or without railings (i.e., needs no human assistance or assistive device).
- ☐ ☐ 1 - Requires use of device (e.g., cane, walker) to walk alone or requires human supervision or assistance to negotiate stairs or steps or uneven surfaces.
- ☐ ☐ 2 - Able to walk only with the supervision or assistance of another person at all times.
- ☐ ☐ 3 - Chairfast, *unable* to ambulate but is able to wheel self independently.
- ☐ ☐ 4 - Chairfast, unable to ambulate and is *unable* to wheel self.
- ☐ ☐ 5 - Bedfast, unable to ambulate or be up in a chair.
- ☐ UK - Unknown

58. (M0710) Feeding or Eating: Ability to feed self meals and snacks. Note: This refers only to process of *eating, chewing,* and *swallowing, not preparing* the food to be eaten.

Prior *Current*

- ☐ ☐ 0 - Able to independently feed self.
- ☐ ☐ 1 - Able to feed self independently but requires:
  - (a) meal set-up; *OR*
  - (b) intermittent assistance or supervision from another person; *OR*
  - (c) a liquid, pureed or ground meat diet.
- ☐ ☐ 2 - *Unable* to feed self and must be assisted or supervised throughout the meal/snack.
- ☐ ☐ 3 - Able to take in nutrients orally *and* receives supplemental nutrients through a nasogastric tube or gastrostomy.
- ☐ ☐ 4 - *Unable* to take in nutrients orally and is fed nutrients through a nasogastric tube or gastrostomy.
- ☐ ☐ 5 - Unable to take in nutrients orally or by tube feeding.
- ☐ UK - Unknown

59. (M0720) Planning and Preparing Light Meals (e.g., cereal, sandwich) or reheat delivered meals:

Prior *Current*

- ☐ ☐ 0 - (a) Able to independently plan and prepare all light meals for self or reheat delivered meals; *OR*
  (b) Is physically, cognitively, and mentally able to prepare light meals on a regular basis but has not routinely performed light meal preparation in the past (i.e., prior to this home care admission).
- ☐ ☐ 1 - *Unable* to prepare light meals on a regular basis due to physical, cognitive, or mental limitations.
- ☐ ☐ 2 - Unable to prepare any light meals or reheat any delivered meals.
- ☐ UK - Unknown

60. (M0730) Transportation: Physical and mental ability to *safely* use a car, taxi, or public transportation (bus, train, subway).

Prior *Current*

- ☐ ☐ 0 - Able to independently drive a regular or adapted car; *OR* uses a regular or handicap-accessible public bus.
- ☐ ☐ 1 - Able to ride in a car only when driven by another person; *OR* able to use a bus or handicap van only when assisted or accompanied by another person.
- ☐ ☐ 2 - *Unable* to ride in a car, taxi, bus, or van, and requires transportation by ambulance.
- ☐ UK - Unknown

61. (M0740) Laundry: Ability to do own laundry – to carry laundry to and from washing machine, to use washer and dryer, to wash small items by hand.

Prior *Current*

- ☐ ☐ 0 - (a) Able to independently take care of all laundry tasks; *OR*
  (b) Physically, cognitively, and mentally able to do laundry and access facilities, *but* has not routinely performed laundry tasks in the past (i.e., prior to this home care admission)
- ☐ ☐ 1 - Able to do only light laundry, such as minor hand wash or light washer loads. Due to physical, cognitive, or mental limitations, needs assistance with heavy laundry such as carrying large loads of laundry.
- ☐ ☐ 2 - *Unable* to do any laundry due to physical limitation or needs continual supervision and assistance due to cognitive or mental limitation.
- ☐ UK - Unknown

62. (M0750) **Housekeeping: Ability to safely and effectively perform light housekeeping and heavier cleaning tasks.**

Prior Current

☐ ☐ 0 - (a) Able to independently perform all housekeeping tasks; *OR*
(b) Physically, cognitively, and mentally able to perform *all* houskeeping tasks but has not routinely participated in housekeeping tasks in the past (i.e., prior to this home care admission).
☐ ☐ 1 - Able to perform only *light* housekeeping (e.g., dusting, wiping kitchen counters) tasks independently.
☐ ☐ 2 - Able to perform housekeeping tasks with intermittent assistance or supervision from another person.
☐ ☐ 3 - *Unable* to consistently perform any housekeeping tasks unless assisted by another person throughout the process.
☐ ☐ 4 - Unable to effectively participate in any housekeeping tasks.
☐ UK - Unknown

63. (M0760) **Shopping: Ability to plan for, select, and purchase items in a store and to carry them home or arrange delivery.**

Prior Current

☐ ☐ 0 - (a) Able to plan for shopping needs and independently perform shopping tasks, including carrying packages; *OR*
(b) Physically, cognitively, and mentally able to take care of shopping, but has not done shopping in the past (i.e., prior to this home care admission).
☐ ☐ 1 - Able to go shopping, but needs some assistance:
(a) By self is able to do only light shopping and carry small packages, but needs someone to do occasional major shopping; *OR*
(b) *Unable* to go shopping alone, but can go with someone to assist.
☐ ☐ 2 - *Unable* to go shopping, but is able to identify items needed, place orders, and arrange home delivery.
☐ ☐ 3 - Needs someone to do all shopping and errands.
☐ UK - Unknown

64. (M0770) **Ability to Use Telephone: Ability to answer the phone, dial numbers, and *effectively* use the telephone to communicate.**

Prior Current

☐ ☐ 0 - Able to dial numbers and answer calls appropriately and as desired.
☐ ☐ 1 - Able to use a specially adapted telephone (i.e., large numbers on the dial, teletype phone for the deaf) and call essential numbers.
☐ ☐ 2 - Able to answer the telephone and carry on a normal conversation but has difficulty with placing calls.
☐ ☐ 3 - Able to answer the telephone only some of the time or is able to carry on only a limited conversation.
☐ ☐ 4 - *Unable* to answer the telephone at all but can listen if assisted with equipment.
☐ ☐ 5 - Totally unable to use the telephone.
☐ ☐ NA - Patient does not have a telephone.
☐ UK - Unknown

MEDICATIONS

65. (M0780) **Management of Oral Medications: *Patient's ability* to prepare and take *all* prescribed oral medications reliably and safely, including administration of the correct dosage at the appropriate times/intervals. *Excludes* injectable and IV medications. (NOTE: This refers to ability, not compliance or willingness.)**

Prior Current

☐ ☐ 0 - Able to independently take the correct oral medication(s) and proper dosage(s) at the correct times.
☐ ☐ 1 - Able to take medication(s) at the correct times if:
(a) individual dosages are prepared in advance by another person; *OR*
(b) given daily reminders; *OR*
(c) someone develops a drug diary or chart.
☐ ☐ 2 - *Unable* to take medication unless administered by someone else.
☐ ☐ NA - No oral medications prescribed.
☐ UK - Unknown

66. (M0790) **Management of Inhalant/Mist Medications: *Patient's ability* to prepare and take *all* prescribed inhalant/mist medications (nebulizers, metered dose devices) reliably and safely, including administration of the correct dosage at the appropriate times/intervals. *Excludes* all other forms of medication (oral tablets, injectable and IV medications).**

Prior Current

☐ ☐ 0 - Able to independently take the correct medication and proper dosage at the correct times.
☐ ☐ 1 - Able to take medication at the correct times if:
(a) individual dosages are prepared in advance by another person, *OR*
(b) given daily reminders.
☐ ☐ 2 - *Unable* to take medication unless administered by someone else.
☐ ☐ NA - No inhalant/mist medications prescribed.
☐ UK - Unknown

67. (M0800) **Management of Injectable Medications: *Patient's ability* to prepare and take *all* prescribed injectable medications reliably and safely, including administration of correct dosage at the appropriate times/intervals. *Excludes* IV medications.**

Prior Current

☐ ☐ 0 - Able to independently take the correct medication and proper dosage at the correct times.
☐ ☐ 1 - Able to take medication at the correct times if:
(a) individual syringes are prepared in advance by another person, *OR*
(b) given daily reminders.
☐ ☐ 2 - *Unable* to take injectable medications unless administered by someone else.
☐ ☐ NA - No injectable medications prescribed.
☐ UK - Unknown

EQUIPMENT MANAGEMENT

68. (M0810) Patient Management of Equipment (includes *ONLY* oxygen, IV/infusion therapy, enteral/parenteral nutrition equipment or supplies): *Patient's ability* to set up, monitor and change equipment reliably and safely, add appropriate fluids or medication, clean/store/dispose of equipment or supplies using proper technique. (NOTE: This refers to ability, not compliance or willingness.)

- ☐ 0 - Patient manages all tasks related to equipment completely independently.
- ☐ 1 - If someone else sets up equipment (i.e., fills portable oxygen tank, provides patient with prepared solutions), patient is able to manage all other aspects of equipment.
- ☐ 2 - Patient requires considerable assistance from another person to manage equipment, but independently completes portions of the task.
- ☐ 3 - Patient is only able to monitor equipment (e.g., liter flow, fluid in bag) and must call someone else to manage the equipment.
- ☐ 4 - Patient is completely dependent on someone else to manage all equipment.
- ☐ NA - No equipment of this type used in care **[If NA, go to *M0803*]**

69. (M0820) Caregiver Management of Equipment (includes *ONLY* oxygen, IV/infusion therapy, enteral/parenteral nutrition, ventilator therapy equipment or supplies): *Caregiver's ability* to set up, monitor and change equipment reliably and safely, add appropriate fluids or medication, clean/store/dispose of equipment or supplies using proper technique. (NOTE: This refers to ability, not compliance or willingness.)

- ☐ 0 - Caregiver manages all tasks related to equipment completely independently.
- ☐ 1 - If someone else sets up equipment, caregiver is able to manage all other aspects.
- ☐ 2 - Caregiver requires considerable assistance from another person to manage equipment, but independently completes significant portions of task.
- ☐ 3 - Caregiver is only able to complete small portions of task (e.g., administer nebulizer treatment, clean/store/dispose of equipment or supplies).
- ☐ 4 - Caregiver is completely dependent on someone else to manage all equipment.
- ☐ NA - No caregiver
- ☐ UK - Unknown

EMERGENT CARE

70. (M0830) Emergent Care: Since the last time OASIS data were collected, has the patient utilized any of the following services for emergent care (other than home care agency services)? (Mark all that apply.)

- ☐ 0 - No emergent care services **[If No emergent care and patient discharged, go to *M0855*]**
- ☐ 1 - Hospital emergency room (includes 23-hour holding)
- ☐ 2 - Doctor's office emergency visit/house call
- ☐ 3 - Outpatient department/clinic emergency (includes urgicenter sites)
- ☐ UK - Unknown

71. (M0840) Emergent Care Reason: For what reason(s) did the patient/family seek emergent care? (Mark all that apply.)

- ☐ 1 - Improper medication administration, medication side effects, toxicity, anaphylaxis
- ☐ 2 - Nausea, dehydration, malnutrition, constipation, impaction
- ☐ 3 - Injury caused by fall or accident at home
- ☐ 4 - Respiratory problems (e.g., shortness of breath, respiratory infection, tracheobronchial obstruction)
- ☐ 5 - Wound infection, deteriorating wound status, new lesion/ulcer
- ☐ 6 - Cardiac problems (e.g., fluid overload, exacerbation of CHF, chest pain)
- ☐ 7 - Hypo/Hyperglycemia, diabetes out of control
- ☐ 8 - GI bleeding, obstruction
- ☐ 9 - Other than above reasons
- ☐ UK - Reason unknown

DATA ITEMS COLLECTED AT INPATIENT FACILITY ADMISSION OR AGENCY DISCHARGE ONLY

72. (M0855) To which Inpatient Facility has the patient been admitted?

- ☐ 1 - Hospital **[Go to *M0890*]**
- ☐ 2 - Rehabilitation facility **[Go to *M0903*]**
- ☐ 3 - Nursing home **[Go to *M0900*]**
- ☐ 4 - Hospice **[Go to *M0903*]**
- ☐ NA - No patient facility admission

73. (M0870) Discharge Disposition: Where is the patient after discharge from your agency? (Choose only one answer.)

- ☐ 1 - Patient remained in the community (not in hospital, nursing home, or rehab facility)
- ☐ 2 - Patient transferred to a noninstitutional hospice **[Go to *M0903*]**
- ☐ 3 - Unknown because patient moved to a geographic location not served by this agency **[Go to *M0903*]**
- ☐ UK - Other unknown **[Go to *M0903*]**

74. (M0880) After discharge, does the patient receive health, personal, or support Services or Assistance? (Mark all that apply.)

- ☐ 1 - No assistance or services received
- ☐ 2 - Yes, assistance or services provided by family or friends
- ☐ 3 - Yes, assistance or services provided by other community resources (e.g., meals-on-wheels, home health services, homemaker assistance, transportation assistance, assisted living, board and care)

Go to *M0903*

75. (M0890) If the patient was admitted to an acute care Hospital, for what Reason was he/she admitted?

- ☐ 1 - Hospitalization for *emergent* (unscheduled) care
- ☐ 2 - Hospitalization for *urgent* (scheduled within 24 hours of admission) care
- ☐ 3 - Hospitalization for *elective* (scheduled more than 24 hours before admission) care
- ☐ UK - Unknown

76. (M0895) Reason for Hospitalization: (Mark all that apply.)

- ☐ 1 - Improper medication administration, medication side effects, toxicity, anaphylaxis
- ☐ 2 - Injury caused by fall or accident at home
- ☐ 3 - Respiratory problems (SOB, infection, obstruction)
- ☐ 4 - Wound or tube site infection, deteriorating wound status, new lesion/ulcer
- ☐ 5 - Hypo/Hyperglycemia, diabetes out of control
- ☐ 6 - GI bleeding, obstruction
- ☐ 7 - Exacerbation of CHF, fluid overload, heart failure
- ☐ 8 - Myocardial infarction, stroke
- ☐ 9 - Chemotherapy
- ☐ 10 - Scheduled surgical procedure
- ☐ 11 - Urinary tract infection
- ☐ 12 - IV catheter-related infection
- ☐ 13 - Deep vein thrombosis, pulmonary embolus
- ☐ 14 - Uncontrolled pain
- ☐ 15 - Psychotic episode
- ☐ 16 - Other than above reasons

Go to *M0903*

77. (M0900) For what Reason(s) was the patient Admitted to a Nursing Home? (Mark all that apply)

- ☐ 1 - Therapy services
- ☐ 2 - Respite care
- ☐ 3 - Hospice care
- ☐ 4 - Permanent placement
- ☐ 5 - Unsafe for care at home
- ☐ 6 - Other
- ☐ UK - Unknown

78. (M0903) Date of Last (Most Recent) Home Visit:

__ __/__ __/__ __ __ __
month day year

79. (M0906) Discharge/Transfer/Death Date: Enter the date of the discharge, transfer, or death (at home) of the patient.

__ __/__ __/__ __ __ __
month day year

☐ UK - Unknown

Appendix

C

Advanced Practice Nurse Legislation

TABLE A-2 Summary of Advanced Practice Nurse (APN) Legislation: Prescriptive Authority*

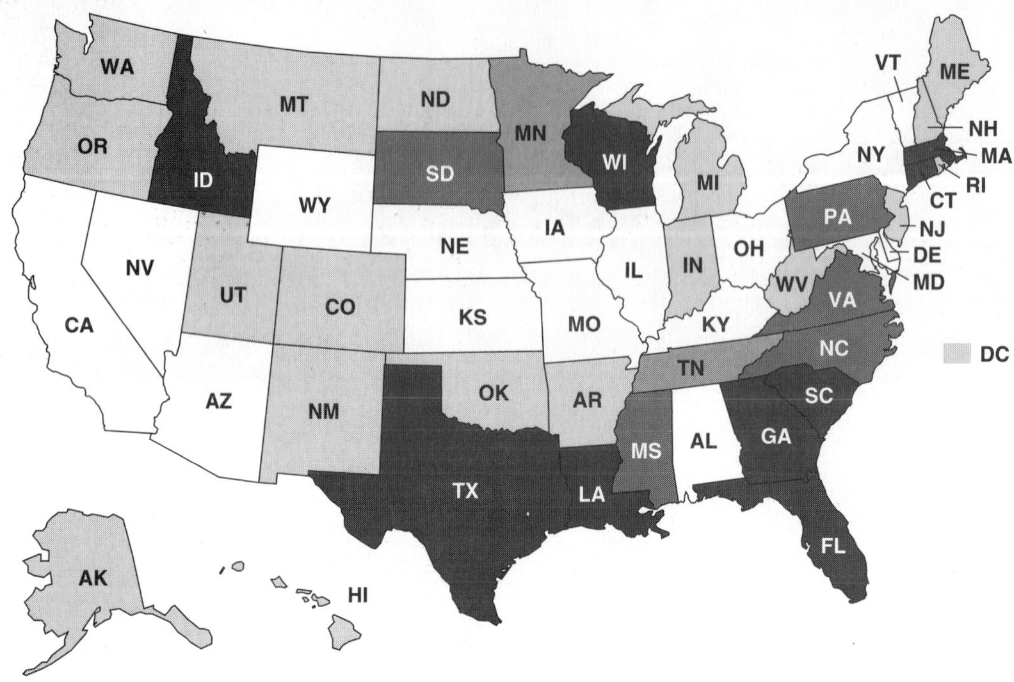

- States with nurse practitioner† title protection and the board of nursing has sole authority in scope of practice with no statutory or regulatory requirements for physician collaboration, direction, or supervision: **AK, AR, CO, DC, HI, IN, ME, MI, MT, ND, NH, NJ, NM, OK, OR, RI, UT, WA, WV**
- States with nurse practitioner† title protection and the board of nursing has sole authority in scope of practice, but scope of practice has a requirement for physician collaboration: **AL, AZ, CA, DE, IA, IL, KS, KY, OH, MD, MO, NE, NV, NY, VT, WY**
- States with nurse practitioner† title protection and the board of nursing has sole authority in scope of practice, but scope of practice has a requirement for physician supervision: **CT, FL, GA, ID, LA, MA, SC, TX, WI**
- States with nurse practitioner† title protection but the scope of practice is authorized by the board of nursing and the board of medicine: **MS, NC, PA, SD, VA**
- States without nurse practitioner† title protection where APNs function under a broad nurse practice act: **MN, TN**

KEY:

* This table provides a state-by-state summary of the degree of independence for all aspects of the NP scope of practice including diagnosing and treating (except prescribing). See Table 2 for a state-by-state analysis of the degree of independence for the prescriptive authority aspect of the NP scope of practice.

† The information may apply to other APNs (clinical nurse specialists, nurse midwives, and nurse anesthetists). See State Survey for details.

[Note that Washington, D.C. is included as a state in this table.]

TABLE A-2 Summary of Advanced Practice Nurse (APN) Legislation: Prescriptive Authority*

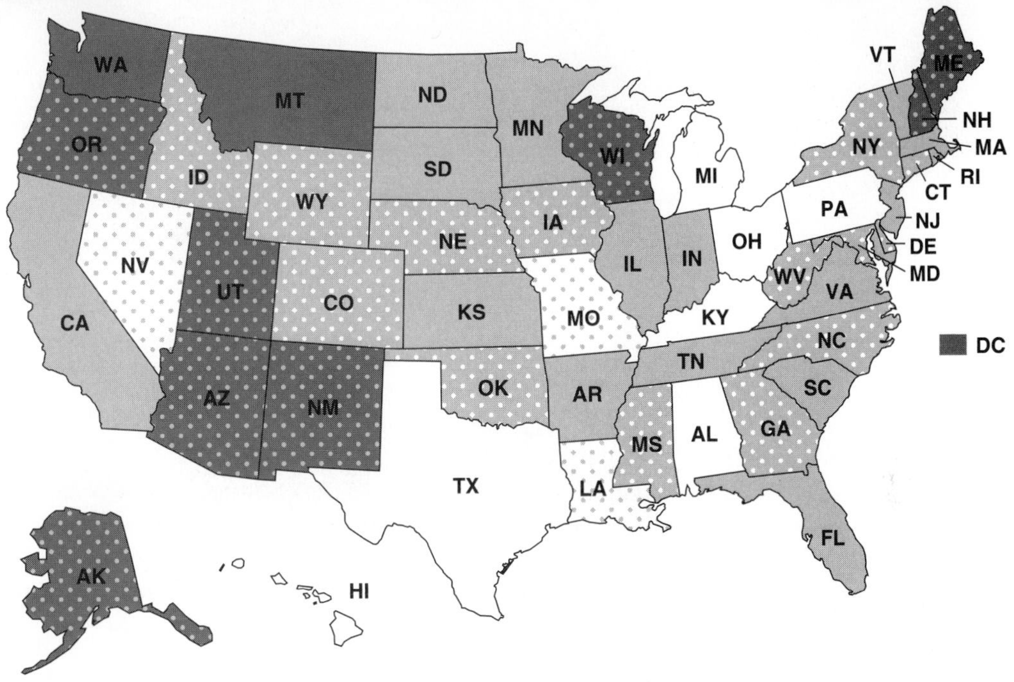

States where nurse practitioners† can prescribe (including controlled substances) independent of any required physician involvement in prescriptive authority: **AK, AZ, DC, ME, MT, NH, NM, OR, UT**, WA**, WI**

States where nurse practitioners† can prescribe (including controlled substances) with some degree of physician involvement or delegation of prescription writing: **AR, CA, CO, CT, DE, FL***, GA, IA, ID, IL***, IN, KS‡, MA, MD, MN, MS‡, NC, ND, NE, NJ, NY, OK, RI, SC‡, SD, TN***, VA, VT, WV, WY**

States where nurse practitioners† can prescribe (excluding controlled substances) with some degree of physician involvement or delegation of prescription writing: **AL, HI, KY, LA, MI, MO, NV, OH‡, PA***, TX**

States where nurse practitioners† have no statutory or regulatory prescribing authority: (None)

States where nurse practitioners also have the authority to dispense drug samples according to statute or rules and regulations: **** **AK, AZ, CO, CT, DE, GA, IA, ID, LA, ME, MD, MN, MO, MS, NC, NE, NH, NM, NV, NY, OK, OR, WI, WV, WY**

KEY:

* This table provides a state-by-state analysis of the degree of independence for the prescriptive authority aspect of the NP scope of practice. For analysis of the degree of independence for the other aspects of the NP scope of practice (including diagnosing and treating) see Table 1.

† The information may apply to other APNs (clinical nurse specialists, nurse midwives, and nurse anesthetists). See State Survey for details.

‡ In narrowly specified situations

** Schedule IV and/or V only

*** Pending approval of R&R

**** In many states the authority by NPs to distribute/dispense samples is not legislatively specified in the statute or R&R, but it has become the community standard as accepted practice.

[Note that Washington, D.C. is included as a state in this table.]

Index

D

O

Q

R

S

T

U